General Surgery/GI Words and Phrases

H·E·A·L·T·H
PROFESSIONS
INSTITUTE

Health Professions Institute • Modesto, California • 2001

General Surgery/GI Words and Phrases

Developed by

H•E•A•L•T•H PROFESSIONS HPI INSTITUTE

Sally C. Pitman
Editor & Publisher
Health Professions Institute
P. O. Box 801
Modesto, CA 95353-0801
Phone 209-551-2112
Fax 209-551-0404
Web site: http://www.hpisum.com
E-mail: hpi@hpisum.com

Printed by
Parks Printing & Lithograph
Modesto, California

ISBN 0-934385-36-X
Last digit is the print number: 9 8 7 6 5 4 3 2 1

In loving memory

of Rose Moore

Preface

In today's fast-paced, high-tech society, the quest to improve healthcare documentation is an ongoing challenge. Medical breakthroughs, new surgical techniques, and advances in pharmacology have given way to thousands of new medical terms. Every procedure must be documented in detail, each surgery described accurately, and every drug spelled correctly.

To stay abreast of the ever-changing world of healthcare documentation, it is vital to have direct access to the most accurate, comprehensive, up-to-date references. To this end we have produced *General Surgery/GI Words and Phrases,* truly a milestone in excellence and value.

General Surgery/GI Words and Phrases combines terminology from general surgery practice—a vast field in and of itself—with a multitude of terms from gastroenterology. Over 60,000 entries make word researching easier and more accurate for the production-oriented healthcare professional who needs help with general surgery instruments and devices; anatomic landmarks; dressings and bandages; wound management; gastroenterology practice (conditions, diseases, diagnosis, treatment); gastrointestinal surgery; hernia surgery; bariatric surgery; minimally invasive surgery; endoscopic and laparoscopic surgery; intra-abdominal transplantation; colorectal surgery; surgical oncology; trauma surgery; endocrinology practice (conditions, diseases, diagnosis, treatment); endocrine surgery; breast conditions and surgery; and breast devices.

A special feature in this edition is the Appendix with Tables of Arteries, Muscles, and Veins. Medical transcriptionists especially will appreciate listings of these common anatomic structures in both English and their Latin equivalents.

General Surgery/GI Words and Phrases is extensively cross-referenced to assure greater success in finding a desired word or phrase. Terms were gathered from thousands of actual surgical and gastrointestinal transcripts, from medical journals and textbooks, and through extensive research on the Internet.

Research for this second edition was done primarily by Linda C. Campbell, CMT; Georgia Green, CMT; and Diane S. Heath, CMT. Our warmest gratitude is also extended to those readers who called or wrote with comments and suggestions; this book is better because of their feedback.

Sally C. Pitman, M.A.
Editor & Publisher

How to Use This Book

The words and phrases in this book are alphabetized letter by letter of all words in the entry, ignoring punctuation marks and words or letters in parentheses. The possessive form ('s) is omitted from eponyms for ease in alphabetizing. Numbers are alphabetized as if written out, with the exception of subscripts and superscripts which are ignored.

Eponyms appear alphabetically as well as under the nouns they modify. For example, *Wise areola mastopexy breast augmentation (WAMBA)* is found alphabetically in the W's as well as under the main entries *mammoplasty* and *operation*. *Gastrografin* is found in the G's as well as under *imaging agent* and *medications*. The names of hundreds of medications used in general surgery and gastroenterology included in this book appear under the entry *medications*. Names of instruments appear under individual main entries like *catheter* and *forceps*, and in addition various kinds of technology are listed under the broad terms *device* and *system*.

In medical dictation physicians may arbitrarily refer to an operative procedure as an *approach*, *method*, *operation*, *procedure*, *repair*, or *technique*, or by the type of procedure, such as *gastrostomy* and *herniorrhaphy*. Thus, all procedures are listed alphabetically by the eponym, such as *Payne-DeWind jejunoileal bypass*, as well as under the type of procedure and under the main entry *operations*.

Many anatomical terms are found in the book, but no attempt was made to be comprehensive. The Appendix includes Tables of Arteries, Muscles, and Veins, with both English and Latin forms in tabular form for quick reference.

Main entries with a lengthy list of subentries include the following:

anesthesia
bandage
biopsy
blade
cannula
carcinoma
catheter
clamp
device
disease
dressing
elevator
endoscope
flap
forceps
graft
hernia
hook
imaging
incision
knife
laser
lesion
medications
nail
needle
operation
plate
retractor
rongeur
scissors
stent
suture
syndrome
system
test
tube
tumor
view

A, a

AA (acetabular anteversion)
AA (Alcoholics Anonymous)
AAA (aromatic amino acid)
AAA ("triple A") (abdominal aortic aneurysm)
Aagenaes syndrome (cholestasis-lymphedema syndrome)
AAI (axial acetabular index)
Aaron sign
Aarskog syndrome
AASLD (American Association for the Study of Liver Diseases)
Aastrom CPS (cell-production system)
abarelix
abate, abatement
Abbe operation
ABBI (advanced breast biopsy instrumentation) system
Abbokinase (urokinase)
Abbott esophagogastrostomy
Abbott gouge
Abbott-Miller tube
Abbott pump
Abbott-Rawson double-lumen gastrointestinal tube
Abbott tube
Abbreviated Injury Scale (AIS)
ABC (airway, breathing, circulation)
ABC (argon beam coagulator)
ABCD (amphotericin B colloid dispersion)
abdomen
  accordion
  acute
  acute surgical
  apertures of
  boardlike rigidity of
  boatlike
  boat-shaped
  concave
  diffusely tender
  distended
  doughy
  dull to percussion
  exquisitely tender
  fascia of
  flabby
  flat
  flat plate of
  free air in
  guarding of
  hyperdistended
  hyperresonant
  nondistended
  postlymphangiography
  postsurgical

abdomen *(cont.)*
  protuberant
  prune-belly
  resonant
  roof of
  rotund
  scaphoid
  silent
  soft
  splinting of
  surgical
  tight
  tympanitic
abdomen closed in anatomical layers
abdomen was deflated and laparoscope removed
abdominal abscess (see *abscess*)
abdominal angina
abdominal aorta
abdominal aortic aneurysm (AAA)
abdominal aortic artery
abdominal aortic plexus
abdominal aponeurosis
abdominal apron
abdominal bandage
abdominal binder
abdominal brace position
abdominal canal
abdominal cavity
abdominal colectomy
abdominal colic
abdominal compartment syndrome (ACS)
abdominal contents
abdominal cramp
abdominal distention
abdominal exploration
abdominal fat
abdominal fat pad
abdominal fissure
abdominal fistula
abdominal flap
abdominal fluid wave
abdominalgia, periodic
abdominal girth
abdominal impalement
abdominal incision dehiscence
abdominal iron deposition
abdominal kidney
abdominal lap (laparotomy) pad
abdominal lavage
abdominal lymph node
abdominal lymphatics
abdominal mass
abdominal migraine (cyclic vomiting syndrome)
abdominal muscle
abdominal muscle deficiency syndrome (prune-belly syndrome)
abdominal ostium
abdominal pad
abdominal panniculus
abdominal paracentesis
abdominal-perineal resection
abdominal peritoneum
abdominal pool
abdominal pregnancy
abdominal pull-through
abdominal pulse
abdominal raphe
abdominal rectopexy
abdominal reflex
abdominal region
abdominal retractor
abdominal rigidity
abdominal ring
abdominal sac
abdominal-sacral colpoperineopexy
abdominal scissors
abdominal scoop
abdominal section
abdominal situs inversus
abdominal stoma
abdominal stool
abdominal tap
Abdominal Trauma Index (ATI)
abdominal trocar
abdominal ultrasound

abdominal vascular accident
abdominal view
abdominal viscus (pl. viscera)
abdominal wall, elevation of
abdominal wall fistula
abdominal wall hernia
abdominal wall venous pattern
abdominal x-ray (AXR)
abdominal x-ray and computed tomography (AXR/CT)
abdominal zone
abdominis rectus muscle
abdominis transversus muscle
abdominocardiac reflex
abdominogenital
abdominojugular reflux
abdominopelvic abscess
abdominopelvic cavity
abdominopelvic mass
abdominopelvic viscera
abdominoperineal or abdominal-perineal resection (APR)
abdominoperineal proctectomy
abdominoscrotal
abdominothoracic arch
abdominovaginal
abdominovesical
ABD pad dressing
Abel scissors
Aberdeen knot suture
Abernethy sarcoma
aberrant goiter
aberrant pancreas
aberrant umbilical stomach
aberrant vessel
ABGs (arterial blood gases)
A bile
Ablatherm HIFU (high-intensity focused ultrasound) system
ablation
  celiac alcohol
  endoscopic
  endoscopic mucosal
  heater probe

ablation *(cont.)*
  laparoscopic uterine nerve
  laser
  laser uterosacral nerve (LUNA)
  Livewire TC
  percutaneous
  photothermal laser
  radioiodide
  radioiodine
  thermal
  thyroid
ablation catheter
ablation of tumor
ablative laser therapy
ablator
  Concept
  R.F. tissue
  Sonablate 200 tissue
ablepharon-macrostomia syndrome (AMS)
ABMTR (Autologous Bone Marrow Transplant Registry)
abnormal bleeding
abnormal clotting
abnormal feeding blood vessel
abnormality (pl. abnormalities)
  anatomic
  bleeding
  clotting
  DNA ploidy
  electrolyte
  mucosal
  persistent breast
  skeletal
  small-bowel congenital
abnormal mammographic findings
ABP (acute biliary pancreatitis)
abraded wound
Abrami disease
Abrams biopsy needle
Abrams needle
Abramson catheter
Abrikosov tumor

abscess (pl. abscesses)
abdominal
abdominopelvic
actinomycotic brain
acute
amebic or amoebic
amebic liver
amoebic or amebic
anal
anorectal
appendiceal
arthrifluent
Aspergillus cerebral
atraumatic
bacterial
bone
bowel
brain
breast
Brodie metaphyseal
cerebral
chronic subareolar
collar button
colonic
crypt
cuff
daughter
debridement of
deep
deep interloop
drainage of palate
draining
echinococcal
encapsulated brain
entamebic
enteroperitoneal
epidural
epiploon
extradural
extraperitoneal
fluctuant
frontal
fungal
gallbladder wall

abscess *(cont.)*
gas-forming liver
growth plate
hepatic
Highmore
horseshoe
incision & drainage (I&D) of
interloop
intersphincteric
intra-abdominal
intractable
intradural
intrahepatic
intramesenteric
intramural
intramuscular
intraosseous
intraperitoneal
ischiorectal
kidney
liver
local
localized
lumbar epidural
mesenteric
metaphyseal
midpalmar
missile track
necrotic
nonpuerperal breast
omental
Paget
pancreatic
paracolic
pararectal
parasitic
parotid
parumbilical
pelvic
pelvirectal
perianal
periappendiceal
pericecal
pericholecystic

abscess *(cont.)*
  pericolic
  pericolonic
  periesophageal
  perihepatic
  perirectal
  peritoneal
  periumbilical
  pilonidal
  postoperative
  Pott
  psoas
  puerperal breast
  pyogenic
  pyogenic liver
  rectal
  retrocecal
  retroperitoneal
  retroperitoneal-iliopsoas
  retrorectal
  serous
  simple liver amebic
  soft tissue
  spinal epidural (SEA)
  splenic
  subaponeurotic
  subdiaphragmatic
  subdural
  subgaleal
  subhepatic
  submucosal
  subperiosteal
  subphrenic
  subungual
  superficial
  supralevator
  suture
  thecal
  thenar space
  traumatic (of spleen)
  tubo-ovarian
  wound
abscess formation
Abscession fluid drainage catheter
absence of rugal folds
absent abdominal muscle syndrome
absent bowel sounds
absent gag reflex
absent peristalsis
Absolok endoscopic clip applicator
Absolok locking PDS clip
Absolok Plus clip
absolute alcohol sclerosant
absolute diet
absolute granulocyte count
absorbable cellulose cotton
absorbable collagen sponge
absorbable dusting powder
absorbable endoclip
absorbable gelatin film
absorbable gelatin sponge
absorbable pin
absorbable polyparadioxanone pin
absorbable rod
absorbable sponge
absorbable surgical suture
absorbable suture
absorbent gauze
absorbent (lymph) gland
absorption, impaired gastric
absorptive area of small intestine
abuse, laxative
a.c. (L. *ante cibum*, before meals)
acalculous cholecystitis
acanthocytosis
acanthosis, glycogenic
acanthosis nigricans
acanthotic lesion
acarbose
ACAT (automated computerized axial
  tomography)
Accel stopcock
access
  body
  minimally invasive surgical
  peripheral I.V.
  remote
  surgical

access *(cont.)*
  transjugular
  transjugular liver
  transcervical tubal
  transcutaneous
  transperitoneal aortic
  vascular
  venous
  ventricular
accessible lesion
accessory breast
accessory gland
accessory nipple
accessory pancreas
accessory pancreatic duct
accessory spleen
accessory trocar
accommodation reflex
accordion abdomen
accordion sign
Accu-Chek Advantage blood glucose monitor
Accu-Chek Complete blood glucose monitor
Accu-Chek Compass glucose management software
Accu-Chek Easy blood glucose monitor
Accu-Chek Instant blood glucose monitor
Accu-Chek Instant Plus blood glucose monitor
Accu-Chek Simplicity blood glucose monitor
Accu-Chek II Freedom blood glucose monitor
Accu-Chek Voicemate blood glucose monitor
Accucore II core biopsy needle
accuDEXA bone mineral density assessment device
Accu-Flo dura film
Accu-Flo ventricular catheter
AccuGuide injection monitor
AccuLase excimer laser
Accu-Line guide
Acculink self-expanding (carotid) stent
Acculite Contour Tip endoprobe
AccuPort seal
Accuprep HPF powder
AccuProbe 600 cryotherapy probe
AccuSpan tissue expander
Accutom low-speed diamond saw
Accuzyme enzymatic debriding ointment
Ace adherent bandage
Acephen (acetaminophen) analgesic suppository
Aceta (acetaminophen)
Aceta with Codeine (codeine phosphate; acetaminophen)
acetabular cup detaching rod
acetabular cup push (pushing) rod
acetabular guide
acetabular knife
acetabular reamer
acetabular reconstruction plate
acetabuloplastic round chisel
acetaminophen overdose
acetaminophen poisoning
acetohexamide
achalasia
  classic
  cricopharyngeal
  esophageal
  pelvirectal
  sphincteral
  vigorous
Achard-Thiers syndrome
Achiever balloon dilatation catheter
achlorhydria
  gastric
  histamine-resistant
achlorhydric
acholangic biliary cirrhosis
acholic stool
acholuric jaundice
achondroplastic dwarfism
achylia gastrica

achylia pancreatica
acid
  arachidonic
  aromatic amino (AAA)
  bile
  branched chain amino (BCAA)
  carbonic
  caustic
  chenodeoxycholic
  choleic
  conjugated bile
  essential fatty (EFA)
  fecal bile (FBA)
  folinic
  gastric
  hepatoiminodiacetic (HIDA)
  hydrochloric
  intraesophageal
  intraluminal
  isovaleric
  medium chain fatty (MCFA)
  short chain fatty (SCFA)
  ursodeoxycholic
acid base imbalance
acid clearance test (ACT)
acid cell
acid dyspepsia
acidemia, isovaleric
acid-fast bacillus (AFB)
acid-fast bacteria
acid-fast organism
acid gland
acid hypersecretion
acidification of stool test
acidophilic adenoma
acidophilic body
acidophilus capsule
acidophilus milk
Acidose-Aqua
acidosis
  compensated
  diabetic
  hyperchloremic metabolic
  hypochloremic metabolic
acidosis *(cont.)*
  hypokalemic metabolic
  hypovolemia-induced metabolic
  ketoacidosis
  lactic
  metabolic
  normochloremic
  persistent
  pure respiratory
  renal tubular
  respiratory
  severe
  starvation
  uncompensated
acid-pepsin reflux esophagitis
acid peptic disease
acid peptic disorder
acid peptic juice
acid peptic ulcer
acid perfusion test
acid reflux disease
acid reflux test
acid regurgitation
acid-related disorder (ARD)
acid suppression
Acidulin (glutamic acid hydrochloride)
acid water, electrolyzed
Acier stainless steel suture
acinar cell
acinarization
acinar tissue
Acinetobacter calcoaceticus var. *lwoffi* (formerly *Mima polymorpha*)
acinous adenoma
acinous cell carcinoma
Aciphex (rabeprazole sodium) proton pump inhibitor
Ackland mouth gag
Acland-Banis arteriotomy set
Acland clamp-applying forceps
Acland microvascular clamp
ACL drill guide
ACL graft
ACMI Martin endoscopy forceps

ACMI monopolar electrode
ACMI rigid laparoscope
ACMI ulcer measuring device
AC137 analog of human amylin used with insulin
acorn-tipped bougie
acorn treatment
acoustic papilla
acoustic shadowing (in ultrasonography)
acoustic window
acquired benign adrenal androgenic overactivity
acquired disorder of coagulation
acquired esophagocele
acquired hemolytic jaundice
acquired hernia
acquired hypothyroidism
acquired immunodeficiency syndrome (AIDS)
acquired lactose deficiency
acquired lesion
acquired megacolon
acquired reflex
ACR (adenomatosis of colon and rectum)
Acra-Cut wire pass drill
acral lentiginous melanoma
Acremonium falciform
Acremonium kiliense
Acremonium recifei
acrodermatitis enteropathica (AE)
Acro-Lase Plus
AcroMed VSP plate
acromegaly
acroparesthesia
AcryDerm border island dressing
AcryDerm Sheet dressing
AcryDerm Strands dressing
ACS (abdominal compartment syndrome)
ACS Concorde catheter
ACS Endura coronary dilation catheter
ACS Hi-Torque Balance Middleweight guidewire
ACS Multi-Link OTW (over-the-wire) Duet stent
ACS:180 BR breast cancer screening test
ACS OTW (over-the-wire) Lifestream coronary dilatation catheter
ACS OTW (over-the-wire) Photon catheter
ACS RX Comet coronary dilatation catheter
ACS RX Multi-Link coronary stent
ACS SULP II balloon
ACS Tourguide II guiding catheter
ACT (acid clearance test)
ACT (activated clotting time)
Actalyke ACT (activating clotting test)
ACTH (adrenocorticotropic hormone) deficiency
Acticoat burn dressing
Acticoat foam dressing
Acticon neosphincter implantable prosthesis
ACTID (analgesic cell therapy implantable device)
Actidose Aqua (activated charcoal)
Actidose with Sorbital (activated charcoal; sorbital)
Actifoam collagen sponge
Actigall (ursodiol-ursodeoxycholic acid)
Actimmune (interferon gamma-1b)
actinomycotic brain abscess
Actiprep skin preparation
Actiq lozenge ("lollipop") oral transmucosal fentanyl citrate
activated attapulgite
activated charcoal
activated clotting time (ACT)
activated coagulation time
activated partial thromboplastin time (APTT)
activated thromboplastin time (ATT)
active bowel sounds
active duodenal ulcer
Active Life barrier
active source of bleeding

actively bleeding varices
activity tolerance
Actos (pioglitazone hydrochloride)
Actron (ketoprofen) pain reliever
Acucise retrograde procedure
ACU-derm wound dressing
ACU-dyne ointment
ACU-dyne wash
Acufex bioabsorbable Suretac suture and anchor
Acufex convex rasp
Acufex curved basket forceps
Acufex distractor pin
Acufex double-lumen cannula
Acufex gouge
Acufex mallet
Acufex nerve hook
Acufex probe
Acufex rasp
Acufex rotary biting basket forceps
Acufex rotary punch
Acufex scissors
Acufex TAG rod
Acufex T-fix suture anchor
Acufex tibial guide
Acumed suture anchor
AcuNav ultrasound catheter
acupuncture anesthesia
acupuncture laser
Acuson Aspen ultrasound system
acute abdomen
acute abdominal series
acute abdominal vascular disease
acute abscess
acute alcoholism
acute appendicitis
acute biliary pancreatitis (ABP)
acute cholangitis
acute cholecystitis
acute diverticulitis
acute erosive gastritis (AEG)
acute fatty liver of pregnancy
acute gallstone pancreatitis
acute gastritis
acute gastroenteritis (AGE)
acute hemorrhagic gastritis
acute hemorrhagic pancreatitis
acute hepatocellular degeneration
acute hypersensitivity reaction
acute idiopathic inflammatory bowel disease
acute infectious colitis
acute infectious diarrhea
acute infectious gastroenteritis
acute intermittent porphyria (AIP)
acute interstitial pancreatitis
acute juvenile cirrhosis
acute malaria
acute mononucleosis-like hepatitis
acute obstructive cholangitis
acute pancreatitis
acute parenchymatous hepatitis
acute peptic ulcer
acute porphyria
acute proctitis
acute prostatitis
acute sclerosing hyaline necrosis (ASHN)
acute self-limited colitis (ASLC)
acute septic splenitis
acute surgical abdomen
acute tubular necrosis
acute viral hepatitis (AVH)
Acutrainer for urinary incontinence
Acutrim
acyl-CoA dehydrogenase deficiency, long-chain
ad lib. (L. *ad libitum*, freely; at pleasure)
ADA (American Diabetes Association)
ADA (American Dietetic Association)
Adair-Allis forceps
Adair breast clamp
Adair clamp
Adair forceps
Adair tenaculum
Adams-DeWeese vena caval clip
Adams saw

adapter
  Carlens tube
  clip
  diamond Ohio
  DISS body
  dual irrigation
  Lamis
  open laparoscopy cannula
  VCS clip
Adaptic dressing
Adaptic packing
adaptive colitis
ADCC (antibody-dependent cell-mediated cytotoxicity)
Adcon-A
Adcon-C
Adcon-I
Adcon-L gel
Adcon-P adhesion control barrier
Adcon-P solution
Adcon-T/N gel
Addison disease
addisonian crisis
Addison point
AddOn-Bucky imaging device
adefovir dipivoxil
ADEKs multivitamin pediatric supplement
adelomorphous cell
adenitis, mesenteric
adenocarcinoma
  annular
  colloid
  esophageal
  exophytic
  gastric
  giant cell
  infiltrating
  malignant mucoid
  papillary
  prostate
  scirrhous
  tubular
  ulcerating
adenocystic carcinoma
adenoid cystic carcinoma
adenoid pattern
adenoid squamous cell carcinoma
adenoma
  acidophilic
  acinous
  ACTH-producing
  adnexal
  adrenocortical
  apocrine
  basal cell
  basophilic
  benign liver
  benign solitary
  bile duct (BDA)
  bronchial
  canalicular
  chromophil
  chromophobe
  colloid
  colonic
  embryonal
  eosinophil
  fibroid
  follicular
  Fuchs
  gallbladder
  gonadotropin-producing
  growth hormone-producing
  hepatic
  hepatocellular (HCA)
  Hürthle (Huerthle) cell
  islet cell
  lactating
  Leydig cell
  liver cell
  macrofollicular
  microfollicular
  moderately differentiated
  monomorphic
  mucinous
  nephrogenic
  nipple

adenoma *(cont.)*
null cell
ovarian tubular
oxyphil
pancreatic
papillary cystic
Pick tubular
pituitary
pleomorphic
polypoid
poorly differentiated
prolactin-producing
prostatic
renal cortical
sessile
solitary benign
testicular tubular
thyroid
thyrotropin-producing
tubular
tubulovillous
undifferentiated
villoglandular
villous
well-differentiated
adenoma prevention with celecoxib (APC) study
adenomatosis of colon and rectum (ACR)
adenomatous goiter
adenomatous hyperplasia (AH)
adenomatous polyp
adenomatous polyposis coli (APC)
adenomatous polyposis coli, familial
adenomatous polyposis coli gene
adenomyoma of gallbladder
adenomyomatosis
adenopapillomatosis, gastric
adenopathy
axillary
cervical
inguinal
lymph node

adenopathy *(cont.)*
palpable
paraductal
splenic hilar
adenosquamous carcinoma
adenoviral p53 gene
adenovirus, enteric
adenovirus infection
adenovirus test kit
Adenovirus EIA test kit
Adept (icodextrin) antiadhesion solution
ADH (alcohol dehydrogenase)
ADH (antidiuretic hormone)
adhesion
attic
bandlike
banjo-string
bleb-like
cell-cell
dense
fibrinous
fibrous
filmy
freeing up of
hard
intra-abdominal
intraperitoneal
lysis of
meningeal
mesenteric
omental
pelvic
pericholecystic
peritoneal
postop
primary
secondary
takedown of
taking down of
thick
thin
tight
violin-string

adhesive (see also *bandage*; *cement*; *dressing*; *glue*)
  APR cement fixation
  Aron Alpha
  autologous fibrin tissue (AFTA)
  BEMA (bioerodible mucoadhesive)
  benzoin
  Biobrane
  Bioerodible Mucoadhesive (BEMA)
  BioGlue surgical
  CicaCare topical gel sheeting
  Coe-pak paste
  Comfeel skin
  CoSeal resorbable synthetic sealant
  CoStasis
  Coverlet
  Cover-Roll gauze
  Colly-Seel
  cyanoacrylate (Superglue) tissue
  Dermabond topical skin
  Dynastat
  EMLA anesthetic disc
  Fibrijet
  fibrin glue
  fibrin sealant
  FloSeal matrix hemostatic sealant
  FocalSeal-S surgical sealant
  gelatin-resorcin-formalin tissue glue
  HemaMyst aerosol
  Hemaseel APR fibrin
  Hemaseel HMN biological tissue glue
  HemaSyst sealant
  Histoacryl Blue (HAB) tissue adhesive
  Histoacryl glue (cyanoacrylate) tissue
  hydroxyapatite (HA)
  Implast bone cement
  Indermil topical tissue
  isobutyl 2-cyanoacrylate (IBC) tissue
  ligand
  LPPS hydroxyapatite
  medical

adhesive *(cont.)*
  methyl methacrylate
  Palacos cement
  Proceed hemostatic surgical sealant
  ReliaSeal skin barrier
  Simplex
  Soothe-N-Seal
  Superglue (cyanoacrylate) tissue
  Surfit
  Tisseel "surgical glue"
  Vitex tissue
  Zimmer low viscosity
adhesive bandage
adhesive band
adhesive dressing
adhesive plastic drape
adhesive tape
ADICOL insulin delivery system
Adipex-P (phentermine HCl)
adipose fold
adipose graft
adipose tissue
adiposis dolorosa
adiposogenital dystrophy
adjacent organ invasion
adjunctive chemotherapy
adjunctive suppressive medical therapy
adjustable angle guide
adjustable nail
adjustable saline breast implant
adjustable silicone gastric banding
adjuvant chemotherapy
adjuvant radiotherapy
adjuvant systemic therapy
adjuvant therapy
Adler Eagle Vision laparoscope
Adler P.L.U.S. laparoscope
admitting diagnosis
adnexal carcinoma
ADOPT (diabetes outcome progression) trial
adrenal cortex hyperfunction
adrenal cortex hypofunction
adrenal gland

adrenal medulla
adrenal medulla graft
adrenal medullary insufficiency
adrenal pseudocyst
adrenal pseudohermaphroditism
adrenal tumor
adrenalectomy
  bilateral total
  complete
  laparoscopic
  partial
adrenocortical carcinoma
adrenogenital syndrome
adrenoleukodystrophy (ALD)
Adriamycin (doxorubicin)
Adrucil (fluorouracil)
Adson-Anderson cerebellar retractor
Adson aneurysm needle
Adson baby forceps
Adson baby retractor
Adson bayonet dressing forceps
Adson bipolar forceps
Adson brain-exploring cannula
Adson brain suction tube
Adson-Brown clamp
Adson-Brown tissue forceps
Adson cerebellar retractor
Adson chisel
Adson clamp
Adson clip applier
Adson clip-introducing forceps
Adson cranial rongeur
Adson dissecting hook
Adson dressing forceps
Adson drill guide
Adson dura protecting forceps
Adson dural hook
Adson dural knife
Adson dural needle holder
Adson dural protector guide
Adson forceps
Adson ganglion scissors
Adson hemilaminectomy retractor
Adson hemostatic forceps
Adson hook
Adson hypophyseal forceps
Adson laminectomy chisel
Adson lightweight plain forceps
Adson lightweight toothed forceps
Adson micro tissue forceps
Adson-Mixter neurosurgical forceps
Adson nerve hook
Adson periosteal elevator
Adson retractor
Adson right-angle knife
Adson rongeur forceps
Adson saw guide
Adson scalp needle
Adson suction tube
Adson tissue forceps
Adson-Toennis scissors
Adson twist drill
Adson wire saw
adsorbent
adult chronic immune thrombocytopenic purpura
adult-onset (now type 2) diabetes mellitus
adult-onset obesity
adult polycystic disease
adult respiratory distress syndrome (ARDS)
adult sigmoidoscope
adult-to-adult living related donor liver transplant
advanced breast biopsy instrumentation (ABBI) system
Advance formula
advancement
  mucosal
  rectal sleeve
  transanal pouch
advancement flap graft
advancement of rectal flap
advance to regular diet
AdvaSeal
adventitial forceps
adverse event profile

adynamic ileus
adynamic intestinal obstruction
adynamic paralytic ileus
AE (acrodermatitis enteropathica)
AEG (acute erosive gastritis)
Aerobacter (old name for *Enterobacter*)
AER Plus (automatic endoscope reprocessor) infection
aerobic bacteria
aerobic culture
aerobilia
aerophagia
Aeroplast dressing
AeroView optical intubation system
AERx (morphine sulfate)
AERx diabetes management system
AERx electronic inhaler
AERx pain management system
Aesculap ABC cervical plate
Aesculap bipolar cautery forceps
Aesculap saw
AESOP (Automated Endoscopic System for Optimal Positioning)
AESOP 2000 surgical robot system
AESOP 3000 surgical robot system
Aestiva/5 MRI anesthesia machine
AFB (acid-fast bacillus) smear
afebrile
afferent
  spinal
  vagal
afferent jejunostomy
afferent limb
afferent loop
afferent loop syndrome
afferent vessels of kidney
Afipia felis
AFP (alpha-fetoprotein) globulin
AGA (American Gastroenterological Association)
agalsidase beta
agammaglobulinemia
aganglionic bowel
aganglionic segment of colon
aganglionosis, congenital
Agaricus (mushroom)
AGE (acute gastroenteritis)
AGE (advanced glycosylation end product)
agency, organ procurement
agenesis, congenital sacral
agent (see also *imaging agents*)
  5-ASA
  antitubulin
  immunosuppressive
  lymphocyte-depleting
  prokinetic
  wetting
ageusia
aggressive malignancy
agnogenic intestinal infarction
agonal clot
agonal infection
Agoral (mineral; phenolphthalein)
Agris-Dingman submammary dissector
AH (adenomatous hyperplasia)
AHD (arteriohepatic dysplasia)
Ahn thrombectomy catheter
AIDS (acquired immunodeficiency syndrome)
AIDS-related complex (ARC)
Ailee needle
Ailee suture
Ainsworth modification of Massie nail
AIOD (aortoiliac obstructive disease)
AIO (all-in-one) parenteral solution
AIP (acute intermittent porphyria)
air
  bowel loop
  colonic
  expired
  free
  Hampton
  inspired
  intramural colonic
  intraperitoneal
  Ohio
  Oxequip

air *(cont.)*
  room
  subcutaneous
  swallowed
airborne infection
air collection
air contrast barium enema
air cyst
air density
air-dried smear
air drill
air embolism
air enema
air exchange
air-filled loop
air-fluid level
Airis II open MRI system
airless lung
Airlift balloon retractor
air-powered cutting drill
air-powered saw
Air Pulse Sensory Stimulator
air sac
airsick
airsickness
airspace-filling pattern
airway
  Berman oropharyngeal
  COPA cuffed oropharyngeal
  disposable
  esophageal gastric tube (EGTA)
  esophageal obturator
  Guedel disposable
  Guedel plastic
  Guedel rubber
  Harrell Y
  LMA-Unique
  oropharyngeal
  pharyngeal
airway, breathing, circulation (ABC)
airway obstruction
airway pattern
AJ (ankle jerk)
Ajmalin liver injury
A-K diamond knife
akinesia, rectal
Akros extended-care mattress
ALA (alpha lipoic acid)
Alagille syndrome
Alamag (aluminum hydroxide; magnesium hydroxide)
Alamag Plus (aluminum hydroxide; magnesium hydroxide; simethicone)
alanine aminotransferase (ALT) (formerly SGPT) liver function test
Al-Anon
Alan-Parks rectal speculum
alar fold
alar plate
AlaSTAT latex allergy test
Alatest Latex-specific IgE allergen test kit
Albarran deflecting level
albatross syndrome
Albee bone graft
albendazole
Albenza Tiltab (albendazole)
Albert suture
Albright syndrome
albuminoid liver
albumin, serum
alcohol consumption
alcohol dehydrogenase (ADH)
alcoholic cirrhosis
alcoholic consumption
alcoholic fatty liver
alcoholic fibrosis
alcoholic gastritis
alcoholic hepatitis
alcoholic hyalin
alcoholic hypoglycemia
alcoholic ketoacidosis
alcoholic liver disease
alcoholic pancreatitis
Alcoholics Anonymous (AA)
alcoholic varices

alcoholism
  acute
  chronic
  gamma
ALD (adrenoleukodystrophy)
ALD (alcoholic liver disease)
Aldactone (spironolactone)
Aldara cream 5%
Alden loop gastric bypass
Alderkreutz tissue forceps
aldesleukin
aldolase
aldosterone-producing carcinoma
aldosterone-secreting carcinoma
aldosteronism
Aldrete needle
Aldurazyme
Alenic Alka (aluminum hydroxide; magnesium trisilicate)
Alenic Alka Extra Strength (aluminum hydroxide; magnesium carbonate)
Alexa 1000 noninvasive breast diagnostic system
Alexagram breast lesion diagnostic test
Alexander biopsy forceps
Alexander chisel
Alexander-Farabeuf rasp
Alexander gouge
Alexander rasp
alexandrite (solid-state) laser
AlexLazr or AlexLAZR laser
"alfa and new sling" configuration of gracilis muscle
Alferon N (interferon alfa-n3)
Alfred M. Large clamp
algesimeter (pain monitor), Aly
Algicon
AlgiDERM alginate wound dressing
AlgiDERM calcium alginate gel dressing
alginate wound dressing
AlgiSite alginate wound dressing
alglucerase
AlgoMed drug infusion system
Algosteril alginate wound dressing
Alibra (alprostadil/prazosin HCl)
alignment guide
alignment pin
alignment rod
alimentary canal
alimentary hypoglycemia
alimentary lipemia
alimentary mucosa
alimentary obesity
alimentary system
alimentary tract
alimentary tract smear
alimentation
  enteral
  forced
  parenteral
  peripheral intravenous
  rectal
  total parenteral
Aliminase
AlitraQ formula
alitretinoin
alkaline esophagitis
alkaline gastritis
alkaline phosphatase (ALP)
alkaline reflux gastritis
Alka-Mints (calcium carbonate)
Alka-Seltzer (sodium bicarbonate; citric acid; aspirin; phenylalanine)
Alkets (calcium carbonate)
Alldress composite wound dressing
Allen anastomosis clamp
Allen-Brown vascular access shunt
Allen clip applier
Allen intestinal clamp
Allen intestinal forceps
Allen-Kocher clamp
Allen stirrups
allergic colitis
allergic gastritis
allergic granulomatous angiitis
allergic ileitis
allergic jejunitis

allergic sigmoiditis
allergy
  cow's milk protein
  food
  insulin
  latex
  wheat gliadin
Allevyn foam dressing
Allevyn nonadherent dressing
alligator forceps
alligator grasper
alligator grasping forceps
alligator jaws forceps
alligator scissors
Allis-Adair clamp
Allis atraumatic tissue forceps
Allis clamp
Allis forceps
Allison gastroesophageal reflux repair
Allison lung retractor
Allis-TC tissue forceps
Allis tissue forceps
Alliston GE reflux correction procedure
Allis-Willauer forceps
AlloDerm processed tissue graft
Allofix freeze-dried cortical bone pin
allogenic (also allogeneic)
allogenic bone graft
allogenic peripheral blood mononuclear cells
allogenous bone graft
allograft
  functioning
  hepatic
  intestinal
  pancreatic
AlloMatrix injectable putty bone graft substitute
Allon system
allostimulation
allotransplantation
  islet
  liver
Allovectin-7 (DNA/lipid complex)
Allport multiple clip applier
Allport retractor
Alm self-retaining retractor
Alm wound retractor
Almacone II (aluminum hydroxide; magnesium hydroxide; simethicone)
Aloe Vesta perineal dressings
Alogsteril (sterile alginate) dressing
Aloka 650 ultrasound system
Alond (zopolrestat)
alosetron HCl
ALP (alkaline phosphatase)
$alpha_1$ (also alpha-1)
$alpha_1$-antitrypsin deficiency disease
$alpha_1$-antitrypsin globulin
$alpha_2$ (also alpha-2)
$alpha_2$-antiplasmin functional assay
alpha chain disease
alpha chain syndrome
alpha-D-galactosidase enzyme
alpha-fetoprotein (AFP) globulin
alpha-Gal antibody
alpha-Gal epitope
alpha-galactosidase deficiency
alpha heavy chain disease
alpha lipoic acid (ALA)
AlphaNine
alpha sigmoid loop
alpha *Streptococcus viridans*
alprostadil
Alprox-TD (alprostadil)
ALPS (autologous leukapheresis, processing, and storage)
Alramucil (psyllium hydrophilic mucilloid)
ALRT1550 capsules
Alstrom syndrome
ALT (alanine aminotransferase) (formerly SGPT)
ALTE (apparent life-threatening event)
Altemeier repair of rectal prolapse
altered mucosal defenses
altered nutrition
altered thought processes due to advanced cirrhosis

altered tissue perfusion
ALternaGEL (aluminum hydroxide gel)
alternating blue and white mattress suture
alternating pressure mattress
Alteromonas putrefaciens
Altex polypropylene mesh
ALT (alanine aminotransferase) (formerly SGPT) liver function test
Altracin (bacitracin)
altumomab pentetate
Alu-Cap (aluminum hydroxide gel)
Aludrox (aluminum hydroxide; magnesium hydroxide; simethicone)
aluminum carbonate gel
aluminum hydroxide gel
aluminum sulfate
Alu-Tab (aluminum hydroxide gel)
alveolar cell carcinoma
alveolar mucosa
alveolar pattern
alveolar soft-part sarcoma (ASPS)
alvine calculus
Aly algesimeter
Alzate catheter
AMA (antimitochondrial antibody)
Amaryl (glimepiride) tablets
Amazr catheter
ambulant edema
ambulatory anesthesia
ambulatory surgery center
AMC needle
amebiasis, indigenous
amebic (also amoebic)
amebic abscess
amebic appendicitis
amebic colitis
amebic cyst
amebic granuloma
amebic hepatitis
amebic liver abscess
amebic ulcer
amelanotic melanoma
ameloblastic carcinoma
ameloblastic sarcoma
American ACMI flexible sigmoidoscope
American Association for the Study of Liver Diseases (AASLD)
American Association for the Surgery of Trauma Organ Injury Scale
American Cancer Society (ACS)
American College of Gastroenterology (ACG)
American Diabetes Association (ADA)
American Dietetic Association (ADA)
American Digestive Health Foundation (ADHF)
American Endoscopy mechanical lithotriptor
American Gastroenterological Association (AGA)
American Hernia Society (AHS)
American Liver Foundation (ALF) hepatitis screening
American Pancreatology Association (APA)
American Society for Gastrointestinal Endoscopy (ASGE)
American Society of Colon and Rectal Surgeons (ASCRS)
Amicus separator blood collection device
amifostine
Amin-Aid powdered feeding
amine precursor uptake and decarboxylation cell
Aminofusin L Forte amino acid solution
aminoglutethimide
Amino Mel Hepa
aminopyrine breath test
aminosalicylic acid
aminosidine
aminosterol
Aminosyn (multiple essential and nonessential amino acids)
Aminosyn M
Aminosyn II

Amitone (calcium carbonate)
AML (angiomyolipoma) solid renal
  tumor
ammonia
  blood
  serum
  urinary
ammonium molybdate tetrahydrate
ammonia N 13 test
amniotic fluid
amniotic fold
amoebic (see *amebic*)
amoebic cyst (also amebic)
Amoena breast prosthesis
amorphous material
Amphojel (aluminum hydroxide gel)
amphotericin B
ampicillin
Ampique
Amplatz dilator
Ampligen
ampulla of Vater
ampulla, rectal
ampullary carcinoma
ampullary stenosis
ampullary tumor
ampullectomy
ampulloma
amputating saw
amputation knife
amputation retractor
AMS (ablepharon-macrostomia
  syndrome) Endoview camera
Amset R-F rod
Amsterdam stent
Amussat operation
amylase
  ascitic
  pancreatic
  P-type (pancreatic)
  salivary
  serum
  S-type (salivary)
  urinary
amylase/creatinine clearance ratio
amyloglucosidase
amyloid degeneration of liver
amyloid kidney
amyloidosis, hepatic
amylo-1,6-glucosidase deficiency
  (Forbes disease)
amylopectinosis
amyotrophy, diabetic
ANA (antinuclear antibody)
Anaconda stent and delivery system
anaerobe, obligate
anaerobic bacteria
anaerobic culture
anakinra
anal abscess
anal anastomosis
anal atresia
anal bulging
anal canal
anal cellulitis
anal cleft
anal column
anal condyloma
anal crypt
anal dilatation
anal dilator
anal disk
anal endoscopy
anal epithelial neoplasia
analeptic enema
anal fascia
anal fissure
anal fistula
analgesia, patient-controlled
anal gland
anal ileostomy with preservation
  of sphincter
anal intermuscular septum
anal intersphincteric groove
anal manometry
anal mapping
anal membrane
analog, nucleoside

analogous tissue
anal orifice
anal papillae
anal pit
anal plate
anal pouch angle
Analpram-HC (hydrocortisone acetate; pramoxine)
anal procidentia
anal prolapse
anal protrusion
anal pruritus
anal reflex
anal region
anal retractor
anal sac
anal seton
anal sinus
anal spasm
anal speculum
anal sphincter
anal sphincteroplasty
anal sphincter squeeze pressure
anal sphincter tone
anal squamous dysplasia
anal squamous intraepithelial lesion
anal stenosis
anal stretch
anal stricture
anal triangle
anal valve
anal vein
anal verge
anal wink
analysis (pl. analyses)
  automated image
  fecal
  gastric
  Monte Carlo
  multivariate
analyzer
  automated blood cell
  BiliChek
  bilirubin

analyzer *(cont.)*
  Body Logic Pro body fat
  BVA-100 blood volume
  ChromaVision digital
  HemoCue
  Hitachi Model 737 multichannel
  LARA
  Piccolo blood
  Sequential Multiple (SMA)
  Sequential Multiple Analyzer C (SMAC)
anaphylactic shock
anaplastic carcinoma of thyroid gland
anaplastic tumor
anasarca
Anaspaz (hyoscyamine sulfate)
Anastaflo stent
anastamose
anastomosed
anastomosing fiber
anastomosing veins
anastomosis (pl. anastomoses)
  anal
  arteriolovenular
  arteriovenous
  Braun
  coloanal
  crucial
  end-to-end
  end-to-end invaginating
  end-to-side
  extracorporeal
  gastroduodenal
  gastrojejunal
  handsewn
  heel-toe
  ileoanal
  ileorectal
  intracorporeal
  LAMA (laser-assisted microvascular anastomosis)
  LAMA (laser-assisted microanastomosis)
  LeDuc

anastomosis *(cont.)*
  longitudinal
  low pelvic
  microvascular
  portacaval
  primary
  side-to-side
  supraoptic
  tension-free
  two-layer
anastomosis clamp
anastomosis of arteries
anastomotic area, portal systemic
anastomotic branch
anastomotic dehiscence
anastomotic fiber
anastomotic leakage
anastomotic stoma
anastomotic ulceration
anastomotic vein
anastrozole
anatomic abnormality
anatomical dead space
anatomical landmark
anatomical layer
anatomical root
anatomical snuffbox
anatomical sphincter
anatomical tooth
anatomical tubercle
anatomic diagnosis
anatomic landmark
anatomic nervous system
anatomic pathology
anatomy, anomalous
Anatrast (barium sulfate)
Ancef (cefazolin sodium)
ancestral organ
anchor (also suture anchor)
  Acufex bioabsorbable suture
  Acufex T-fix suture
  Acumed suture
  Anchorlok soft tissue
  Anspach suture

anchor *(cont.)*
  AxyaWeld bone anchor system
  Bio-Anchor suture
  Biologically Quiet mini-screw suture
  Bio-Phase suture
  BioROC
  Bio-Sphere suture
  Bio-Statak suture
  Catera suture
  ConTack
  ConvaTec Flextrak gastrostomy
  Cope suture
  Corkscrew suture
  fascia
  FASTak suture
  Fastin
  GLS suture
  GII EasyAnchor
  GII Snap-Pak
  Harpoon suture
  In-Tac bone-anchoring system
  intraosseous suture
  knotless suture
  Mainstay urologic soft tissue
  MicroMite suture
  Micro QuickAnchor
  Mini GLS
  Mini QuickAnchor
  Mini-Revo Screw suture
  Mitek bone
  Mitek GII suture
  Mitek knotless suture
  Mitek Superanchor
  Mitek suture
  Multitak SS suture
  OBL RC5 soft tissue
  Ogden
  Panalok RC absorbable soft tissue
  Parachute corkscrew suture
  PeBA suture
  Radial Osteo Compression (ROC) soft tissue
  ROC EZ

anchor *(cont.)*
ROC XS
Sherlock threaded suture
SmartAnchor suture
Statak suture
StatLock Universal Plus
Stryker wedge suture
SuperAnchor suture
suture
T
Tacit threaded
TAG suture
T-fix suture
traction
UltraFix MicroMite suture
anchoring suture
Anchorlok soft tissue anchor
anchor plate
Ancure system for minimally invasive repair of abdominal aortic aneurysm
ancylostomiasis (also ankylostomiasis)
Andersen disease
Anderson-Adson scalp retractor
Anderson clamp
Anderson forceps
Andractim (dihydrotestosterone gel)
André hook
Andrews gouge
Andrews Pynchon suction tube
Androderm testosterone transdermal patch
Androgel (testosterone)
androgen therapy
Androsorb
anemia
autoimmune hemolytic
congenital hemolytic
iron-deficiency
microcytic
pernicious
sickle cell
splenic
anergy, clonal
aneroid manometry
anesthesia
acupuncture
ambulatory
axillary
balanced
basal
Bier block
block
bolus
brachial
caudal
cervical
circle absorption
circuit
closed
closed circuit
combined
compression
conduction
continuous epidural
continuous-flow catheter
continuous spinal
crossed
diagnostic
differential spinal
dissociated
dissociative
dolorosa (painful)
electric
endotracheal
epidural
endotracheal
extradural
field block
fractional epidural
fractional spinal
general
general endotracheal
general mask
girdle
glove
gustatory
high spinal
hyperbaric

anesthesia *(cont.)*
hyperbaric spinal
hypnosis
hypobaric spinal
hypotensive
hypothermic
hysterical
induced under
induction
infiltration
inhalation
inhalation mask
insufflation
intercostal
intramedullary
intranasal
intraoral
intraosseous
intraspinous
intravenous (IVA)
intravenous regional
intravenous sedation
ischiorectal fossa block
isobaric spinal
I.V., IV (intravenous)
local
low spinal
lumbar epidural
MAC (monitored anesthesia care)
mask
nerve block
Nerve Block Infusion Kit
nonrebreathing
ON-Q anesthesia delivery system
open
open drop
oropharyngeal
outpatient
painful
paracervical block
paravertebral
patient-controlled (PCA)
peridural
perineural

anesthesia *(cont.)*
periodontal
Ponka technique for local
postoperative
presacral
pressure
pudendal
rapid-acting
Raplon (rapacuronium bromide)
rebreathing
rectal
refrigeration
regional
retrobulbar
sacral
saddle
saddle block
segmental
semiclosed
semiopen
spinal
splanchnic
stocking
stocking glove
subarachnoid
supraclavicular block
surgical
tactile
therapeutic
thermal
to-and-fro
topical
topical oropharyngeal
total intravenous (TOPA)
total spinal
Tracrium (atracurium besylate)
transdermal
traumatic
unilateral
variable-dose patient-controlled
vecuronium bromide
visceral

anesthesia adjunct
anesthetic hepatitis

aneuploid tumor
AneuRX graft
AneuRX stent
aneurysm, abdominal aortic (AAA)
aneurysmal dilatation
aneurysmal sac
aneurysm clip applier
aneurysm needle
Angelchik antireflux ring prosthesis
Angell James hypophysectomy forceps
Angell James reverse-action hypophysectomy forceps
angiitis, granuloma
angina
  abdominal
  intestinal
  mesenteric
  pseudomembranous
  Vincent
angina dyspeptica
angiocatheter
Angiocath PRN catheter
angiocentric immunoproliferative lesion
angiocholecystitis
Angiocidin
angiodysplasia
  intestinal
  jejunal
angioedema, hereditary
Angiografin contrast agent
angiogram, cystic duct
angiographic catheter
angiographic variceal embolization
AngioLaz Medi-Vu endoscope
angiolithic sarcoma
angioma (pl. angiomata)
  capillary
  cavernous
  cherry
  hemangioma
  lymphangioma
  petechial
  spider
  telangiectatic
AngioMark contrast agent
angiomatosis
angioneurotic edema
AngioOptic microcatheter
angioprokinetic effect
angiosarcoma, hepatic
AngioStent
Angiovist
Angiozyme
angle
  anal pouch
  anorectal
  cardiohepatic
  epigastric
  hepatic-renal
  hepatorenal
  splenic-renal
  splenorenal
angled awl
angled-down forceps
angled jaw rongeur
angled peripheral vascular clamp
angled pituitary rongeur
angled pleural tube
angled probe
angled rasp
angled retractor
angled-up forceps
angle of His
angle suture
angular bone rongeur
angular elevator
angular hinge clamp
angularis body
angular knife
angulated lesion
angulus of stomach
anhaustral colonic gas pattern
anhemolytic strep (streptococcus)
anhepatic jaundice
anhepatic stage of liver transplantation
anicteric hepatitis
anicteric sclerae
anicteric skin

aniline cancer
animal bite infection
anismus
anisotropine methylbromide
Ankeney sternal retractor
ankle jerk (AJ)
ankle region
anlage of pancreas
annamycin
annular adenocarcinoma
annular esophageal stricture
annular pancreas
anococcygeal raphe
anoderm-preserving hemorrhoidectomy
Anogesic (nitroglycerin ointment)
anomaly
  cloacal
  Cruveilhier-Baumgarten
  vascular
anomaly of Zahn
anoperineal fistula
anoplasty (see *operation)*
anorectal abscess
anorectal angle
anorectal fistula
anorectal impalement
anorectal junction
anorectal line
anorectal lymph node
anorectal malformation
anorectal manometry
anorectal melanoma
anorectal mucosal prolapse
anorectal myomectomy
anorectal ring
anorectal sphincter
anorectal wall
anorectic
anorectoplasty
anorectovaginoplasty
anorexia
anorexia-cachexia syndrome
anorexia nervosa
anorexic
anoscope (also *endoscope, proctoscope, rectoscope, speculum*)
  ACMI
  Alan-Parks
  Arakawa
  Bensaude
  Blond
  Brinkeroff
  disposable
  di-wing
  Enproct disposable
  Fansler-Ives
  front-lifting hood
  Gabriel
  Galencia disposable
  Heine
  Hirschman
  Ives
  Ives-Fansler
  Jasan
  Karl Storz
  Kelly
  KleenSpec disposable
  Medix
  Naunton Morgan
  Newman
  Pratt
  Romanoscope
  Sani-Scope
  Sapimed
  Sklar disposable
  slotted
  St. Mark's
  Storz
  Strauss
  tri-wing
  two-valved
  UniSpec disposable
  video
  Welch Allyn
anoscopy
anosigmoidoscopy
anovestibular fistula
Anspach power drill

Anspach reamer
Anspach suture anchor
antacid
  liquid
  pain relieved by
  phosphate-binding
  p.r.n. (as needed)
antagonism, drug
antagonist, histamine-2 (H_2) receptor
antecolic anastomosis
antecolic gastrojejunostomy
antegrade femoral nail
antegrade scrotal sclerotherapy
antelmycin (also anthelmycin)
antemesenteric corner
antemortem clot
antenatal diagnosis
antepartum constipation
anterior abdominal wall
anterior abdominal wall syndrome
anterior band of colon
anterior colon resection
anterior forceps
anterior iliac crest graft
anterior rectopexy
anterior rectus fascia
anterior rectus sheath
anterior resection clamp
anterior sliding tibial graft
anterior superior iliac spine
anterior surface of pancreas
anterior view
anterior wall antral ulcer
anterolateral thoracotomy incision
anteromedial incision
antero-oblique position
anthelmintic
anthelmycin (also antelmycin)
anthracene-type laxative
anthraquinone of cascara
anthrax colitis
Anthron heparinized catheter
anthropometry
antiangiogenesis
Antibacterial Personal Catheter
antibiotic
  broad-spectrum
  perioperative
  postoperative
  preoperative
  prophylactic
antibiotic-associated colitis (AAC)
antibiotic-induced diarrhea
antibody
  alpha-Gal
  anticolonic
  antidelta IgM
  anti-HA (anti-hepatitis A)
  anti-HAV (anti-hepatitis A virus)
  anti-HB (anti-hepatitis B)
  anti-HB_c (anti-hepatitis B core)
  anti-HB_c-IgM (anti-hepatitis B core-IgM)
  anti-HB_e (anti-hepatitis B "e")
  anti-HB_s (anti-hepatitis B surface)
  anti-HCV (anti-hepatitis C virus)
  anti-interleukin (IL)-2 receptor
  antimitochondrial (AMA)
  antinuclear (ANA)
  anti-pig
  anti-VEGF (vascular endothelial growth factor)
  cA2 monoclonal
  CEA-Cide (^{131}I-labeled humanized antibody against carcinoembryonic antigen)
  cold-hemolytic
  C100-3 hepatitis C virus
  Cotara
  CytoTAb purified monoclonal
  detection
  HACA (human antichimeric antibody)
  HB_cAb (hepatitis B core antibody)
  HB_eAb (hepatitis B "e" antibody)
  HB_sAb (hepatitis B surface antibody)
  HCV (hepatitis C virus) (formerly non-A, non-B)

antibody *(cont.)*
  Herceptin (trastuzumab) monoclonal
  human antihepatitis B
  infliximab monoclonal
  islet cell
  LeuTech radiolabeled
  OST-577 human antihepatitis B
  serum HCV-specific
  transglutaminase
antibody-dependent cell-mediated cytotoxicity (ADCC)
antibody-mediated attack (hyperacute rejection)
antibody-mediated immune reaction (type III)
antibody-mediated immunity
antibody to HCV (anti-HCV)
anticholinergic drug
anticholinergic therapy
anticoagulant-treated blood
anticolonic antibody
Anticort
antidelta IgM antibody
antidiarrheal
antiemetic drug
antiendomysial antibody test
antifibrin antibody imaging
antigastrin therapy
antigen
  Australian
  CA 19-9
  delta (delta-Ag)
  endogenous
  enterobacterial common (ECA)
  exogenous
  HbAg, HB Ag ("H-bag") (hepatitis B antigen)
  HB_eAg (soluble "e" antigen in hepatitis B antigen)
  HB_sAg (hepatitis B surface antigen)
  HDAg (hepatitis D antigen)
  hepatitis-associated
  hepatitis B antigen (HbAg)
  hepatitis B_e (anti-HBe)

antigen *(cont.)*
  histocompatibility
  Histoplasma capsulatum polysaccharide antigen (HPA)
  HLA (human lymphocyte antigen)
  HSP (heat shock protein)
  human lymphocyte antigen (HLA)
  PCNA (proliferating cell nuclear)
antigen-antibody complex
antigen-antibody ratio
antigenemia
antigen load
antigenic properties of blood
antigenic triggering of immune inflammation
antigen-presenting cell (APC)
anti-HA, anti-HAV antibody (antibody to hepatitis A virus)
anti-HB antibody
anti-HB_c antibody
anti-HB_e antibody
anti-HB_e antigen
anti-HB_s antibody
anti-HB_c-IgM antibody
anti-HB_e-positive chronic hepatitis
anti-HCV antibody
anti-interleukin (IL)-2 receptor antibody
antilymphocyte globulin
antilymphocyte induction therapy
antimesenteric border of distal ileum
antimesenteric fat pad
antimesocolic side of the cecum
antimicrobial prophylaxis
antimicrobial therapy
Antiminth (pyrantel pamoate)
antimitochondrial antibody (AMA)
antimotility drug
antinauseant
antineoplastic drug
antinuclear antibody (ANA)
antiperistaltic operation
anti-pig antibody
antiprostaglandin
Anti-Pr-3 ELISA autoimmune test

antireflux mechanism
antireflux operation
antireflux regimen
antireflux surgery for esophageal stricture
antireflux therapy
antireflux valve
antirejection medication
anti-Schiff stain
antischistosomal drug
antisecretory drug therapy
antisense technology
antiseptic dressing
Antispas (diclyclomine HCl)
antispasmodic drug
anti-Tamm-Horsfall protein
anti-TNF (anti-tumor necrosis factor) therapy
antitubulin agent
anti-VEGF (vascular endothelial growth factor) antibody
Antivert (meclizine)
antivibratory glove
antiviral therapy
antral edema
antral G cell hyperplasia
antral gastric cell
antral gastritis
antral mucosa
antral pouch
antral sphincter
antral stasis
antral stenosis
antral stricture
antral ulcer
antrectomy
Antrenyl (oxyphenonium bromide)
Antrocol (atropine sulfate; phenobarbital)
antrotomy
antrum
  cardiac
  gastric
  prepyloric

antrum *(cont.)*
  pyloric
  retained
antrum of stomach
antrum of Willis
Anucort HC (hydrocortisone acetate)
Anumed (bismuth subgallate)
anus
  artificial
  ectopic
  high imperforate
  imperforate
  low imperforate
  patulous
  preternatural
Anusol (pramoxine HCl; zinc oxide)
Anusol-HC (hydrocortisone acetate)
anvil portion of EEA stapler
anvil-shaft assembly of stapling device
Anvirzel
anxiety-related diarrhea
Anzemet (dolasetron mesylate)
AO blade plate
AO condylar blade plate
AO contoured T plate
AODM (adult-onset diabetes mellitus) (now type 2)
AO hook plate
AOI blade plate
A-OK ShortCut knife
AO reconstruction plate
AO reduction forceps
AO semitubular
AO slotted medullary nail
AO small-fragment plate
aorta
  abdominal
  coarctation of
  dissecting
  esophageal artery of
  supraceliac
  thoracic
aortic aneurysm clamp
aortic arch

aortic bifurcation
aortic clamp
aortic hiatus
aortic occlusion clamp
aortic orifice
aortic root perfusion needle
aortic sac
aortic valve stenosis
aortoduodenal fistula
aortoenteric fistula
aortoesophageal fistula
aortofemoral bypass graft (AFBG)
aortohepatic arterial graft
aortosigmoid fistula
AP (anteroposterior)
APA (American Pancreatology Association)
APC (adenoma prevention with celecoxib) study
APC (adenomatous polyposis coli) gene
APC (argon plasma coagulation)
APECED syndrome
  APE (autoimmune polyendocrinopathy)
  C (candidiasis)
  ED (ectodermal dysplasia)
aperient
aperistalsis, esophageal
aperitive
apertures of abdomen
apex (pl. apices)
  bladder
  duodenal bulb
  external ring
  fibrous
  fibula
  heart
  ischiorectal fossa
  lingual
  lung
  nose
  prostate
apex cordis
apex pulmonis
Apex Plus excimer laser
AP (anteroposterior) film
aphtha (pl. aphthae)
aphthoid ulcer
aphthous ulcer
apical duodenal ulcer
apical infection
apical lordotic view
apical segment
apical suture
apical view
apicoposterior segment
Apligraf (graftskin)
AP (anteroposterior) nail
apocrine carcinoma
apocrine gland
apocrine metaplasia
Apo-Domperidone (domperidone maleate)
Apollo3 triple-lumen papillotome
Apomate radiopharmaceutical imaging agent
apomorphine
aponeurosis of internal oblique muscle
aponeurosis of external oblique muscle
aponeurosis, transversus abdominis
aponeurotic layer
apophyseal pouch
apoplectic pancreatitis
apoptosis (programmed cell death)
apoptotic index
apoptotic potential
apparatus (see *device*)
apparent death
apparent life-threatening event (ALTE)
appearance
  bat-wing
  beads-on-a-string
  beefy
  cobblestone
  collar-button (in colon)
  corkscrew
  dewy
  granular

appearance *(cont.)*
  ground-glass
  hobnailed
  honeycomb(ed)
  lead pipe
  macroscopic
  meaty
  moth-eaten
  mottled
  nutmeg
  onion peel
  onionskin
  orange peel
  signet ring
  speckled
  steamy
  string-of-beads
  tigroid
  whorled
appearance infarct
appendage clamp
appendage, epiploic
appendectomy
  emergency
  emergent
  incidental
  inversion-ligation
  laparoscopic
  laser-assisted
  McBurney
  negative
  percutaneous
appendiceal abscess
appendiceal colic
appendiceal concretion
appendiceal constriction
appendiceal fecalith
appendiceal fistula
appendiceal hyperplasia
appendiceal intussusception
appendiceal lumen
appendiceal mass
appendiceal mucocele
appendiceal retractor
appendiceal stercolith
appendiceal stump
appendicitis
  acute
  amebic
  chronic
  complex
  early
  fulminating
  gangrenous
  helminthic
  inflamed
  lumbar
  nonperforated
  obstructive
  perforated
  perforated acute
  recurrent
  relapsing
  segmental
  stercoral
  subacute
  subperitoneal
  suppurative
  traumatic
appendicitis obliterans
appendicocele
appendicoenterostomy
appendicolith
appendicolithiasis
appendicolysis
appendicopathy
appendicovesicotomy
appendicular artery
appendicular colic
appendicular lymph node
appendicular muscle
appendicular skeleton
appendicular vein
appendix (pl. appendices)
  auricular
  cecal
  ensiform
  epiploic

appendix *(cont.)*
  gangrenous
  hot
  indurated
  inflamed
  inflammation
  mesentery of
  Morgagni
  nonperforated
  normal
  orifice of
  paracecal
  perforated
  preileal
  retrocecal
  retrocolic
  retroileal
  right auricular
  ruptured
  serpentine
  subcecal
  suppurative
  testis
  ventricle of larynx
  vermiform
  vesicular
  xiphoid
appendix fibrosa
appendix of epididymis
appendix of testis
appendolithiasis
apperceptive mass
appetite juice
apple-core configuration of mass
apple-core lesion
apple-peel bowel
apple-peel syndrome
appliance (see *barrier; device; pouch*)
  Bard colostomy
  closed-end ostomy
  ConvaTec colostomy
  Dansac DuoSoft pouch
  Dansac Nova ostomy
  Divine colostomy

appliance *(cont.)*
  Erlangen magnetic colostomy
  Gentle Touch colostomy
  Hollister
  Hollister Karaya
  Karaya ring ileostomy
  loop ostomy
  Nu-Comfort
  Nu-Flex
  Nu-Hope ostomy
  Nu-Self
  ostomy
  Remedy
applicator (see also *applier; forceps*)
  cotton
  cotton-tipped
  Eder cotton
  Endo Clip
  Farrell cotton
  Frankenfeldt cotton
  Olympus rotatable clip
applier (see also *applicator*; *forceps)*
  Absolok clip
  Adson clip
  Allen clip
  Allport multiple clip
  aneurysm
  Aslan clip
  Auto Suture Endo Clip
  bayonet clip
  clip
  Cyanamid clip
  double clip
  Duraclose clip
  Endo clip
  Endo Hernia
  endoscopic
  Ethicon clip
  Filshie clip
  Hulka clip
  Imagyn endoscopic clip
  laparoscopic clip
  Ligaclip ERCA endoscopic clip
  ligating clip

applier *(cont.)*
- Mayfield miniature clip
- Mayfield temporary aneurysm clip
- mini
- Mirage ostomy
- Multifire Endo Hernia clip
- MUR (Multiuse Reposable) clip
- multiple ligating clip
- Olympus clip
- Olympus rotatable clip
- One Shot vascular clip
- PermaClip endoscopic clip
- Reflex ELC clip
- reposable clip
- Richard Allen clip
- right-angle
- rotatable
- Sovereign Multifire clip
- Stahl clip
- Sur-Fit AutoLock
- Sur-Fit Natura ostomy
- Surgiclip
- USSC clip
- Vari-angle clip
- VCS clip
- VitaClip
- Weck clip

applying forceps
Appolito suture
Appraise blood glucose monitor
approach
- axillary
- cervical
- double seton modified surgical
- extraperitoneal
- inframammary
- Kugel
- laparoscopic
- preperitoneal
- retroperitoneal
- sacroperineal
- sternal split
- supraduodenal
- takedown abdominal

approach *(cont.)*
- transabdominal
- transabdominal preperitoneal
- transanal
- transcoccygeal
- transsacral
- transthoracic
- transumbilical

approximated
approximating forceps
approximation
- skin
- tissue
- wound

approximation suture
approximator clamp
"appy" (appendectomy) tape
APR (abdominoperineal or abdominal-perineal resection)
APR cement fixation adhesive
Apra (CT-2584 mesylate)
APRL (Army Prosthetics Research Laboratory)
apron (panniculus)
- abdominal
- fatty
- vascular

AP (anteroposterior) supine view
Aptosyn (exisulind)
APTT (activated partial thromboplastin time)
APUD (amine precursor uptake and decarboxylation) cell
APUDoma
AP (anteroposterior) view
Aquacel Hydrofiber wound dressing
Aquacel Hydrofiber wound packing
Aquaphor gauze dressing
Aquasorb transparent hydrogel dressing
Aquilion CT scanner
arachadonic acid
arachnoid fibrosis
arachnoid knife
arachnoid-shaped Beaver blade

Arakawa anoscope
arbaprostil
arborization of ducts
ARC (AIDS-related complex)
arcade, ileocolic
arch, aortic
arch cookie (pad)
archimedean hand drill
architectural atypia
architecture
  hepatic
  lobular
arcitumomab (CEA-Scan) imaging agent
arclofenin hepatic function test
Arco-Lase (amylase; protease; lipase; cellulase)
Arco-Lase Plus
arc reflex
arcuate artery of kidney
arcuate line
ARD (acid-related disorder)
ARDS (adult respiratory distress syndrome)
area gastrica (pl. areae gastricae)
area of mucosal irregularity
areola (pl. areolae)
areola of breast
areolar gland
areolar lesion
areolar tissue
ArF (argon fluorine) excimer laser
argentaffin cell
argentaffin reaction test
Arglaes antimicrobial barrier film dressing
argon beam coagulator (ABC)
argon/krypton laser
argon laser
argon plasma coagulation (APC)
Argyle chest tube
Argyle Medicut R catheter
Argyle-Salem sump tube
Argyle Sentinel Seal chest tube
argyrophil (or argyrophilic) cell
Aria coronary artery bypass graft
Arias syndrome
Aries-Pitanguy correction of mammary ptosis
Arimidex (anastrozole)
A ring, esophageal
A ring of esophagus
arm
  MINI 6600 C-arm
  PinPoint stereotactic
  robotic
arm abducted to 90 degrees
Armanni-Ebstein kidney
Armanni-Ebstein lesion
arm board
Armenian syndrome
Armstrong plate
Army bone gouge
Army-Navy retractor
Aromasin (exemestane)
aromatic amino acid (AAA)
aromatic cascara fluid extract
aromatic cascara sagrada
Aron Alpha adhesive
Aronson esophageal retractor
Aroplatin
Arrequi laparoscopic knot pusher
Arrestin (trimethobenzamide HCl)
arrhythmia mapping system catheter
Arrowgard Blue Line catheter
Arrow-Howes multilumen catheter
Arrow Twin Cath catheter
Arruga needle
Arruga-Nicetic forceps
arsenic, inorganic
arsenic trioxide (ATO)
ArtAssist compression dressing
arteria lusoria
arterial arcade of jejunum
arterial blood
arterial blood gases
arterial line
arterial missile embolism

arterial obstruction
arterial stenosis
arterial thrombosis
arteries were skeletonized
arteriogram
arteriography
arteriohepatic dysplasia (AHD)
arteriolar necrosis
arteriosclerotic kidney
arteriovenous (AV) fistula
arteriovenous malformation (AVM)
arteritis, necrotizing
artery (see Table of Arteries in
  Appendix)
artery forceps
Arthrex coring reamer
Arthrex femoral guide
Arthrex tibial guide
arthrifluent abscess
Arthrinium
arthritis panel
Arthrocare Wand probe
Arthroderma
arthropathy, neurogenic
arthroplasty gouge
arthropod-borne virus
ArthroProbe laser
arthroscopic blade
arthroscopic cannula
arthroscopic knife
arthroscopic probe
arthroscopic scissors
arthroscopy basket
arthroscopy grasping forceps
ArthroSew suture
Arthrotek RC needle
Arthrotek rigid laparoscope
ArthroWand
articular cartilage autograft
articular fluid
articulating dissector
artificial anus
artificial bezoar
artificial gut
artificial kidney
artificial sphincter
Artiflex bandage
aryepiglottic fold
aryepiglottis
arytenoid gland
Asacol (mesalamine)
ASAP antimicrobial solution
ascariasis, biliary
Ascaris lumbricoides
ascending cholangitis
ascending colon
Ascent guiding catheter
Asch forceps
ascites
  bile
  blood-tinged
  bloody
  chylous
  cloudy
  dialysis-related
  exudative
  fatty
  hemorrhagic
  hydremic
  milky
  myxedema
  nephrogenic
  pancreatic
  progressive
  pseudochylous
  refractory
  straw-colored
  tense
  transudative
ascites drainage tube
ascites trocar
ascitic amylase
ascitic fluid (see *fluid*)
Ascriptin A/D
ASCRS (American Society of Colon
  and Rectal Surgeons)
ASCUS (atypical squamous cells
  of uncertain significance)

ASE (axilla, shoulder, elbow) bandage
AS-800 artificial sphincter
Aselli pancreas
aseptic necrosis
aseptic technique
aseptic wound
Asepto irrigation syringe
ASGE (American Society of Gastro-intestinal Endoscopy)
Asherson syndrome
ASHN (acute sclerosing hyaline necrosis)
ASIF chisel
ASIF right-angle blade plate
Askin tumor
Ask-Upmark kidney
Aslan clip applier
ASLC (acute self-limited colitis)
aspartate transaminase (AST) (formerly SGOT) liver function test
A-Spas S/L (hyoscyamine sulfate)
Aspen laparoscopy electrode
Aspen ultrasound system
Aspergillus cerebral abscess
aspirate
 bilious
 bone marrow
 gastric
 NG (nasogastric)
aspirating needle
 large-bore slotted
 mediastinoscopy
aspiration
 cervical
 cyst
 fine-needle
 hematoma
 iliac crest bone
 needle
 percutaneous
 peritoneal
 puncture
aspiration associated with gastrostomy feeding
aspiration biopsy
aspiration biopsy cytology
aspiration needle
aspiration syringe
aspirator
 Cavitron ultrasonic
 Cavitron surgical
 Cooper Cavitron surgical
 CUSA (Cavitron ultrasonic surgical aspirator)
 CUSA EXcel surgical
 Dissectron ultrasonic
 Lysonix 2000 soft tissue
 Millennium ultrasonic
 PSI-TEC
 Selector ultrasonic
 ultrasonic surgical
 Vabra
aspirin-induced gastritis
asplenia syndrome
ASPS (alveolar soft-part sarcoma)
assay (see also *test*)
 alpha-2 antiplasmin functional
 Bioclot protein S
 bladder tumor (BTA)
 BTA stat bladder tumor
 BTA TRAK bladder tumor
 CA15-3 RIA
 CA27.29 antigen
 coagulation factor
 ELISA (enzyme linked immuno-sorbent assay)
 Emit 2000 cyclosporine specific
 EndoCab ELISA
 enzyme-linked immunosorbent
 ER-ICA (estrogen receptor immuno-chemical assay)
 Escherichia coli O157:H7
 FLU OIA
 Glycacor
 Heprofile ELISA
 Innofluor FPIA (fluorescence-polarization immunoassay)
 intact molecule

assay *(cont.)*
intragraft polymerase chain reaction (PCR)
IOS immunoassay system
Limulus amoebocyte lysate (LAL) chromogenic endotoxin
MATRIX
N High Sensitivity CRP (C-reactive protein)
OncoChek immunoassay
OnCyte
plasma assay coagulation panel
PP-CAP IgA enzyme immunoassay
PreVue *Borrelia burgdorferi* antibody detection
PTH
PyloriProbe
recombinant immunoblot (RIBA)
RIBA (recombinant immunoblot assay)
RIBA HCV 3.0 SIA (strip immunoblot assay)
sandwich radioimmunoassay
SIA (strip immunoblot assay)
steroid-binding
strip immunoblot assay (SIA)
thyrocalcitonin assay
Truquant BR radioimmunoassay
Velogene rapid VRE
assay of altered DNA exfoliated into stool
assessment of bowel function
assessment, preoperative
ASSI (Accurate Surgical and Scientific Instruments) device
ASSI No-scalpel vasectomy fixator ring clamp
Assure blood glucose monitoring system
AST (aspartate aminotransferase) liver function test (formerly SGOT)
asterixis
asteroid body
ASTRA profile
astrovirus gastroenteritis
Astwood-Coller staging system for carcinoma
asymmetric mural thickening
asymmetrical breast prosthesis
asymmetry, breast
asymptomatic appendicitis
asymptomatic cholelithiasis
asymptomatic gallstone
Atabrine
ataxia, late-onset
atelectasis, postoperative
atelectatic lung
Atgam (lymphocyte immune globulin; antithymocyte)
atherectomy catheter
AtheroCath Bantam coronary atherectomy catheter
AtheroCath catheter
atheromatous ulcer
atherosclerotic lesion
Athlete coronary guidewire
athyrotic cretinism
ATI (Abdominal Trauma Index)
Atkinson scoring system for dysphagia
Atkinson silicone rubber tube
Atlantic Ileostomy Catheter
Atlas 2.0 diagnostic ultrasound system
AtLast blood glucose monitor
ATL UM 9 HDI Colorflow ultrasound system
atmospheres of pressure in balloon catheter
ATO (arsenic trioxide; $As2O_3$)
atonic consti pation
atonic esophagus
atony
colonic
gastric
intestinal
sphincter
atorvastatin calcium
atovaquone/proguanil

ATPase (adenosine triphosphatase)
  inhibitors
atracurium besylate
Atraloc needle
Atrauclip hemostatic clamp
AtrauGrip forceps
atraumatic abscess
atraumatic forceps
atraumatic grasper
atraumatic suture
atraumatic vascular clamp
atresia
  anal
  biliary
  congenital
  congenital biliary
  duodenal
  esophageal
  extrahepatic biliary (EBA)
  intestinal
  intrahepatic (IHA)
  posterior choanal
  prepyloric
atrial retractor
atriocaval shunt
atrioventricular orifice
Atrisol aerosol
Atrocholin
atrophic cirrhosis
atrophic gastritis
atrophic-hyperplastic ulcer
atrophic kidney
atrophy
  crypt
  gastric
  healed yellow
  intestinal villous
  mammary
  mucosal
  muscular
  villous
  yellow
atropine sulfate
ATS (autotransfusion) catheter
attachment
  mesenteric
  peritoneal
  point of
Attain parenteral nutritional therapy
attapulgite
attenuated
attic adhesion
atypia, architectural
atypical gallbladder disease
atypical squamous cells of uncertain
  significance (ASCUS)
Auchincloss modified radical
  mastectomy
auditory mucosa
Auerbach mesenteric plexus
AU5 Harmonic ultrasound system
Aufranc awl
Aufranc cobra retractor
Aufranc cup
Aufranc gouge
Aufranc hook
Aufranc periosteal elevator
Aufranc psoas retractor
Aufranc reamer
Aufricht dissecting scissors
Aufricht glabellar rasp
augmentation, breast
augmentation mammoplasty
augmentation of anesthesia
Augustine boat nail
Aura desktop ENT laser
auricular appendix
auricular perichondritis
Aurora diode soft tissue laser
Aurora MR breast imaging system
auscultation of bowel sounds
Austin awl
Austin Moore chisel
Austin Moore extractor
Austin Moore hook
Austin Moore pin
Austin Moore rasp
Austin Moore reamer

Australian antigen
Auth atherectomy catheter
Autoblock safety syringe
autochthonous graft
autochthonous malaria
autoclavable
Autoclix fingerstick device
autocount sponge
autocrine mediator of bone metastasis
autodigestion
autoerotic rectal trauma
Autofuse Byron infiltration pump
autogenous bone graft
autogenous dermal graft
autogenous fascial heterograft
autogenous inlay graft
autogenous soft tissue graft
autograft harvesting
AutoGuard-P catheter
autoimmune attack
autoimmune disease
autoimmune disorder
  diabetes mellitus
  hypoadrenalism
  hypoparathyroidism
  pernicious anemia
  thyroiditis
autoimmune hemolytic anemia
autoimmune hepatitis
autoimmune hypoglycemia
autoimmune polyendocrinopathy (APE)
autoimmune process
autoimmune thyroiditis
autoinoculation
auto-Lancet
AuTolo Cure Process
autologous blood
autologous bone marrow transplant (AuBMT)
Autologous Bone Marrow Transplant Registry (ABMTR)
autologous clot
autologous crest bone graft
autologous fat graft
autologous leukapheresis, processing, and storage (ALPS)
autologous rectus abdominis fascia
autologous reverse graft
autologous transfusion
autologous tumor cells
autologous vein-covered stent
automated blood cell analyzer
Automated Cellular Imaging System (ACTS)
automated computerized axial tomography (ACAT)
Automated Endoscopic System for Optimal Positioning (AESOP)
automated image analysis
automated islet-cell shaking device
automatic knot-tying device
automatic skin retractor
automatic staple
autonomously hyperfunctioning nodule
autonomy, nutritional
autopepsia
autopsy knife
auto-reinforced polyglycolide rod
autosomal dominant disease
autosomal dominant genetic trait
autosomal dominant polycystic disease
autosomal recessive disorder
autosomal recessive genetic trait
AutoSonix system
autosplenectomize
autostapler, TA-55
autostapling device
Auto Suture ABBI system
Auto Suture Multifire Endo GIA 30 stapler
Auto Suture One-Shot anastomotic device
Auto Suture Premium CEEA stapler
Auto Suture Premium TA-55 surgical stapler
Auto Suture Soft Thoracoport obturator
Auto Suture SurgiStitch
Auto Suture suture

autosuture technique
Auto Suture universal retractor base
autotransfusion system
autotransplantation, parathyroid, to forearm
autotransplant, islet
Autovac autotransfusion system
Autovac LF autotransfusion system
Auvard speculum
auxiliary transplant
AV (arteriovenous) fistula
Avakine (infliximab)
Avandia (rosiglitazone maleate)
avascular necrosis (AVN)
AVA 3Xi advanced venous access device
AVCO aortic balloon
Avelox (moxifloxacin)
AVH (acute viral hepatitis)
avian leukosis virus
avian malaria
Avicine therapeutic cancer vaccine
Avitene "flour" dressing
Avitene Hemostat
Avitene macrofibrillar collagen hemostatic material
Avitene Ultrafoam collagen hemostatic sponge
AVM (arteriovenous malformation)
avulsed wound
avulsion of appendiceal tip
awl
  angled
  Aufranc
  Austin
  bone
  curved
  DePuy
  Ender
  Küntscher (Kuentscher)
  Mark II Kodros radiolucent
  pointed
  reaming

awl *(cont.)*
  rectangular
  Rush
  square-shaped
  Swanson lunate
  Swanson scaphoid
  T-handled
  Zuelzer
axial hiatal hernia
axial plate
axial sesamoid view
axial wall
Axid (nizatidine)
Axid AR ("acid reducer")
axilla (pl. axillae)
axillary adenopathy
axillary anesthesia
axillary approach in surgery
axillary artery
axillary contents
axillary dissection
axillary envelope
axillary fat pad
axillary fold
axillary fossa
axillary line
axillary lymphadenectomy
axillary lymphadenopathy
axillary lymph node
axillary node dissection
axillary region
axillary tail
axillary vein
axillary view
axiom double sump tube
axis
  bowel
  celiac
  enteroinsular
  hypothalamic-pituitary
  hypothalamic-pituitary-adrenal
Axokine (ciliary neurotrophic factor [CNTF])

AXR (abdominal x-ray)
AXR/CT (abdominal x-ray and computed tomography)
AxyaWeld Bone Anchor System
Ayers needle holder
Aylett operation
Ayre brush
Ayre knife
Ayre spatula
Ayre tube
ayw1, ayw2, ayw3, ayw4, ayr (hepatitis B surface antigen subdeterminants)
AZA (azathioprine)
azathioprine
azotemia
aztreonam
Azulfidine (sulfasalazine)
Azulfidine EN-tabs
azygos vein
azygous system

B, b

Babcock atraumatic tissue forceps
Babcock clamp
Babcock grasping forceps, double-action
Babcock intestinal forceps
Babcock retractor
Babcock stainless steel suture wire
Babcock-TC tissue forceps
Babcock wire-cutting scissors
Babesia divergens
Babinski percussion hammer
baby Adson forceps
baby Allis tissue forceps
baby Babcock tissue forceps
baby Balfour abdominal retractor
baby Deaver retractor
baby Doyen intestinal forceps
baby Gelpi retractor
baby Harrington retractor
baby Jones towel clip
baby Metzenbaum dissecting scissors
baby Mollison retractor
baby Payr pylorus clamp
baby Poole suction tube
baby Reynolds dissecting scissors
baby Roux retractor
Babytherm IC gel mattress
baby Tischler biopsy forceps
baby Yankauer suction tube
Bacher flexible biopsy forceps
bacillary colitis
bacillary diarrhea
bacillary dysentery
bacillary necrosis
bacillus Calmette-Guérin (BCG)
Bacillus cereus
bacitracin ointment
Backhaus clamp
Backhaus dilator
Backhaus forceps
Backhaus knife
Backlund biopsy needle
back pain
backup of portal pressure
backward-cutting knife
backwash ileitis
Bacon bone rongeur
Bacon cranial rongeur
Bacon rasp
Bacon rongeur forceps
Bacon thoracic shears
BACTEC system
bacteremia
  community-acquired
  fulminant
  persistent

bacteremia *(cont.)*
  polymicrobial
  transient
bacteria (pl. of bacterium)
  acid-fast
  Acinetobacter
  aerobic
  anaerobic
  Calymmatobacterium
  Campylobacter
  Candida
  Chauveau
  coliform
  colonic
  corkscrew-shaped
  corynebacteria
  Cryptococcus
  defense against
  Enterobacter
  fibrillary
  fungus-like
  gas-forming
  gram-negative
  gram-positive
  Haemophilus
  helical
  intestinal
  intracellular
  Klebsiella
  Lactobacillus
  luminal
  mesophilic
  Nocardia
  pathogenic
  Proteus
  Pseudomonas
  pus-forming
  pyogenic
  Salmonella
  Serratia
  Shigella
  spiral-shaped
  toxigenic
  Toxoplasma
bacteria-impervious seal
bacteria in stool
bacteria in urine
bacterial abscess
bacterial cellular protein
bacterial cholangitis
bacterial cirrhosis
bacterial co-infection
bacterial colitis
bacterial colony
bacterial colonization
bacterial culture
bacterial culture media
bacterial dissociation
bacterial enterocolitis
bacterial esophagitis
bacterial flora
bacterial food poisoning
bacterial gastroenteritis
bacterial infection
bacterial lipopolysaccharide
bacterial meningitis
bacterial metabolism
bacterial myocarditis
bacterial nephritis
bacterial overgrowth
bacterial pericarditis
bacterial peritonitis
bacterial pneumonia
bacterial pneumonitis
bacterial protein
bacterial toxemia
bacterial toxin
bacterial vaginosis
bacterial virus
bactericidal antibiotic
bactericidal oxygen radical
bacteriocholia
bacteriologic smear, AFB (acid-fast bacillus)
bacteriostatic, mafenide acetate
bacteriostatic water
bacterium (see *bacteria*)
bacteriuria

Bacteroides bividius
Bacteroides capillosus
Bacteroides distasonis
Bacteroides fragilis
Bacteroides nodosus
Bacteroides praeacutus
Bacteroides putredinis
Bacteroides splanchnicus
Bacteroides thetaiotamicron
Bacteroides ureolyticus
Bacteroides vulgatus
Bactigen *Salmonella-Shigella* slide test
Bactrim (trimethoprim, sulfamethoxazole)
Baculovirus Expression Vector System (BEVS)
Badgley laminectomy retractor
Badgley plate
BA-EDTA (bile acid-EDTA) solution
Baer bone-cutting forceps
Baer bone rongeur
Baermann stool filter
Baermann stool test
Baer rib shears
bag (see also *appliance*; *pouch*)
  bile
  bowel
  colostomy
  Endopouch Pro specimen
  Endosac specimen
  Hollister
  ileostomy
  intestinal
  Karaya seal stoma
  Lahey
  Lapides
  Marlen
  ostomy
  Perry
  Petersen
  pneumatic
  Ponsky Endo Sock retrieval
  Rutzen ileostomy
  stomal
  Whitmore
bag and mask
bag breathing
Bagby angled compression plate
BAGF (brachioaxillary bridge graft fistula)
bagged
Baggish biopsy forceps
Bahnson aortic clamp
Baho endoscope
Bailey aortic clamp
Bailey aortic valve-cutting forceps
Bailey-Dubow nail
Bailey-Gibbon rib contractor
Bailey-Gigli saw
Bailey-Gigli saw guide
Bailey rib contractor
Bailey wire saw
Bainbridge intestinal clamp
Bainbridge intestinal forceps
Baird forceps
Bakamjian flap
Baker intestinal decompression tube
Baker jejunostomy tube
Bakes common duct dilator
Bakes probe
Bak-Pac portable ultrasound scanner
BAL (bronchoalveolar lavage)
balanced anesthesia
balanced diet
balanced electrolyte solution (BES)
balanced salt solution (BSS)
balance, equal fluid
balantidial colitis
BalAsa (balsalazide disodium) (now Colazal)
bald gastric fundus
Baldy-Webster operation
Balfour abdominal retractor
Balfour center blade
Balfour retractor
Balfour self-retaining retractor
Ballance sign
ball-and-socket towel forceps
Ballantine clamp
Ballantine forceps

Ballantine hemilaminectomy retractor
Ballenger-Hajek chisel
Ballenger sponge-holding forceps
Ballenger swivel knife
ballerina-foot pattern
ball guide pin
ballistic wound
Ballobes gastric balloon
balloon
  ACS SULP II
  AVCO aortic
  Ballobes gastric
  banana-shaped
  bifoil
  BioEnterics gastric
  Blakemore
  Blue Max
  Brandt cytology
  DURAglide stone removal
  DURAglide 3 stone removal
  Duralon occlusion
  esophageal
  Extra View
  Extractor three-lumen retrieval
  Fogarty
  Garren-Edwards
  gastric
  Gau gastric
  Grüntzig (Gruentzig)
  Hartzler angioplasty
  Hartzler Micro II
  Hunter-Sessions
  hydrostatic
  Inoue
  intra-aortic (IAB)
  intragastric
  kissing
  Kontron intra-aortic
  low-compliance hydrostatic
  LPS
  Mansfield
  mercury-containing
  Microvasive endoscopic
  Microvasive Mini Button low-profile

balloon *(cont.)*
  Microvasive Rigiflex TTS
  Monorail
  Origin
  PDB laparoscopic
  PEG
  Percival gastric
  Percor DL-II (dual-lumen)
    intra-aortic
  Percor-Stat intra-aortic
  PET
  preperitoneal distention (PDB)
  pulsation
  Quantum
  rectal
  Rigiflex TTS
  Sci-Med Express Monorail
  scintigraphic
  self-positioning
  Sengstaken
  Sengstaken-Blakemore tamponade
  slave
  Soto USCI
  Stack autoperfusion
  Taylor gastric
  traction
  transendoscopic
  trefoil
  TTS (through-the-scope)
  Wilson-Cook gastric
balloon biliary catheter
balloon catheter
balloon catheter fenestration
balloon cholangiogram
balloon decompression
balloon dilating catheter
balloon dilation
balloon dissector
balloon-expandable flexible coil stent
balloon-expandable intravascular stent
balloon expulsion test
balloon extraction technique
balloon fenestration procedure
ballooning degeneration of hepatocytes

ballooning of hepatocytes
balloon occlusion
balloon pump
balloon reflex manometry
balloon sphincterotome
balloon tamponade of varices
balloon-tipped catheter
balloon-tipped end-hole catheter
Ball operation for treatment of pruritus ani
ballotable liver
ballottement, abdominal
ball-point guide pin
ball reamer
ball-tip electrode
ball-tip guide pin
ball-tipped Küntscher (Kuentscher) guide
ball-wedge catheter
balm of Gilead
Balneol
balsalazine
balsalazide disodium
Balser fatty necrosis
BAMBI (breast augmentation mammoplasty by injection)
Banalg (methyl salicylate; camphor; menthol)
banana Beaver blade
banana knife
banana-shaped balloon
band
  anterior
  colon
  fascial
  free
  gastric
  Harris
  Ladd
  Lane
  Marlex
  mesocolic
  musculoaponeurotic
  omental
band *(cont.)*
  peritoneal
  ReliefBand NST
  silicone elastomer
bandage (see also *dressing*)
  Ace
  Ace adherent
  adhesive
  Artiflex
  ASE (axilla, shoulder, elbow)
  Band-Aid
  Barton
  butterfly
  capeline
  Cellona
  Champ elastic
  chip mat
  "chocolate bar"
  Clean Seals
  collodion
  Comperm
  Comperm PD
  Comperm tubular elastic
  compression
  Comprilan
  Conco Gauze
  cotton elastic
  Cover-Roll
  cravat
  crepe
  Daverbinde K
  Dema-Band
  Dema Pad
  demigauntlet
  Desault
  Dressinet netting
  Durelast
  E Cotton
  elastic
  elastic wrap
  Elastic Foam
  elastomer
  Elastomull
  Elastoplast

bandage *(cont.)*
Esmarch
Fabco gauze
figure-of-8 interscapular
Flex-Foam
Flexilite conforming elastic
Flex-Master
FlexTube
foam roll
foam sheet
Fractura Flex
gauntlet
Gibney
Gibson
gray foam
gum rubber Martin
Hamilton
hand piece
Heliodorus
Hippocrates
Hueter
Hydron burn
Idealbind
immobilizing
Isoband
Kerlix
Kling elastic
K.T. Medical
Komprex
Komprex-Binde
LiquiBand topical wound-closure glue
Liquiderm liquid
Luekosilk
malleable metal finger splint
Martin sheet rubber
Mollelast
"muff"
nonadhesive
Nu Gauze sterile gauze
Ortho-Trac adhesive
Ortho-Vent nonadhesive
Pavlik
POP (plaster of Paris)

bandage *(cont.)*
pre-cut foam
PRN
Profore four-layer
Redigrip pressure
replantation
restrictive
Ribble
Richet
Rosidal
Sayre
scultetus
self-adhering
Silverlon wound packing strips
sling and swathe
Snugs
spica
spiral
starch
stockinette
Tg
Transelast
Tricodur compression support
Tricodur Epi (elbow) compression
Tricodur Omos (shoulder) compression
Tricodur Talus (ankle) compression
Tricofix
Tru-Support EW (elastic wrap)
Tru-Support SA (self-adhering)
Tubigrip
tubular elastic
tubular stockinette
tumescent absorbent bandage (TAB)
two-inch gauze
Velpeau
Webril
bandage and utility scissors
bandage scissors
Band-Aid
Band-Aid dressing
band and cut
band and snare
band circling needle

bandeau defect
Bandeau post-augmentation bra, The
banded bag
banding
  adjustable silicone gastric
  gastric
  hemorrhoidal
band ligation of esophageal varices
band-ligator device
bandlike adhesion
band sigmoidopexy
band slippage
band-snare technique
Bane mastoid rongeur
Bane rongeur forceps
Bane-Hartmann bone rongeur
Bangerter muscle forceps
banjo curet
banjo-string adhesion
Bankart lesion
Bankart shoulder retractor
Banks bone graft
Bantam coagulator
Bantam irrigation set
Bantam wire-cutting scissors
Banthine (methantheline bromide)
Banti disease
Banti syndrome
BAO:MAO (basal:maximal acid output ratio)
bar, cricopharyngeal
barbed staple
barber chair position
barber pole sign (on x-ray)
Barbidonna #2
Bard BTA test
Bard colostomy appliance
Bard Composix mesh graft material
Bard-Davol trumpet valve
Bardeleben bone-holding forceps
Bardeleben rasp
Bard Eliminator 1 balloon dilator
Bard endoscopic suturing system
Bard Extra Ileo B pouch
Bard flexible endoscopic injection system
Bard gastrostomy button
Bard gastrostomy catheter
Bard gastrostomy feeding tube
Bard Integrale pouch
Bard Memotherm colorectal stent
Bard-Parker blade
Bard-Parker knife
Bard Protective Barrier for ostomy skin
Bard Safety Excalibur catheter introducer
Bard Safety Excalibur PICC introducer
Bard Sperma-Tex preshaped mesh
Bard Visilex mesh graft
Bard XT bifurcated stent
bare area of liver
bare area of stomach
bariatric operation
bariatric surgery
Baricon contrast medium for GI imaging
barium
  residual
  retained
barium enema (BE)
barium enema with air contrast
barium esophagram
barium meal
barium sediment in urine
barium sulfate ($BaSO_4$)
barium sulfate-impregnated shunt
barium sulfate suspension
barium suspension, oral
barium swallow
Barnes-Neville forceps
Barnes perineorrhaphy scissors
Barnhill adenoid curette
Barobag contrast for GI imaging
Baro-cat contrast for GI imaging
Baroflave contrast medium
Baron suction tube
Baros adjunct for GI imaging
Barosperse contrast for GI imaging

barotrauma
Barouk microstaple
Barraquer cilia forceps
Barraquer Colibri forceps
Barraquer needle
Barraquer needle holder
Barraquer suture-removing forceps
Barr body analysis
Barr crypt hook
Barr D/E fistula probe
barrel guide
barrel reamer
barrel-shaped stone
Barr-Epstein virus
Barrett disease
Barrett epithelium
Barrett esophagus (BE)
Barrett intestinal forceps
Barrett mucosa
Barrett placenta forceps
Barrett syndrome
Barrett tenaculum forceps
Barrett ulcer
Barr fistula hook
Barr fistula probe
Barr hook
barrier (see also *appliance; dressing; mesh; ointment; pouch*)
  Active Life skin
  BioMesh surgical mesh
  CenterPointLock skin
  Coly-Seel ostomy
  ConvaTec skin
  CoStop surgical adhesion
  cut-to-fit skin
  Cymed colostomy
  gastric mucosal
  Gore-Tex surgical mesh
  Guidor surgical mesh
  Interceed surgical adhesion
  MicroSkin skin
  Nu-Hope skin
  Resolut surgical mesh
  SecureLife skin
barrier *(cont.)*
  SprayGel adhesion
  stockinette
barrier pack
Barr nail
Barron hemorrhoidal band
Barron hemorrhoidal ligator
Barron scalpel
Barr rectal probe
Barr rectal retractor
Barr rectal speculum
Barr-Shuford rectal speculum
Barsky skin hook
Barth curette
Barth hernia
Bartholin gland
Barton bandage
Bartonella bacilliformis
Barton obstetrical forceps
Bartter syndrome
basal acid secretion
basal anesthesia
basal cell
basal cell carcinoma
basal cell nevus syndrome
basal cell papilloma
basal granular cell
Basaljel (aluminum carbonate gel, basic)
basal:maximal acid output ratio (BAO:MAO)
basaloid carcinoma
basal plate
basal secretory flow rate (BSFR)
basal sphincter
bascule volvulus
baseball stitch
baseball suture
base deficit
Basedow disease
Basedow goiter
base excess
baseline, gastric
baseline mammogram

baseline tenting
baseline view
base material
basement membrane
base of appendix
base of tongue
base plate, bipod
base radical
basic fibroblast growth factor (bFGF)
basidiobolomycosis
basilar skull fracture
basilar suture
basiliximab
basket
  biliary stone
  CBD (common bile duct)
  Dormia stone
  four-wire
  gallstone
  intraductal biliary
  Pursuer CBD helical stone
  Pursuer CBD mini helical
  Segura CBD
  Segura stone
  six-wire
  sphincterotomy
basket extraction technique
basket forceps
basket impaction
basket retrieval
basket rongeur
basket sphincterotome
basket-type crushing forceps
basket weave pattern
$BaSO_4$ (barium sulfate)
basophil, basophile
basosquamous cell carcinoma
Bassen-Kornzweig syndrome (acanthocytosis)
Bassini herniorrhaphy
Bassini inguinal hernia repair
  modified
  standard
basting suture
Batchelor plate
bathroom privileges (BRP)
bath, sitz
bathygastry
BAT (B-mode acquisition and targeting) system
batten graft
battery-driven hand drill
battledore (racquet-shaped) incision
Battle incision
Battle operation
Battle sign
bat-wing appearance
bat-wing catheter
Bauer and Black hernia belt
Bauer forceps
Bauhin gland
Bauhin, valve of
Baumgarten-Cruveilhier cirrhosis
Baumgartner needle holder
Baum wall unit
Baxter K-modified hose
Baxter mini-K thermia pump
Baylor sump tube
bayonet bipolar forceps
bayonet bone file
bayonet clip applier
bayonet forceps
bayonet fracture position
bayonet knife
bayonet rongeur
bayonet saw
bayonet-shaped forceps
bayonet-shaped hook
bayonet-shaped scissors
bayonet-type incision
B bile
B Braun/McGaw
BCAA (branched chain amino acids)
BCAA/AAA plasma ratio
B cell (fetal liver and bone marrow derived)
B-cell lymphoma
BCG (bacillus Calmette-Guérin)

BCT (breast-conserving therapy)
BDA (bile duct adenoma)
BDD (body dysmorphic disorder)
B-D Easy A1c test kit
BD Insyte Autoguard shielded I.V. catheter (also Autoguard-P)
BD Sensability breast self-examination aid
B-D Weiss epidural needle with fixed wings
BE (barium enema)
BE (Barrett esophagus)
Beacham amniotome
beach chair position
beach chair shoulder drape
Beacon Technology System (BTS)
beaded hepatic duct
beaded hip pin
beaded reamer guide pin
beading sign
beads
  PPMA (polymethyl-methacrylate-copolymer)
  Septopal
beads-on-a-string appearance
beaker cell
Beall circumflex artery scissors
Beamer injection stent system
Beamer Plus ABC unit
Beano (alpha-D-galactosidase enzyme)
bear-claw ulcer
Beardsley esophageal retractor
Bear-E-Bag Pediatric contrast medium
Bear-E-Yum GI contrast medium
Bearn-Kunkel-Slater syndrome
Beasley-Babcock forceps
Beath needle
Beath pin
Beath view
Beaver blade
  arachnoid shape
  banana
  cataract
  discission
  keratome

Beaver blade *(cont.)*
  retrograde
  rosette
  sickle shape
Beaver cataract blade
Beaver-DeBakey blade
Beaver-DeBakey knife
Beaver keratome blade
Beaver saw
BEB (blind esophageal brushing)
becaplermin
Beck aortic clamp
Becker breast implant
Becker external drain
Becker One-Piece cannula
Becker suture
Becker tissue expander/breast prosthesis
Becker Toomey syringe cannula
Beckman-Adson laminectomy blade
Beckman-Adson laminectomy retractor
Beckman-Eaton laminectomy blade
Beckman-Eaton laminectomy retractor
Beckman nasal speculum
Beckman pH probe
Beckman retractor
Beckman thyroid retractor
Beckman-Weitlaner laminectomy retractor
Beck miniature aortic clamp
Beck-Potts clamp
Beck triad
Beck vascular clamp
Beckwith syndrome
Beckwith-Wiedemann chromosome region
Beckwith-Wiedemann syndrome
Béclard hernia
Becton Dickinson introducer
Becton Dickinson Teflon-sheathed needle
Becton Dickinson Vacutainer
bed
  bladder
  capillary
  gallbladder

bed *(cont.)*
  hepatic
  liver
  nail
  pancreatic
  portal vascular
  stomach
  ulcer
Bedel drape
Bedford syndrome
Bedge antireflux mattress
Beebe wire-cutting scissors
beef-lung heparin
beefy appearance
beefy texture
bee pollen
Beer cilia forceps
B.E. Glass abdominal retractor
Behçet disease
Behçet syndrome
Behrend cystic duct forceps
Bel-Phen-Ergot SR (belladonna alkaloids; phenobarbital; ergotamine tartrate)
belching
Bellacane elixir (atropine sulfate; scopolamine hydrobromide; hyoscyamine sulfate; phenobarbital)
Bellacane SR (sustained release) (belladonna alkaloids; phenobarbital; ergotamine tartrate)
Belladenal
Bellafoline
Bell/ans tablets (sodium bicarbonate)
Bellatal (phenobarbital)
bell-clapper deformity
Belle-Amie breast prosthesis
Bellergal-S (belladonna extract; phenobarbital; ergotamine tartrate)
bellows, inflating sigmoidoscopic
Bell suture
Bellucci alligator forceps
Bellucci alligator scissors
"belly button" augmentation mammoplasty
Belsey antireflux operation
Belsey IV fundoplasty
Belsey Mark IV antireflux procedure
Belsey Mark IV 240° fundoplication
Belsey two-thirds wrap fundoplication
belt
  Bauer and Black hernia
  spigelian hernia
belt loop gastropexy
Belzer organ preservation unit
Belzer solution
BEMA (bioerodible mucoadhesive)
bendable metallic rod
Benedict-Talbot body surface area method
BeneFix (coagulation factor IX [recombinant])
Benelli mastopexy
Bengash-type needle
Bengolea artery forceps
benign adenomatous polyp
benign bile duct tumor
benign biliary stricture
benign breast condition
benign breast disease (BBD)
benign cyst
benign disease
benign epidermal tumor
benign fibrocystic disease of breast
benign gastric ulcer
benign hamartoma
benign hyperplastic gastropathy
benign in appearance
benign inflammatory thyroid
benign juvenile melanoma
benign liver adenoma
benign lymphoepithelial lesion
benign neoplasm
benign papillary stenosis
benign paroxysmal peritonitis
benign pigmented lesion
benign polyp
benign postoperative jaundice
benign primary tumor

benign prostatic hypertrophy or hyperplasia (BPH)
benign recurrent intrahepatic cholestasis
benign solitary adenoma
benign squamous papilloma
benign subcutaneous cyst
benign tertian malaria
benign thyroid nodule
benign tumor
benign ulcer
benign uveal melanoma
benign vascular tumor of the liver
Benique catheter guide
Benjamin-Havas fiberoptic light clip
Bennett bone elevator
Bennett bone retractor
Bennett self-retaining retractor blade
Bennett tibia retractor
Bensaude proctoscope
Bensaude rectal speculum
Benson pylorus separator
Benson pylorus spreader
bent inner tube
bent malleable retractor
bent-tine, forklike retractor
bentiromide test
bentonite flocculation test
Bentyl (dicyclomine HCl)
benzalkonium chloride
benzidine
benzimidazoles, substituted
benzocaine
benzodiazepine
benzoin adhesive
benzquinamide
benztropine; benztropine mesylate
Beppu score
Berci-Shore choledochoscope
Berens clamp
Berens esophageal retractor
Berens muscle clamp
Berens muscle forceps
Berger disease
Berger magnifying loupe
Bergstrom cannula
Berkeley-Bonney self-retaining 3-blade abdominal retractor
Berkson-Gage calculation of breast cancer survival rates
Berliner percussion hammer
Berman airway
Berman aortic clamp
Berman oropharyngeal airway
Bernard-Sergent syndrome
Bernstein acid perfusion test
Bernstein esophageal acid infusion test
Berry sternal needle holder
Berry-TC wire-twisting forceps
Beset right-angle colon clamp
Bessauds-Hilmand-Augier syndrome
Bessey-Lowry unit for alkaline phosphatase
beStent Rival coronary stent system
Best gallstone forceps
Best intestinal clamp
Best right-angle colon clamp
beta-adrenergic blockade
beta blockade therapy
beta blocker
Beta-Cath system catheter
beta cell function
beta cell protective agent
beta cells of pancreatic islets
beta cell tumor of pancreas
Betadine (povidone-iodine)
Betadine dressing
Betadine gel
Betadine scrub
Betadine-soaked Owen gauze dressing
Betadine soap
Betadine solution
Betadine Surgi-Prep
beta hCG (human chorionic gonadotropin)
beta hemolytic strep (streptococcus)
Beta LT (beta-alethine)
beta-lactamase enzyme
beta 1 and beta 2 agonist

beta-naphthylamine
Betathine (beta-alethine)
betazole stimulation test
betel cancer
bethanechol
Bethea sheet holder
Bethune-Coryllos rib shears
Bethune periosteal elevator
Bethune rib shears
Bethune rongeur
Bevan abdominal incision
Bevan gallbladder forceps
beveled chisel
beveled knife
beveled speculum
beveled thin-walled needle
BEVS (Baculovirus Expression Vector System)
Bexxar (tositumomab, ^{131}I tositumomab)
Beyer paracentesis needle
Beyer forceps
Beyer rongeur
Beyer-Stille bone rongeur
bezoar formation
BFDR (bronchospasm, flushing, diarrhea, right-sided heart failure)
bFGF (basic fibroblast growth factor)
Biafine WDE (wound dressing emulsion)
biarticular bone shears
biarticular bone-cutting forceps
bias stockinette wrap
Biaxin XL (clarithromycin) extended-release tablets
BIB (biliointestinal bypass)
bicanalicular sphincter
BiCAP (Bipolar Circumactive Probe)
BiCAP bipolar diathermy
BiCAP cautery
BiCAP electrocoagulation probe
BiCAP endoscopic probe
BiCAP hemostatic system
Bicarbolyte
bicarbonate (HCO_3^-)
bicarbonate concentration
bicarbonate, sodium
biceps jerk (BJ)
bichloroacetic acid
Bickel intramedullary nail
Bickel intramedullary rod
BiCOAG bipolar forceps
bicortical iliac bone graft
bicortical ilial strip graft
bidomal shield template
Bier amputation saw
Bier block anesthesia
Bier lumbar puncture needle
Bierman needle
Biermer disease
Biesenberger technique of mastopexy
Biethium ostomy rod
bifid hook
Bifidobacterium bifidum
biflanged drill
bifoil balloon
bifoil balloon catheter
bifrontal incision
bifurcated cable
bifurcation
  aortic
  bile duct
  common bile duct
  hepatic
  iliac vessel
bifurcation lesion
bifurcation tumor
Big Bag 3000
Bigelo calvarium clamp
Bihrle dorsal clamp
bikini skin incision
BiLAP bipolar cautery
BiLAP bipolar cutting and coagulating probes
BiLAP bipolar needle electrode
bilateral adrenal hemorrhage
bilateral adrenalectomy
bilateral cortical necrosis
bilateral hernia

bilateral herniorrhaphy
bilateral hyperplasia
bilateral incarcerated scrotal hernia
bilateral inguinal hernia
bilateral inguinofemoral lymphadenectomies
bilateral mammogram
bilateral mastectomies
bilateral nodular dysplasia
bilateral pleural tube
bilateral recurrent laryngeal nerve damage
bilateral right-sidedness sequence
bilateral subcostal incision
bilateral total adrenalectomy
bilateral ureteral obstruction (BUO)
bilateral vagotomy
bilayer patch hernia repair
bilayer polypropylene mesh
bile
  A
  B
  C
  canaliculus
  clear
  cloudy
  conjugated
  extrahepatic
  gallbladder
  inspissated
  limy
  lithogenic
  liver
  stagnant
  supersaturated
  thick
  turbid
  viscid
  viscous
  white
bile acid
  conjugated
  fecal
  oxidized
  total
bile acid binder
bile acid breath test
bile acid-EDTA (BA-EDTA) solution
bile acid pool
bile acid sequestrant
bile acid tolerance test
bile antigen
bile ascites
bile bag
bile capillary
bile concretion
bile duct
  common (CBD)
  extrahepatic
  infundibulum of
  interlobular
  preampullary portion of
  sphincter of
bile duct abscess
bile duct adenoma (BDA)
bile duct calculus
bile duct carcinoma
bile duct colic
bile duct cystadenocarcinoma
bile duct dyskinesia
bile duct epithelium
bile duct gland
bile duct hamartoma
bile duct injury
bile duct lumen
bile duct obstruction
bile duct pressure
bile duct proliferation
bile duct stasis
bile duct stone
bile duct stricture
bile-induced gastritis
bile lake
bile leakage
bile papilla
bile peritonitis
bile pigment in basal ganglia
bile plug
bile reflux
bile reflux gastritis

bile salt-binding resin
bile salt diarrhea
bile salt-losing enteropathy
bile salts in the skin
bile sludge
bile solubility test
bile spillage, intraoperative
bile-stained fluid
bile-stained vomitus
bile stasis
bile supersaturated with cholesterol
bile-tinged fluid
Bilezyme
bilharzial carcinoma
"bili" (see *bilirubin*)
biliary atresia
  distal
  extrahepatic
biliary balloon catheter
biliary balloon probe
biliary calculus
biliary canal
biliary cirrhosis
biliary cirrhotic liver
biliary colic
biliary conduit
biliary-cutaneous fistula
biliary decompression
biliary dilation; dilatation
biliary duct
biliary ductule
biliary-duodenal fistula
biliary-duodenal pressure gradient
biliary dyskinesia
biliary dyspepsia
biliary endoprosthesis
biliary endoscopy
biliary-enteric anastomosis
biliary-enteric bypass
biliary-enteric fistula
biliary fistula
biliary gland
biliary manometry
biliary mud
biliary obstruction, malignant
biliary pancreatitis
biliary passage
biliary peritonitis
biliary piecemeal necrosis
biliary plexus
biliary radicle (*not* radical)
biliary reconstruction
biliary saturation index
biliary scintiscan
biliary sludge
biliary sphincter
biliary sphincterotomy and stent placement
biliary stasis
biliary stenosis
biliary stent
biliary stone disease
biliary stricture, long-segment intrahepatic
biliary structure
biliary tract disease
biliary tract infection
biliary tract stone
biliary tree
BiliChek bilirubin analyzer
Biligrafin contrast medium
Bili mask
bilioenteric fistula
biliointestinal bypass (BIB)
biliopancreatic bypass (BPB)
biliopancreatic shunt
Biliopaque
bilious aspirate
bilious colic
bilious diarrhea
bilious emesis
biliousness
bilious pneumonia
bilious remittent malaria
bilious stool
bilious vomiting
bilirubin ("bili")
  conjugated
  direct
  elevated

bilirubin *(cont.)*
  fat-soluble
  indirect
  serum
  total
  unconjugated
  urine
  water-soluble
bilirubin analyzer
bilirubinate stone
bilirubinemia
bilirubin encephalopathy
bilirubin glucuronide deconjugation
bilirubin glucuronosyltransferase deficiency
bilirubin metabolism
bilirubin pigment gallstone
bilirubinometer
bilirubinuria
Biliscopin contrast medium
biliverdin
Bilivist contrast medium
Bill axis traction handle
Billingham-Bookwalter retractor
Billingham hemorrhoidal grasping forceps
Billroth anastomosis
Billroth forceps
Billroth gastroenterostomy
Billroth I (truncal vagotomy, antrectomy, gastroduodenostomy)
Billroth I anastomosis
Billroth I gastroduodenostomy
Billroth II (truncal vagotomy, antrectomy, gastrojejunostomy)
Billroth II anastomosis
Billroth II gastrojejunostomy
Billroth II-type gastrectomy
Billroth retractor
Billroth tumor forceps
bilobed gallbladder
bilobed polypoid lesion
bilocular stomach
biloma
Bilopaque contrast for cholecystography
Biloptin contrast medium
Bilos pin
Biltricide
bimoclomol
binder (see also *bandage*; *dressing*)
  Dale abdominal
  Expand-a-Band breast
  scultetus
binder test
binge drinker
bingeing
binge-purge behavior (bulimia)
binocular loupe
binocular microscope
bioabsorbable suture
Bio-Anchor suture anchor
Biobrane adhesive
Biobrane glove
Biobrane/HF graft
BioBypass
biocavity laser
Biocell RTV saline-filled breast implant
biochemical abnormalities
biochemical cure
biochemical response
Bioclot protein S assay
Bioclusive dressing
Bioclusive transparent dressing
biodegradable pin
biodegradable plate
biodegradable rod
BioDimensional breast implant
bioelectrical impedance
BioEnterics gastric balloon
Bio-Enzabead test
bioerodible mucoadhesive (BEMA)
Biofield diagnostic system
Biofield test
Biofix system pin
Bio-Form glove
Biofreeze with Ilex analgesic ointment
BioGlue surgical patch
Biograft bovine heterograft

Bio-Hep-B vaccine
Biolex wound cleanser
Biolex wound gel dressing
biologic aggressiveness
biological response modifier
  interferon
  interleukin-2
  lymphocyte-activated killer cell
  monoclonal antibody
  tumor necrosis factor
biologically active thyroid cancer
Biologically Quiet Mini-Screw suture anchor
BioLogic-DT liver dialysis system
BioLogic-HT system (now ThermoChem-HT system)
biomedical glue
BioMesh surgical barrier
Bionx SmartNail
Biopatch foam wound dressing
Biopatch antimicrobial dressing
Bio-Phase suture anchor
BioPolyMeric graft
biopsy
  aspiration
  blind percutaneous liver
  bone
  bone marrow
  brain
  breast
  brush
  channel and core
  CKC (cold knife cone)
  cold
  colposcopically directed punch
  core
  core needle
  CT (computed tomography)
  CT-directed needle
  CT-guided needle aspiration
  diathermic loop
  direct-vision liver
  Dunn
  endoscopic

biopsy *(cont.)*
  ERCP-guided
  EUS-guided fine-needle aspiration
  excisional
  fine-needle aspiration (FNA)
  forage core
  freehand CT-guided
  full-thickness rectal
  guided transcutaneous
  hot
  image-guided pancreatic core
  incisional
  laparoscopic
  large-needle
  large-particle
  lift-and-cut
  liver
  mammogram-guided core
  Mammotest breast
  Mammotest Plus breast
  Mammotome breast
  Menghini liver
  Michele vertebral
  mirror image breast
  muscle
  needle core
  nerve
  onion bulb changes on
  open brain
  open liver
  optical
  Optical Biopsy system
  outpatient percutaneous liver
  pancreatic
  PEBB (percutaneous excisional breast)
  percutaneous
  percutaneous fine-needle
  percutaneous liver
  percutaneous needle muscle
  periodic liver
  plugged liver
  point-in-space stereotactic
  punch

biopsy *(cont.)*
  random needle
  scan-directed
  serial liver
  shave
  SiteSelect breast
  small bowel endoscopic
  snare loop
  Sonopsy 3-D ultrasound
  StereoGuide stereotactic needle core
  stereotactic aspiration
  stereotactic brain
  stereotactic breast
  stereotactic core needle (SCNB)
  stereotactic needle
  strip
  suction
  sural nerve
  synovial
  targeted brain
  temporal artery
  TNB (transthoracic needle)
  transfemoral liver
  transjugular liver
  transnasal
  transpapillary
  transvenous liver
  Tru-Cut needle (TCNB)
  ultrasonography-guided fine-needle aspiration
  ultrasound-guided anterior subcostal liver
  ultrasound-guided echo
  ultrasound-guided needle
  ultrasound-guided stereotactic
  vertebral body
  Vim-Silverman needle
  wedge
  wedge hepatic (or liver)
biopsy and brushings
biopsy cannula
biopsy excisors
biopsy cup forceps
biopsy needle
biopsy of breast, needle core
biopsy of cyst wall
biopsy of kidney
biopsy of pancreas
biopsy punches
biopsy specimen
biopsy suction curette
biopsy trephine
Biopty cut needle for breast biopsy
Biörck syndrome
BioROC absorbable suture anchor
Biosafe PSA4 test
BioSorb resorbable urology stent
BioSorb suture
Biostent stent
BioStinger
biosurgery
Biosyn synthetic monofilament suture
biotinylated IL-10 monoclonal antibody
Biotrack coagulation monitor
Bio-Tract proprietary strain of *Lactobacillus salivarius*
BioTwist
BioVue PICC catheter
BiPAP S/T-D 30 ventilatory support
BiPAP S/T-D ventilatory support
biparietal suture
biplanar aortography
biplane sector probe
bipod base plate
bipod suspension apparatus
bipolar cable
bipolar cautery (BiCAP)
bipolar cautery forceps
bipolar cautery probe
bipolar cautery scissors
bipolar coagulation
bipolar connecting cables
bipolar electrocoagulation
bipolar forceps
bipolar probe
bipolar urological loop
BiQ bipolar hand instrument

BI-RADS (Breast Imaging Reporting and Data System)
Bircher bone clamp
Bircher cartilage clamp
Bircher-Ganske cartilage forceps
Bircher meniscus knife
bird-beak configuration or narrowing
bird-breeder's lung
bird's nest lesion
biricodar dicitrate
BIS Sensor
BIS Sensor Plus
bisacodyl tannex
Bisco-Lax (bisacodyl)
Bishop chisel
Bishop clamp
Bishop gouge
Bishop-Harmon forceps
Bishop-Koop ileostomy
Bishop saw
Bismatrol (bismuth subsalicylate)
bismuth compounds
bismuth subcarbonate
bismuth subgallate
bismuth subsalicylate
Bismuth classification of benign bile duct stricture, types I-V
Bisound AP 3000 Colorflow ultrasound system
bisoxatin; bisoxatin acetate
BiSure laparoscopic forceps
bite down
bite of tissue
bite, surgical
bithionol
Bitin (bithionol)
bivalve (noun); bivalved (verb)
Bivona tracheostomy tube
BJ (biceps jerk)
BK DNA virus
Black and Decker drill
black blood clot
black death
Black-Draught syrup (casanthranol; senna extract)
Black-Draught tablets (senna concentrate)
black faceted stone
black liver disease
black lung
black pigment gallstone
Black rasp
black stone
black suture
black tarry stool
black widow spider bite
bladder bed
bladder carcinoma classification
bladder decompression
bladder fistula
bladder incontinence
bladder injury
bladder neck spreader
bladder neck support prosthesis
bladder pheochromocytoma
BladderScan
bladder scissors
bladder sound
bladder spatula
bladder stone
bladder tumor
bladder tumor assay (BTA)
blade (see also *knife*)
  arachnoid shape
  arthroscopic
  banana
  Bard-Parker
  Beaver cataract
  Beaver discission
  Beaver keratome
  Beaver-DeBakey
  Beckman-Adson laminectomy
  Beckman-Eaton laminectomy
  Bennett self-retaining
  carotid
  cartilage shaver
  Caspar
  cataract
  chisel
  chondroplasty

blade *(cont.)*
- copper
- craniotome
- crescentic
- Curdy
- deep
- Dennis
- discission
- double-edged razor
- Doyen vaginal retractor
- drill
- Dyonics arthroscopic
- Feild (not Field)
- full curve
- Gigli saw
- Gomel
- guillotine
- Hebra
- Hibbs
- Incisor arthroscopic
- K
- keratome
- knife
- laminectomy
- laryngoscope
- LaserSonics EndoBlade
- LaserSonics Nd:YAG LaserBlade
- LaserSonics Surgiblade
- malleable
- McIntosh laryngoscope
- meniscal trimmer
- meniscectomy
- Meyerding laminectomy
- Meyerding-Scoville
- MicroAire
- mini meniscus
- MVR
- notchplasty
- oscillating
- partial curve
- Paufique
- PowerCut drill
- RAD Airway laryngeal
- razor

blade *(cont.)*
- retractor
- retrograde
- ring-cutter
- Rosenkranz deep retractor
- rosette
- saw
- scalpel
- Scoville
- sickle-shaped
- skin
- spinal retractor
- spoon
- S/P surgical
- Superblade
- Surgiblade sterile scalpel
- Swann-Morton surgical
- Synovator arthroscopic
- synovectomy
- Taylor spinal retractor
- Temperlite saw
- 3M Maxi Driver
- tongue
- tracheal
- triradial resector
- UltraCision ultrasonic knife
- UltraClean electrosurgical

bladebreaker knife
blade handle
blade holder
blade plate
blade plate driver
blade-safe
Blair chisel
Blair elevator
Blair palate hook
Blair saw guide
Blair silicone drain
Blaivas classification of urinary incontinence
Blake drain
Blake gallstone forceps
Blakemore-Sengstaken tube
Blakemore tube

Blakesley suction flow forceps
Blake wound drain
Blalock-Niedner clamp
Blalock pulmonary clamp
Blalock-Taussig clamp
blanching of mucosa
blanching spider telangiectasias
bland diet
bland food
Blandin gland
bland thrombosis
blastic lesion
bleb-like adhesion
bleed (noun)
  GI
  herald
  slow
  variceal
BLEED (bleeding, low BP, elevated PT, erratic mental status, disease [comorbid]) classification
bleeder
bleeding
  abnormal
  active source of
  colorectal
  concomitant
  dysfunctional uterine (DUB)
  excessive
  external
  gastrointestinal tract
  GI (gastrointestinal)
  retroperitoneal
  intra-abdominal
  massive
  massive lower GI
  occult
  painless rectal
  pinpoint gastric mucosal defect
  portal hypertension-induced variceal
  postcoital
  postmenopausal
  purpuric
  rectal
bleeding *(cont.)*
  recurrent
  refractory
  variceal
  widespread
bleeding abnormality
bleeding controlled with direct pressure
bleeding controlled with electrocautery
bleeding diathesis
bleeding esophageal ulcer
bleeding esophageal varices
bleeding esophagogastric varices
bleeding from gastroduodenal artery
bleeding gastric varices
bleeding gums
bleeding into cyst
bleeding into joint
bleeding into parenchyma
bleeding into pericardial sac
bleeding lesion
bleeding per rectum
bleeding points were cauterized
bleeding polyp
bleeding time
  Duke
  Ivy
  Mielke
  Simplate
bleeding time coagulation panel
bleeding ulcer
bleeding vessel, embolization of
blenderized diet
BLEND waveform desiccation
Blickman Health Industries
blind clamping
blind enema
blind esophageal brushing (BEB)
blind gut
blindness
blind limb
blind loop syndrome
blind medullary nail
blind needle insufflation
blind percutaneous liver biopsy

blind pouch
blind stump
blind upper esophageal pouch
BlisterFilm transparent dressing
bloat; bloated
bloating, gas
Bloch-Paul-Mikulicz operation
block
  intercostal nerve
  ischiorectal fossa
  neuroplexus
blockade
block anesthesia
blocked shunt tube
blocked sweat gland
Blom-Singer tracheoesophageal fistula
Blond anoscope
blood
  anticoagulant-treated
  antigenic properties of
  arterial
  autologous
  bright red
  capillary
  gross
  Hemolink blood substitute
  hemolyzed
  Hextend blood substitute
  intraperitoneal
  iron-binding capacity of
  laky
  mass of congealed
  microscopic
  mixed venous
  nonoxygenated
  occult
  oozing
  oxygenated
  oxygen-carrying capacity of
  PentaLyte
  peripheral
  platelet-poor (PPB)
  PolyHeme blood substitute
  sludged

blood *(cont.)*
  spurting
  stagnation of
  transfusion of incompatible
  typed and crossmatched
  venous
  whole
blood admixed with stool
blood-borne organism
blood cell filtration, Hemasure r/LS
  circulating
blood clot (see *clot*)
blood coagulation
blood culture
  defibrinated
  degenerated
  dissecting (from the retroperitoneal)
  donor
  extravasated
  fecal occult
  frank
blood flow
  increased collateral
  reduced transhepatic
blood gas
  arterial
  base excess
  bicarbonate (bicarb)
  HCO_3^-(bicarbonate)
  $PaCO_2$
  PaO_2
  pCO_2
  pH
  pO_2
blood gas on oxygen (FiO_2—fractional
  percentage of inspired oxygen)
blood gas on room air
blood glucose, fasting
blood glucose monitor
  Accu-Chek Advantage
  Accu-Chek Complete
  Accu-Chek Easy
  Accu-Chek Freedom II
  Accu-Chek Instant

blood glucose monitor *(cont.)*
  Accu-Chek Instant Plus
  Accu-Chek Simplicity
  Accu-Chek Voicemate
  Appraise
  Assure
  AtLast
  Chemstrip MatchMaker
  Companion 2
  Diasensor 1000
  Digital Response
  Duet
  ExacTech
  ExpressView
  FastTake
  FreeStyle
  FreeStyle glucose
  Glucochek Pocketlab II blood
  Glucometer DEX system
  Glucometer Elite
  Glucometer Elite R
  Glucometer Elite XL
  Glucometer Encore
  Glucometer II
  Gluco-Protein OTC self-test
    glucose system
  GlucoWatch
  Glycosal
  In Charge
  Medisense Pen 2
  One Touch Basic
  One Touch FastTake
  One Touch Profile
  One Touch II
  One Touch Ultra
  Precision QID
  Precision Xtra
  Prestige Smart System (PSS)
  Select GT
  self (SBGM)
  Sof-Tact
  Supreme II
  SureStep
  SureStep Pro

blood glucose monitor *(cont.)*
  TD Glucose
  Tracer
  Visidex
  Visidex II
Bloodgood syndrome
blood in cyst aspirate
blood in stool
  gross
  microscopic
  occult
blood in toilet bowl
blood irradiator, portable
bloodless field
bloodless operation
bloodless zone of necrosis
blood mixed with stool
blood on surface of stool
blood on toilet paper
blood outflow line
blood passed with stool
blood pool
blood pressure, orthostatic
blood pressure titration
blood sludge
blood smear
blood-stained effusion
blood-streaked stool
blood substitute
  HemAssist (hemoglobin
    crosfumaril)
  Hemolink
  Hemopure
  Oxygent (emulsified perflubron)
  PolyHeme (human hemoglobin
    cross-linked with glutaral)
blood-sucking intestinal parasite
blood-tinged ascites
blood-tinged discharge
blood-tinged fluid
blood-tinged sputum
blood transfusion, mismatched
blood urea level
blood urea nitrogen (BUN)

blood vessel invasion
blood volume
blood volume expander
  Plasbumin-5
  Plasbumin-25 (human albumin)
  Plasmanate
  Plasma-Plex
  Plasmatein
  Protenate
blood volume expansion
blood vomitus
Bloodwell forceps
bloody ascites
bloody aspirate
bloody diarrhea
bloody discharge
bloody fluid
bloody nipple discharge
bloody peritoneal fluid
bloody spinal fluid
bloody stools
bloody vomitus
Bloom syndrome
Blount anvil retractor
Blount blade plate
Blount disease
Blount hip retractor
Blount knee retractor
Blount knife
Blount staple
blowhole ileostomy
blowing wound
blown pupil
blowout of suture ties
blue and white mattress suture
blue and white Tycron suture
Blue Cushion anesthesia face mask
blue diaper syndrome
blue dot sign
Blue FlexTip catheter
Blue Goo (Iamin hydrating gel) dressing
blue line Murphy tracheal tube
blue liver
Blue Max balloon
blue rubber-bleb nevus syndrome
blue rubber nevus syndrome
blue stone
bluish discoloration
Blumberg sign of peritonitis
Blumenthal bone rongeur
Blumenthal lesion
Blumenthal rongeur
Blumer rectal shelf
Blumgart technique for hepatico-jejunostomy
blunt abdominal trauma
blunt and sharp dissection
blunt caliper
blunt dissection
blunt elevator
blunt grasping forceps, double-action
blunt hook
blunting of valve
blunt injury
blunt nerve hook
blunt-nose grasper
blunt-point suture
Bluntport disposable laparoscopic trocar
blunt probe
blunt rupture of liver
blunt rupture of spleen
blunt tapered T-handled reamer
blunt-tip cannula
blunt-tipped scissors
blunt trauma
blunt trocar
blurred pericecal fat (on CT scan)
B lymphocyte (B cell)
BM (bone marrow)
BM (bowel movement)
BMI (body mass index) (pl. indices)
B-mode acquisition and targeting (BAT)
B-mode ultrasonography
BMP (bone morphogenic protein)
BMT (bone marrow transplant, bone marrow transplantation)
boardlike rigidity of abdomen
Boas point of gastric ulcer

Boas sign of gastric ulcer
Boas test of gastric ulcer
boatlike abdomen
boat nail
boat-shaped abdomen
Bobechko hook
Bochdalek, foramen of
Bochdalek hernia
Bodenhammer rectal speculum
Bodnar retractor
body
  acidophilic
  asteroid
  Barr
  Councilman
  esophageal
  foreign
  gallbladder
  Heinz
  Howell-Jolly
  inclusion
  Lafora
  Mallory
  malpighian
  Pappenheimer
  pancreas
  psamomma
  Schaumann
  stomach
  vermiform
body access instrumentation
body cell mass
body composition
body density
body dysmorphic disorder (BDD)
body fat calipers
body fluid
body habitus
body hair loss
body mass index (or indices) (BMI)
body of gallbladder
body of pancreas
body of stomach
body wall
Boeck, sarcoid of
Boehler (Böhler)
Boehler bone rongeur
Boehler calcaneal view
Boehler lumbosacral view
Boehler plaster cast breaker
Boehler plaster shears
Boehringer suction regulator
Boerema anterior gastropexy
Boerema hernia repair
Boerhaave syndrome (esophageal rupture)
Boettcher artery forceps
Bogros space
Böhler (Boehler)
Böhler clamp
Böhler pin
Bohlman pin
Boies forceps
Bolivian hemorrhagic fever virus
bolster
  cotton
  Dacron velour
bolster suture
bolus anesthesia
bolus challenge test
bolus dressing
bolus feeding
bolus of cotton
bombesin
Bondek absorbable suture
bone abscess
bone awl
bone biopsy
bone biopsy needle
bone-biting forceps
bone-breaking forceps
Bone Bridge suture passer
Bone Bullet suture anchor
bone chip graft
bone chisel
bone curette
bone-cutting instrument
bone drill

bone elevator
bone extension clamp
bone extractor
bone flap fixation plate
bone gouge
bone graft punch
bone graft substitute
bone-grasping forceps
bone-holding clamp
bone-holding forceps
bone hook
bone mallet
bone marrow (BM)
bone marrow aspirate
bone marrow augmentation, donor-specific
bone marrow biopsy
bone marrow dysfunction
bone marrow transplant, bone marrow transplantation (BMT)
bone metastasis
bone morphogenic protein (BMP)
bone-nibbling rongeur
bone peg graft
BonePlast
bone plate
bone plug extractor
bone punch
bone punch forceps
bone reamer
bone-retinaculum-bone autograft
bone retractor
bone round needle
bone saw
bone-splitting forceps
bone staple
bone-tendon-bone graft
bone tumor
bone wax
bone wire guide
Bonfiglio bone graft
Bonine (meclizine)
Bonner position
Bonney forceps
Bonney insufflator
Bonney needle
Bonney stress incontinence test
Bonn scissors
bony landmarks
bony plate
Bookler swivel-ball laparoscopic instrument holder
Bookwalter retractor
boomerang needle holder
BOOP (bronchiolitis obliterans with organizing pneumonia)
Boorman gastric cancer typing system (types 1–4)
boot
  O_2 Boot
  pneumatic compression
  Unna
borborygmus (pl. borgorygmi)
border, antimesenteric (*not* ante-)
border cell
borderline malignancy
bore needle
borescope
  ITI rigid
  KLI rigid
borescope endoscope
Borge clamp
boring pain
Bornholm disease
Borrelia burgdorferi
bosselated stone
Bosworth drill
Bosworth spine plate
Botox injection
Botox sphincter injection
botryoid sarcoma
bottle and specimen forceps
bottle, DISS suction
bottle-nose forceps
bottle-nose grasper
botulinum toxin
botulism
Bouchard disease

Bouge needle
bougie
  acorn-tipped
  Celestin dilator
  Clutton urethral
  EndoLumina
  esophageal
  filiform
  French
  Hegar
  Hurst mercury
  Jackson esophageal
  large-diameter
  Lister
  Maloney
  mercury-filled
  mercury-weighted
  Savary
  tapered rubber
  Trousseau esophageal
  Van Buren urethral
bougie and catheter
bougienage
  esophageal
  peroral
bougie à boule
Bouin fixative solution
Bouin fluid
Bouin solution
bound down with adhesions
Bourne test
Boutin thoracoscope
Bouveret syndrome
bovie; bovied (verb)
Bovie 2100 coagulating electrosurgical device
Bovie electrocautery
Bovie knife
bovine collagen graft
bovine heterograft
bovine immunoglobulin concentrate
bovine pericardium graft
bovine pericardium strip
bowel
  aganglionic
  apple-peel
  dead
  friable
  gangrenous
  infarcted
  intussuscepted
  ischemic
  knuckle of
  large
  necrotic
  nonviable
  small
  strangulated
bowel abscess
bowel adherent to omentum
bowel axis
bowel bag
bowel contents
bowel continuity
bowel dilatation
bowel disease with protein loss
bowel elimination disorder
bowel entrapment (internal hernia)
bowel evacuant (see *bowel prep; enema*)
bowel function, assessment of
bowel gas
bowel gas pattern
bowel grasper
bowel habits
bowel incontinence
bowel infarction
bowel intussusception
bowel loop
bowel loop air
bowel lumen
bowel mass, intramural
bowel mobilization
bowel movement (BM)
bowel necrosis
bowel obstruction
  functional
  mechanical

bowel packed out of the way
bowel perforation
bowel prep (see also *enema*)
  Ceo-Two suppository
  ChloraPrep One-Step
  Colonlite
  CoLyte
  Davol
  Dulcolax
  Emulsoil
  Evac-Q-Kit
  Fleet
  Go-Evac
  GoLYTELY
  inadequate
  ipepac syrup
  magnesium citrate
  magnesium sulfate
  NuLytely
  OCL
  syrup of ipecac
  Tridrate Bowel Evacuant Kit
  Visicol
  X-Prep
bowel preparation (bowel prep)
bowel pseudo-obstruction
bowel rest
bowel retractor
bowel scissors
bowel sounds
  absent
  active
  crescendoing
  decreased
  diminished
  gurgling
  high-pitched
  hyperactive
  hypoactive
  low-pitched
  musical
  negative
  normal
  normoactive (NABS)
bowel sounds *(cont.)*
  positive
  quiet
  return of
  rumbling
  tinkling
bowel stenosis
bowel stoma
bowel tones
bowel wall, compromised
bowel wall hematoma
bowel wall involvement
Bowen chisel
Bowen disease of anal canal
Bowen periosteal elevator
Bowen syndrome
Bowlby tracheal dilator
bowler hat sign
Bowles scope
Bowles stethoscope
Bowman probe
Bowman scissors
Bowman tube
bow-shaped spatula
bow-type saw
box chisel
boxer's punch or fracture (of fifth metacarpal)
boxwood mallet
Boyce modification of Sengstaken-Blakemore tube
Boyce sign
Boyd dual-onlay bone graft
Boyden sphincter
Boyden test meal
Boyes-Goodfellow hook
Boyes-Goodfellow retractor
Boyes muscle clamp
Boyle uterine elevator
Boynton needle
Boynton needle holder
Bozeman (knee-elbow) position
Bozeman sponge-holding forceps
Bozeman-Thomson Walker needle holder

Bozicevich test
BPB (biliopancreatic bypass)
BPB (bone-patellar ligament-bone) autologous graft
BPB (bone-patellar tendon-bone) autologous graft
BPI (bactericidal/permeability-increasing) protein
BPM (Laserflo blood perfusion monitor)
BPS spinal angiographic catheter
bra
 Caromed postaugmentation
 "Laser Bra" procedure (see *L.I.F.T.*)
 postaugmentation mammoplasty
 The Bandeau postaugmentation
BRACAnalysis test for detection of hereditary breast and ovarian cancer
brace drill
brace-type reamer
brachial anesthesia
brachial plexus
brachial plexus root retractor
brachioaxillary bridge graft fistula (BAGF)
brachiocephalic vein
brachiosubclavian bridge graft fistula (BSGF)
Brachmann-de Lange syndrome
Bracht-Wachter lesion
BrachySeed iodine ^{125}I
brachytherapy, gamma
Braden score
Bradley disease
bradyarrhythmia
braided Nurolon suture
braided silk suture
braided suture
braided tape
brain abscess
brain biopsy
brain clip forceps
brain death
brain-exploring cannula
brain forceps
brain metastasis
brain retractor
brain scissors
brain spatula forceps
brain suction tube
brain swelling
brain tumor forceps
Braithwaite knife
Bralon braided nylon suture
Bramber head mirror
branched chain amino acid (BCAA)
brancher deficiency glycogenosis
brancher enzyme deficiency
brancher glycogen storage disease
branches of superior mesenteric artery
branchial cleft cyst
branchial fistula
branchial pouch
branching pattern
branchiogenous cyst
branch of celiac axis
Brand tendon-holding forceps
Brand tendon-passing forceps
Brand tendon-tunneling forceps
Brandt cytology balloon
Brandt syndrome
Branhamella catarrhalis (formerly *Neisseria catarrhalis*)
Branham sign
brash
 sour
 water
BRAT (bananas, rice cereal, apple-sauce, toast) diet
BRATS (bananas, rice, apples, toast, saltines) diet
Braun anastomosis
Braun depressor
Braun episiotomy scissors
Braun hook
Braun-Jaboulay gastroenterostomy
Braun skin graft
Braun-Stadler scissors

Braun tenaculum forceps
BRBPR (bright red blood per rectum)
BRCA (breast cancer [gene]) mutation
BRCA1 (breast cancer one) gene
BRCA2 (breast cancer two) gene
breadlike material
BreakAway absorptive wound dressing
breakaway pin
breakdown product
breaker
  blade
  Boehler plaster cast
  Castroviejo blade
  Swiss-pattern blade
breakfast, Ewald
break-screw extractor
breast
  accessory
  fibroadenoma of
  fibrocystic
  proemial
  shotty
breast abscess
BreastAlert differential temperature sensor (DTS)
breast asymmetry
breast atrophy
breast augmentation (see *mammoplasty*)
breast binder, Expand-A-Band
breast biopsy system, Mammotest
breast bolster
breast bone (also, breastbone)
breast calcifications
breast cancer (carcinoma)
  cystosarcoma phyllodes
  in situ
  inflammatory
  intraductal
  invasive
  metastatic
  Paget disease
breast cancer genes
  BRCA1
  BRCA2
breast cancer metastasis
Breast Cancer Prevention Trial
breast carcinoma (see *breast cancer*)
BreastCheck device
breast-conserving surgery
  lumpectomy
  partial mastectomy
  quadrantectomy
  wide-excision
breast-conserving therapy (BCT) (lumpectomy, axillary dissection, and radiation therapy)
breast contour
breast cyst
breast degeneration
BreastExam device for breast cancer detection
breast examination, B-D Sensability Breast Self-Examination Aid
breast feeding
breast fibroadenoma
breast fibrocystic disease
breast form—see *breast implant; prosthesis*
Breast Imaging and Reporting System (BI-RADS) of the American College of Radiology
breast implant (also see *prosthesis*)
  adjustable saline
  Amoena
  asymmetrical
  Becker
  Belle-Amie
  Biocell RTV saline-filled
  filled
  BioDimensional
  calcified
  Contour Profile
  Cronin breast
  custom
  Discrene
  Dow Corning
  encapsulated
  explantation of

breast implant *(cont.)*
gel-filled
Hartley
Leading Lady
McGhan
Mentor
moulage for
Nearly Me
NovaGold breast
NovaSaline inflatable saline
NovaSaline pre-filled
Perras-Papillon
silicone gel
Siltex silicone gel
Spectrum
Spenco
subcutaneous
subpectoral
symmetrical
teardrop
3M
Trilucent
Trulife silicone
Yours Truly
breast implant insertion, delayed
breast induration
breast inflammation
breast lump
breast mass
benign
fat necrosis
fibroadenoma
malignant
sclerosing adenosis
solid
breast microcalcifications
breast milk jaundice
breast neoplasm
breast pain
breast parenchyma
breast prosthesis
breast pump
breast reconstruction
fleur de lis pattern
free flap (gluteus maximus muscle to internal mammary vessels)
Kiricuta
lateral transverse thigh flap or "saddle bags"
latissimus dorsi myocutaneous flap
Rubens flap
transverse rectus abdominis myocutaneous flap
breast reconstruction donor sites for autogenous tissue
breast reconstruction during mastectomy
breast reconstruction pattern, fleur de lis
breast reconstruction with latissimus dorsi flap
breast reduction
Lejour-type
short-scar technique
tumescent technique
vertical pedicle technique
wet technique
wet technique with liposuction
breast scanning system
DOBI (Dynamic Optical Breast Imaging System)
Aurora MR breast imaging system
BI-RADS (Breast Imaging Reporting and Data System)
Miraluma nuclear breast imaging
Sonopsy 3-D ultrasound breast biopsy system
TransScan TS2000
Trex digital mammography system (TDMS)
breast self-examination
breast skin changes
breast skin satellite metastasis
breast symmetry
breast tenderness
breast thickening
breast tumor
breast ultrasound

Breath Bag
breath hydrogen test
breathing, compromised
breathing pattern
breath sounds, decreased
breath test (also see *test*)
  aminopyrine
  bile acid
  C-glycolic acid breath test
  Helicobacter pylori
  Horizons C-13 urea breath test
    for *H. pylori*
  hydrogen
  lactose
  lactose breath hydrogen test
  rice-flour
  urea
  UBT (urea breath test) for *H. pylori*
Breck pin
bregmatomastoid suture
Breisky-Navratil retractor
Breisky retractor
Bremer AirFlo Vest
Brennemann syndrome
Brennen biosynthetic surgical mesh
Brenner tumor
Brescia-Cimino AV fistula
Breslow classification of malignant
  melanoma
Breuerton view
BrevaRex (monoclonal antibody
  B43.13) vaccine for solid tumors
Brevi-Kath epidural catheter
Brevital Sodium; Brietal Sodium
  (methohexital sodium)
Brewer speculum
Bricker ureteroileostomy
Brickner position
bridge
  colostomy
  fascial
  loop ostomy
  mucosal
  telescope
bridge graft
bridge to transplant
bridge to transplantation
Bridge forceps
bridging fibrosis
bridging necrosis
bridging suture
bridle suture
Brigham brain tumor forceps
bright red blood per rectum (BRBPR)
bright red vomitus
brimstone liver
B ring of esophagus
Brinkerhoff proctoscope
Brinkerhoff rectal speculum
Bristow periosteal elevator
Bristow rasp
British Digestive Foundation
Brittain chisel
brittle bones
brittle diabetes mellitus
brittle mass
BRK series transseptal needle
broach
broach probe
broad-based polyp
broad-spectrum antibiotics
Broca pudendal pouch
Brochman suction tube
Brock clamp
Brockenbrough needle
Brockenbrough transseptal needle
Broden x-ray view
Broders index of malignant tumors
Brodie metaphyseal abscess
Brodie probe
Broesike fossa (parajejunal)
bromocriptine mesylate
Bromo-Seltzer (sodium bicarbonate;
  citric acid; acetaminophen)
bromosulfophthalein (BSP) test
Brompton's Cocktail
Brompton's Mixture
bronchial carcinoid

bronchial mucosa
bronchial polyp
bronchial sponge
bronchial stenosis
bronchioalveolar carcinoma
bronchiolar edema
bronchiolitis obliterans with organizing pneumonia (BOOP)
bronchioloalveolar carcinoma
Bronchitrac L catheter
bronchoalveolar lavage (BAL)
bronchobiliary fistula
Broncho-Cath endobronchial tube
Broncho-Cath endotracheal tube
Broncho-Cath with carinal hook
bronchocavitary fistula
bronchoesophageal fistula
bronchoesophageal forceps
bronchoesophageal scissors
bronchogenic carcinoma
bronchopleural fistula
bronchopulmonary segment
bronchoscopic smear
bronchospasm
bronchus forceps
bronze diabetes (iron storage disease)
bronze edema
bronze liver
Brooke-Bookwalter retractor
Brooke ileostomy
Brooker femoral nail
Brooker-Wills nail
Brook stitch scissors
Brophy periosteal elevator
Brophy scissors
Broviac catheter
brow-down skull view
Brown-Adson tissue forceps
Brown-Cushing forceps
Brown dietary method for colon preparation
Browne pneumatic impactor
Brown-McHardy pneumatic dilator
Brown needle holder
brown pigment gallstone
Brown rasp
brown stones
brown stool
Brown tissue forceps
brown tumor
brow-up skull view
Broxine (broxuridine) radiosensitizer
broxuridine radiosensitizer
BRP (bathroom privileges)
Brucella abortus
Brucella canis
Brucella melitensis
Brucella suis
brucellosis
Bruel-Kjaer 3535 ultrasound scanner
Bruening chisel
Bruening-Citelli rongeur
bruisability, easy
bruit, Cruveilhier-Baumgarten
Brunetti chisel with guard
Brun metacarpal saw
Brunner gland
Brunner gland adenoma
Brunner gland of duodenum
Brunner intestinal forceps
Brunner modified incision
Brunner palmar incision
Brunner rib shears
brunneroma
Bruns curette
Brunschwig artery forceps
Brunschwig operation
Bruns shears
Bruser skin (knee) incision
brush
  ERCP
  facial cannula
  Olympus cytology
brush and biopsy
brush biopsy
brush border of intestine
brush cytology
brushings and biopsy

brushings and washings
Bryan laparoscope
Bryan rigid laparoscope
BSA (body surface area)
BSD-2000 (*Lactobacillus salivarius*)
BSFR (basal secretory flow rate) test
BSGF (brachiosubclavian bridge graft fistula)
BSP (bromosulfophthalein) test
BTA stat bladder tumor assay
BTA TRAK bladder tumor assay
BTI-322 monoclonal antibody
bubble (see *balloon*)
  duodenal
  Garren-Edwards gastric (GEG)
  gastric
  intragastric
bubonocele
buccal frenulum
buccal gland
buccal mucosa
buccal region
buccal ulcer
Buck elevator
Buck-Gramcko gouge
Buck-Gramcko retractor
Buckley chisel
Buck neurological percussion hammer
Buck periosteal elevator
Buck scissors
Bucky imaging device
Bucky view
Bucladin-S
buclizine; buclizine HCl
bucrylate sclerosant
bucrylate (or bucrilate) tissue adhesive
Bucy chordotomy (or cordotomy) knife
Bucy-Frazier coagulating suction cannula
Bucy laminectomy rongeur
Budd-Chiari syndrome
Budd cirrhosis
Budd disease
Budde-Greenberg-Sugita retractor
Budd jaundice
Budd syndrome
budesonide
buffalo hump
buffer local instillation
buffer system
Buffets II (acetaminophen; aspirin; caffeine; aluminum hydroxide)
Buie fistula clamp
Buie fistula forceps
Buie fistula probe
Buie pile clamp
Buie position
Buie rectal forceps
Buie rectal probe
Buie rectal scissors
Buie rectal suction tip
Buie rectal suction tube
Buie-Smith retractor
Buie sigmoidoscope
Buie suction tube
Build Up enteral feeding
buildup of secretions
bulb and Air-Flo control valve
bulbar peptic ulcer
bulb, duodenal
bulbocavernous gland
bulbourethral gland
bulb suction
bulge
bulging of mucosa
bulimia nervosa
bulimorexia
bulk laxative
bulky dressing
bulky stools
bulky tumor
bulldog clamp
bulldog clamp-applying forceps
bulldog forceps
bullet driver
bullet-nose grasper
bullet-nose grasping, tissue well, double-action forceps

bullous appearance
bullous dermatitis
bullous-like edema
Bullseye guide
bull's-eye lesion
Bumex (bumetanide)
Bumm placenta curette
bumper (bolster)
BUN (blood urea nitrogen)
bunching suture
bundle suture
bunion retractor
Bunnell crisscross suture
Bunnell dissecting probe
Bunnell dressing
Bunnell forwarding probe
Bunnell hand drill
Bunnell probe
Bunnell tendon needle
Bunnell wire pullout suture
Bunyavirus infection
BUO (bilateral ureteral obstruction)
bupivacaine; bupivacaine HCl
Burch colposuspension
Burch iliopectineal ligament
    urethrovesical suspension
Burch laparoscopic procedure
burden, disease
Burdick paper
Burford-Finochietto retractor
Burford retractor
Burhenne biliary duct stone extraction
Burhenne steerable catheter
buried bumper syndrome
buried interrupted suture
buried-knot suture
buried penis
buried suture
buried vaginal island
Burke biopsy forceps
Burkitt lymphoma
burn
    chemical
    contact
burn *(cont.)*
    electrical
    first-degree
    flame
    scald
    second-degree
    third-degree
burn classification
burn debridement
burned-out mucosa (on x-ray)
burned-out pancreas
Burnett syndrome
burning pain
burning vulvar syndrome
burn scar carcinoma
burn wound
Burns plate
Buro-Sol (aluminum sulfate)
Burow solution (aluminum sulfate)
burp; burping
bursoscopy, supragastric
Burton headlight
Burton Nova exam light
Burton reflector light
Burton ultraviolet light
Busch suture scissors
Busch umbilical scissors
Buscopan
busulfan
Busulfex (busulfan)
butenafine
Butibel (belladonna extract; butabarbital
    sodium)
Butler bayonet forceps
butterflies in the stomach
butterfly bandage
butterfly needle
butterfly pattern
butterfly sponge
butter meal
buttocks
button
    Bard gastrostomy
    gastrostomy

button *(cont.)*
  Medicina percutaneous
  MIC-Key gastrostomy
  one-stage gastrostomy
  stoma
button electrode
buttonhole puncture technique for hemodialysis needle insertion
button hook
button of duodenum
button suture
Button gastrostomy feeding device
Button-One Step gastrostomy feeding device
buttonpexy fixation for stomal prolapse
buttress plate
buttress the sphincter
buttressed hook
butyrylcholinesterase
BVA-100 blood-volume analyzer
BVM (bag-valve-mask) device
BV-1 needle
BV130-5 needle
BV-175-6 needle
BV-175-8 needle
BV-2 needle
Bx Velocity coronary artery stent
Bx Velocity sirolimus-coated stent
Bx Velocity stent
Byler disease
bypass (see *operation*)
  Alden loop gastric
  aortofemoral
  Aria coronary
  biliary enteric
  biliointestinal (BIB)
  biliopancreatic (BPB)

bypass *(cont.)*
  cardiac
  cardiopulmonary
  carotid artery
  coronary artery
  duodenoileal (DIB)
  end-to-end jejunoileal
  end-to-side jejunoileal
  exclusion
  femoral-popliteal artery
  femoropopliteal artery
  gastric
  gastric loop
  Greenville gastric
  Griffen Roux-en-Y
  Hallberg biliointestinal
  hepatorenal
  jejunal
  jejunoileal (JIB)
  intestinal
  laparoscopic gastric
  laparoscopic Roux-en-Y gastric
  Litwak aortic
  long-limb gastric artery
  lymphaticovenous
  mini gastric
  operative biliary
  partial ileal
  Payne-DeWind jejunoileal
  Roux-en-Y biliary
  Roux-en-Y gastric
  Scopinaro pancreaticobiliary
  Scott jejunoileal
  transected vertical gastric
  venovenous
  vertical gastric

C, c

CAB (combined androgen blockade)
cabergoline
CABG (coronary artery bypass)
cable
  bifurcated
  bipolar
  bipolar connecting
  fiberoptic light
  monopolar
cable graft
Cabot CCD 3000 endoscopic camera
Cabot cystoscope
Cabot insufflator
Cabot laparoscope
Cabot rigid laparoscope
Cabot trumpet valve
cachectic-appearing
cachectic diarrhea
cachexia
  malignant
  pituitary
CAD (continuous analgesia delivery)
cadaveric donor
cadaveric liver
cadaveric organ
caddy (dark sandy mud) stool
CadPlan cancer planning therapy
cafe coronary syndrome
caffeinated beverage
caffeine gut
CA 15-3 RIA (radioimmunoassay)
  serum tumor marker
CAGEIN (catheter-guided endoscopic
  intubation)
CAH (chronic active hepatitis)
Cairns artery forceps
Cairns hemostatic forceps
Cairns-Oliver hook
Cairns ribbon retractor
cake kidney
"cake mix" kit for hematopoietic
  progenitor assay
Calandruccio side plate
calcaneal pin
calcaneal region
calcaneal stance position
calcareous material
calcareous pancreatitis
calcar reamer
calcifediol
calcification
  breast
  clustered
  focal
  linear
  multiple

calcification *(cont.)*
  questionable
  suspicious
calcified breast implant
calcified gallbladder
calcified lesion
calcified outline of cyst
calcified scar tissue in gallbladder wall
calciform cell
calcifying pancreatitis
Calcijex (calcitriol)
calcineurin inhibitor
Calcitite graft
calcitonin level
calcitonin, serum
calcitriol
calcium (Ca)
calcium alginate dressing
calcium bilirubinate stone
calcium carbonate
calcium gluconate
calcium lactate
calcium metabolism regulation
calcium polycarbophil
calcium supplementation
calculator, body mass index (BMI)
calculous cholecystitis
calculous gallbladder disease
calculus
  alvine
  bile duct
  biliary
  cholesterol
  common duct
  decubitus
  ductal
  gallbladder
  gastric
  hepatic
  hepatic duct
  impacted
  intestinal
  jackstone calculus
  mammary

calculus *(cont.)*
  metabolic
  mulberry
  nephritic
  nonopaque
  pancreatic
  pocketed
  prostatic
  radiopaque
  renal
  salivary
  staghorn
  stomach
  stonelike
calculus cirrhosis
Calcutript lithotriptor
Calderol (calcifediol)
caliber of stool
calibrate
calibrated pin
calibrated pin guide
calibration of the cardia
calibration tube
Caliciviridae
calicivirus gastroenteritis
calipers
  blunt
  body fat
  Castroviejo
  CV
  Harpenden
  Lange skin-fold
  Mitutoyo digital
  Thomas walking
  Townley femur
  vernier
  weight-relieving
Callaway formula for calorie intake
Calman carotid artery clamp
Calman ring clamp
Calmette-Guérin bacillus
Calm-X (dimenhydrinate)
Calogen LCT emulsion
caloric supplement

Calot node
Calot triangle
Caltagirone chisel
Caluso PEG (percutaneous endoscopic gastrostomy) tube
calvarial free bone graft
calvarium clamp
Calymmatobacterium granulomatis (formerly *Donovania granulomatis*)
Calypso Rely catheter
Camalox
cambendazole
camera
  AMS Endoview
  Concept 8160 IntraVision Lumi-Trac endoscopic
  Dyonics Vision 325z endoscope
  EndoMate
  Endoview endoscopy
  Enview
  Fujinon FG-135 endoscopic
  MedCam Pro Plus video
  Olympus OM-2N endoscopic
  Olympus OTV-S2 Hi-Resolution Soakable Surgical color endoscopic
  Olympus SCA-3 endoscopic
  Pentax endoscopic
  Polaroid endocamera EC-3
  StereoScope
  still
  Storz 9050B AutoexposureColor endoscopic
  Storz KSA-2S SuperCam endoscopic
  Storz laparoscopic video
  Stryker 590 color endoscopic
camera light source
camera trocar
Cameron-Haight periosteal elevator
Cameron-Miller electrocoagulation unit
Cameron-Miller electrode
Cameron-Miller monopolar probe
Cameron-Miller suction-coagulator
Camey ileocystoplasty
Camey reservoir
Camino ICP (intracranial pressure) catheter
Camino microventricular bolt catheter
Campbell gouge
Campbell nerve root retractor
Campbell onlay graft
Campbell periosteal elevator
Campbell reamer
Campbell rongeur
Camper fascia
Camptosar (irinotecan hydrochloride) injection
Campylobacter coli
Campylobacter concisus
Campylobacter fennelliae
Campylobacter fetus enteritis
Campylobacter hyointestinalis (Vibrio coli)
Campylobacter intestinalis
Campylobacter jejuni
Campylobacter lari
Campylobacter pylori (Helicobacter pylori)
Canada-Cronkhite syndrome
Canakis pin
canal
  abdominal
  alimentary
  anal
  biliary
  femoral
  Hering
  inguinal
  Nuck
  pleuroperitoneal
  stomach
canalicular cholestasis
canalicular sphincter
canaliculus, bile
Canasa (mesalamine)
cancelling A's (mental test for hepatic encephalopathy)

cancellous bone graft
cancellous chip bone graft
cancer (see *carcinoma*)
cancer embolism
cancer-inducing virus
cancerization
cancer of cervix
cancer of head of pancreas
cancer prophylaxis
Cancidas (caspofungin acetate)
Candela 405 nm pulsed-dye laser
Candela SPTL laser
Candida albicans esophagitis
candidal esophagitis
candidal infection
candida mucositis
candidiasis
  disseminated
  esophageal
  intestinal
Candistat-G
Candistroy
C&S (culture and sensitivity)
Candy Cane One-Piece cannula
Candy Cane superficial cannula
CA 19-9 (carbohydrate antigen) test
CA 19-9 tumor marker
canker sore
cannabinol
cannister, Guardian suction
cannula
  Acufex double-lumen
  Adson brain-exploring
  arthroscopic
  Becker One-Piece
  Becker Toomey syringe
  Bergstrom
  biopsy
  blunt-tip
  brain-exploring
  Bucy-Frazier coagulating suction
  Bucy-Frazier suction
  Candy Cane One-Piece
  Candy Cane superficial

cannula *(cont.)*
  Chieftan aspirating
  Clagett S
  coagulating
  coagulating suction
  Cohen
  Coleman infiltration
  Concorde
  cone biopsy
  Congreve
  cystic duct
  DeRoyal
  Dohrmann-Rubin
  Dorsey ventricular
  Duke
  Dyonics
  Elsberg brain
  Elsberg ventricular
  Endotrac
  Entree thoracoscopy
  ERCP
  Eriksson muscle biopsy
  exploring
  Fischer ventricular
  Ford Hospital ventricular
  Fournier One-Piece
  Fournier Toomey syringe
  Franklin-Silverman biopsy
  Frazier brain-exploring
  Frazier ventricular
  Gilliland etching
  Grinfeld cannula
  Hasson blunt-end cannula
  Hasson laparoscopy
  Hasson open laparoscopy
  Hasson SAC (stable access)
  Haynes brain
  high-flow
  inflow
  infusion
  intraventricular
  Iotec
  Jarcho self-retaining uterine
  J-hook

cannula *(cont.)*
- Kahn uterine trigger
- Kanavel brain-exploring
- Keel Cobra Toomey syringe
- Killian antrum
- LaparoSAC single-use
- large-bore inflow
- large egress
- Las Vegas One-Piece
- Leech Wilkinson
- Mayo-Ochsner suction
- Mayo subclavian
- McCain TMJ
- Mercedes
- Mercedes One Piece
- Mercedes tip
- Mercedes Toomey syringe
- microirrigating
- Mladick
- Mladick concave
- Mladick liposuction
- MultAport
- Neal fallopian
- Nelson
- Olympus monopolar
- One Piece
- outflow
- Pereyra improved ligature
- perfusion
- polyethylene
- portal
- Portnoy ventricular
- Provis
- Ray ventricular
- reusable
- Rumel tourniquet flex
- Scott attic
- Scott ventricular
- Sedan-Vallicioni
- Simple Suction Probe
- single-use
- slotted
- small egress
- soft tissue shaving (liposhaver)

cannula *(cont.)*
- SpaceSEAL cannula
- spatula One-Piece
- spatula-tip Toomey syringe
- standard One-Piece
- Stöckert
- suction
- suprapatellar
- Teflon ERCP
- thoracoscopy
- USCI
- ventricular
- Veress

cannula grommet
cannula reducer
cannula system
cannulated drill
cannulated Henderson reamer
cannulated nail
cannulated pin cutter
cannulation catheter
- common bile duct
- cystic duct
- retrograde
- selective

Canny Ryall retractor
canstatin
Cantil (mepenzolate bromide)
Cantlie line
Cantor tube
CA1-18 tumor marker
CA 72–4 gastric cancer antigen tumor marker
cap
- duodenal
- endoscopic suction

cap-and-anchor plate
Caparosa wire-crimping forceps
CAPD (continuous ambulatory peritoneal dialysis)
capecitabine, UFT (uracil plus tegafur), leucovorin (UFT/LV) chemotherapy regimen
capeline bandage

capillary angioma
capillary bed
capillary blood
capillary endothelial cell
capillary fill
capillary leak
capillary sludging
Capio CL transvaginal suture-capturing device
capitonnage
Capmul 8210 (glyceryl 1-mono-octanoate)
Capner gouge
capsaicin
Capset (calcium sulfate) bone graft barrier
capsular cirrhosis
capsular contracture following breast reconstruction
capsular incision
capsular invasion
capsular release forceps
capsule
  enteric-coated
  Glisson
  hepatic
  liver
  splenic
capsulectomy, periprosthetic
capsulitis, thyroid
Captopril test
caput medusae
Carafate (sucralfate)
CaraKlenz wound cleanser dressing
carbantel; carbantel lauryl sulfate
carbohydrate complex, refined
carbohydrate-deficient glycoprotein syndrome (CDGS), type 1a
carbohydrate polymer gel wound dressing
carbon dioxide (CO_2)
carbon dioxide content
carbon dioxide insufflator
carbon dioxide laser
carbon dioxide pneumoperitoneum
carbon fiber
carbon fiber graft
carbon fiber synthetic ligament
carbonic acid concentration
carbon steel surgical blade
carbon tetrachloride poisoning
carbon-tungsten rasp
carbonyl iron
carboplatin-coated plastic biliary stent
Carbo-Seal
carboxypeptidase
carboxypolypeptidase
carcinoembryonic antigen (CEA)
carcinogenicity
carcinoid syndrome
carcinoid tumor
carcinoma (also *cancer*; *sarcoma*; *tumor*)
  acinous cell
  adenocystic
  adenoid cystic
  adenoid squamous cell
  adenosquamous
  adnexal
  adrenocortical
  aldosterone-producing
  aldosterone-secreting
  alveolar cell
  ameloblastic
  ampullary
  aniline
  apocrine
  basal cell
  basaloid
  basosquamous cell
  betel
  bile duct
  bilharzial
  biologically active thyroid
  bladder
  breast
  bronchioalveolar
  bronchioloalveolar
  bronchogenic

carcinoma *(cont.)*
burn scar
cerebriform
chimney-sweep's
cholangiocarcinoma
cholangiocellular
cholangitis
chorionic
choroid plexus
clear cell
clear cell hepatocellular
clay pipe
colloid
colon
colorectal
columnar cuff
comedo
contact
corpus
cortisol-producing
cribriform
cutaneous metastatic breast
cylindrical
cystic
dendritic
disseminated
ductal
duct cell
Dukes (not Duke's)
dye worker's
eccrine
embryonal
embryonal cell
encephaloid gastric
endometrial
epidermal
epidermoid
excavated gastric
exophytic
extrahepatic abdominal
extrahepatic bile duct
familial pancreatic
fibrolamellar hepatocellular (FL-HCC)

carcinoma *(cont.)*
follicular
gallbladder
gastric
gastric stump
gelatinous
genital
giant cell
glandular
glans
granulosa cell
hepatic
hepatic cell
hepatocellular (HCC)
hepatocholangiolitic
hereditary
hereditary nonpolyposis colorectal (HNPCC)
high-grade angioinvasive follicular
hormone-sensitive breast
Hürthle (Huerthle) cell
hypernephroid
infantile embryonal
infiltrating ductal
infiltrating lobular
infiltrative
inflammatory breast
intraductal
intraepidermal
intraepithelial nonkeratizing
invasive
invasive breast
invasive ductal
invasive lobular
juvenile embryonal
kidney
Kulchitsky cell
large cell
laryngeal
latent
lenticular
leptomeningeal
lobular
Lucké

carcinoma *(cont.)*
- lung
- melanotic
- medullary
- melanotic
- meningeal
- Merkel cell
- metastatic
- metatypical
- microinvasive
- micropapillary
- microscopic multifocal medullary
- microtrabecular hepatocellular
- mixed hepatocholangiocellular
- moderately well-differentiated
- mucinous
- mucoepidermal
- mucoepidermoid
- mucous
- mule-spinner's
- nasopharyngeal
- neuroendocrine skin
- noninfiltrating lobular
- non-small cell lung
- oat cell
- occult
- oral
- oropharyngeal
- osteoid
- ovarian
- Paget
- pancreatic
- pancreatic ductal
- papillary gastric
- paraffin
- parathyroid
- perforated
- periampullary
- pitch worker's
- polypoid
- poorly differentiated
- preinvasive
- prickle cell
- primary

carcinoma *(cont.)*
- primary bile duct
- primary hepatic
- primary intraosseous
- protruded gastric
- rectosigmoid
- renal cell
- residual
- retinoblastoma hereditary human
- scar
- schistosomal bladder
- schneiderian
- scirrhous
- sclerosing hepatic (SHC)
- sclerosing well-differentiated
- sebaceous
- sessile nodular
- sigmoid
- signet ring
- small cell
- small cell anaplastic
- small cell lung
- small round cell
- spindle cell
- squamous cell (SCC)
- staging of cervical
- string cell
- submucosal
- superficial gastric
- swamp
- systemic effects
- tar
- T cell
- terminal duct
- thyroid
- transitional cell
- tubular
- undifferentiated squamous cell
- uterine cervix
- uterine corpus
- verrucous
- villous
- well-differentiated
- yolk sac

carcinoma arising from epidermal cells
carcinoma de novo
carcinoma en cuirasse
carcinoma ex mixed tumor
carcinoma ex pleomorphic adenoma
carcinoma in situ
  ductal (DCIS)
  lobular (LCIS)
carcinomatosis
  diffuse
  disseminated
carcinomatous implant
carcinomatous pericarditis
carcinosarcoma
cardia
  gastric
  patulous
cardiac allograft vascular disease (CAVD)
cardiac antrum
cardiac arrhythmias
cardiac catheter
cardiac cirrhosis
cardiac edema
cardiac function, compromised
cardiac impression on liver
cardiac lung
cardiac mucosa of stomach
cardiac obstruction
cardiac of stomach
cardiac orifice
cardiac polyp
cardiac reflex
cardiac retraction clip
cardiac segment
cardiac sphincter (stomach)
cardiac stomach
cardiac tamponade
cardiac valvular lesion
cardiac valvular stenosis
Cardiac Assist intra-aortic balloon catheter
Cardima Pathfinder microcatheter
cardinal suture
Cardiocap 5 patient monitor
cardiochalasia
cardioesophageal (CE) junction
cardioesophageal mucosal junction
cardioesophageal sphincter
cardiograms, serial
Cardio-Green (CG) (indocyanine green)
cardiohepatic angle
cardiohepatic triangle
Cardiomed Bodysoft epidural catheter
Cardiomed endotracheal ventilation catheter
Cardiomed thermodilution catheter
cardiomyotomy
  Heller
  laparoscopic
  stomach
  videolaparoscopic
cardioplegic needle
cardiopulmonary bypass
cardiospasm
Cardio Tactilaze peripheral angioplasty laser catheter
cardiovascular silk suture
CARDS O.S. mono test
CaREpair endoscope repair
Cariel gel dressing
carina
Carlens tube adapter
Carmalt (Walter) splinter forceps
Carmalt artery forceps
Carmalt clamp
Carmalt forceps
Carmalt hemostat
C-arm fluoroscope
carminative
CARN 750 (now CarraVex injectable)
Carnett sign
carnitine deficiency
  myopathic
  primary
  secondary
carnitine deficiency secondary to MCAD deficiency

Caroid (bisacodyl)
Caroli disease
Caroli syndrome
Caromed postaugmentation bra
carotene
carotid artery clamp
carotid artery injury
carotid blade
carotid bruit
carotid fork
carotid retractor
carotid sheath
carotid wall
carpal tunnel glove
carpal tunnel stretch
carpal tunnel view
Carpenter syndrome
CarraFilm transparent film dressing
CarraGauze wound strips dressing
CarraSmart foam dressing
CarraSmart self-adhesive foam dressing
Carra Sorb H wound dressing
Carra Sorb M freeze-dried gel dressing
Carrasyn hydrogel wound dressing
Carrasyn V dressing
Carrasyn wound gel dressing
Carrasyn wound gel spray dressing
CarraVex injectable
Carrel patch
carrier, hepatitis
Carr-Locke snare
Carr-Locke stent remover
Carroll-Bennett retractor
Carroll bone-holding forceps
Carroll dressing forceps
Carroll hand retractor
Carroll-Legg periosteal elevator
Carroll skin hook
Carroll tendon retriever
Carroll tendon-pulling forceps
Carroll tissue forceps
carsick
carsickness
Carson Zero Tip balloon dilator
Carter-Horsley-Hughes syndrome
Carter pillow for immobilization and
  elevation in replantation procedures
Carter-Rowe view
Carter-Thomason suture passer
Carticel autologous cultured chondro-
  cytes
Cartilade (shark cartilage)
cartilage
  cricoid
  shark
cartilage clamp
cartilage-derived inhibitor (CDI)
cartilage forceps
cartilage graft
cartilage knife
cartilage scissors
cartilage shaver blade
cartilaginous growth plate
cartwheel pattern
casanthronol
cascade, metastatic
cascade stomach
caseation
Casec calcium supplement
caseous necrosis
CASH (classic abdominal Semm
  hysterectomy)
Casoni skin test
CASP (contoured anterior spinal) plate
Caspar alligator forceps
Caspar blade
Caspar cervical plate
Caspari suture punch
caspofungin acetate
Castanares facelift scissors
Castaneda anastomosis clamp
Castaneda vascular clamp
cast breaker
Casten classification of groin hernias
  (stage 1–3)
Casten hernia staging
castlike tube
castor oil

Castroviejo blade breaker
Castroviejo caliper
Castroviejo-Colibri forceps
Castroviejo marker
Castroviejo-Mayo needle
Castroviejo-Mayo needle holder
Castroviejo needle
Castroviejo needle holder
Castroviejo scissors
Castroviejo-TC needle holder
cast saw
cast spreader
cast syndrome
catabolic activity
catabolism, tissue
cataract blade
cataract knife
cataract needle
Catarex surgical device for cataract
removal
catarrhal colitis
catarrhal gastritis
catch in chest on inspiration
cat's eye calculi
cat-eye syndrome
catecholamine crisis
catecholamine-induced vasoconstriction
catecholamine production
catechol
Catera suture anchor
catgut suture
cathartic
cathartic abuse
cathartic colon
cathartic (see also *bowel prep*)
magnesium citrate
magnesium sulfate
syrup of ipecac
catheter
ablation
Abramson
Abscession fluid drainage
Accu-Flo ventricular
ACE

catheter *(cont.)*
Achiever balloon dilatation
ACS (Advanced Catheter or Cardiac
Systems)
ACS angioplasty
ACS balloon
ACS Concorde
ACS Endura coronary dilation
ACS JL4 (Judkins left 4 French)
ACS mini
ACS OTW (over-the-wire)
Lifestream coronary dilatation
ACS OTW (over-the-wire) Photon
ACS RX Comet coronary dilatation
ACS RX coronary dilatation
ACS Tourguide II guiding
AcuNav ultrasound
Ahn thrombectomy
AL-1
AL II guiding
Alzate
Amazr
Amplatz cardiac
Amplatz femoral
Amplatz right coronary
Angiocath
Angiocath PRN
Angiocath PRN flexible
angiographic
angiographic balloon occlusion
Angio-Kit
Angiomedics
AngioOptic microcatheter
angiopigtail
angioplasty balloon
angled balloon
angulated
Anthron heparinized antithrombo-
genic
Antibacterial Personal
aortogram
Arani double-loop guiding
Argyle Medicut R
arrhythmia mapping system

catheter *(cont.)*
Arrow pulmonary artery
Arrow Twin Cath
Arrow Twin Cath multilumen
peripheral
Arrow-Berman balloon
ARROWgard Blue
ARROWgard central venous
Arrow-Howes multilumen
arterial embolectomy
AR-2 diagnostic guiding
Ascent guiding
atherectomy
atherectomy, peripheral
AtheroCath
AtheroCath Bantam coronary
atherectomy
Atlantic ileostomy
Atlas LP PTCA balloon dilatation
Atlas ULP balloon dilatation
Atri-Pace I bipolar-flared pacing
Auth atherectomy
AutoGuard-P
AV-Paceport thermodilution
Axiom DG balloon angioplasty
bail-out
Baim pacing
Baim-Turi monitor/pacing
ball-wedge
balloon
balloon biliary
balloon dilatation
balloon dilating
balloon embolectomy
balloon flotation
balloon septostomy
balloon-flotation pacing
balloon-tipped angiographic
balloon-tipped end-hole
balloon-tipped flow-directed
pulmonary artery
Bard guiding
Bardic cutdown
bat-wing

catheter *(cont.)*
Baxter
BD Insyte Autoguard-P shielded I.V.
Benique
Berman angiographic
Bernstein
Beta-Cath system
bicoudate
bifoil balloon
biliary balloon
BioEnterics gastric balloon suction
BioVue PICC
bipolar pacing electrode
bipolar temporary pacemaker
Block right coronary guiding
Blue FlexTip
Blue Max triple-lumen
BPS spinal angiographic
Brevi-Kath epidural
Brockenbrough mapping
Brockenbrough modified bipolar
Brockenbrough transseptal
bronchial
Bronchitrac L
bronchospirometric
Broviac
Broviac atrial
Buchbinder Omniflex
Buchbinder Thruflex
Burhenne steerable
Calypso Rely
Camino ICP (intracranial pressure)
Camino microventricular bolt
cannulation
cardiac
Cardiac Assist intra-aortic balloon
Cardima Pathfinder microcatheter
Cardio Tactilaze peripheral
angioplasty laser
Cardiomarker
Cardiomed Bodysoft epidural
Cardiomed endotracheal ventilation
Cardiomed thermodilution
Castillo

catheter *(cont.)*
Cath-Finder
Cathlon I.V.
Caud-A-Kath epidural
CCOmbo
central venous (CVC)
Cheetah angioplasty
Chemo-Port
Chilli cooled ablation
cholangiography
ChronoFlex
CliniCath peripherally inserted
Closure System by VNUS
Cloverleaf
coaxial
Cobra
Cobra over-the-wire balloon
cobra-shaped
coil-tipped
Comfort Cath I or II
Conceptus Soft Seal cervical
Conceptus Soft Torque uterine
Conceptus VS (variable softness)
Concord Portex epidural
conductance
constantly perfused side-hole
Constellation mapping
Cook arterial
Cook pigtail
Cook TPN
Cool Tip
Cordis Brite Tip guiding
Cordis Ducor I (or II, III) coronary
Cordis Ducor pigtail
Cordis high-flow pigtail
Cordis Predator PTCA balloon
Cordis Son-II
Cordis Trakstar PTCA balloon
coronary dilatation
coronary guiding
coronary sinus thermodilution
corset balloon
coudé
Cournand cardiac

catheter *(cont.)*
Cragg-McNamara valved infusion
CR Bard
Critikon
CrossSail coronary dilatation
cryoablation
cutdown
Cutting Balloon microsurgical dilatation
CVP (central venous pressure)
Dacron
Dale Foley
Datascope
Datascope DL-II percutaneous translucent balloon
decapolar
deflectable quadripolar
diagnostic
Diasonics
dilatation balloon
dilating
DLP cardioplegic
Doppler coronary
Dormia stone basket
Dorros brachial internal mammary guiding
Dorros infusion/probing
Dotter
Dotter caged balloon
Dotter coaxial
Double J indwelling
Double J ureteral
double-lumen
double-lumen femoral vein
double-lumen subclavian vein
Dow Corning ileal pouch
drainage
Ducor balloon
Duette
dummy seed
Du Pen long-term epidural
DURAglide stone removal
DVI Simpson atherocath
DynamicDeca steerable

catheter *(cont.)*
EAC (expandable access catheter)
EchoMark
EchoMark angiographic
Edwards diagnostic
eight-lumen esophageal manometry
El Gamal coronary bypass
Elecath thermodilution
electrode
electrophysiologic (EP)
11 French JCL 3.5 guiding
Elite
embolectomy
Encapslon
end-hole
EndoCPB (endovascular cardiopulmonary bypass)
Endosound endoscopic ultrasound
Endotak C lead
enhanced torque 8F (8 French) guiding
EnSite cardiac
EP (electrophysiologic)
epidural
Eppendorf
ERCP (endoscopic retrograde cholangiopancreatography)
Erythroflex
Erythroflex hydromer-coated central venous
esophageal balloon
e-TRAIN 110 AngioJet
Evert-O-Cath
eXamine cholangiography
expandable access (EAC)
Express
Express PTCA
extraction
ExtreSafe
extrusion balloon
FACT (Focal Angioplasty CatheterTechnology)
Falcon coronary
FAST (flow-assisted, short-term) balloon

catheter *(cont.)*
Fast-Cath introducer
FasTracker
female
femoral guiding
Feth-R-Kath epidural
Finesse large-lumen guiding
Flexguard Tip
Flexxicon Blue dialysis
flotation
flow-directed
flow-oximetry
fluid-filled
Fogarty adherent clot
Fogarty arterial embolectomy
Fogarty balloon
Fogarty balloon biliary
Fogarty-Chin extrusion balloon
Fogarty embolectomy
Fogarty graft thrombectomy
Fogarty irrigation
Fogarty occlusion
Fogarty venous thrombectomy
Foley
Foltz
Force balloon dilatation
FR4 guiding
Freezor cryocatheter
French
French 5 (5 French) angiographic
French MBIH
French mushroom-tip
Ganz-Edwards coronary infusion
Gensini coronary
Gentle-Flo suction
Gold Probe bipolar hemostasis
Goodale-Lubin cardiac
Gorlin pacing
Gould PentaCath 5-lumen thermodilution
graft-seeking
Greenwich
Grollman
Grollman pigtail

catheter *(cont.)*
Groshong
Groshong double-lumen
Groshong PICC
Grüntzig (Gruentzig)
Grüntzig arterial balloon
Grüntzig Dilaca
guide
guiding
Halo
Hanafee
Hartzler ACX-II or RX-014 balloon
Hartzler LPS dilatation
Hartzler Micro II
Hartzler Micro XT dilatation
headhunter visceral angiography
HealthShield
HealthShield antimicrobial mediastinal wound drainage catheter
HealthShield wound drainage
helical-tip Halo
helium-filled balloon
hep lock
hexapolar
Hickman
Hickman indwelling right atrial
Hidalgo
Hieshima coaxial
high-fidelity
high-fidelity microtipped
high-flow
high-pressure
high-speed rotation dynamic angioplasty
HNB angiographic
Hohn central venous
hot-tip
Hurwitz dialysis
HydraCross TLC PTCA
Hydrolyser microcatheter
hydrostatic balloon
hyperthermia
IAB (intra-aortic balloon)
ICP (intracranial pressure)

catheter *(cont.)*
Illumen-8 guiding
ILUS (intraluminal ultrasound)
indwelling
Infiniti
InfusaSleeve II
Inoue balloon
Insyte AutoGuard
interstitial
intra-aortic balloon
intra-aortic balloon double-lumen
intra-arterial chemotherapy
Intracath
intracoronary guiding
intracoronary perfusion
Intran disposable pressure measurement
intratumoral
intravascular ultrasound (IVUS)
intravenous pacing
intraventricular
Intrepid PTCA angioplasty
ITC balloon
ITC radiopaque balloon
IVUS (intravascular ultrasound)
Jackman orthogonal
Jackson-Pratt
jejunostomy
Jelco I.V.
Jelco intravenous
Jelco winged I.V.
JL4 (Judkins left 4 cm curve)
JL5 (Judkins left 5 cm curve)
JR4 (Judkins right 4 cm curve)
Judkins 4 diagnostic
Judkins left 4 cm (JL4)
Judkins left coronary
Judkins right 4 cm (JR4)
Judkins right coronary
Judkins USCI
Kaye tamponade balloon
KDF-2.3
Kensey
Kensey atherectomy

catheter *(cont.)*
Kidney Internal Splint/Stent (KISS)
Kifa
King multipurpose coronary graft
kinking of CNS
Kinsey atherectomy
Kish urethral illuminated
KISS (Kidney Internal Splint/Stent)
Koala pressure
Konton
Kontron balloon
large-bore
large-lumen
laser
Lawrence Add-A-Cath
L-Cath peripherally inserted neonatal
left coronary
left heart
left Judkins
left ventricular sump
Lehman
Lehman ventriculography
LeMaitre biliary
Leonard
LeVeen
Lifestream coronary dilatation
Livewire duo-decapolar steerable
Livewire TC ablation
Longdwel Teflon
Lo-Profile balloon
Lo-Profile II balloon
Lo-Profile steerable dilatation
low-pressure
low-speed rotation angioplasty
LPS
Lumaguide
Malecot
Malinckrodt
Mallinckrodt angiographic
MammoSite RTS (radiation therapy system)
manometer-tipped cardiac
Mansfield

catheter *(cont.)*
Mansfield Atri-Pace 1
Mansfield orthogonal electrode
Mansfield Scientific dilatation balloon
Marathon guiding
Mark IV Moss decompression-feeding
Max Force
McGoon coronary perfusion
McIntosh double-lumen
Medi-Tech
Medi-Tech balloon
Medicut
Medina ileostomy
medium-pressure
Medtronic balloon
Mercator atrial high-density array
Mewi-5 sidehole infusion
Micro-Guide
micromanometer-tip
MicroMewi multi-sidehole infusion
midstream aortogram
Mikro-tip micromanometer-tipped
Millar micromanometer
Millar MPC-500
Millar pigtail angiographic
Millenia balloon
Miller septostomy
Mini-Profile dilatation
Mirage over-the-wire balloon
Mitsubishi angioscopic
Molina needle
Mon-a-therm Foley
Monorail angioplasty
Monorail balloon
Moss decompression feeding
MPF
MS Classique balloon dilatation
Mullins transseptal
multi-electrode impedance
Multi-Med triple-lumen infusion
multifiber
multiflanged Portnoy (for hydrocephalus shunts)

catheter *(cont.)*
- multilumen
- multipolar impedance
- multipurpose
- Multipurpose-SM
- mushroom
- MVP
- Mylar
- nasobiliary
- Navi-Star
- Naviport
- Naviport deflectable tip guiding
- NBIH
- Nelaton solid-tip red latex
- Neo-Sert umbilical vessel
- nephrostomy-type
- NeuroVasx (Sub-Microinfusion)
- Nexus 2 linear ablation
- NIH (National Institutes of Health)
- NIH cardiomarker
- NIH left ventriculography
- 9 Fr JL 4 guiding (9 French Judkins left 4 guiding)
- nontraumatizing
- NoProfile balloon
- NovaCath multi-lumen infusion
- Nutricath
- Nycore
- octapolar
- Oligon
- OmniCath atherectomy
- Omniflex balloon
- On-Command (male and female)
- one-hole angiographic
- OptiQue sensing
- Optiscope
- Optiva I.V.
- Oracle Focus
- Oracle Megasonics
- Oracle Micro
- Oracle Micro Plus
- Oreopoulos-Zellerman
- over-the-wire balloon
- oximetric

catheter *(cont.)*
- Pace bipolar pacing
- Paceport
- Pacewedge dual-pressure bipolar pacing
- pacing
- P.A.S. (peripheral access system) Port catheter
- P.A.S. Port Fluoro-Free
- Passage catheter
- Pathfinder
- Pathfinder microcatheter system
- Pathfinder mini microcatheter
- PA Watch position-monitoring
- PBN
- PEG
- PE Plus II balloon dilatation
- Percor DL balloon
- Percor DL-II balloon
- Percor-Stat-DL
- percutaneous
- percutaneous transhepatic biliary drainage (PTBD)
- percutaneous transhepatic pigtail
- perfusion
- Periflow peripheral balloon
- peripherally inserted central (PICC)
- peritoneal
- peritoneal dialysis (PDC)
- PermCath double-lumen ventricular access
- pervenous
- Pezzer
- Phantom 5 Plus balloon
- Phoenix ventriculostomy
- PIBC (percutaneous intra-aortic balloon counterpulsation)
- PIC (peripherally inserted)
- PICC (peripherally inserted central)
- Pico-ST II
- pigtail
- Pipelle endometrial suction
- Polaris RF
- polyethylene

catheter *(cont.)*
PolyFlo peripherally inserted central (PICC)
Polystan
Polystan venous return
Port-A-Cath
portal
Portnoy ventricular
Positrol II
preformed
preshaped
probing
ProCross Rely over-the-wire balloon
Profile Plus dilatation
Proflex 5 dilatation
Pro-Flo
Pro-Flo XT
PRO infusion
Pruitt-Inahara balloon-tipped perfusion
PTBD (percutaneous transhepatic biliary drainage)
PTCA (percutaneous transluminal coronary angioplasty)
Pudenz peritoneal
pulmonary artery
pulmonary flotation
pulmonary triple-lumen
pusher
quadripolar electrode
quadripolar steerable electrode
Quanticor
Quinton
Quinton Mahurkar dual-lumen peritoneal
Raaf Cath vascular
radial artery
radiopaque Teflon biliary dilating
Raimondi peritoneal
Raimondi spring
Raimondi ventricular
Ranfac cholangiographic
Rashkind balloon
Rashkind septostomy balloon

catheter *(cont.)*
Rebar microcatheter
recessed balloon septostomy
red Robinson
red rubber
Reddick cystic duct cholangiogram
Reddick-Saye screw
Redifurl TaperSeal IAB
Release-NF
Reliance urinary control insert
remote access perfusion (RAP)
Rentrop infusion
Response electrophysiology
retroperfusion
RF (radiofrequency-generated thermal) balloon
right coronary
right heart
right Judkins
Rigiflex TTS balloon
Ring
Rivas vascular
Robinson
Rodriguez
Rodriguez-Alvarez
Rosch-Uchida transjugular liver access needle-catheter
Royal Flush angiographic flush
Rumel
Sable
Sarns wire-reinforced
SCA-EX ShortCutter
Schneider
Schneider-Shiley
Schoonmaker femoral
Schoonmaker multipurpose
Schwarten balloon
Schwarten balloon dilatation
Sci-Med SSC Skinny
SCOOP 1
SCOOP 2
Scott silicone ventricular
Seletz nonrigid ventricular
sensing

catheter *(cont.)*
Seroma-Cath wound drainage
serrated
SET three-lumen thrombectomy
Shaldon
shaver
Shaw
Sheldon
Sherpa guiding
Shiley guiding
Shiley-Ionescu
SHJR4s (side-hole Judkins right, curve 4, short)
side-hole
sidewinder
Silastic
silicone
silicone rubber Dacron-cuffed
Silicore
Simmons-type (sidewinder)
Simplus PE/t dilatation
Simpson
Simpson atherectomy
Simpson peripheral AtheroCath
Simpson-Robert
Simpson Ultra Lo-Profile II balloon
single-stage
Skinny
Skinny dilatation
sliding rail
Slinky
Smec balloon
snare
Soaker
Softip arteriography
Softip diagnostic
Soft Torque uterine
Softouch guiding
Soft-Vu Omni flush
solid-state esophageal manometry
Solo catheter with Pro/Pel coating
SoloPass
Sones cardiac
Sones Cardio-Marker

catheter *(cont.)*
Sones catheter
Sones Hi-Flow
Sones Positrol
Sones woven Dacron
Speedy balloon
SPI-Argent II peritoneal dialysis
SpineCATH intradiscal
split sheath
Spyglass angiography
Stack perfusion coronary dilatation
Stamey-Malecot
standard Lehman
steerable electrode
Steerocath
Stertzer brachial guiding
Stertzer guiding
stimulating
St. Jude 4F Supreme electrophysiology
straight flush percutaneous
subarachnoid
subclavian
subcutaneous ventricular reservoir
subdural drainage
Sub-Microinfusion
Suction Buster
SULP II
sump
Supreme electrophysiology
SureCuff
Sure-Flex dilatation
surgically implanted hemodialysis (SIHC)
Swan-Ganz
Swan-Ganz balloon-flotation pulmonary artery
Swan-Ganz flow-directed
Swan-Ganz Guidewire TD
Swan-Ganz Pacing TD
Swan-Ganz pulmonary artery
Swan-Ganz thermodilution
swan-neck
Swartz SL Series Fast-Cath introducer

catheter *(cont.)*
Syntel latex-free embolectomy
TAC atherectomy
Tactilaze angioplasty laser
Targis microwave
Taut cystic duct
Teflon
temporary pacing
Tenckhoff peritoneal dialysis
Tennis Racquet
tetrapolar esophageal
thermistor
thermodilution
thermodilution balloon
thermodilution pacing
thermodilution Swan-Ganz
thoracic
thrombectomy
Thruflex PTCA balloon
Tiemann
Tis-U-Trap endometrial suction
toposcopic
Torcon NB selective angiographic
Tourguide guiding
Tracker
Tracker-10
Tracker-18 Soft Stream
TrakBack ultrasound
transcutaneous extraction
transducer-tipped
transjugular access
transluminal extraction (TEC)
transseptal
transtracheal oxygen
transvenous pacemaker
trefoil balloon
Triguide
triple-lumen central venous
triple-lumen manometric
triple thermistor coronary sinus
tripolar
tripolar electrode
T-TAC (transcervical tubal access)
TTS (through the scope)

catheter *(cont.)*
twist drill
Tygon
Uldall (not Udall) subclavian hemodialysis
ULP (ultra-low profile)
Ultra 8 balloon
UltraLite flow-directed microcatheter
ultra low-profile fixed-wire balloon dilatation
umbilical artery (UAC)
UMI
Ureflex
UroMax II
USCI Bard
USCI guiding
USCI Mini-Profile balloon dilatation
valvuloplasty balloon
Van Andel
Van Tassel pigtail
vanSonnenberg-Wittich
Vantex central venous
Variflex
Vas-Cath
Vector and VectorX large-lumen guiding
venous
venous thrombectomy
venting
Ventra
ventricular
ventriculography
Ventureyra ventricular
Verbatim balloon
Veripath peripheral guiding
vessel-sizing
VIPER PTA
Visa II PTCA
Vision PTCA
Vitalcor venous
Vitesse Cos laser
Vitesse E-II
VNUS Restore

catheter *(cont.)*
- Voda
- Von Andel
- Vygon Nutricath S
- Was-Cath
- washing
- water-infusion esophageal manometry
- Webster coronary sinus
- Webster orthogonal electrode
- Wexler
- whistle-tip ureteral
- Williams L-R guiding
- Wilton-Webster coronary sinus
- Witzel enterostomy
- Workhorse percutaneous transluminal angioplasty balloon
- Wurd
- X-trode electrode
- XL-11
- Xpeedior
- Xpeedior 60
- Z-Med
- Zucker
- Zuma guiding

catheter balloon valvuloplasty
catheter-directed thrombolysis and endovascular stent placement
catheter entrapment
catheter-guided endoscopic intubation (CAGEIN)
catheter introducer, Bard Safety Excalibur
catheter-introducing forceps
catheterization (see also *catheter*)
- bile duct
- cardiac
- coronary artery
- cystic duct
- double-lumen
- endoscopic
- endoscopic transpapillary
- hepatic vein
- indwelling
- percutaneous
- percutaneous transhepatic
- portal vein
- Seldinger cystic duct
- selective
- transhepatic
- transnasal bile duct
- transpapillary
- two-lumen
- urinary
- venous

catheter sepsis
catheter tip placement
catheter vitrector
Cath-Finder catheter tracking system
Cath-Secure hypoallergenic tape
CathLink implantable vascular access device
Cathlon I.V. catheter
CathTrack catheter locator system
cation
Catlin amputating knife
CAT (computerized axial tomography) scan
cA2 monoclonal antibody
caudad
Caud-A-Kath epidural catheter
caudal anesthesia
caudal dysplasia sequence
caudal hook
caudal pancreatic artery
caudal regression syndrome
caudate lobe of liver (also quadrate)
caudocephalad projection
cause-and-effect relationship
caustic acid (poison)
caustic alkali (poison)
caustic digestive enzymes
caustic ingestion
cauterization
cauterize

cautery (electrocautery)
  Aesculap bipolar
  BiCAP
  BiLAP
  BiLAP bipolar
  bipolar
  Bovie
  ClearCut 2 electrosurgical handpiece
  Cloward
  Concept handheld
  Electroloop
  Endocut
  endoscopic laser
  hook
  Hotsy
  insulated
  looped
  Malis
  Mira
  insulated
  NeoKnife
  Neo-Med
  Olympus BiQ bipolar
  Op-Temp
  RollerLOOP
  Scheie ophthalmic
  snare
  wet field
cautery bend
cautery hook
cautery knife
cautery pencil
caval fold
CAVD (cardiac allograft vascular disease)
CaverMap surgical device
cavernous angioma
cavernous hemangioma
CAVH (chronic active viral hepatitis)
CAVH (continuous arteriovenous hemofiltration)
CAVH-B (chronic active viral hepatitis, type B)
CAVH-NAB (chronic active viral hepatitis, non-A, non-B)
caviar lesion
Cavilon barrier ointment
cavitary fluid
Cavitron ultrasonic surgical aspirator (CUSA)
cavity
  abdominal
  peritoneal
  retroperitoneal
  thoracic
  wound
cavity wall
CAVU (continuous arteriovenous ultra-filtration)
cavum conchal cartilage graft
C-bar web-spacer
C-bloc continuous nerve block system
CBC (complete blood count):
  hematocrit
  hemoglobin
  MCH (mean corpuscular hemoglobin)
  MCHC (mean corpuscular hemoglobin concentration)
  MCV (mean corpuscular volume)
  red blood cell count (RBC)
  white blood cell count (WBC)
CBC with a left shift
CBC with diff (differential)
CBD (common bile duct) stone
CBDE (common bile duct exploration)
CBG (corticosteroid-binding globulin)
CB erbium/2.94 laser
C bile
CBP (chronic bacterial prostatitis)
CBP (copper-binding protein)
C cell
CCD Apex autoclavable camera head
CCFA (Crohn's and Colitis Foundation of America)
CCK (cholecystokinin)
CCK-PZ (cholecystokinin-pancreozymin)
C-cholyl-glycine breath excretion test
C clamp

CCOmbo catheter
CCP (colitis cystica profunda)
CCS (colitis cystica superficialis)
CCS (Composite Cultured Skin)
CD (celiac disease)
CD (Crohn disease)
CDA (chenodeoxycholic acid)
CDAD (*Clostridium difficile*-associated diarrhea)
CDAI (Crohn disease activity index)
CDC (Centers for Disease Control and Prevention)
CDC (Crohn disease of colon)
CDCA (chenodeoxycholic acid)
CDE (common duct exploration)
CD-45RB monoclonal antibody
CDGS (carbohydrate-deficient glycoprotein syndrome), type 1a
CDI (cartilage-derived inhibitor)
CDIS (controlled distention irrigation system)
CDI 2000 blood gas monitoring system
CDS (choledochoduodenostomy)
Cd-texaphyrin photosensitizing agent
CdTOX A OIA kit
CDUS (color-flow Doppler ultrasound)
CE (cardioesophageal) junction
CEA (carcinoembryonic antigen) test
CEA and CA 19-9 (pancreatic tumor markers)
CEA-Cide (^{131}I-labeled humanized antibody against carcinoembryonic antigen)
CEAP (clinical manifestations, etiologic factors, anatomic involvement, and pathophysiologic features) classification
CEA-Scan (arcitumomab) imaging agent
CEA-^{99m}Tc carcinoembryonic antigen
Cebotome drill
cecal appendix
cecal bascule
cecal diverticulitis
cecal fold
cecal hernia
cecal serosa
cecal volvulus
  mesenterico-axial (cecal bascule)
  organo-axial (true volvulus)
cecitis
cecopexy
cecorrhaphy
cecostomy
  percutaneous catheter
  tube
CECT (contrast enhancement of computed tomographic) head and body imaging
cecum, coned
cecum twisted in a clockwise direction (cecal volvulus)
Cedax (ceftibuten)
Cedecea davisae
Cedecea lapagei
Cedecea neteri
cedelizumab monoclonal antibody
CEEA (curved end-to-end anastomotic)
CEEA 21, 25, 28, 31 stapling device
cefadroxil
cefazolin
cefdinir
cefotetan
cefoxitin
ceftibuten
Ceftin (cefuroxime)
cefuroxime
Celebra (celecoxib) (now Celebrex)
Celebrex (celecoxib)
celecoxib
Celestin dilator bougie
Celestin esophageal tube
Celestin graduated dilator
Celestin intraluminal tube
Celestin latex rubber tube
Celestin procedure
celiac alcohol ablation
celiac artery aneurysm

celiac artery compression syndrome
celiac axis
celiac clamp
celiac crisis
celiac dimple
celiac disease (CD)
celiac gland
celiac infantilism
celiac lymph node
celiac node
celiac rickets
celiac sprue disease
celiac trunk
celiacography
celiotomy
  exploratory
  staging
celiotomy and resection of pancreatic
  tumor
celiotomy incision
cell
  acid
  acinar
  adelomorphous
  antral gastric
  APUD (amine precursor uptake
    and decarboxylation)
  argentaffin
  argyrophil
  B
  basal granular
  beaker
  border
  Cajal, interstitial
  calciform
  capillary endothelial
  central
  centroacinar
  chalice
  chief
  Davidoff
  delomorphous
  dendritic reticular
  ECL (enterochromaffin-like)

cell *(cont.)*
  enterochromaffin
  fat
  fat-storing liver
  foam
  G
  gastric pacemaker
  gastrin-secreting
  Gaucher
  gelbe
  giant
  goblet
  ground-glass
  Heidenhain
  helle
  helper T
  interstitial
  Ito
  killer T
  Kulchitsky
  Kupffer
  L
  mucous neck
  mucus-secreting
  Namalwa
  natural killer (NK)
  non-alpha, non-beta pancreatic islet
  nuclear-tagged
  oxyntic
  pacemaker (gastric)
  pale
  pancreatic islet
  Paneth
  parietal
  peptic
  phagocytic stellate
  Pick
  plasma
  PP
  ptyocrinous
  pulpar
  S
  signet-ring
  silver

cell *(cont.)*
  small granule
  specialized columnar
  spindle
  stellate
  suppressor T
  T
  target
  undifferentiated
  von Kupffer
  xanthoma
  zymogenic
cell atypia
cell-cell adhesion
CellCept (mycophenolate mofetil [MMF])
cell death
cell growth regulation program
cell-mediated delayed immune reaction (type IV)
cell-mediated immune inflammation
cell-mediated immune reaction
cell-mediated immunity
Cellolite patty material
Cellona bandage
Cell Recovery System (CRS)
Cell Saver
Cell Saver 5
Cell Saver Haemolite autotransfusion system
celltrifuge
cell turgidity
cellular debris
cellular immunity
cellular polyp
cellular xenograft rejection
cellular xenotransplantation
cellulitis
  anal
  perirectal
  rectal
  wound
cell wall
celomic pouch
celosomia
Celsior organ preservation solution
Cement Eater drill
cement, Implast bone cement
cement tube
Cenflex central monitoring system
Centara (priliximab)
Centauri Er:YAG laser system
centering balloon light guide
centering drill
CenterPointLock skin barrier
Centers for Disease Control and Prevention (CDC)
central cell
central cirrhosis
central cone technique reduction
central hyaline sclerosis
central hyperalimentation
central lesion
central line infection
central lymph node
central necrosis
central nervous system (CNS)
central scar
central venous catheter (CVC)
central venous pressure line
centrilobar pancreatitis
centrilobular necrosis
centrilobular pancreatitis
centrilobular region of liver
centroacinar cell
centrum retractor
Ceo-Two suppository (sodium bicarbonate; potassium bitartrate)
cephalad
cephalic phase of acid secretion
cephalin-cholesterol flocculation test
cephalosporin
Cephulac
ceramic insulated coating
cerclage suture
cerebellar retractor
cerebral abscess
cerebral death

cerebral edema
cerebral malaria
cerebral radiation (CRN) necrosis
cerebriform carcinoma
cerebrohepatorenal syndrome
cerebroside lipidosis (Gaucher disease)
cerebrospinal fluid
cerebrotendinous xanthomastosis
Ceredase (alglucerase)
ceremidetrihexosidase
Cerezyme (imiglucerase)
ceroid-laden macrophage
ceroid-like histiocytic granuloma
Certican (everolimus)
Certiva vaccine
ceruloplasmin, serum
cervical adenopathy
cervical anesthesia
cervical aortic arch
cervical aspiration
cervical disk retractor
cervical drill
cervical esophagogastrostomy
cervical esophagotomy
cervical incision
cervical laminectomy punch
cervical laminectomy rongeur
cervical locking plate
cervical mallet
cervical motion tenderness
cervical node dissection
cervical polyp
cervical punch forceps
cervical roll
cervical stenosis
cervical stump
cervical support pillow
cervical ulcer
CESD (cholesterol ester storage disease)
Cestoda (genus, tapeworm)
cestode (pl. cestodes) (tapeworm)
Cetacaine (benzocaine; tetracaine; butamben)
cetraxate HCl
cetuximab
CFC BioScanner System
CF-HM colonoscope
CF-HM endoscope
CFIDS (chronic fatigue and immune dysfunction syndrome)
CF-LB3R colonoscope
CF-200Z Olympus colonoscope
CF-UM3 echocolonoscope
CG (Cardio-Green)
C-glycolic acid breath test
CGM (coffee-grounds material)
C graft
Chaffin-Pratt drain
CHAG (coralline hydroxyapatite Goniopora)
Chagas disease
chain suture
chain-of-lakes deformity
chain-of-lakes filling defect
chain-of-lakes sign
chalice cell
chalk stone
chamfer reamer
Champ elastic bandage
champagne shield template
Champion (nitinol coronary) stent
Champion Trauma Score (CTS)
Championnière bone drill
Chandler bone elevator
Chandler knee retractor
Chandler spinal perforating forceps
change in bowel habits
channel and core biopsy
channel, pyloric
char (following laser treatment)
CharcoAid (activated charcoal)
CharcoAid 2000
charcoal, activated
Charcoal Plus (activated charcoal)
CharcoCaps (charcoal)
Charcodote (activated charcoal)
Charcot cirrhosis

Charcot triad of symptoms (fever/chills, right upper quadrant pain, jaundice)
Charcot triangle
Chardonna-2 (belladonna extract; phenobarbital)
CHARGE (coloboma, heart, atresia of the choanae, retardation of growth and development, genital and urinary anomalies, and ear anomalies [also tracheoesophageal fistula])
CHARGE association
CHARGE syndrome
Charnley centering drill
Charnley compression clamp
Charnley deepening reamer
Charnley expanding reamer
Charnley femoral condyle drill
Charnley femoral prosthesis neck punch
Charnley horizontal retractor
Charnley incision
Charnley knee retractor
Charnley pin
Charnley pin retractor
Charnley rasp
Charnley reamer
Charnley retractor
Charnley self-retaining retractor
Charnley suction drain
Charnley suture forceps
Charnley taper reamer
Charnley tissue forceps
Charnley trochanter reamer
Charnley vertical retractor
Charnley wire-holding forceps
Charriere amputating saw
Charriere bone saw
Chaufford point
Chauveau bacterium
Cheatle-Henry hernia
Cheatle slit for takedown of colostomy
Cheatle sterilizing forceps
Check-Flo introducer
cheese handler's lung
cheesy necrosis
Cheetah angioplasty catheter
cheilosis
Chelsea-Eaton anal speculum
chem air
chem panel (chemistry)
Chem-7
Chem-10
chemical denaturing in vivo
chemical esophagitis
chemical exposure
chemical gastritis
chemical paralysis
chemical peritonitis
chemistries
chemistry panel
Chemo-Port catheter
chemoprevention
chemoprotective agent
chemoradiation
chemoradiotherapy, external beam radiotherapy and 5-FU
chemosis
chemotactic effects
chemotherapy (see also *medication*)
  adjunctive
  adjuvant
  combination
  intraperitoneal hyperthermic IPHC)
  multi-drug
  palliable
  primary
  systemic
chemotherapy-induced vomiting
chemotherapy protocol
chemotherapy regimen
Chemstrip MatchMaker blood glucose monitor
Chenix (chenodiol)
chenodeoxycholic acid (CDCA)
chenodiol
Chenofalk
Cherchevski disease
Cherney incision

Cherney lower transverse abdominal incision
Cheron dressing forceps
cherry (small dissecting sponge)
cherry angioma
Cherry-Austin drill
Cherry brain retractor
Cherry-Crandall method for testing serum lipase
cherry dissector sponge
cherry endosponge
Cherry extractor
Cherry-Kerrison laminectomy forceps
Cherry-Kerrison laminectomy rongeur
Cherry laminectomy retractor
cherry-pit sponge
cherry-red endobronchial lesions of Kaposi sarcoma
cherry sponge
CHESS (comprehensive health enhancement support system)
chest drainage unit
chest tube
chest wall fixation
chest wall invasion
chevron incision
chew-and-spit test
Cheyne periosteal elevator
CHF (congenital hepatic fibrosis)
CHF (congestive heart failure)
Chiari-Budd syndrome
Chiari disease
Chiba aspiration biopsy needle
Chiba cholangiography needle
Chiba percutaneous cholangiogram
chicken fat clot
Chick nail
chiclero ulcer
chief cell
chief-cell hyperplasia
chief (primary) complaint
Chieftan aspirating cannula
Chilaiditi sign
Chilaiditi syndrome
Child classification of cirrhosis
Child classification (A–C) of esophageal varices
Child classification (A–C) of hepatic reserve
Child classification of hepatic risk criteria
Child classification of liver disease
Childe approximating forceps
Childe hernia director
Child hepatic risk criteria
childhood thyroid irradiation
Child pancreaticoduodenostomy
Child-Pugh bleeding esophageal varices grading scale
Child-Pugh class A–C (used in hepatic disease)
Children's Hospital hand drill
Children's Hospital intestinal forceps
Child-Turcotte classification (used in hepatic surgery)
Childs-Phillips bowel plication
Chilli cooled ablation catheter
chills and fever
chills, shaking
chimney-sweep's cancer
CHIMPANZEES (calcium, hyperparathyroidism/hyperthyroidism/hypocalciuric/hypercalcemia, immobility/iatrogenic, metastasis/milk alkali syndrome, Paget disease, Addison disease/acromegaly, neoplasm, Zollinger-Ellison syndrome, excessive vitamin D, excessive vitamin A, sarcoid)
chin lift
Chin-Up Strip
chip graft
chip mat bandage
Chirocaine (levobupivacaine)
chiropractic film
chisel (see also *gouge*)
  acetabuloplastic round
  Adson

chisel *(cont.)*
    Adson laminectomy
    Alexander
    ASIF
    Austin Moore
    Ballenger-Hajek
    beveled
    Bishop
    Blair
    bone
    Bowen
    box
    Brittain
    Bruening
    Brunetti
    Buckley
    Caltagirone
    Cinelli-McIndoe
    Cloward cervical
    Cloward spinal fusion
    cold
    Converse
    Cottle
    Dautrey
    Derlacki
    D'Errico lamina
    Farrior-Dworacek
    Fomon
    Freer
    gouge
    Hajek
    Hibbs
    hollow
    Lambert-Lowman
    laminectomy
    Lexer
    Lowman-Hoglund
    Lucas
    Martin cartilage
    meniscotomy
    Metzenbaum
    Meyerding
    Miles bone
    mortising

chisel *(cont.)*
    neurosurgical
    Partsch
    Passow
    Pick
    Puka
    Schwartze
    seating
    Sheehan
    Simmons
    Smillie cartilage
    Smillie meniscotomy
    Smith-Petersen
    square hollow
    Stille bone
    straight
    swan-neck
    Trautmann
    U.S. Army bone
    USA pattern
    West bone
chisel blade
chisel edge elevator
chisel elevator
chisel-tip wire
chitosan
Chlamydia pneumoniae
Chlamydia psittaci
Chlamydia trachomatis
Chloraprep preoperative skin preparation
ChloraPrep One-Step
Chloresium (chlorophyllin copper complex)
chloride (Cl^-)
chloride ion
chloride, vinyl
chlormethazine
chloroform poisoning
chlorophyllin
Chloroplast membrane sulfolipids (blue-green algae) nutritional supplement
chloroprocaine

chlorpromazine-induced cholestasis
choana (pl. choanae)
choanal polyp
C HOBBS (calcium, hematocrit, O_2, base deficit, BUN, sequestration)
"chocolate bar" bandage
Cho/Dyonics two-portal endoscopic system
cholagogue
cholangiocarcinoma
cholangiointrahepatic
cholangioperipheral
Cholangiocath
cholangiocatheter
  cystic duct
  saline-filled
cholangiocellular carcinoma
cholangiofibromatosis
cholangiogram, cholangiography
  balloon
  Chiba percutaneous
  cholangiography
  common duct
  contrast selective
  CT
  cystic duct
  drip infusion
  endoscopic retrograde (ERC)
  fine-needle percutaneous
  fine-needle transhepatic
  intraoperative laparoscopic
  intravenous (IVC)
  operative
  percutaneous transhepatic (PTC)
  postoperative T-tube
  serial
  thin-needle percutaneous
  transhepatic (THC)
  T-tube (TTC)
cholangiography instruments and accessories
cholangiohepatitis
  Oriental
  recurrent pyogenic (RPC)
cholangiohepatoma
cholangiole
cholangiolitis
  extrahepatic
  gangrenous
  intrahepatic
  paratyphoidal
cholangioma
cholangiopancreatography, endoscopic retrograde (ERCP)
cholangiophytiasis
cholangioscope
  intraductal
  peroral
cholangiovenous communication
cholangiovenous reflux
cholangitic abscess
cholangitic biliary cirrhosis
cholangitis
  acute
  acute obstructive
  ascending
  bacterial
  chronic nonsuppurative destructive
  fibrous obliterative
  granulomatous
  intrahepatic sclerosing
  lymphoid
  nonsuppurative
  pleomorphic destructive
  postendoscopic
  primary sclerosing (PSC)
  progressive suppurative
  pyogenic
  recurrent pyogenic
  sclerosing
  secondary
  septic
  suppurative
  viral
cholangitis carcinoma
Cholebrine contrast medium
cholecystectomy (see also *operation*)
  laparoscopic
  laser laparoscopic (LLC)
  mini laparoscopic

cholecystectomy *(cont.)*
  micro laparoscopic
  open
  prophylactic
  three-trocar technique
  transcylindrical
cholecystectomy and wedge resection of overlying liver
cholecystectomy clamp
cholecystectomy with incidental appendectomy
cholecystenteric fistula
cholecystitis
  acalculous
  acute
  asymptomatic
  calculous
  chronic
  emphysematous
  erythromycin-induced
  follicular
  gangrenous
  gaseous
  perforated
  suppurative
  typhoidal
  uncomplicated acute
  xanthogranulomatous
cholecystitis with cholelithiasis
cholecystobiliary fistulization
cholecystocholangiography
cholecystocholedochal fistula
cholecystocholedocholithiasis
cholecystocolonic fistula
cholecystoduodenal fistula
cholecystoduodenal ligament
cholecystoduodenocolic fistula
cholecystoduodenocolic fold
cholecystoduodenostomy, Jenckel
cholecystoenteric fistula
cholecystoenterostomy, direct
cholecystogram, oral (OCG)
cholecystojejunostomy
cholecystokinetic food
cholecystokinin (CCK)
cholecystokinin-pancreozymin (CCK-PZ)
cholecystokinin stimulation test
cholecystolithiasis
cholecystoscopy, percutaneous transhepatic
choledochal basal pressure
choledochal-colonic fistula
choledochal cyst
choledochal region
choledochal sphincter
choledochal stent
choledochitis, suppurative
choledochocele
choledochocholedochostomy, side-to-side anastomosis
choledochoduodenal area
choledochoduodenal fistula
choledochoduodenal junction
choledochoduodenal junctional stenosis
choledochoduodenostomy (CDS)
choledochofiberscope (see *endoscope)*
choledochojejunostomy
  end-to-side
  loop
  retrocolic end-to-side
  Roux-en-Y
choledocholith
choledocholithiasis
choledocholithotripsy
choledochopancreatic ductal junction
choledochoscope
  Berci-Shore
  flexible fiberoptic
  Jasan JFE
  Machida
  Olympus CHF-CB30
  Olympus CHF-P20
  Olympus CHF-P20Q
  Pentax ECN-1530 choledochonephroscope
  Pentax FCN-15H flexible

choledochoscopy
  Berci-Shore
  T-tube tract
choledochostomy
choledochotomy, longitudinal
choledochous cyst
choledochous duct
choledochus (noun)
choleic acid
cholelithiasis
  asymptomatic
  chronic
  weight loss-induced
cholelithic dyspepsia
cholelithiasis, cholesterol
cholelitholysis
cholelithotomy
cholelithotripsy
cholemia
  familial
  Gilbert
cholemesis
choleperitoneum
choleperitonitis
cholera morbus
cholera, pancreatic
choleric jaundice
cholescintigram
cholescintigraphy
Cholestagel (now Welchol)
cholestasis
  benign recurrent intrahepatic (of pregnancy)
  canalicular
  chlorpromazine-induced
  drug-induced
  extrahepatic
  familial
  familial intrahepatic
  hepatocellular
  intrahepatic
  intrahepatic in pregnancy (ICP)
  methyltestosterone-induced
  tolbutamide-induced
cholestasis-lymphedema syndrome (Aagenaes syndrome)
cholestasis with peripheral pulmonary stenosis
cholestatic cirrhosis
cholestatic jaundice
cholestatic liver disease
cholestatic syndrome
cholestatic viral hepatitis
Cholestech L.D.X. test
cholesterol
  blood
  dietary
  HDL
  LDL
  serum
  total
  VLDL
cholesterol calculus
cholesterol ester storage disease (CESD)
cholesterol gallstone
cholesterol precipitate
cholesterol stone
cholesterolosis of gallbladder
cholesterolosis of mucosal surface
CholesTrak test
Cholestron PRO test
Cholestron test
cholestyramine resin
Choletec (^{99m}Tc mebrofenin) imaging agent
choline chloride
Cholografin contrast medium
Cholografin Meglumine (iodipamide meglumine)
chondroplasty blade
chondroplasty knife
Chooz (calcium carbonate)
CHOP chemotherapy
chordotomy (cordotomy) knife
chorionic carcinoma
choristoma
choroid plexus carcinoma

choroid plexus papilloma
choroidal hemangioma
choroidal layer of the eye
Christensen interlocking nail
Christie gallbladder retractor
Christmas tree appearance of pancreas (on x-ray)
Christmas tree reamer
Christmas tree sign
Christopher-Williams overtube
Christoudias fascial closure device
chromatin pattern
ChromaVision digital analyzer
chromic catgut suture
chromic gut suture
chromic interrupted suture
chromium (Cr)
chromium picolinate supplementation (in diabetes)
chromium polynicotinate
chromium-51 (^{51}Cr)-tagged red blood cells
Chromobacterium violaceum
chromoscopy
chromosome 14_q tumor marker
chromosome 23
  inverted duplication
  partial tetrasomy
  partial trisomy
chronic acholuric jaundice
chronic active hepatitis (CAH)
chronic active viral hepatitis (CAVH)
chronic active viral hepatitis B (CAVH-B)
chronic active viral hepatitis C (CAVH-C)
chronic active viral hepatitis non-A, non-B (CAVH-NAB) (now CAVH-C)
chronic aggressive hepatitis
chronic alcoholic cirrhosis
chronic alcoholic hepatic cirrhosis
chronic alcoholic liver disease
chronic alcoholic pancreatitis
chronic alcoholism
chronic appendicitis
chronic atrophic duodenitis
chronic atrophic gastritis
chronic bacillary diarrhea
chronic bacterial prostatitis (CBP)
chronic calcific pancreatitis
chronic calcifying pancreatitis
chronic cholecystitis
chronic congestive splenomegaly
chronic constipation
chronic cystic gastritis
chronic cystic mastitis
chronic dermatitis
chronic diarrhea
chronic diverticulitis
chronic Epstein-Barr virus infection
chronic erosive gastritis
chronic familial jaundice
chronic fatigue and immune dysfunction syndrome (CFIDS)
chronic fibrosing hepatitis
chronic fibrous thyroiditis
chronic fissure refractory to conservative treatment
chronic follicular gastritis
chronic gastritis type B
chronic granulomatous disease
chronic hemolysis
chronic hepatitis
chronic hyperparathyroid state
chronic idiopathic intestinal pseudo-obstruction (CIIP)
chronic idiopathic jaundice
chronic infection
chronic inflammation of pancreas
chronic inflammatory process
chronic intermittent colitis
chronic interstitial hepatitis
chronic intestinal pseudo-obstruction (CIP)
chronic ischemic colitis
chronic ischemic enteritis
chronic ischemic enterocolitis

chronic laxative abuse
chronic lobular hepatitis (CLH)
chronic lymphocytic leukemia (CLL)
chronic lymphocytic thyroiditis
chronic mononucleosis
chronic myelogenous leukemia
chronic nonsuppurative destructive cholangitis
chronic obstructive pancreatitis
chronic pancreatitis
chronic peptic esophagitis
chronic peptic ulcer
chronic persistent hepatitis (CPH)
chronic progressive hepatitis
chronic proliferative peritonitis
chronic prostatitis
chronic regurgitation
chronic relapsing pancreatitis
chronic renal disease
chronic scab
chronic sclerosing hyaline fibrosis
chronic stool retention
chronic stricture of the small bowel
chronic subareolar abscess
chronic thyroiditis
chronic ulcer
chronic ulcerative colitis (CUC)
chronically inflamed gallbladder
Chronicle implantable hemodynamic monitor
ChronoFlex catheter
chrontropy
Chronulac (lactulose)
CHRYS CO_2 laser
Chrysalin
Chrysosporium parvum
chuck drill
Chuinard autogenous bone graft
CHUK (conserved helix-loop-helix ubiquitous kinase) protein
Church scissors
Chvostek sign
chyle cyst
chyliferous vessel
chylomicron retention disease
chylopoietic disease
chylous ascites
chylous ascitic fluid
chylous fluid
chylous hydrotherapy
chyme
Chymex (bentiromide)
chymosin
chymotrypsin
CI (cardiac index)
Ciaglia Blue Rhino tracheostomy set
Ciaglia percutaneous tracheostomy introducer
CicaCare topical gel sheeting
cicatricial kidney
cicatricial stricture
cicatricial tissue
cicatrix (cicatrices)
cicatrization
Cicherelli bone rongeur
Cidecin (daptomycin for injection)
Cidex OPA disinfectant solution
cidofovir gel dressing
cigarette drain
CIIP (chronic idiopathic intestinal pseudo-obstruction)
cilansetron
ciliary fold
ciliary neurotrophic factor (CNTF)
cimetidine HCl
Cincinnati incision
Cincinnati subzero unit
cinedefecogram
cinefluorography
cinefluoroscopy
cine-esophagogram
cine-esophagoscope
cine-esophagoscopy
cine-esophagram
cinegastroscopy
Cinelli-McIndoe chisel
cineradiography
cine view

Cintor bone rongeur
CIP (chronic intestinal pseudo-obstruction)
Cipro (ciprofloxacin)
ciprofloxacin
circle
circle absorption anesthesia
circle straight cutting
circomyotomy
Circon-ACMI electrohydraulic lithotriptor probe
Circon bipolar instrument
Circon continuous-flow resectoscope
Circon Corporation video camera system
Circon rigid laparoscope
Circon videohydrothoracoscope
CircPlus compression dressing
circuit anesthesia
circuit without filter
circular cherry-red lesion
circular fold
circular myotomy
circular saw
circular self-retaining retractor
circular stapler
circular suture
circular tape
circular wire suture
circulating antibody
circulating blood
circulating blood volume
circulating endotoxin
circulating T_3 and T_4
circulation
  bile acid
  collateral
  cutaneous collateral
  enterohepatic
  hyperkinetic
  portal
  portal-systemic; portosystemic
  systemic
circulator fold
circulatory decompensation
circulatory overload
Circulon dressing
Circulon System Step 1 (and Step 2) venous ulcer kit dressing
circumanal gland
circumareolar incision
circumcostal gastropexy
circumference
circumferential incision
circumferentially
circumferential suture
circumferential suture ligation
circumferentially sutured onlay patch
circumflex scissors
circumoral numbness and tingling
circumscribing incision
circumumbilical incision
circumvallate papilla
cirrhosis
  acholangic biliary
  acute juvenile
  alcoholic
  atrophic
  bacterial
  Baumgarten-Cruveilhier
  biliary
  Budd
  calculus
  capsular
  cardiac
  central
  Charcot
  cholangitic biliary
  cholestatic
  chronic alcoholic
  coarsely nodular
  congenital
  congestive
  congestive liver
  Cruveilhier-Baumgarten
  cryptogenic
  decompensated
  decompensated alcoholic

cirrhosis *(cont.)*
- dietary
- diffuse septal
- end-stage
- extrahepatic
- fatty
- fatty micromedionodular
- florid
- focal biliary
- frank
- glabrous
- Glisson
- Hanot
- hemochromatotic
- hepatic
- hepatolienal
- hobnail
- hypertrophic
- Indian childhood
- insular
- intrahepatic
- juvenile
- Laënnec
- liver
- lung
- macrolobular
- macronodular
- malarial
- medionodular
- metabolic
- microlobular
- micronodular
- monolobular
- multilobular
- nodular
- nonalcoholic
- nutritional
- obstructive biliary
- passive congestive
- pericholangiolitic biliary
- periportal
- pigment
- pigmentary
- pipestem

cirrhosis *(cont.)*
- portal
- posthepatic
- posthepatitic
- postnecrotic
- primary biliary (PBC)
- progressive familial
- pulmonary
- secondary biliary
- septal
- splenomegalic
- stasis
- stomach
- syphilitic
- Todd
- toxic
- trabecular
- unilobular
- vascular
- xanthomatous biliary

cirrhosis of liver
cirrhosis of lung
cirrhosis of stomach
cirrhotic
cirrhotic gastritis
cirrhotic inflammation
cirrhotic liver
CIS (Colon Injury Score)
cisplatin/epinephrine gel
cisterna chyli
Citelli punch forceps
Citra pH (sodium citrate)
Citralax (magnesium citrate; magnesium sulfate)
citrate
citrate of magnesia
citrate test
Citrobacter amalonaticus
Citrobacter diversus
Citrobacter freundii
Citrocarbonate (sodium bicarbonate; sodium citrate)
Citrotein liquid feeding
Citrucel (methylcellulose)

Citrucel Sugar Free (methylcellulose; phenylalanine)
CK (conductive keratoplasty)
CKC (cold knife cone) biopsy
CKPT (combined kidney-pancreatic transplant)
Cl^- (chloride)
CLA (conjugated linoleic acid)
C lactose test
Cladosporium
Clagett Barrett esophagogastrostomy
Clagett S cannula
clammy
clamp (see also *clip*)
  Acland
  Adair
  Adair breast
  Adams-DeWeese vena caval
  Alfred M. Large
  Allen anastomosis
  Allen intestinal
  Allen-Kocher
  Allis
  Allis-Adair
  anastomosis
  Anderson
  angled peripheral vascular
  angular hinge
  anterior resection
  aortic
  aortic aneurysm
  aortic occlusion
  appendage
  approximator
  ASSI No-scalpel vasectomy fixator ring clamp
  Atrauclip hemostatic
  atraumatic vascular
  Atraumax
  Babcock
  baby Payr pylorus
  Backhaus towel
  Bahnson
  Bailey aortic

clamp *(cont.)*
  Bainbridge intestinal
  Ballantine
  Beck
  Beck-Potts
  Benjamin-Havas fiberoptic light
  Berens muscle
  Berman aortic
  Best right-angle colon
  Bigelo calvarium
  Bihrle dorsal
  Bircher bone/cartilage
  Bishop
  Blalock-Niedner
  Blalock pulmonary
  Blalock-Taussig
  Böhler (Boehler)
  bone extension
  bone-holding
  Borge
  Boyes muscle
  Brock
  Buie pile
  bulldog
  C
  Calman carotid artery
  Calman ring
  calvarium
  cardiac retraction clip
  Carmalt
  carotid artery
  cartilage
  Castaneda anastomosis
  Castaneda vascular
  celiac
  Charnley compression
  cholecystectomy
  Clark clamp
  coarctation
  colon resection
  Cooley anastomosis
  Cooley aortic
  Cooley-Beck
  Cooley bulldog

clamp *(cont.)*
Cooley coarctation
Cooley cross-action bulldog
Cooley-Derra anastomosis
Cooley iliac
Cooley partial occlusion
Cooley patent ductus
Cooley pediatric
Cooley renal
Cooley-Satinsky
Cooley vascular
Cooley vena cava catheter
Cope crushing
Cope modification of Martel intestinal
Cosgrove Flex
Crafoord aortic
Crafoord coarctation
Crile appendix
Crile-type
Crutchfield carotid artery
Cunningham
curved
curved Cooley
curved Mayo
Dandy
Daniel colostomy
Dardik
Davidson vessel
Davis aneurysm
DeBakey aortic aneurysm
DeBakey arterial
DeBakey atraumatic bulldog
DeBakey-Bahnson vascular
DeBakey-Bainbridge
DeBakey-Beck
DeBakey bulldog
DeBakey coarctation
DeBakey colon resection
DeBakey cross-action bulldog
DeBakey-Derra anastomosis
DeBakey-Harken
DeBakey-Howard
DeBakey-Kay

clamp *(cont.)*
DeBakey patent ductus
DeBakey pediatric
DeBakey peripheral vascular bulldog
DeBakey-Reynolds anastomosis
DeBakey ring-handled bulldog
DeBakey-Semb
DeBakey sigmoid anastomosis
DeBakey tangential occlusion
DeBakey vascular
DeMartel vascular
DeMartel-Wolfson anastomosis
Demos tibial artery
Dennis
Derra vena cava
Derra vestibular
DeWeese vena cava
Dieffenbach bulldog
Diethrich bulldog
Diethrich micro bulldog
Dingman bone and cartilage
Dingman cartilage
Dixon-Thomas-Smith
double
double-occluding
Doyen intestinal
Duval lung-grasping
Earle hemorrhoid
Edna towel
Endo Babcock
exclusion
Fehland colon resection
Fergusson
Filshie female sterilization
Fogarty
Fogarty-Chin
Fogarty Hydrogrip
Foss intestinal
Fukushima C-
Furniss anastomosis
Furniss-Clute
Gant
Garcia aorta
Gardner neurosurgical skull

clamp *(cont.)*
Gerbode patent ductus
Glassman atraumatic bowel
Glover bulldog
Glover coarctation
Glover patent ductus
Glover vascular
Goldblatt
Goldstein Microspike approximator
Grant aneurysm
Greenberg
Gregory baby profunda
Gregory carotid bulldog
Gregory DeBakey bulldog
Gregory external
Gross coarctation occlusion
Grover
Gusberg hysterectomy
Gutgemann
Guyonn-Pean kidney
Gwilliam
Haberer intestinal
Halifax interlaminar
Harken auricle
Harrington hook
Harrington rod
Harvey Stone
Hayes anterior resection
Heaney
Heifitz
Hemoclip
Hem-o-lok
hemorrhoidal
hemostatic
Hendrin ductus
Henley vascular
Herrick kidney
Hirschman pile
Hoen
hook
Hopkins aortic
Hufnagel aortic
Humphries aortic
Hurwitz esophageal

clamp *(cont.)*
hyperinsulinemic-euglycemic
glucose
infant skull
interlaminar
intestinal
intestinal crushing
intracranial
Jackson bone extension
Jacobson bulldog
Jacobson-Potts vascular
Jahnke anastomosis
Jarvis pile
Javid carotid artery
Johns Hopkins bulldog
Johns Hopkins coarctation
Jones thoracic
Kantrowitz thoracic
Kapp-Beck
Kapp-Beck-Thomson
Kartchner carotid artery
Kay aorta
Kay-Lambert
Kelly
Kelsey pile
Kern bone-holding
Kindt carotid artery
Kinsella-Buie lung
Kleinschmidt appendectomy
Klintmalm
Koala vascular
Kocher
Lahey
Lambert aortic
Lambert-Kay aorta
Lambert-Kay vascular
Lambert-Lowman bone
Lamis patella
Lane bone
Lane bone-holding
Lane intestinal
Lane twin stomach
Lang Stevenson intestinal
Lee microvascular

clamp *(cont.)*
- Leland-Jones vascular
- Lewin bone-holding
- Liddle aorta
- Ligaclip
- Linnartz intestinal
- Locke
- long Péan
- Lowman bone
- Lowman bone-holding
- Lowman-Gerster bone
- Lowman-Hoglund bone-holding
- Maingot
- Martel
- Martin cartilage
- Martin meniscus
- Martin muscle
- Mason vascular
- Masters intestinal
- Masters-Schwartz liver
- Mastin muscle
- Matthew cross-leg
- Mattox aorta
- Mayfield neurosurgical skull
- Mayfield three-pin skull
- Mayo
- Mayo-Guyon kidney pedicle
- Mayo-Robson intestinal
- McCleery-Miller intestinal
- McDougal prostatectomy
- McLean pile
- M.D. Anderson
- Meeker gallbladder
- meniscus
- metal
- metallic
- Michel aortic
- micro cross-action bulldog
- Microspike approximator
- microvascular
- Mikulicz
- Mixter
- Mixter right-angle
- Mogen circumcision

clamp *(cont.)*
- Morris aorta
- mosquito
- Moynihan towel
- Muller pediatric
- Multiclip
- muscle biopsy
- Neuromeet nerve approximator
- Niedner anastomosis
- noncrushing bowel
- noncrushing vascular
- Noon AV fistula
- Nussbaum intestinal
- occluding
- occlusion
- Olsen cholangiogram
- Omed bulldog vascular
- O'Hanlon intestinal
- O'Neill
- Parham-Martin fracture
- Parker-Kerr intestinal
- partial occluding
- partial occlusion
- partially occluding vascular
- patch-clamp
- patellar
- patent ductus
- Payr gastrointestinal
- Payr pyloric
- Pean
- pediatric bulldog
- pediatric vascular
- pedicle
- Pemberton sigmoid
- Pemberton spur-crushing
- Pennington
- Perneczky aneurysm clamp
- Petz
- pin
- Poppen-Blalock carotid
- Poppen-Blalock-Salibi
- Potts aortic
- Potts coarctation
- Potts patent ductus

clamp *(cont.)*
- Potts-Niedner
- Potts-Satinsky
- Potts-Smith aortic occlusion
- Presbyterian Hospital tubing
- Presbyterian tube-occluding
- Price muscle biopsy
- Quick Bend flex
- Raney
- Rankin
- Rayport muscle biopsy
- rectal occlusion
- Redo intestinal
- Reinhoff
- Reynolds vascular
- Right Clip
- right-angle
- rod
- Roosevelt
- Rosenkranz universal
- rubber-shod
- Rumel myocardial
- Rumel thoracic
- saddle
- Salibi carotid artery
- Sarot bronchus
- Satinsky aortic
- Satinsky vascular
- Satinsky vena cava
- Schlein
- Schnidt (not Schmidt)
- Schumaker aortic
- Schwartz temporary intracranial artery
- Scudder intestinal
- Secu
- Sehrt
- self-retaining
- Selman
- Selverstone carotid
- Selverstone carotid artery
- Senning bulldog
- serrefine
- Sevrain cranial

clamp *(cont.)*
- Shoemaker intestinal
- side-biting
- sigmoid anastomosis
- single
- skull
- sliding
- Slocum meniscal
- Smith bone
- sponge
- spoon
- spur-crushing
- stainless steel
- Steinhauser bone
- Stetten intestinal
- Stille-Crawford
- Stille vessel
- Stockmann
- Stone-Holcombe intestinal
- Stone intestinal
- straight
- Strelinger colon
- St. Vincent tube occluding
- Subramanian
- Sugita right-angle aneurysm
- supraceliac aortic cross-
- suprarenal aortic cross-
- Swan aortic
- "sweetheart" (Harrington)
- swivel
- Thompson carotid artery
- Thomson Walker
- three-point skull
- tissue occlusion
- towel
- trochanter-holding
- tubing
- tube-occluding
- twin stomach
- Ulrich bone-holding
- vascular
- Verbrugge bone
- Veridien
- V. Mueller bulldog

clamp *(cont.)*
  Vorse-Webster
  VSF (Vermont spinal fixator)
  Walton cartilage
  Wangensteen anastomosis
  Wangensteen patent ductus
  Weber aortic
  Weck
  Wertheim
  Wertheim-Cullen
  Winston
  Winston-Acland
  wire fixation
  Wirthlin splenorenal
  Wister vascular
  Wolfson intestinal
  Wylie carotid artery
  Wylie hypogastric
  Yasargil carotid
  Z
  Zachary Cope-DeMartel
  Zeppelin
  Zinnanti Z
clamp-and-sew technique
clamp-applying forceps
clamped, cut, and ligated
clamshell incision
Clark clamp
Clark classification I–V
Clarke-Hadefield syndrome
Classen-Demling papillotome
classic abdominal Semm hysterectomy (CASH)
classic achalasia
classic coffee bean sign
classic hyperthyroidism
classic triad of palpitations, headache, episodic diaphoresis (PHE)
classic triad of Rigler
classification (also *grade; stage*)
  Abbreviated Injury Scale (AIS)
  American Association for the Surgery of Trauma Organ Injury Scale

classification *(cont.)*
  Bismuth bile duct stricture, types I-V
  bladder carcinoma classification
  Blaivas classification of urinary incontinence
  BLEED (bleeding, low BP, elevated PT, erratic mental status, disease [comorbid])
  Boorman gastric cancer typing system (types 1-4)
  Breast Imaging and Reporting Data System of the American College of Radiology (BI-RADS)
  Breslow
  Broders index of malignant tumors
  burn
  carcinoma of bladder
  Casten
  CEAP (clinical manifestations, etiologic factors, anatomic involvement, pathophysiologic features)
  Child classification of cirrhosis
  Child esophageal varices (A–C)
  Child hepatic dysfunction
  Child hepatic reserve (A–C)
  Child hepatic risk criteria
  Child liver disease
  Child-Pugh class A–C used in hepatic disease
  Child-Turcotte hepatic surgery
  Couinaud liver anatomy
  cytoprotective agent
  Dagradi esophageal variceal
  diabetes mellitus
  Dubin and Amelar varicocele
  Dukes Astler-Coller, modified
  Dukes carcinoma
  ECOG (Eastern Cooperative Oncology Group) performance status
  Edmondson Grading System
  Edmondson-Steiner histologic grading of hepatocellular carcinoma

classification *(cont.)*
Flint Colon Injury Scale (FCIS)
Forrest gastroduodenal ulcer
gastric mucosal pattern
Gilbert
Gilbert-Rutkow-Robbins
Glasgow Coma Scale (GCS)
Goldberg Anorectic Attitude Scale
Graham scale for drug-induced gastric damage
GSRS (gastrointestinal symptom rating scale)
GVHD (graft-versus-host disease) grading
Halverson
Halverson-McVay hernia
Hara gallbladder inflammation
Hepatitis Activity Index
Hinchey diverticulitis grade
Ishak chronic hepatitis C (0-6)
Japanese gastric carcinoma
Jewett
Karnofsky rating scale
Kasugai chronic pancreatitis
KESS constipation scoring system
Knodell chronic hepatitis C
Kodsi scale of candidal esophagitis
Lanza scale for drug-induced mucosal damage
Lauren gastric carcinoma
Marseille pancreatitis
Masuka modified thymic carcinoma
Mayo Clinic primary biliary cirrhosis
McVay
METAVIR chronic hepatitis C (0-4)
Ming gastric carcinoma
Niemeier
Nyhus
PAIS (Psychosocial Adjustment to Illness Scale)
Ponka hernia
Pressure Ulcer Scale for Healing (PUSH) tool

classification *(cont.)*
Pugh
Pugh-Child bleeding esophageal varices grading scale
PUSH (Pressure Ulcer Scale for Healing) tool
Ranson acute pancreatitis
ROME I (and II) diagnostic criteria for irritable bowel syndrome
Rutkow-Robbins-Gilbert
Savary-Miller grading scale
Symptom Distress Scale
thiazolidinedione
TNM carcinoma
Van Heuven diabetic retinopathy
Visick grading system for post-gastrectomy carcinoma recurrence
White diabetes mellitus
World Health Organization (WHO) gastric carcinoma
Zollinger

class of drugs (see *drug class*)
claudication
Claus breast cancer model
clavate papilla
clavicle pin
clavipectoral fascia
clawed pedicle hook
claw forceps
claw grasping forceps, 2 x 3 teeth, double-action
clay-colored stools
clay pipe cancer
CLC 2000 swabable intravenous connector
clean wound
Clean & Clear oil-absorbing sheets
Clean Seals waterproof bandage
cleanser (also see *medications*)
Betadine soap
Betadine scrub
Biolex wound
Dey-Wash skin wound

cleanser *(cont.)*
  DiabKlenz wound
  Hibiclens (chlorhexidine gluconate; alcohol)
  MicroKlenz wound
  Operand (povidone; iodine)
  Puri-Clens wound
  Sea-Clens wound
  Shur-Clens wound
  Skinvisible hypoallergenic hand lotion
  Surgi-Kleen skin
  Techni-Care surgical scrub
  UltraKlenz wound
  Zepiran
cleansing, intestinal
clearance, ineffective airway
clear bile
clear cell carcinoma
clear cell hepatocellular carcinoma
ClearCut 2 electrosurgical handpiece
clear effluent
clear fluid
clear-liquid diet
clear margins of tumor
clear otorrhea
clear rhinorrhea
ClearSite absorbent hydrogel wound dressing
ClearSite border dressing
ClearSite borderless dressing
ClearSite Hydro Gauze dressing
clear tap
ClearVac smoke evacuation system
ClearView CO_2 laser
"cleavoplasty" augmentation mammoplasty
cleft lip
clenched fist view
clenoliximab
Cleveland bone-cutting forceps
Cleveland bone rongeur
CLH (chronic lobular hepatitis)
clidinium bromide
Clik-Tite connector
clindamycin
clinical diagnosis
clinical parameters
clinical pathologic classification
clinical pathology
clinical picture
CliniCath peripherally inserted catheter
Clinifeed Iso enteral feeding
Clinimix E (amino acid with electrolytes in dextrose with calcium)
Clinipad Corporation
Clinistix reagent strips
Clinitest-negative stool
Clinitest-positive stool
Clinitest stool test
Clinoril (sulindac)
clip (see also *clamp*)
  Absolok locking PDS
  Absolok Plus
  Acland
  Adson scalp
  aneurysm
  aneurysm window
  Atrauclip
  baby Jones towel
  Biemer-Clip aneurysm
  brain
  Braun-Yasargil right-angle
  Children's Hospital scalp
  cobalt alloy aneurysm
  Codman aneurysm
  Cologne
  Cologne pattern scalp
  Drake aneurysm
  fenestrated Drake
  Filshie
  Heifitz
  Hem-o-lok ligating
  Hemoclip
  hemostasis
  hemostatic
  Horizon
  Housepan aneurysm

clip *(cont.)*
- Ingraham-Fowler tantalum
- Jones towel
- Khodadad
- Lapra-Ty absorbable suture
- Lapro-Clip
- Lapro-Clip ligating
- LeRoy-Raney scalp
- Liga
- Ligaclip
- Ligaclip hemostatic
- ligating
- M.A.R.C.
- Mayfield aneurysm
- MCAS (modular clip application system)
- McFadden temporary aneurysm
- McKenzie brain
- McKenzie hemostasis
- McKenzie silver
- Michel wound
- microclip
- MicroMark
- modular clip application system (MCAS)
- Multiclip
- Olivecrona aneurysm
- pin
- Raney hemostasis (hemostatic)
- Raney scalp
- ring angled
- scalp
- Schwartz aneurysm
- Schwartz micro
- Secu ("C-Q")
- Shardle towel
- silver
- skin
- sponge stopper
- Sugita aneurysm
- Sundt encircling
- Sundt-Kees aneurysm window
- supracondylar medial
- surgical

clip *(cont.)*
- surgical steel skin
- Sutured-Clip
- temporary vessel
- titanium aneurysm
- towel
- vari-angle aneurysm
- VCS
- vessel
- Weck
- Yasargil vessel

clip applier (see *applier; applicator*)
clip-applying forceps
clip-bending forceps
clip-cutting forceps
clip-inserting forceps
clip-introducing forceps
clipped, doubly
clipping of aneurysm
clipping of cystic artery
clip-removing forceps
cloacal anomaly
cloacogenic zone
cloagenic carcinoma
clockwise direction
Clomycin (polymyxin B sulfate; bacitracin; neomycin sulfate; lidocaine)
clonal anergy of T cells
clonal deletion
clonidine gel
clonidine hydrochloride injection
clonorchiasis
Clonorchis sinensis
C-loop of duodenum
Cloquet gland
Cloquet hernia
clorsulon
clortermine
clortermine HCl
closantel
closed anesthesia
closed circuit anesthesia
closed drainage system

closed-end ostomy pouch
closed hemorrhoidectomy
closed Küntscher (Kuentscher) nail
closed loop
closed loop bowel obstruction
closed loop intestinal obstruction
closed loop strangulation of bowel
closed nail
closed neck dissector
closed pin
closed suction
closed-system irrigation
closed unlocked nail
closed wound
Closer suture
Closer, The
CloseSure procedure kit
close-up view
Clostridium bifermentans
Clostridium botulinum
Clostridium botulinum toxin
Clostridium butyricum
Clostridium cadaveris
Clostridium difficile
Clostridium difficile-associated diarrhea
  (CDAD)
Clostridium histolyticum
Clostridium innocuum
Clostridium novyi
Clostridium paraputrificum
Clostridium perfringens
Clostridium putrificum
Clostridium ramosum
Clostridium septicum
Clostridium sordellii
Clostridium sphenoides
Clostridium subterminale
Clostridium tertium
Clostridium tetani
Clostridium tertium
Clostridium welchii
closure
  crural
  fascial

closure *(cont.)*
  Graham
  ileostomy
  latex
  marlex
  primary
  secondary
  single-layer continuous
  Smead-Jones
  transmural
  two-layer latex
  V-to-Y
  water-tight
  wound
Closure catheter/radiofrequency
  generator
Closure endovascular coagulation
  system
closure of colostomy
closure of fistula
closure of perforation
Closure System by VNUS catheter
clot
  agonal
  antemortem
  black blood
  blood
  chicken
  chicken fat
  currant jelly
  distal
  evacuating
  external
  fresh blood
  friable
  heart
  internal
  laminated
  marantic
  organized
  passive
  plastic
  postmortem
  proximal

clot *(cont.)*
  retraction of
  sentinel blood
  spider-web
  stratified
  washed
CLOtest (*Campylobacter*-like organism)
cloth shears
clothespin spinal fusion graft
clot lysis test
clot retraction coagulation panel
clot retraction test
clotting, abnormal
clotting abnormality
clotting factors
clotting parameters
clotting time (also, coagulation)
  activated
  Lee-White
  plasma
clotting time coagulation panel
clot tube
cloudy ascites
cloudy bile
cloudy fluid
clove-hitch suture
cloverleaf deformity
cloverleaf intramedullary nail
cloverleaf Küntscher (Kuentscher) nail
cloverleaf pin extractor
cloverleaf plate
Cloward blade retractor
Cloward brain retractor
Cloward hook
Cloward cervical chisel
Cloward cervical retractor
Cloward-Cushing vein retractor
Cloward drill
Cloward drill guide
Cloward dural hook
Cloward dural retractor
Cloward-English laminectomy rongeur
Cloward hammer
Cloward-Harper laminectomy rongeur
Cloward-Hoen hemilaminectomy retractor
Cloward-Hoen laminectomy retractor
Cloward intervertebral disk rongeur
Cloward large cervical rongeur
Cloward lumbar lamina retractor
Cloward nerve root retractor
Cloward osteophyte elevator
Cloward periosteal elevator
Cloward pituitary rongeur
Cloward punch forceps
Cloward rongeur forceps
Cloward skin retractor
Cloward small cervical retractor
Cloward spinal fusion chisel
Cloward tissue retractor
club-shaped bacillus
clustered calcifications
Clutton bladder sound
Clutton urethral bougie
clysma
Clysodrast (bisacodyl tannex)
CMBC (cutaneous metastatic breast cancer)
C-mount
CMV (cytomegalovirus) enteritis
CMV inclusion
CMV prophylaxis
CMV-IGIV (cytomegalovirus immune globulin, intravenous)
CMV-positive donor
CNS (central nervous system) tumor
CNS depression
CNTF (ciliary neurotrophic factor)
CO (cardiac output)
CO_2 (carbon dioxide)
CO_2 embolus
CO_2 gas filter
CO_2 Guard gas filter for laparoscopy
CO_2 insufflation
CO_2 laser
CO_2 laser vaporization
CO_2 medium

CO_2 needle
CO_2 tubing
coag (coagulation)
coagulase-negative staphylococcus
coagulase test
coagulate bleeding vessel
coagulated protein
coagulating cannula
coagulating current
coagulating forceps
coagulating suction cannula
coagulation (see also *cautery*)
  acquired disorder of
  argon plasma
  BiLap
  bipolar
  blood
  Bovie
  congenital disorder of
  diffuse intravascular (DIC)
  disseminated intravascular (DIC)
  electric
  endovascular
  ILC (interstitial laser)
  interstitial laser
  massive
  monopolar
  multipolar
coagulation defect
coagulation electrode
coagulation factor
  I (fibrinogen)
  II (prothrombin)
  III (tissue thromboplastin)
  IV (calcium)
  V (proaccelerin)
  VI (stable)
  VII (proconvertin)
  VIII (antihemophilic)
  IX (plasma thromboplastin component)
  IX recombinant
  X (Stuart-Prower)
  XI (plasma thromboplastin antecedent)
coagulation factor *(cont.)*
  XII (Hageman)
  XIII (fibrin stabilizing)
coagulation factor assay
coagulation necrosis
coagulation of tissue
coagulation panel
  bleeding time
  clot retraction
  clotting time
  partial thromboplastin time
  plasma assay
  platelet count
  prothrombin time
coagulation study
coagulation suction, insulated
coagulation time (also, clotting)
  activated
  Lee-White
  plasma
coagulation time test
coagulator (also see *electrocautery; forceps*)
  argon beam (ABC)
  argon plasma
  Bovie
  Coaguloop
  Cosman
  Cutting LOOP
  Delasco electrocoagulator
  Endopath EZ-RF linear cutter and coagulation device
  Hydromer
  LaparoSonic coagulating shears
  LigaSure vessel sealing system
  Modulap
  Olympus SonoSurg ultrasonic cutter/coagulator
  Pivotal
  PROloop
  smart loop
  SonoSurg ultrasonic cutter/coagulator
Coaguloop system

coagulopathy, consumption
COAG waveform desiccation
Coakley antrum trocar and wash tube
coalesce
coalescence
coalition view
coal-miner's lung
coaptation bioplar forceps
coaptation plate
coapting suture
coarctation clamp
coarctation of the aorta
coarse nodularity
coarsely nodular cirrhosis
coated suture
coated Vicryl Rapide (polyglactin 910) suture
Cobactin E (*Lactobacillus acidophilus*)
Coballoy twist drill
Cobalt Knife
cobalt-60 gamma knife
Coban dressing
Cobb periosteal elevator
Cobb spinal elevator
Cobb spinal gouge
Cobbett knife
cobblestone appearance of mucosa
cobblestone mucosa
cobblestone pattern of hepatocytes
cobblestoning of colon
cobblestoning of mucosa
cobblestoning on endoscopic exam
cobblestoning sign
Cobelli gland
Cobe stapler
Coblation-Channeling operation
Coblation technology
cobra grasping forceps, double-action
cobra retractor
Cobra rat-tooth grasping forceps
cobra-head plate
CO/BSA (cardiac output/body surface area = cardiac index)
coccidial colitis
Coccidioides immitis
coccidioidomycosis
coccidiosis
cockscomb papilloma
cocktail, immunosuppressant
codeine
Codivilla bone graft
Codman-Harper laminectomy rongeur
Codman-Kerrison laminectomy rongeur
Codman-Leksell laminectomy rongeur
Codman-Schlesinger cervical laminectomy rongeur
Codman wire pass drill
Coe-pak paste adhesive
coffee bean sign of cecal volvulus
coffee-grounds emesis
coffee-grounds vomitus
Coffey ureterointestinal anastomosis
Cohen cannula
Cohen periosteal elevator
Cohen rongeur
Cohen syndrome
Coherent CO_2 surgical
Coherent UltraPulse 5000C laser
CO/HR (cardiac output/heart rate = stroke volume)
coil
  Gianturco wool-tufted wire
  Stylet internal esophageal MRI
coil gland
coil of intestine
coil of jejunum
coinfection with hepatitis B
coin lesion of lung
Colace (docusate sodium)
Colanis maneuver
Colapinto transjugular liver biopsy needle
Colaris test
Co-Lav (polyethylene glycol electrolyte solution; electrolytes)
Colax (phenolphthalein; docusate sodium)
Colazal (balsalazide disodium)

Colazide (balsalazide disodium)
Colclough-Scheicher laminectomy
  rongeur
cold abscess
cold agglutinin pneumonia
cold agglutinins
cold biopsy
cold chisel
cold compressive dressing
cold cone biopsy
cold cup biopsy
cold defect
cold erythema
cold-hemolytic antibody
cold laser
cold light source
cold nodule
cold spot
colectomy
  abdominal
  hand-assisted laparoscopic
  laparoscopic
  left
  partial
  prophylactic
  subtotal
  total abdominal (TAC)
  transverse
Coleman infiltration cannula
colesevelam HCl
Cole sign
Colestid (colestipol)
colestipol
Cole tube
coli (see *Escherichia coli*)
colibacillemia
colibacillosis, enteric
Colibri forceps
colic
  abdominal
  appendiceal
  appendicular
  bile duct
  biliary
colic *(cont.)*
  bilious
  common duct
  Devonshire
  episodic
  esophageal
  flatulent
  gallbladder
  gallstone
  gastric
  hepatic
  hysterical
  infantile
  intestinal
  kidney
  lead
  liver
  mucous
  nephritic
  Painter
  pancreatic
  psychogenic
  saturnine
  spasmodic
  vermicular
colic artery
colic flexure
colic impression on the liver
colicky abdominal pain
colicky pain
colic omentum
colic patch
colic plexus
colic sphincter
colic surface
colic vein
coliform bacillus (pl. bacilli)
coliform bacteria
colipase
colistimethate
colistin
colitis (see also *enterocolitis*)
  acute infectious
  acute self-limited (ASLC)

colitis *(cont.)*
- adaptive
- allergic
- amebic
- anthrax
- antibiotic-associated
- bacillary
- bacterial
- balantidial
- *Campylobacter*
- catarrhal
- chronic intermittent
- chronic ischemic
- chronic ulcerative (CUC)
- coccidial
- collagenous
- Crohn
- croupous
- dietetic
- enterocolitis
- exudative
- familial ulcerative
- focal
- fulminant
- fulminating ulcerative
- functional
- gangrenous
- giardial
- granulomatous
- granulomatous transmural
- hemorrhagic
- idiopathic
- infectious
- infective
- intractable ulcerative
- ischemic
- left-sided
- left-sided ulcerative
- lymphocytic
- membranous
- microscopic
- mucous
- nondysenteric
- noninfectious

colitis *(cont.)*
- phlegmonous
- progesterone-associated
- pseudomembranous (PMC)
- psychogenic
- radiation
- radiation-induced
- regional
- *Salmonella*
- *Shigella*
- single-stripe (SSC)
- staphylococcus
- thromboulcerative
- toxic
- transmural
- trichomonal
- tuberculous
- ulcerative (UC)
- universal
- universal ulcerative
- *Yersinia enterocolitica*

colitis cystica profunda (CCP)
colitis cystica superficialis (CCS)
collagen accumulation
collagen-alginate wound dressing
collagen arranged in swirls
collagen deposition
collagen hemostat
collagen hemostatic material
collagenolysis
collagenous colitis
collagenous sprue
collagen suture
collagen synthesis inhibitor
collagen vascular disease
CollagENT wand
Collagraft bone graft matrix
collapsible pin
collar-button abscess
collar-button appearance in colon
collar-button-like ulcer
Collastat hemostatic sponge
CollaTape
collateral circulation

Colleague 3 (triple channel) infusion pump
CollectFirst autotransfusion system
collection, air
collection of pus
Collier needle holder
collimator
 ConforMAX MMLC (mini-multileaf collimator)
 MCAT (modular coded aperture technology)
 Millennium MLC-120 multileaf
Collin abdominal retractor
Collin amputating knife
Collin-Duval lung grasping forceps
Collin dynamometer
Collin tissue-grasping forceps
Collingwood Stewart hernia ring forceps
Collins intestinal forceps
Collins intestinal retractor
Collins rib shears
Collins solution
colliquative diarrhea
colliquative necrosis
Collis antireflux operation
Collis gastroplasty
Collis-Nissen fundoplication
Collis-Nissen gastroplasty
Collis-Taylor retractor
Collison drill
Collison forceps
Collison plate
colloid adenocarcinoma
colloidal bismuth subcitrate
colloid cancer
colloid carcinoma
colloid formation
colloid goiter
collodion dressing
colloid material
colloid shift on liver-spleen scan
Collyer pelvimeter
Colly-Seel wafer-type skin barrier for ostomy skin
coloanal anastomosis
coloanal anastomosis with colonic reservoir
ColoCare test for fecal occult blood
colocolic intussusception
colocolostomy
Colocort (hydrocortisone enema)
colocutaneous fistula
coloenteric fistula
Cologel
Cologne clip
Colomed enema
colon
 anterior band of
 ascending
 cathartic
 descending
 distal
 elongated
 free band of
 functional shrunken
 giant
 hepatic flexure of
 iliac
 inflammation of
 irritable
 lateral reflection of
 lead pipe
 left
 loops of redundant
 megacolon
 mesosigmoid
 midsigmoid
 pelvic
 perforated
 perisigmoid
 rectosigmoid
 right
 saccular
 sigmoid
 spastic
 transverse
colon adenocarcinoma
colon and mesocolon

colon bacillus
colon cancer
colon conduit
colon cutoff sign
Colon Injury Score (CIS)
colon interposition
colonic abscess
colonic adenoma
colonic air
colonic atony
colonic bacteria
colonic balloon volume
colonic crypt region
colonic distention
colonic diverticulitis
colonic diverticulum
colonic fistula
colonic flora
colonic hypersecretion
colonic inertia
colonic lavage
colonic loop
colonic mesenteric plexus
colonic motility
colonic myenteric plexus
colonic necrosis
colonic obstruction
colonic patch
colonic perforation
colonic pit
colonic polyp
colonic pseudo-obstruction (Ogilvie syndrome)
colonic solitary ulcer syndrome
colonic transit study
colonic transit test
colonic tube
colonic tuberculosis
colonic varices
colonic volvulus
colonization infection
Colonlite bowel prep
colon mass

colonoscope (see also *endoscope*)
- ACMI
- CF-HM
- CF-LB3R
- CF-MB-M
- Fujinon EVC-M video
- MIS Source
- Olympus CF
- Olympus CF-140I video
- Olympus CF-140L video
- Olympus CF-140S video
- Olympus CF-1T10L flexible therapeutic
- Olympus CF-1T20L flexible therapeutic
- Olympus CF-20L flexible
- Olympus CF-30L flexible
- Olympus CF-ITS2 fiberoptic
- Olympus CF-MB/LB
- Olympus CF-P
- Olympus CF-Q160AL/I innoflex video
- Olympus CF-UHM
- Olympus CF-VL
- Olympus DF-HM magnifying
- Olympus PCF pediatric
- Olympus PCF-10 flexible pediatric
- Olympus PCF-140I pediatric video
- Olympus PCF-140L pediatric video
- Olympus PCF-160AL/I video
- Olympus SIF-M
- Pentax EC-3430F video
- Pentax EC-3430L video
- Pentax EC-3440F video
- Pentax EC-3440L video
- Pentax EC-3830 video
- Pentax EC-3830L video
- Pentax EC-3830TL video
- Pentax EC-3840L video
- Pentax EC-3840T video
- Pentax FC-38LV fiberoptic
- Pentax FC-38MV fiberoptic
- variable-stiffness

colonoscopic polypectomy
colonoscopy
  complete
  incomplete
  real-time
  stomal
  virtual
colonoscopy per rectum
colonoscopy per stoma
colon polyp
colon resection clamp
colon syndrome
colon tumor
Colopath test
colopexy
Coloplast Flange Mini Caps
Coloplast Flange pouch
Coloplast Mini pouch
Coloplast ostomy irrigation set
Coloplast skin barrier
coloplasty pouch
coloplasty procedure
coloproctitis
coloproctostomy
color and caliber of stool
Colorado microdissection needle
Colorado tick fever virus
colorectal bleeding
colorectal cancer (CRC)
colorectal cancer screening
colorectal carcinoma
colorectal disease
colorectal malignancy
colorectal mucosa
colorectal polyp
colorectal segment
Colormate TLc BiliTest System
colorrhaphy
Col-R-Sponge sponge
ColoScreen occult blood test
ColoScreen Self Test
ColoScreen Slide Test
Coloshield
colosigmoid resection
colostomy (see also *appliance*; *bag; barrier; mesh; pouch*)
  blow hole decompressing
  da Silva
  decompression
  descending loop
  Devine
  diverting
  diverting proximal
  divided-stoma
  double-barrel (or barreled)
  dry
  end
  end-loop
  end-sigmoid
  exteriorization
  Hartmann
  ileoascending
  ileosigmoid
  ileotransverse
  Lazaro da Silva technique
  loop
  Mikulicz
  permanent
  permanent end
  resective
  sigmoid-end
  sigmoid-loop rod
  temporary end
  terminal
  transverse
  transverse-loop rod
  Turnbull
  wet
colostomy bag
colostomy bridge
colostomy closure
colostomy rod
Colovage (polyethylene glycol-electrolyte solution)
colovaginal fistula
COLO-Vax
colovesical fistula
colpohysteroscope

colpoperineopexy, abdominosacral
colpopexy
colporrhaphy, posterior
colposcope
colposcopic diagnosis
colposcopically directed punch biopsy
colposuspension needle
colposuspension suture
column, anal
columnar cell lined
columnar cuff cancer
columnar epithelium
columnar-lined esophagus
columnar metaplasia
column of Morgagni
Colver tonsil-seizing forceps
Coly-Mycin M
Coly-Mycin S
Coly-Seel ostomy barrier
Colyte (polyethylene glycol-electrolyte solution)
coma
- diabetic
- hepatic
- hyperosmolar
- hyperosmolar nonketotic
- insulin
- myxedema
- nondiabetic insulin
- nonketotic
- nonketotic hyperglycemic-hyperosmolar (NKHHC)

Comamonas terrigena
CombiDerm absorbent cover dressing
Combidex imaging agent
combination chemotherapy
combined androgen blockade (CAB)
combined anesthesia
combined Collis gastroplasty-fundoplication operation for scleroderma reflux esophagitis
combined defect
combined hemorrhoids
combined hernia
combined liver and intestinal transplantation
combined modality therapy
comblike redness sign
combretastatin
comedo carcinoma
Comeg rigid laparoscope
Comfeel Plus dressing
Comfeel Purilon dressing
Comfeel Ulcus occlusive dressing
Comfort Cath I or II catheter
Commando procedure (glossectomy)
commensally (without harm)
commode, bedside
common bile duct (CBD)
common bile duct exploration (CBDE)
common bile duct obstruction
common bile duct stone
common cavity phenomenon
common cold virus
common duct
common duct calculus
common duct cholangiogram
common duct colic
common duct dilator
common duct exploration
common duct obstruction
common duct scoop
common duct sound
common duct stone
common gall duct
common hepatic artery
common hepatic duct
common iliac artery
common iliac node
common variable hypogammaglobulinemia
communicable infectious disease
communicating pseudocyst
community-acquired bacteremia
community-acquired infection
community-acquired pneumonia
comorbidity
Compaction pliers

comparison film
compartment, preperitoneal
compartment syndrome
Compazine suppositories (prochlorperazine)
compensated acidosis
compensated dysphagia (for solid foods)
Compere threaded pin
Comperm bandage
Comperm PD bandage
Comperm tubular elastic bandage
competency of repair
competent ileocecal valve
competent valve
Compleat-B liquid feeding
Compleat modified formula
complete adrenalectomy
complete bowel obstruction
complete hemostasis
complete hernia
complete mastectomy
complete obstruction
complete rupture
complete thymectomy
complete thyroidectomy
complete wrap (Nissen operation)
complex
  esophagogastric
  gastroduodenal artery
  Meyenburg
  nipple-areola
  von Meyenburg
complex anorectal fistula
complex appendicitis
complex IV deficiency
complex lesion
complex regional pain syndrome (CRPS)
compliance
complicated residual hepatolithiasis with biliary stricture
complication
  concomitant obesity
  postsplenectomy
complication *(cont.)*
  surgery
  trocar wound site
Comply
composite graft
composite procedure
composition, body
Composix mesh
compound cyst
compound gland
compound volvulus
comprehensive health enhancement support system (CHESS)
compressed carbon dioxide gas
compressed malignant cells
compression
  extrinsic
  mechanical variceal
  vena cava
compression anesthesia
compression bandage
compression hook
compression of the hepatoduodenal ligament
compression plate
compression rod
compression stay suture
compression tape
compression wrap dressing
compressive dressing
compressive symptoms
Comprilan bandage
comprimeter
Compro (prochlorperazine)
compromise of blood supply
compromised bowel wall
compromised breathing
compromised cardiac function
Compton clavicle pin
computed tomography (CT) scan
computed tomography laser mammography (CTLM)
computer-assisted microsurgery
computerized axial tomography (CAT)

computerized lithotriptor
computerized peristaltic pump
computerized phonoenterography
Computerized Thermal Imaging system
computerized treatment planning
Comvax (*Haemophilus* purified capsular polysaccharide; *Neisseria meningitidis* OMPC; hepatitis B virus vaccine)
concave abdomen
concave obturator
concave sheath
concave wound
concealed hemorrhage
concealed vomiting
concentration, extracellular
concentration of lipopolysaccharide-binding protein
concentric hiatal hernia
concentric layers of epithelial cells
concentric lesion
concentric needle electrode
concentrically laminated mass
Concept 8160 IntraVision Lumi-Trac endoscopic camera
Concept ablator
Concept endoscope
Concept handheld cautery
Concept/Linvatec laparoscope
Concept rigid laparoscope
Conceptus Soft Seal cervical catheter
Conceptus Soft Torque uterine catheter
Conceptus VS (variable softness) catheter
Conco elastic bandage
Conco gauze bandage
concomitant acute alcoholic hepatitis
concomitant bleeding
concomitant complications of obesity
concomitant health problems
concomitant injury
concomitant spinal cord injury
Concorde cannula
Concord Portex epidural catheter

concretion
  appendiceal
  bile
  calculus
  fecal
  gallbladder
  intestinal
  preputial
  prostatic
  salivary
  tophic
concurrent chemotherapy and radiation therapy
conditioning
  interceptive
  semantic
condition, pathological hypersecretory
conduction anesthesia
conductive keratoplasty (CK)
conduit
  aortic
  arterial
  artificial
  autologous
  biliary
  Bricker
  bypass
  circumferential
  colon
  colonic
  continent
  flow
  free jejunal
  homograft
  jejunal
  ileal
  intestinal
  Kock
  mucosa-lined
  obstructed
  peristaltic
  prosthetic
  radial
  sigmoid

conduit *(cont.)*
- silicone
- substitute
- surgical
- synthetic
- thoracic
- transdermal
- T-shaped
- ureteroileal
- urinary
- valve

condylar plate
condylocephalic nail
condyloma (pl. condylomata)
- anal
- flat
- genital
- penile
- perianal
- vaginal
- venereal

condyloma acuminatum
condyloma latum
cone biopsy
cone biopsy cannula
cone biopsy needle
coned-down appearance of colon
coned-down view
cone laminectomy retractor
cone-nose forceps
cone retractor
cone scalp retractor
cone skull punch
cone skull punch forceps
cone suction tube
cone ventricular needle
cone view
cone wire-twisting forceps
confined to mucosa
confined to muscularis
confined to serosa
confirmatory needle biopsy
confluent
Conform dressing
Conforma 3000 photon beam therapy system
Conformant contact-layer wound dressing
ConforMAX MMLC (mini-multileaf collimator)
confusion, mental
congenital adrenal hyperplasia
congenital anomaly
congenital atresia
congenital biliary atresia
congenital cardiac malformation
congenital cavernous malformation of the splenic vein
congenital choledochal cyst
congenital choledochal dilatation
congenital cirrhosis
congenital cystic liver disease
congenital dilatation of intrahepatic bile duct
congenital disorder of coagulation
congenital diverticulum
congenital erythropoietic porphyria
congenital esophageal stenosis
congenital familial nonhemolytic jaundice
congenital goiter
congenital hemangioma
congenital hemolytic anemia
congenital hemolytic jaundice
congenital hepatic fibrosis (CHF)
congenital hernia
congenital hourglass stomach
congenital hypertrophic pyloric stenosis
congenital hypothyroidism
congenital lactose malabsorption
congenital lesion
congenital lipomatosis of pancreas
congenital malaria
congenital malrotation of the gut
congenital megacolon
congenital pulmonary arteriovenous fistula
congenital pyloric stenosis

congenital sacral agenesis
congenital splenomegaly
congenital sucrose intolerance
congenital sucrose-isomaltose
  deficiency (CSID)
congenital sucrose-isomaltose
  malabsorption
congenital thyroid deficiency
congenital virilizing adrenal hyperplasia
congenital zinc deficiency
congested kidney
congestive cirrhosis
congestive heart failure (CHF)
congestive hepatomegaly
congestive liver cirrhosis
congestive splenomegaly
Congo red dye
Congreve cannula
congruous cup-shaped reamer
conical cecum
conical mass
conical papilla
conical reamer
conical tectal plate
conical trocar
conization knife
conjoined tendon (also conjoint)
conjoining of the aponeurosis
  to the internal oblique
conjoint tendon (also conjoined)
conjugate forward gaze position
conjugated bile acid
conjugated bilirubin
conjugated hyperbilirubinemia
conjugated linoleic acid (CLA)
conjunctival icterus
Conley pin
Conmed Corporation
Conn syndrome
connecting plate
Conn pneumatic tourniquet
connective tissue disease (overlap
  syndrome)
connector
  banana plug
  Olympus
  tubing
Connell suture
Conray contrast medium
conscious sedation
Conseal ostomy irrigation set
consented
conservative measures
conservative therapy
conservative treatment with close
  observation
considerable fibrosis
consistency of stool
consolidated graft
constantly perfused side-hole catheter
Constellation mapping catheter
Constilac (lactulose)
constipated
constipation
  antepartum
  atonic
  chronic
  drug-induced
  functional
  gastrojejunal
  geriatric
  intermittent
  lifelong
  new-onset
  normal transit (NTC)
  outlet
  postpartum
  proctogenous
  refractory
  spastic
constipation and diarrhea, alternating
constipation due to ganglioneuromatosis
constipation-predominant irritable
  bowel syndrome
constricting pain
constriction, appendiceal
constrictive lesion

Constulose (lactulose)
consumption
  alcoholic
  dietary
  ethanol (EtOH)
consumption coagulopathy
ConTack suture anchor
contact cancer
contact laser hemorrhoidectomy
contact-layer wound dressing
contagious infectious disease
contaminated wound
contamination
  fecal
  peritoneal
ConTE-Pak-4 (multiple trace elements)
contents
  abdominal
  bowel
  digestive tract
  enteric
  gastric
  intestinal
  intraluminal
  refluxed gastric
contents of axilla
contiguous loop
contiguous spread
contiguous structures
continence, fecal
continent ileal pouch
continent ileal reservoir
continent ileostomy
continent of stool
continent supravesical bowel urinary diversion
continued blood per NG tube
continued clinical exploration
continuous ambulatory peritoneal dialysis (CAPD)
continuous analgesia delivery (CAD)
continuous compression
continuous drainage
continuous drip feeding
continuous electrocardiogram monitoring
continuous epidural anesthesia
continuous-flow catheter anesthesia
continuously perfused probe
continuous NG suction
continuous pull-through technique
continuous running suture
continuous spinal anesthesia
continuous suture
continuous thoracic epidural analgesia
Continuum total knee base plate
contour, breast
contoured tilting compression mammography
contoured T-plate
Contour Profile breast implant
Contour scalp retractor
contracted kidney
contractile capacity of esophageal body
contractile stricture
contractility
contraction (pl. contractions)
  esophageal
  gallbladder
  hypotensive esophageal
  intestinal muscle
  longitudinal muscle
  peristaltic
  phasic
  primary
  secondary
  tertiary
  tonic
contraction alkalosis
contraction band necrosis
contraction of gallbladder, decreased
contraction-relaxation cycles
contractive ring dysphagia
contractor
  Bailey rib
  Bailey-Gibbon rib
  Lemmon rib
  rib
  Sellors rib

contralateral breast
contralateral hernia
contralateral subtotal thyroid lobectomy
contrast agent (see *contrast medium*)
contrast echocardiography
contrast enema
contrast enhancement of computed tomographic (CECT) imaging
contrast esophagography
contrast medium (pl. media)
  Amipaque
  Angiografin
  Angiovist
  Baricon
  barium sulfate
  Baro-cat
  Baroflave
  Barosperse
  Biligrafin
  Biliscopin
  Bilivist
  Bilopaque
  Biloptin
  Cholebrine
  Cholografin
  Conray
  diatrizoate meglumine
  extravasated
  Gastrografin
  Gastrovist Hexabrix
  Hippuran
  Hypaque
  Hypaque-Cysto
  iocetamic acid
  iodinated
  iodipamide meglumine
  iohexol
  iopamidol
  iopanoic acid
  iothalamate
  ipodate
  Isovue
  Kinevac
  MD-60

contrast medium *(cont.)*
  meglumine diatrizoate
  meglumine iotroxate
  metrizamide
  metrizoate
  Niopam
  Omnipaque
  Oragrafin
  Pantopaque
  rectal
  Reno-M-Dip
  Renografin
  sodium diatrizoate with Menoquinon
  sodium iodipamide
  sodium iothalamate
  Solu-Biloptin
  Telepaque
  Thoratrast
  Tomocat
  tyropanoate
  Urografin
contrast-enhanced CT scan
contrast selective cholangiogram
contrast study
control, glycemic
controlled distention irrigation system (CDIS)
controlled fistula with duodenostomy tube
contused wound
convalescent phase of hepatitis
ConvaTec Active Life Stoma Cap
ConvaTec colostomy pouch
ConvaTec Durahesive Wafer ostomy
ConvaTec Flextrak gastrostomy anchor
ConvaTec Little One Sur-Fit pouch
ConvaTec skin barrier
ConvaTec Sur-Fit two-piece pouch
conventional concentric electromyography
conventional cutting-sternum needle
Converse chisel
Converse needle holder

Converse periosteal elevator
Converse-TC needle holder
conversion of T_4 to T_3
conversion to ileostomy
conversion to laparotomy
Converspaz
convert from laparoscopic to open procedure
convertible slipknot suture
Convertor drape
Convertor setup
Converzyame
convex border of
convex rasp
ConXn (recombinant human relaxin, H_2)
Cook aspiration biopsy needle
cookie (pad)
  arch
  Gelfoam
  navicular shoe
  scaphoid shoe
cookie cutter
Cook introducer
Cook Oasis biliary stent
Cook rectal speculum
Cook TPN catheter
Cook-Wilson gastric balloon
Cooley anastomosis clamp
Cooley aortic clamp
Cooley atrial retractor
Cooley-Baumgarten aortic forceps
Cooley-Baumgarten wire twisters
Cooley-Beck clamp
Cooley bulldog clamp
Cooley coarctation clamp
Cooley cross-action bulldog clamp
Cooley-Derra anastomosis clamp
Cooley graft suction tube
Cooley iliac clamp
Cooley intracardiac suction tube
Cooley partial occlusion clamp
Cooley patent ductus clamp
Cooley pediatric clamp
Cooley renal clamp
Cooley rib retractor
Cooley rib shears
Cooley-Satinsky clamp
Cooley vascular clamp
Cooley vascular forceps
Cooley vena cava catheter clamp
Cool Tip catheter
Coombs test, direct
Cooper Cavitron surgical aspirator
Cooper hernia
Cooper ligament
Cooper ligament repair
Cooper Surgical cystoscope
Cooper Surgical Marro Nu-Tip
Cooper Surgical trocar
COPA cuffed oropharyngeal airway
Cope (aspirin; caffeine; magnesium hydroxide; aluminum hydroxide)
Cope biopsy needle
Cope crushing clamp
Cope modification of Martel intestinal clamp
Cope needle
Cope suture anchor
copious amounts of saline
copious irrigation
copious peritoneal lavage
copious rice-water diarrhea
copious watery diarrhea
copper-binding protein (CBP) test
copper blade
copper mallet
copper-vapor pulsed laser
Corbett bone rongeur
cord
  hepatic
  spermatic
Cordis-Hakim shunt
Cordis Predator PTCA balloon catheter
Cordis Trakstar PTCA balloon catheter
cord lipoma
Cordonnier ureteroileal loop
cordotomy (chordotomy) knife

cordotomy hook
Cordox
cord structure
core biopsy
core needle biopsy
core of tumor
core probe
Core aspiration/injection needle
Core audible trocar
Core cannula system
Core CO_2 insufflation needle
Core Entree Plus laparoscopic trocar and cannula system
Core Entree II laparoscopic trocar system
Core laparoscopic aspiration/injection needle
Core laparoscopic dilator
Core laparoscopic Kittner dissector
Core laparoscopic smoke eliminator
Core reposable trumpet
Core shielded laparoscopic trocar
Core suction/irrigation probe
Core trocar
Corey forceps
Cori disease
corkscrew appearance
corkscrew dural hook
corkscrew esophagus
corkscrew femoral head extractor
corkscrew-shaped bacteria
corkscrew suture anchor
corneal shield sponge
corneal ulcer
CorneaSparing LTK system laser
Cornelia de Lange syndrome
corner, antemesenteric
corner mouth lift
cornflake esophageal motility test
corona mortis
coronal incision
coronal scalp incision
coronal suture
coronary arteriole vasodilation
coronary artery lesion
coronary artery of stomach
coronary artery scissors
coronary artery vasoconstriction
coronary ligament
coronary stent
coronary vein
coronavirus gastroenteritis
Corpak feeding tube
corpus carcinoma
correction of electrolytes
corrective soft dressing
Correctol (bisacodyl)
Correctol Extra Gentle (docusate sodium)
corrosive esophagitis
corrosive gastritis
corrugated reamer
corrugated tubing
corset effect
Corson needle electrode
CorTek laparoscope
CorTek semirigid microlaparoscope
Cortenema (hydrocortisone)
Cortenema retention enema
cortex drill
Corticaine
cortical bone graft
cortical drill
cortical plate
cortical strut graft
corticoadrenal insufficiency
corticocancellous bone graft
corticocancellous chip graft
corticorelin ovine triflutate
corticosteroid
corticosteroid-based immunosuppression
corticosteroid-binding globulin (CBG)
corticotropin-releasing factor (CRF)
Cortifoam (hydrocortisone acetate)
cortisol analog
cortisol-binding globulin
cortisol-producing carcinoma

cortisol-secreting tumor
cortisol secretion
Coryllos-Doyen periosteal elevator
Coryllos rasp
Coryllos retractor
Coryllos rib shears
Corynebacterium genitalium
CoSeal resorbable synthetic vascular
  sealant
CoSeal surgical sealant
Cosgrove Flex clamp
Cosman coagulator
cosmetic conventional cutting suture
cosmetic reverse cutting suture
costal margin
costal rasp
CoStasis enterocolic hemostatic sealant
CoStasis surgical hemostat
costocolic fold
CoStop surgical adhesion barrier
costopleural reflection
costovertebral angle (CVA) tenderness
costovertebral angle tenderness (CVAT)
cot death
Cotara
Cotazym-S (lipase; protease; amylase)
Cotrel-Dubousset hook
Cottle chisel
Cottle-Kazanjiann rongeur
Cottle-MacKenty elevator
Cottle-MacKenty rasp
Cottle mallet
Cottle retractor
Cottle saw
Cottle style
Cottle suction tube
cotton, absorbable cellulose
cotton applicator
cotton carrier
cotton dressing
cotton elastic bandage
cotton suture
Cotton cartilage graft
coudé catheter
Couinaud liver disease grading
  classification
Coumadin (warfarin sodium)
coumarin green tunable dye laser
  lithotripsy
coumarin pulsed-dye laser
Councilman body (in viral hepatitis)
Councilman lesion
Count EZ sponge counter bag
counterirritant
counter rotating saw
count, sponge and needle
coupled suture
Cournand arteriogram needle
Cournand-Grino arteriogram needle
Cournand needle
Courvoisier gallbladder
Courvoisier gastroenterostomy
Courvoisier law
Courvoisier sign
Courvoisier-Terrier syndrome
couvade syndrome
Covaderm composite wound dressing
Covaderm Plus adhesive barrier
  dressing
Coventry staple
Coverlet adhesive surgical dressing
Cover-Roll adhesive gauze dressing
CoverTip safety syringe
Cowden disease
cow kidney
COX (cytochrome C oxidase) deficiency
  French-Canadian type
  infantile mitochondrial myopathy
  Leigh disease
  subacute necrotizing encephalo-
    myopathy
COX-1-sparing agent
COX-2 (cyclo-oxygenase-2) inhibitor
Cox-Uphoff International tissue
  expander (CUI)
Coxiella burnetii
coxsackievirus
CPAP (continuous positive airway
  pressure)

CPAP valve
CPAS-free (caffeine, alcohol, pepper, spicy foods) diet
CPC connector
C-peptide (protein)
CPH (chronic persistent hepatitis)
CPK (creatine phosphokinase)
C-plasty
Cr (chromium)
Crabtree dissector
cracked nipple
Crafoord aortic clamp
Crafoord coarctation clamp
Crafoord forceps
Crafoord thoracic scissors
Cragg endoluminal
Cragg Endopro System I stent
Cragg-McNamara valved infusion catheter
Craig biopsy needle
Craig scissors
Craig vertebral body biopsy instrument set
cramping
crampy abdominal pain
Crane mallet
cranial angled view
cranial bone fixation plate
cranial bone graft
cranial drill
cranial rongeur
cranial rongeur forceps
cranial suture
craniocaudad view
craniocaudal view
craniocerebral penetrating wound
craniopharyngioma
craniotome blade
craniotomy saw
craterlike (with jagged edges) ulcer
crater, ulcer
cravat bandage
Crawford aortic retractor
Crawford dural elevator
Crawford needle
CRC (colorectal cancer)
CRD canister
crease
  inframammary
  midline abdominal
  palmar
  skin
  torso
  wound
crease wound
creatinine
creatinine clearance
creatorrhea
Credé maneuver
creeping of mesenteric fat
Crego elevator
Crego-McCarroll pin
Crego retractor
cremasteric fascia
cremasteric fascial fibers
cremasteric fiber
cremasteric reflex
cremasteric sheath
cremasteric vessel
Creon
crepe bandage
crepitus
crescendoing bowel sounds
crescent knife
crescent of the cardia
crescentic blade
CREST syndrome
Crestor (rosuvastatin)
cretinism
  athyrotic
  endemic
  goitrous
CRF (corticotropin-releasing factor)
CRH (corticotropin-releasing hormone)
crib death
cribriform fascia
cribriform carcinoma
cribriform pattern

cribriform plate
Cricket stapler
cricoid cartilage
cricoid myotomy
cricopharyngeal achalasia
cricopharyngeal bar
cricopharyngeal dilation
cricopharyngeal diverticulum
cricopharyngeal myotomy
cricopharyngeal sphincter
cricopharyngeus muscle
cricopharyngeus myotomy
cricothyroid membrane
cricothyroid muscle
cricothyroidotomy
Crigler-Najjar syndrome
Crile appendix clamp
Crile artery forceps
Crile bile duct forceps
Crile clamp
Crile forceps, curved
Crile gasserian ganglion knife
Crile hemostat
Crile hemostatic forceps
Crile hook and dissector
Crile nerve hook
Crile-Rankin forceps
Crile retractor
Crile stone hook
Crile thyroid retractor
Crile-type clamp
Crile-Wood needle
Crile-Wood needle holder with
  tungsten carbide inlay
crisis
  addisonian
  celiac
  thyroid
  thyrotoxic
crisscross suture
criteria (see *classification*)
critical lesion
Criticare HN (high nitrogen) elemental
  liquid feeding
Cro-Man-Zin (chromium; manganese;
  zinc)
Crohn's and Colitis Foundation
  of America, Inc. (CCFA)
Crohn colitis
Crohn disease (CD)
Crohn disease (regional ileitis)
Crohn disease activity index (CDAI)
Crohn ileitis
Crohn ileocolitis
Crohn regional enteritis
Cronkhite-Canada disease
Cronkhite-Canada syndrome
Crosby-Kugler capsule for biopsy
crossbar
  inner
  outer
crossbridge cycle
cross-circulation
cross-clamp
cross-clamping
crosscut saw
crossed anesthesia
crossed embolism
crossed reflex
crossed-swords technique suture
CrossFlex LC coronary stent
CrossFlexTMLC coronary stent
cross-infection
crossing over (also, crossover)
cross-irrigation of wound
cross-linking
cross-lip pedicle flap
crossmatch
  HLA (human lymphocyte antigen)
  major
  minor
  pretransplant
  type and
crossmatching
crossover (also, crossing over)
cross pin
cross-reacting agglutinin
cross-reacting antibody

cross-reacting material (CRM)
cross-reactivation
cross-reactivity
cross-reference
cross-resistance
CrossSail coronary dilatation catheter
cross-section (noun, verb)
cross-sectional (adj.)
cross-sectional imaging technique
cross-sensitization
cross-table lateral film
cross-table view
"cross-the-heart" augmentation
  mammoplasty
cross-tunneling incision
Crotti-Kocher thyroid retractor
Crotti thyroid retractor
croup-associated virus (CA v.)
croupous colitis
Crowe-Davis mouth gag
Crowe pilot point on Steinmann pin
crown and collar scissors
crowns the liver
CRP (C reactive protein)
CRPS (complex regional pain
  syndrome)
CRS (Cell Recovery System)
Cr,TM,Ho:YAG crystal laser
cruciate four-strand suture
cruciate incision
crural closure
crural repair
crural ring
crura of the external oblique
crus (pl. crura) of diaphragm
crush kidney
crutch-and-belt femoral closed nail
crutched stick-type biliary duct stent
Crutchfield carotid artery clamp
Crutchfield hand drill
Cruveilhier-Baumgarten bruit
Cruveilhier-Baumgarten cirrhosis
Cruveilhier-Baumgarten syndrome
Cruveilhier sign
Cruveilhier ulcer
cryoablation, NeoCure
CRYOcare system
Cryo/Cuff ankle dressing
cryoglobulinemia, essential mixed
CRYOguide
CryoHit
cryoprecipitate
cryosurgery
cryosurgical lesion
cryotherapy
  endoscopic
  flexible gastrointestinal
cryotherapy for hemorrhoids
crypectomy
crypt
  anal
  enamcl
  epithelium
  ileal
  Lieberkühn (Lieberkuehn)
  Morgagni
  tonsillar
crypt abscess
crypt and surface epithelium (from
  colonic biopsy specimens)
crypt atrophy
crypt epithelium
crypt hook
crypt hyperplasia
cryptitis
cryptogenic cirrhosis
cryptogenic infection
cryptogenic septicopyemia
cryptosporidiosis
Cryptosporidium parvum
Cryptosporidium parvum bovine
  colostrum IgG concentrate
crystal, cholesterol monohydrate
crystal tracheostomy tube
crystallized trypsin
crystalloid fluid
crystalloid infusion

crystalloid solution
CSF (cerebrospinal fluid)
CSF glucose
CSF glutamine test
CSF protein
CSF shunt
C-shaped incision
C-shaped microplate
C-shaped plate
CSID (congenital sucrose-isomaltose deficiency)
CSM Stretta system
C-spine traction
CT (computed or computerized tomography)
CT cholangiography
CT-directed hook-wire localization
CT-directed needle biopsy
CTE:YAG (CrTmEr:YAG) laser
CT-guided needle aspiration biopsy
CTLA4-Ig monoclonal antibody
CTLM (CT laser mammography)
CTLV (cross-table lateral view)
CTP-37 theraccine
CT PEG (CT-guided percutaneous endoscopic gastrostomy)
CT-scan-directed needle biopsy
CT scan, dual-energy
CT scan with I.V. contrast
CTS (Champion Trauma Score)
CTS Harvester bipolar scissors
CT-2584 mesylate
Cubbins incision
CUC (chronic ulcerative colitis)
Cuda endoscope
Cuda laparoscope
Cuda retractor
Cuda 0° 10 mm rigid laparoscope
cuff
  gastric
  musculotendinous
  one-tube
  rectal muscle
  rotator
cuff *(cont.)*
  suprahepatic caval
  vaginal
cuff abscess
cuffed endotracheal tube
cuffed fenestrated tube
cuff measurement
CUI (Cox-Uphoff International)
CUI gel breast prosthesis
CUI saline breast prosthesis
CUI tissue expander
Culbertson canal knife
cul-de-sac of Douglas
cul-de-sac smear
culdolaparoscopy
culdoscope
Cullen sign
Culler hook
culprit lesion
culture and sensitivity (C&S)
culture, blood
cultured epithelial autograft
cultured organism
Cunningham clamp
cup
  acetabular
  graduated metal
  Malmstrom
  stone
cup-and-spill stomach
cup forceps
cupped jaw
cup reamer
Curaderm hydrocolloid dressing material
Curafil hydrogel dressing
Curafoam foam wound dressing
Curagel hydrogel dressing
Curasol gel wound dressing
Curasorb calcium alginate dressing
curative operation
curative restorative resection
curative therapy
Curdy blade

^{14}C urea (PYtest)
curettage
  blunt
  sharp
curette
  banjo
  Barnhill adenoid
  biopsy suction
  Bone
  Bruns
  Bumm placenta
  Derlacki
  dermal
  double-ended
  Fox
  Fukushima-Giannotta
  Guilford-Wright micro bone
  Heaney biopsy
  Hibbs-Spratt
  House-Paparella stapes
  House stapes
  Jansen
  Kevorkian-Townsend biopsy
  Kevorkian-Younge
  large sharp
  Lempert fine
  Milan
  Novak suction
  Paparella angled ring
  Paparella mastoid
  Randall suction
  Recamier
  Rheinstadter
  Semm biopsy suction
  serrated
  Sims
  Spratt
  Volkmann
  Williger
  Yankauer
Curity disposable sponge
Curity economy shave prep tray
Curity Oil emulsion dressing
Curity saline dressing
Curity sterile gauze pads
Curlin 2000 Plus infusion pump
Curling duodenal ulcer
Curling esophagus
Curling gastric ulcer
currant jelly clot
currant jelly stools
current
  coagulating
  cutting
Curry hip nail
Curtin incision
curvature of stomach
  greater
  lesser
curve
  duodenum
  Frank-Starling
  sigmoid
curved awl
curved bone rongeur
curved circular stapler
curved clamp
curved Cooley clamp
curved Crile forceps
curved dissecting scissors
curved double-action Metzenbaum scissors
curved end-to-end (CEEA) stapler
curved excavator
curved forceps, Crile
curved gouge
curved incision
curved Kelly forceps
curved Maryland dissector
curved Mayo clamp
curved Mayo scissors
curved micro-grasper
curved mosquito forceps
curved periosteal elevator
curved retractor
curved scissors
curved-tip Metzenbaum
curve of duodenum

curvilinear incision
CUSA (Cavitron ultrasonic surgical aspirator) dissector
CUSA EXcel surgical aspirator
Cusco Swiss pattern vaginal speculum
Cushing angular hook
Cushing bayonet forceps
Cushing bipolar forceps
Cushing brain retractor
Cushing-Brown forceps
Cushing-Cairns forceps
Cushing cranial rongeur
Cushing decompression retractor
Cushing delicate forceps
Cushing disease
Cushing dressing forceps
Cushing dural hook
Cushing dural hook knife
Cushing flat drill
Cushing forceps
Cushing gasserian ganglion hook
Cushing-Gigli saw guide
Cushing-Hopkins periosteal elevator
Cushing hook
Cushing intervertebral disk rongeur
Cushing Little Joker elevator
Cushing monopolar forceps
Cushing nerve hook
Cushing nerve retractor
cushingoid facies
cushingoid state
Cushing perforator drill
Cushing periosteal elevator
Cushing pituitary elevator
Cushing pituitary rongeur
Cushing reflex
Cushing retractor
Cushing rongeur
Cushing rongeur forceps
Cushing saw
Cushing saw guide
Cushing staphylorrhaphy elevator
Cushing suture
Cushing syndrome
Cushing tissue forceps
Cushing ulcer
Cushing vein retractor
Cushing ventricular needle
custocolic fold
custom breast implant
Cutalon nylon polyamide surgical suture
cutaneous enterostomy
cutaneous graft
cutaneous hyperesthesia
cutaneous metastatic breast cancer (CMBC)
cutaneous papilloma
cutaneous punch
cutaneous stoma
cutaneous tumor
cutaneous ulcer
cutaneous wound
cut-back procedure
cut, clamp, and tie
cutdown catheter
cuticle scissors
Cutinova Cavity wound filling material
Cutinova Hydro dressing
cutter (also see *dissector*)
- Circon continuous flow resectoscope
- ClearCut 2 electrosurgical handpiece
- Endopath ETS-FLEX endoscopic articulating linear
- Endopath linear
- Endo Mini Shears
- Endo Shears
- Evershears
- EZ45 thoracic linear
- finger ring
- Lempert malleus
- Modulap
- Neoknife
- Proximate linear
- Quadripolar
- Questus Leading Edge
- Ruskin-Liston bone
- Stille-Liston bone

cutting biopsy needle
cutting Bovie
cutting current
cutting forceps
cutting jig
Cutting Balloon microsurgical dilatation catheter
Cutting LOOP coagulator
cutting needle
CUT waveform desiccation
CVA (costovertebral angle) tenderness
CVAT (costovertebral angle tenderness)
CVC (central venous catheter)
CV caliper
CV forceps
CVI (common variable immunodeficiency)
CVP (central venous pressure) line
CVP right atrium
CXR (chest x-ray)
CY-1899
Cyanamid clip applier
cyanoacrylate tissue adhesive
cyanoacrylate glue
cyanocobalamin radioactive agent
cyanosis
cyanotic kidney
cyclic changes of hyperplasia and colloid formation
cyclic pain
cyclic tenderness
cyclic vomiting
cyclic vomiting syndrome (abdominal migraine)
cyclizine
cyclooxygenase
cyclophilin
cyclophosphamide rescue
cycloserine (L-cycloserine)
cyclosporin A
cyclosporine steroid therapy
CycloTech cyclosporine delivery system
cylindrical carcinoma
cylindrical sponge
cymba conchal cartilage
Cymed colostomy barrier
Cymed Micro Skin one-piece drainage pouch
Cymetra tissue replacement material
CyPat
cyproheptadine
cyst
- air
- amebic, amoebic
- Baker
- benign liver
- benign subcutaneous
- blue dome breast
- branchial cleft
- branchiogenous
- breast
- chocolate
- choledochal
- choledochus
- chyle
- compound
- congenital choledochal
- corpus luteum
- daughter
- duplication
- echinococcal
- echinococcus liver
- enteric
- enterogenous
- epidermal inclusion
- epidermoid
- follicular
- ganglion
- gastric duplication
- granddaughter
- hepatic parasitic
- hydatic liver
- hydatid
- intraluminal
- mesenteric
- milk-filled
- mother
- multilocular

cyst *(cont.)*
  mytoid
  nabothian
  omental
  pancreatic
  parasitic
  pilonidal
  primordial
  Rathke pouch
  retention
  Sampson
  sebaceous
  splenic
  theca-lutein
  thymic
  thyroglossal
  thyroglossal duct
  Tornwaldt
  unilocular
  vitellointestinal
  wolffian
cystadenocarcinoma
  bile duct
  mucinous
  papillary
  pseudomucinous
  serous
cystadenoma
  ductal
  hyperplastic mucinous
  thyroid
cyst aspiration
cyst aspiration needle
cystectomy
cystica polyposa gastritis
cystic artery
cystic cancer
cystic carcinoma
cystic changes
cystic-choledochal junction
cystic degeneration
cystic duct cannula
cystic duct catheterization
cystic duct cholangiogram
cystic duct forceps
cystic duct leak
cystic duct lumen
cystic duct obstruction
cystic duct rupture
cystic duct stone
cysticercosis
cysticercus disease
Cysticercus dellulosae
cystic fibrosis
cystic fistula
cystic fluid
cystic goiter
cystic kidney
cystic lesion
cystic mass
cystic mastitis
cystic medial necrosis
cystic plexus
cystic polyp
cystic structure
cystine stone
cystitis
  acute
  allergic
  bacterial
  honeymoon
  interstitial
  radiation
cystoatrial shunt
cystoduodenostomy
cystogastrostomy, endoscopic
cystohepatic triangle
cystojejunostomy
cystopericystectomy
cystoperitoneal shunt
cystosarcoma phyllodes
cystoscope (see *endoscope*)
Cytadren (aminoglutethimide)
cytarabine liposomal
Cytobrush Plus
cytochrome C oxidase (COX)
  deficiency

CytoGam (cytomegalovirus immune globulin, solvent/detergent treated)
CytoImplant
cytokine induction
cytokine interleukin-10 (IL-10)
cytokine interleukin-8 (IL-8)
Cytolex (pexiganan acetate) (now Locilex)
Cytolex cream (pexiganan acetate)
cytologic diagnosis
cytologic examination
cytologic smear
cytology
  abnormal
  aspiration biopsy (ABC)
  brush
  equivocal pancreatic
  EUS-guided
  fine-needle aspiration (FNAC)
  gastric
  guided-needle aspiration
  peritoneal
  salvage
CytoLyt solution
cytomegalic inclusion virus disease
cytomegalovirus (CMV)
cytomegalovirus hepatitis
cytomegalovirus immune globulin, human
cytomegalovirus mucositis
Cytomel (liothyronine sodium)
cytopathologic examination
cytopathologic preparation
cytopathologist
cytoplasmic granules
cytoplasmic material
cytoprotective agent
cytoreductive surgery
CytoTAb antibody
Cytotec (misoprostol)
cytotoxic antibodies
cytotoxic lymphocyte
cytotoxic lymphocytic proliferation
cytotoxic T cell
Cytovene (oral ganciclovir)
Cytoxan (cyclophosphamide)
Czaja-McCaffrey endoscope
Czaja-McCaffrey rigid stent introducer
Czerny-Lembert suture
Czerny rectal speculum
Czerny retractor
Czerny suture

D, d

dacarbazine
dacliximab monoclonal antibody
Dacron-bolstered suture
Dacron-impregnated silicone rod
Dacron interposition graft
Dacron mesh
Dacron patch
Dacron suture
Dacron synthetic ligament material
Dacron tape
Dacron velour bolster
Dagradi classification of esophageal varices
Dagrofil suture
Dahedi 25 insulin delivery pump
Dahl-Iverson mastitis
Dahlgren cranial rongeur
daily weights
DairyCare
Dairy Ease (lactase enzyme)
Dakin solution
Dale abdominal binder
Dale first rib rongeur
Dale Foley catheter
Dale forceps
DALM (dysplasia with associated lesion or mass)
dalteparin sodium
dam, rubber
damage, macroscopic
danaparoid sodium
danazol
Danbolt-Closs syndrome
Dance sign
Dandy clamp
Dandy forceps
Dandy nerve hook
Dandy neurosurgical scissors
Dandy probe
Dandy hemostatic forceps
Dandy scalp hemostats
Dandy scissors
Dandy trigeminal nerve scissors
Dandy ventricular needle
Dane particle
Daniel colostomy clamp
Daniel iliac bone graft
Dansac DuoSoft pouch
Dansac DuoSoft wafer
Dansac Karaya Seal one-piece drainage pouch
Dansac Nova ostomy appliance
Dansac ostomy irrigation set
Dansac Skin Barrier for ostomy
Dansac Standard Ileo pouch
danthron

daptomycin for injection
Darbid
Dardik Biograft
Dardik clamp
Daricon PB
darifenacin
darkfield microscope
darkfield microscopy
dark green stools
dark stools
dark urine
Darrach elevator
dartos fascia
Darvocet-N 100
da Silva colostomy
Datascope catheter
daughter abscess
daughter cyst
Dautrey chisel
Daverbinde K
David Baker bleph retractor
Davidoff cell
David rectal speculum
Davidson pulmonary vessel clamp
Davidson retractor
Davidson-Sauerbruch-Doyen periosteal elevator
Davidson scapula retractor
Davidson thoracic trocar
da Vinci surgical laparoscopic system
Davis blade
Davis brain retractor
Davis clamp
Davis coagulating forceps
Davis forceps
Davis guide for Gigli saw
Davis monopolar forceps
Davis mouth gag
Davis muscle-pedicle graft
Davis percussion hammer
Davis pin
Davis retractor
Davis ribbon retractor
Davis saw
Davis saw guide
Davis scalp retractor
Davis spatula
Davol prep
Davol sump drain
dawn phenomenon
Dawson-Yuhl gouge
Dawson-Yuhl-Kerrison rongeur forceps
Dawson-Yuhl-Key elevator
Dawson-Yuhl-Leksell rongeur forceps
Dawson-Yuhl periosteal elevator
Dawson-Yuhl suction tube
Daxor quantitative injection syringe kit
Day pin
Day staple
dazopride, dazopride fumarate
DBx diagnostic system
DC softgels (docusate calcium)
DCBE (double-contrast barium enema)
DCC (deleted in colorectal carcinoma) gene
DCIS (ductal carcinoma in situ)
DCP (dynamic compression) plate
DDAVP (desmopressin acetate)
DDS-Acidophilus
dead bowel
deadly agaric (*Amanita phallodes*)
dead pancreatic tissue
dead space
Dean bone rongeur
Dean dissecting scissors
death
- apparent
- black
- brain
- cell
- cerebral
- cot
- crib
- fetal (early, intermediate, late)
- functional
- genetic
- liver
- local

death *(cont.)*
 molecular
 natural
 programmed cell
 SIDS (sudden infant death syndrome)
 somatic
 sudden cardiac
 unsuspected cause of
 voodoo
Deaver incision
Deaver retractor
Deaver scissors
DeBakey-Adson tissue forceps
DeBakey aortic aneurysm clamp
DeBakey arterial clamp
DeBakey arterial forceps
DeBakey AtrauGrip forceps
DeBakey atraumatic bulldog clamp
DeBakey atraumatic colon resection clamp
DeBakey atraumatic tissue forceps
DeBakey-Bahnson vascular clamp
DeBakey-Bainbridge atraumatic intestinal forceps
DeBakey-Bainbridge clamp
DeBakey-Beck clamp
DeBakey bulldog clamp
DeBakey coarctation clamp
DeBakey colon resection clamp
DeBakey-Cooley dissecting forceps
DeBakey-Cooley retractor
DeBakey cross-action bulldog clamp
DeBakey-Derra anastomosis clamp
DeBakey-Diethrich atraumatic tissue forceps
DeBakey-Diethrich vascular forceps
DeBakey dissecting forceps
DeBakey dissecting scissors
DeBakey double-action grasping forceps
DeBakey endarterectomy scissors
DeBakey forceps
DeBakey-Harken clamp
DeBakey-Howard clamp
DeBakey-Kay clamp
DeBakey-Mixter artery forceps
DeBakey needle
DeBakey needle holder with tungsten carbide inlay
DeBakey patent ductus clamp
DeBakey pediatric clamp
DeBakey peripheral vascular bulldog clamp
DeBakey pickups
DeBakey-Reynolds anastomosis clamp
DeBakey ring-handled bulldog clamp
DeBakey scissors
DeBakey-Semb clamp
DeBakey-Semb forceps
DeBakey sigmoid anastomosis clamp
DeBakey tangential occlusion clamp
DeBakey-TC needle holder
DeBakey tissue forceps
DeBakey vascular clamp
DeBakey vascular forceps
debrancher deficiency
debrancher enzyme
debrancher enzyme deficiency
debrancher glycogen storage disease
debrided
debridement of abscess
debridement tissue
debris
 amorphous
 cellular
Debrisan (dextranomer)
debulking of tumor
debulking surgery
decannulation plug
decanting device
decarboxylase
D cell tumor
Decholin (dehydrocholic acid)
DecisionMaker software
decitabine
deck plate
Decker alligator forceps
Decker micro scissors

Decker microsurgical forceps
Decker microsurgical rongeur
Decker microsurgical scissors
Decker pituitary rongeur
declamping
decompensated alcoholic cirrhosis
decompensated cirrhosis
decompensation
  circulatory
  metabolic
decompression
  balloon
  bladder
  duodenal
  endoscopic
  endoscopic biliary
  gastric
  gastrointestinal
  hydrostatic
  intestinal
  percutaneous
  transhepatic (PTD)
  portal
  tube
  variceal
decompression colostomy
decompression jejunostomy
decompression procedure
decompression retractor
decompression therapy, transduodenal endoscopic
decompression tube
decompressive surgery
decompression of varices
deconjugation, bilirubin glucuronide
Decon Mini-Plus kit
decreased afterload
decreased alveolar ventilation
decreased blood flow
decreased blood pressure
decreased bowel sounds
decreased breath sounds
decreased cardiac output
decreased colonic motility
decreased contraction of gallbladder
decreased cytoprotection
decreased gastric acid secretion
decreased gastric emptying
decreased gastric reservoir
decreased GI calcium absorption
decreased GI motility
decreased hematocrit
decreased ileus
decreased libido
decreased lower esophageal sphincter (LES) tone
decreased perfusion of the juxta-glomerular apparatus
decreased peristalsis
decreased pH
decreased pituitary production
decreased preload
decreased shunt fraction
decreased skin turgor
decreased testosterone
decreased uptake with patchy distribution
decreased urinary 17-OCHS
decreased venous return
decreased xylose absorption
decrease in systemic vascular resistance
decrease p.o. protein intake
decubitus calculus
decubitus film
decubitus position
decubitus ulcer
decubitus view
Deddish-Potts intestinal forceps
deep abscess
deep blade
deep blade knife
deep epigastric vessel
deep interloop abscess
deep perineal pouch
deep-purple spleen
deep retention suture
deep section
deep suture

deep tendon reflexes (DTRs)
deep to pectoral minor muscle
deep vein thrombophlebitis (DVT)
deep vein thrombosis (DVT)
deepening reamer
defatting of panniculus
defecate
defecation, painful
defecatory urgency
defecogram
defecography
defect
  bandeau
  cold
  combined
  diaphragmatic
  direct
  fascial
  filling
  frondlike filling
  hernia
  hot
  indirect
  large hernia
  pinpoint gastric mucosal
  postinjury immunologic
  skin
  slitlike
  small hernia
  thoracoscopic repair of diaphragmatic
  ventricular septal wound
defective hemoglobin synthesis
defect of pyrrole metabolism
defense against bacteria
defenses, altered mucosal
deferoxamine mesylate infusion test
defervesce
defervescence of fever
defibrinated blood
deficiency
  acquired lactose
  ACTH
  alpha-galactosidase

deficiency *(cont.)*
  amylo-1,6-glucosidase
  bilirubin glucuronosyltransferase
  brancher
  brancher enzyme
  complex IV
  congenital thyroid
  congenital zinc
  COX (cytochrome C oxidase)
  debrancher
  debrancher enzyme
  essential fatty acid (EFAD)
  glucose-6-phosphorylase
  hepatic phosphorylase
  immune
  isolated thyroid-stimulating hormone
  isovaleric acid CoA dehydrogenase
  isovaleryl CoA carboxylase
  long chain acyl-CoA dehydrogenase
  low density beta lipoprotein
  medium chain acyl-CoA dehydrogenase (MCAD)
  muscle carnitine
  myopathic carnitine
  nutritional
  PEPCK (phosphoenolpyruvate carboxykinase)
  PiZZ $alpha_1$ antitrypsin
  prolactin
  sucrose-isomaltose (SI)
  systemic carnitine
  thyroid
  uridine diphosphate glucuronosyltransferase
  vasopressin
deficit (see also *deficiency*)
  endocrine
  fluid volume
  focal neurologic
  neurologic
  nutritional
defined parenteral exposure
definitive care
definitive diagnosis

definitive surgery
Definity ultrasound contrast agent
deflecting mechanism
defocused (laser) beam
defogging of laparoscopic telescope
  immersion in warm saline
  intra-abdominal irrigation
  intra-abdominal wiping
  use of defogging agent
deformity
  Akerlund duodenal
  bell-clapper
  cloverleaf
  crossbar stomach
  duodenal bulb
  hourglass (on x-ray)
  phrygian cap
  splenic vein
  trefoil
  Whitehead
Defourmentel bone rongeur
defunctionalization
Degas (simethicone)
degenerated blood
degeneration
  acute hepatocellular
  amyloid
  feathery
  fibroid
  hepatolenticular
  lardaceous
  parenchymous
  sarcomatoid
degeneration of pancreas
degenerative liver
deglutition disorder
deglutition mechanism
deglutition reflex
deglutitive pharyngeal chamber
deglutitive tongue biomechanics
deglutitive tongue force modulation
Degos disease
degradable polyglycolide rod
degraded liver
degree of accuracy
degree of encephalopathy
degree of penetrance
degree of specificity
degrees centrigrade
dehisced (verb)
dehiscence
  abdominal incision
  anastomotic
  staple line
  suture line
  wound
DEHOP (diethylhomospermine)
DEHSPM (diethylhomospermine)
dehydration
dehydrocholic acid
dehydroemetine
dehydroepiandrosterone (DHEA)
DEI (diffraction-enhanced imaging)
Dejerine-Davis percussion hammer
Dejerine percussion hammer
Dejerine-Sottas syndrome
Deklene and Deklene II suture
Deknatel suture
Delafield fluid
Delaginiere abdominal retractor
Delasco electrocoagulator device
delayed closure of suture
delayed gastric emptying
delayed hypersensitivity reaction
delayed insertion of breast prosthesis
delayed primary intention healing
delayed splenic rupture
delayed umbilical ring closure
delayed whole gut transit
delayed xenograft rejection (DXR)
DeLee forceps
DeLee-Hillis stethoscope
DeLee suction trap
deletion
  chromosomal
  clonal
Delicot sponge
Deliver 2.0 formula

delomorphous cell
Delorme rectal prolapse repair
delphian lymph node group
delta-Ag (delta antigen)
delta agent hepatitis
delta antigen (HDAg, hepatitis D virus)
delta hepatitis
delta hepatitis superinfection
delta virus
deltoid region
deltoid-splitting incision
deltopectoral fascia
deltopectoral flap
deluxe lightweight quad cane
Dema-Band bandage
Dema Pad bandage
demarcator
DeMarneffe meniscotomy knife
DeMartel appendix forceps
DeMartel clamp
DeMartel dissecting scissors
DeMartel neurosurgical scissors
DeMartel scalp flap forceps
DeMartel vascular clamp
DeMartel vascular scissors
DeMartel wire saw
DeMartel-Wolfson anastomosis clamp
DeMeester score
Demel wire-tightening forceps
Demel wire-twisting forceps
dementia
Demerol
demigauntlet bandage
demineralized bone graft
Demir rigid laparoscope
demise
Demling-Classen sphincterotome
DeMorgan spot
Demos tibial artery clamp
denatured homograft
dendritic cancer
dendritic reticular cell
dengue fever
dengue virus
Denham pin
Denhardt mouth gag
Denis Browne abdominal retractor
Denis Browne intestinal holding forceps
Denis Browne pouch
Dennis blade
Dennis-Brooke ileostomy
Dennis forceps
Dennis intestinal clamp
Dennis intestinal tube
Dennis-Varco pancreaticoduodenostomy
Denonvillier fascia
de novo lesion
de novo presentation
dens (cervical spine) view
dense adhesions
dense breast tissue
density
  body
  radiopaque
DENSPM (diethylnorspermine)
Dent sleeve
dental drill
dental malocclusion
dental polyp
dentate line
dentate margin
dentate suture
dentinal fluid
dentinal papilla
dentoalveolar structures
denuded mucosa
denutrition
Denver hydrocephalus shunt
Denver peritoneal venous shunt
deoxyribonuclease
deoxyspergualin
Depage-Janeway gastrostomy
DePalma stapler
dependent drainage
dependent edema
dePezer gastrostomy tube
depigmented lesion
depilatory forceps

DepoCyt (cytarabine liposomal)
DepoMorphine (morphine sulfate)
deposition of porphyrins
depressed cell-mediated immunity
depression of left mainstem bronchus
depressor
  bone
  Braun
  blood pressure
  lifter-
  pin
  scleral
  tongue
depth of invasion
depth of wound
DePuy awl
DePuy femoral acetabular overlay guide
DePuy nerve hook
DePuy pin
DePuy plate
DePuy rasp
DePuy reamer
de Quervain thyroiditis
deranged electrolyte balance
derangement, metabolic
Derby nail
Dercum disease
Derf needle
Derf needle holder with tungsten carbide inlay
Derf-TC needle holder
Derifil (chlorophyllin)
Derlacki capsule knife
Derlacki chisel
Derlacki curette
Derlacki hook
Derlacki mobilizer
Dermabond dressing
Dermabond topical skin adhesive
Dermabond wound adhesive
DermaFreeze
Dermagraft human-based dermal replacement
Dermagraft-TC (transitional covering)
Dermagran hydrophilic wound dressing
Derma K laser
DermaLase ErCr:YSGG laser system
dermal collagen homograft
Dermalene suture
Dermalon suture
dermal papilla
dermal-subdermal plexus
dermal suture
DermaMend foam wound dressing
DermaMend hydrogel dressing
DermaMend moisture barrier cream dressing
DermaMend polyurethane foam dressing
DermaNet contact-layer wound dressing
DermaScan system
DermaSeptic iontophoresis device
DermaSorb dressing
DermAssist hydrocolloid dressing
DermAssist wound filling material
Dermatell hydrocolloid dressing
dermatitis herpetiformis
dermatitis of the nipple
dermatome pain
dermatomyositis
dermatophytic fungi
Derma 20 laser
Dermol HC (hydrocortisone)
Dermoplast (benzocaine; menthol)
dermotropic virus
Dermuspray (trypsin; Peruvian balsam)
DeRoyal surgical cannula
Derra vena cava clamp
Derra vestibular clamp
D'Errico-Adson retractor
D'Errico bayonet pituitary forceps
D'Errico hypophyseal forceps
D'Errico lamina chisel
D'Errico nerve root retractor
D'Errico perforating drill
D'Errico periosteal elevator
D'Errico pituitary forceps

D'Errico ventricular needle
DES (diffuse esophageal spasm)
Desault bandage
des-carboxy-prothrombin
descending colon
descending duodenum
descending loop colostomy
descending perineum syndrome
descensus ventriculi
descent of testes
Deschamps ligature carrier
Deschamps ligature needle
Deschamps needle
desiccation
  BLEND waveform
  COAG waveform
  electrosurgical
Desilets-Hoffman catheter introducer
Desjardins gall duct forceps
Desjardins gallbladder forceps
Desjardins gallbladder scoop
Desjardins gallstone probe
Desjardins gallstone scoop
Desjardins point
Desjardins probe
Desmarres paracentesis knife
Desmarres retractor
desmoid disease
desmoid tumor
desmoplastic malignant melanoma
desmopressin acetate (DDAVP)
Desormaux endoscope
destruction of digestive enzymes
destruction of parenchyma
DeTakats-McKenzie brain clip forceps
detection antibody
Detecto scale
detorsion of bowel
Deucher abdominal retractor
devascularization, paraesophagogastric
development, impaired thymic
device (see also *system*)
  Accel stopcock
  accuDEXA bone mineral density
    assessment

device *(cont.)*
  AccuGuide injection monitor
  AccuPort seal
  Acticon neosphincter
  ACTID (analgesic cell therapy
    implantable device)
  AddOn-Bucky imaging
  ADMI ulcer measuring
  AdvaSeal
  AER Plus (automatic endoscope
    reprocessor)
  AESOP 2000 (Automated Endo-
    scopic System for Optimal
    Positioning)
  AESOP 3000 endoscopic system
  Aestiva/5 anesthesia machine
  Air Pulse Sensory Stimulator
  Akros extended-care mattress
  Amicus separator blood collection
  Anaconda device
  Ancure system
  Aquilion CT scanner
  argon beam coagulation
  argon laser
  Arrequi laparoscopic knot-pusher
    ligator
  ArthroWand
  Aspen laparoscopy electrode
  ASSI (Accurate Surgical and
    Scientific Instruments)
  automated islet-cell shaking
  automatic knot-tying
  Auto Suture Soft Thoracoport
  Auto Suture universal retractor base
  AVA 3Xi venous access
  Bak-Pac portable ultrasound scanner
  band-ligator device
  Bard flexible endoscopic injection
    system
  B-D Sensability Breast Self-
    Examination Aid
  Beacon Technology System (BTS)
  Bedge antireflux mattress
  Belzer organ preservation unit

device *(cont.)*
BiPAP S/T-D 30 ventilatory support
bipod suspension apparatus
bipolar urological loop
BiQ bipolar hand instrument
BIS Sensor
BIS Sensor Plus
Bovie electrocoagulation unit
Bovie 2100 coagulating electro-surgical
BreastAlert differential temperature sensor (DTS)
breast bolster
BreastCheck
BreastExam
Bremer AirFlo Vest
broach
Bucky imaging
Button and Button-One Step gastrostomy feeding
BVA-100 (blood-volume analyzer)
BVM (bag-valve-mask)
Cameron-Miller electrocoagulation unit
Capio CL transvaginal suture-capturing
Carr-Locke stent remover
Carroll tendon retriever
Carter pillow
Carter-Thomason suture passer
Catarex
catheter vitrector
CathLink implantable vascular access
CaverMap surgical aid
C-bar web-spacer
Cell Saver
Cellolite patty material
Cholestron PRO
Christoudias fascial closure
Cincinnati subzero unit
CLC 2000 swabable intravenous connector
ClearCut 2 electrosurgical handpiece

device *(cont.)*
Closure catheter/radiofrequency generator
Closure endovascular coagulation
Conforma 3000 photon beam therapy
decanting
DermaSeptic iontophoresis
Devine colostomy
DeWitt-Stetten colostomy spur-crushing
DiaScreen
digital x-ray detector
Digitizer Director
DirectRay imaging
Disetronic insulin pen
Dissectron aspirator
Diva laparoscopic morcellator
Dix foreign body
Dormia noose
Draffin bipod suspension apparatus
duodenal decompression
Dynamic PACSPlus
DynaWell
8-lumen silicone recording assembly
ELAD (extracorporeal liver assist)
Elmor tissue morcellator
Endo Babcock surgical grasping
Endo Catch
Endocut cautery
Endo Lumenal Gastroplication
EndoLumina II transillumination
EndoMate Grab Bag
Endopath EZ-RF linear cutter and coagulation
Endopath laparoscopic trocar
Endopath Optiview optical surgical obturator
Endopath TriStar trocar
Endo-P-Probe
endoscopic "sewing machine"
endoscopic suction cap
Endo Mini Shears
Endo Shears

device *(cont.)*
Enterra gastric stimulation
Erbotom F2 electrocoagulation unit
Erlangen magnetic colostomy
esophageal decompression
EU-M30S endoscopic ultra-sonography receiver
Favaloro-Morse rib spreader
First Warning breast cancer screening
Flexiflo Lap G laparoscopic gastrostomy kit
Flexiflo Lap J laparoscopic jejunostomy kit
Fuller shield
Gauderer Genie gastrostomy feeding
Glassman stone extractor
Gottschalk Nasostat
Gould polygraph
G-suit external counterpressure
Haemonetics Cell Saver 5
Hancke/Vilmann biopsy handle instrument
HandPort hand-assist
Harrison-Nicolle polypropylene pegs
Health Buddy health monitoring
Hemasure r/LS red blood cell filtration system
Hemi Sling
HemoCue photometer
hemodialyzer
hemofiltration
HemoSleeve
Hemotherapies Liver Dialysis Unit
HepatAssist bioartificial liver
Hercules 7000 mobile x-ray unit
HERMES Control Center for medical robotics
HERMES surgery monitoring unit
HumatroPen
Hummingbird wand
IMED infusion device
Import vascular-access port with BioGlide

device *(cont.)*
Innervasc
InstaTrak
InstaTrak 3000
IrrigaTORR
Irrijet DS
IsoMed implantable drug pump
IVAC Vital·Check
joker (slang for instrument)
Kao Lectrolyte
Karl Storz N2O Endoflator
Kelly sphincterotome
leading bar
Leonard Arm pneumatic action support
Licox monitoring
Lightstic 180 and 360 fiberoptic medical laser diffuser
LIMA-Lift
LIMA-Loop
Linvatec micro debrider
liposhaver
lithotrite
Littleford/Spector introducer
Liver Dialysis Unit
Lunderquist-Ring torque guide
M2A Swallowable Imaging Capsule
Maddacrawler
malleus nipper
Mammotome breast biopsy
Mandibular Excursiometer
Marlow Primus instrument collection
Masimo SET (signal extraction technology) pulse oximeter
Maxima Forté blood oxygenator
Medi-Jector Choice needle-free insulin injection
MedPulser
MegaDyne all-in-one hand control
MetraTie knot pusher
MicroAire power-assisted lipoplasty device
Microblater ArthroWand

device *(cont.)*
Micro Diamond-Point microsurgery instruments
Micro-Probe micro dissection tip
MINI 6600 C-arm
Mobetron electron accelerator
morcellator
MultApplier
MultAvalue laparoscopic
Navigator
NeedleAid
Neo-Med cautery
Nerve Block Infusion Kit
NeuroSector ultrasound
Neurotone multipurpose
Nibblit laparoscopic
nitinol mesh-covered frame
Nottingham Key-Med introducing
One-Shot anastomotic
On-Q postoperative pain management system
Opal R.F. tissue ablation
Origin Tacker
OsmoCyte pillow
PC Polygraf HR
Pelosi Illuminator
permanent lead introducer
Phillips ultrasound
Pilot suturing guide
Pneumo-Needle reusable
Pneumo Sleeve laparoscopic airlock
PocketDop ultrasound
Ponsky "Pull" gastrostomy feeding
portable blood irradiator
PROloop electrosurgical
Prostar percutaneous closure
Prostar Plus percutaneous closure
Prostar XL percutaneous closure
prosthetic
Protect-a-Pass suture passer
Protocult stool sampling device
Quadripolar electrosurgical unit
Quinton suction biopsy

device *(cont.)*
R.F. tissue ablation
roentgen knife stereotaxic radiosurgical
Roho air-filled mattress
Rolyan Firm D-Ring wrist support
Rotablator
Roth retrieval net
roticulating endograsper
rubber-band loader
Sensability lubricated plastic sheet for breast self-examination
Sepacell RZ-2000 leukoreduction
Skin Skribe skin marker
smoke evacuation unit
Soehendra stent retriever
Sofpulse pulsed magnetic energy
Somogyi (amylase)
Sonotron radiofrequency
Spacemaker
stapling
Step minimally invasive surgical access
Storz cholangiograsper
Storz LaproFlator
Stretta
Surg-I-Loop
SurgiScope robotic surgery
Suture Assistant endoscopic suturing
Suture Assistant knot-tying
suture-welding
SYBIOL (synthetic bio-liver)
Tapertome sphincterotome
targeted cryoablation
Thora-Port
Tissomat application
tissue expander
TissueLink Monopolar Floating Ball
TQa (transcutaneous access flow)
Trachlight
TransScan TS 2000 electrical impedance breast scanning
TransScan 2000 breast mapping

device *(cont.)*
TraumaJet wound debridement
Tru-Area Determination wound-measuring
TULIP (transurethral laser-induced prostatectomy)
20/30 Indeflator Inflation
Ultramark 4 ultrasound
USSC (United States Surgical Corp.)
Valleylab laparoscopic and electrosurgical unit
Valleylab SSE-2 cautery unit
Vasotrax blood pressure/heart rate sensor
VerreScope micro laparoscopic entry
Vibra-Surge ultrasonic
Volkmann spoon
Wilson-Cook (modified) wire-guided sphincterotome
XPS Straightshot
DeVilbiss cranial rongeur
DeVilbiss rongeur forceps
Devine procedure
devitalized bone graft
Devonshire colic
Devrom (bismuth subgallate)
DeWeese vena cava clamp
Dewey obstetric forceps
dewy appearance
dexamethasone sodium phosphate
dexamethasone suppression test
dexanabinol
Dexatrim
dexfenfluramine
dexmedetomidine
Dexon Plus suture
Dexon polyglycolic acid mesh
Dexon suture
Dexon II suture
dexpanthenol
dextran 40 plasma volume expander
dextranomer
dextrinizing time
dextrinosis, limit
dextrorotation
Dextrostix
Dey-Wash skin wound cleanser
Deyerle II pin
Deyerle pin
Deyerle plate
DFDR diamond fraise
DF-2 bacillus
DGHAL (Doppler-guided hemorrhoidal artery ligation)
DG Softgut suture
DGR (duodenogastric reflux)
DHEA (dehydroepiandrosterone)
DHEA sulfate (DHEAS)
DHEAS (DHEA sulfate)
DiaBeta (glyburide)
diabetes induced by beta-cell toxins
diabetes insipidus
acquired
central
idiopathic
primary
secondary
vasopressin-sensitive
diabetes mellitus
adult-onset
brittle
bronze
gestational
IDDM (insulin-dependent diabetes mellitus)
insulin-dependent, associated with acanthosis nigricans
juvenile-onset (now classified as type 1)
lipoatrophic
maturity-onset diabetes of the young (MODY)
neonatal
NIDDM (non-insulin-dependent diabetes mellitus)
non-insulin-dependent
nonclinical

diabetes *(cont.)*
post-transplant diabetes mellitus
type 1 (formerly classified as juvenile or juvenile-onset)
type 2 (formerly classified as adult-onset)
uncontrolled maternal
diabetes secondary to pancreatic disease
diabetic acidosis
diabetic amyotrophy
diabetic colitis
diabetic diet
diabetic enteropathy
diabetic gangrene
diabetic gastroparesis
diabetic gastropathy
diabetic hyperglycemia
diabetic hyperosmolar nonketotic coma
diabetic ketoacidosis (DKA)
diabetic mononeuropathy
diabetic neuropathy
diabetic polyneuropathy
DiabetiSweet sugar substitute
diabetologist
DiabGel hydrogel dressing
DiabKlenz wound cleanser
Diacol
Diagnex Blue gastric acid test
diagnosis (pl. diagnoses)
admitting
antenatal
clinical
colposcopic
cytologic
definitive
differential
discharge
empirical
fetal
final
frozen section
genetic
gross
histologic

diagnosis *(cont.)*
histopathologic
initial
microscopic
neonatal
operative
pathologic
physical
postoperative
preliminary
prenatal
prenatal genetic
preoperative
presumptive
principal
provisional anatomic
tentative
ultrasound
working
diagnosis by exclusion
diagnostic and therapeutic administration
diagnostic anesthesia
diagnostic cascade
diagnostic findings
diagnostic laparoscopy
diagnostic pancreatography
diagnostic peritoneal lavage (DPL)
diagnostic radiology procedures (see *operation*)
Diagnostix sphygmomanometer
Dialock hemodialysis access system
Dialose (docusate sodium)
Dialose Plus (yellow phenolphthalein; docusate sodium)
Dialume (aluminum hydroxide gel)
Dialyflex dialysis fluid
dialysis
BioLogic-DT (now Liver Dialysis Unit)
continuous ambulatory peritoneal (CAPD)
kidney
liver
peritoneal

dialysis-related ascites
diamond fraise
diamond inlay graft
diamond knife sponge
diamond Ohio adapter
Diamond pin cutter
diamond rasp
diamond-shaped incision
diamond-shaped medullary nail
diaper rash
diaphoresis
diaphragm veins
diaphragmatic defect
diaphragmatic hernia
diaphragmatic hiatus
diaphragmatic hump
diaphragmatic injury
diaphragmatic irritation
diaphragmatic rupture
diaphragmatic surface of liver
Diapid (lypressin)
Diar-Aid (loperamide)
diarrhea
  acute infectious
  antibiotic-induced
  anxiety-related
  bacillary
  bile salt
  bilious
  bloody
  cachectic
  chronic
  chronic bacillary
  Clostridium difficile-associated
  colliquative
  copious rice-water
  copious watery
  Dientamoeba
  dysenteric
  enteral
  enterotoxin
  explosive
  familial chloride
  flagellate

diarrhea *(cont.)*
  functional
  gastrogenous
  hemorrhagic
  ileostomy
  infectious
  inflammatory
  intermittent
  intractable
  irritative
  lactose-associated
  lienteric
  liquid
  malabsorptive
  maldigestive
  mechanical
  mucous
  osmotic
  pancreatogenous
  postvagotomy
  rotavirus
  secretory
  serous
  stercoral
  toxic
  traveler's
  unexplained
  unrelenting
  viral
  virulent
  watery
diarrheal disease
diarrhea-predominant irritable bowel syndrome
diarrhea stools
Diascan reagent strips
DiaScreen reagent strips
Diasensor 1000 glucose monitor
Diasorb (activated attapulgite)
diastasis of suture
diastasis recti abdominis
Diastat vascular access graft
diastatic serosal tear
diastolic blood pressure

diastolic cardiac arrest
diastolic hypertension
diathermic loop
diathermic loop biopsy
diathermy dissection of the esophagus
diathermy-excision hemorrhoidectomy
diathermy forceps
diathermy rectal snare
diathermy scissors
diathermy suction tube
diathesis (pl. diatheses), bleeding
diatrizoate meglumine
diazepam
DIB (duodenoileal bypass)
Dibent (dicyclomine)
dibucaine
DIC (diffuse intravascular coagulation)
DIC (disseminated intravascular coagulopathy)
DIC (drip infusion cholangiography)
DIC parameters
dicarboxylicaciduria
dicyclomine HCl
DIDMOAD (diabetes insipidus, diabetes mellitus, optic atrophy, and deafness)
Dieffenbach bulldog clamp
Dieffenbach serrefine
diencephalic syndrome
Dientamoeba diarrhea
Dientamoeba fragilis
diet
  absolute
  ADA (American Diabetes Association or American Dietetic Association)
  balanced
  bland
  blenderized
  BRAT (bananas, rice cereal, applesauce, toast)
  BRATS (bananas, rice, apples, toast, saltines)
  CAPS-free (caffeine, alcohol, pepper, spicy foods)

diet *(cont.)*
  clear liquid
  diabetic
  elemental
  elimination
  exclusion
  fasting
  fluid-restricted
  fractionated
  full liquid
  gastric
  Glutasorb
  gluten-free
  grapefruit
  high-bulk, low-fat
  high-carbohydrate
  high-fiber
  high-protein
  high-residue
  hypercaloric
  hyperprotidic
  lactose-free
  liquid
  liver
  low-calorie
  low-fat
  low-fiber
  low-protein
  low-residue
  low-roughage
  low-sodium
  Meulengracht
  milk
  mixed elemental-fat
  mixed protein-fat
  Moro-Heisler
  ovolactovegetarian
  Portagen
  progressive
  ProSol 20%
  reduced lactose
  regular
  rice-fruit
  Schmidt

diet *(cont.)*
  semielemental
  Sippy
  smooth
  soft bland
  vegetarian
  very low calorie (VLCD)
  Weight Watchers
  Western
  yo-yo
diet ad lib.
dietary cholesterol
dietary cirrhosis
dietary fat
dietary fiber
dietary habits
dietary history
dietary protein
dietary protein restriction
dietary supplementation
dietetic colitis
dietetic ileitis
dietetic jejunitis
dietetic regimen
dietetic sigmoiditis
Diethrich bulldog clamp
Diethrich bulldog clip
Diethrich coronary scissors
Diethrich-Hegemann scissors
Diethrich micro bulldog clamp
Diethrich-TC needle holder
Diethrich valve scissors
Diethrich vascular scissors
diethylcarbamazine
diethylcarbamazine citrate
diethylhomospermine (DEHOP; DEHSPM)
diethylnorspermine (DENSPM)
diethylpropion
dieting plateau
dieting, yo-yo
diet therapy
Dieulafoy disease
Dieulafoy gastric lesion
Dieulafoy lesion of anal canal
Dieulafoy triad
Dieulafoy ulcer
Dieulafoy vascular malformation
difenoximide HCl
difenoxin HCl
differential diagnosis
differential spinal anesthesia
DiffGAM
difficulty breathing
Diffistat-G
diffraction-enhanced (breast) imaging (DEI)
diffuse abdominal pain
diffuse abdominal tenderness
diffuse abscess
diffuse breast involvement
diffuse carcinomatosis
diffuse colloid goiter
diffuse esophageal spasm (DES)
diffuse GI hamartoma polyps
diffuse goiter
diffuse intravascular coagulation (DIC)
diffuse lesion
diffuse lobular fibrosis
diffusely tender abdomen
diffuse microcalcifications
diffuse microvascular thrombosis
diffuse mucosal polyposis
diffuse multinodular goiter
diffuse necrosis
diffuse pain
diffuse pancreatitis
diffuse peritonitis
diffuser
  Lightstic 180 fiberoptic medical laser
  Lightstic 360 fiberoptic medical laser
diffuse septal cirrhosis
diffuse thyroid enlargement
diffuse toxic goiter
diffuse toxic non-nodular goiter
diffuse transmural ganglioneuromatosis

diffuse transmural intestinal ganglioneuromatosis
diffuse varioliform gastritis
diffusion problem
digastric impression
digastric triangle
Di-Gel (aluminum hydroxide; magnesium hydroxide; simethicone)
Di-Gel Advanced Formula (magnesium hydroxide calcium carbonate; simethicone)
DiGeorge syndrome
Digepepsin (pancreatin; pepsin; bile salts)
digestant
digestive enzyme
 Hi-Vegi-Lip (pancreatase; lipase; protease; amylase)
 lipase
 Ku-Zyme HP (amylase; protease; lipase; cellulase)
 Kutrase
 Pancrease MT 20 (lipase; protease; amylase)
 pancreatin
 Pancreatin 8X (pancreatin; lipase; protease; amylase)
 Pancrecarb MS-8 (lipase; protease; amylase)
 pancrelipase
 Pancrezyme 4X (pancreatin; lipase; protease; amylase)
 Papaya Enzyme (papain; amylase)
 Trizyme
 Ultralase MT 12, Ultralase MT 20
 Vita-PMS, Vita-PMS Plus
digestive fluid
digestive tract
digestive tract contents
digestive tract sensorimotor physiology and pathophysiology
Digestozyme (pancreatin; pepsin; dehydrocholic acid)
Digibar 190 (barium sulfate for suspension)
digital examination
digital rectal examination
digital subtraction angiography
digital subtraction film
digital subtraction imaging technique
digital wrist blood pressure monitor
digital x-ray detector
Digital Response (DRx) glucose monitor
digitalization
Digitizer Director
Digitrapper MKIII device
dilatation (see also *dilation*)
 anal
 aneurysmal
 bowel
 ductal
 esophageal
 gastric
 percutaneous transfemoral
 periportal sinusoidal
 pneumatic bag esophageal
 urethral
dilatation of stenotic hepatico-jejunostomy
dilatation of the pouch
dilated bowel
dilated gallbladder
dilated loop of bowel
dilating catheter
dilating forceps
dilating tip trocar
dilating window
dilation (see also *dilatation*)
 balloon
 biliary
 cricopharyngeal
 ductal
 Eder-Puestow
 endoscopic
 endoscopic retrograde balloon
 esophageal
 extrahepatic biliary cystic
 hepatic web

dilation *(cont.)*
  intrahepatic biliary cystic
  percutaneous balloon
  pneumatic balloon catheter
  postoperative ductal
dilation instrument
dilation of gastric outlet
dilation of stomach
dilation of subareolar duct
dilator
  American Dilation System
  Amplatz
  anal
  Bakes common duct
  Bard Eliminator balloon
  Bowlby tracheal
  Brown-McHardy pneumatic
  Carlson Zero Tip balloon
  Celestin graduated
  common duct
  Core laparoscopic
  CRE wireguided controlled radial expansion
  Eder-Puestow metal olive-tipped
  Einhorn
  Endo-Flex balloon
  esophageal
  Ferris biliary duct
  Flex-EZ balloon
  French
  Garrett
  Hegar
  Hegar rectal
  Hobbs
  Hurst bullet-tip
  Hurst mercury-filled
  Hurst-Tucker pneumatic
  Kollman urethral
  Kron bile duct
  Laborde
  Laborde tracheal
  Maloney esophageal
  Maloney mercury-filled

dilator *(cont.)*
  Maloney tapered-tip
  Med-Tech Teflon
  mercury-filled
  mercury-weighted
  Murphy common duct
  Plummer esophageal
  pneumatic balloon
  probe
  rectal
  Rigiflex balloon
  Savary-Gilliard
  Savary tapered thermoplastic
  Sippy esophageal
  Soehendra dilator
  Starck
  Stucker bile duct
  through-the-scope (TTS)
  Trousseau trachea
  Tucker spindle-shaped
  Wilson-Cook esophageal balloon
dilator system
diloxanide furoate
dimenhydrinate
dimercaptosuccinic acid scan
dimethyl iminodiacetic acid scan
dimethyl sulfoxide
diminished bowel sounds
DIMOAD syndrome (diabetes insipidus, diabetes mellitus, optic atrophy, and deafness)
dimple, celiac
dimpling of skin
Dinate (dimenhydrinate)
Dingman bone and cartilage clamp
Dingman bone-holding forceps
Dingman cartilage clamp
Dingman mouth gag
Dingman oral retractor
Dingman osteotome
Diocto-C (casanthranol; docusate sodium)
Diocto-K (docusate potassium)

Diocto-K Plus (casanthronol; docusate potassium)
Dioctolose Plus (casanthronol; docusate potassium)
diode laser
Dioeze (docusate sodium)
DiPAS-positive granule
Dipentum (olsalazine sodium)
diphenoxylate HCl
Diphtheria
diphtheria bacillus
Diphyllobothrium latum
Diplococcus pneumoniae
Diprivan (propofol)
Diquinol (iodoquinol)
Dirame (propiram)
direct and indirect component
direct antagonist
direct bilirubin
DirectBite disposable biopsy forceps
direct cholecystoenterostomy
direct contrast ductography
direct Coombs test
directed biopsy
direct extension
direct extension of tumor
direct hernia
direct hernia defect
direct inguinal hernia
direction
  clockwise
  counterclockwise
directional endotracheal tube
direct laryngoscopy
direct ligation of esophageal varices
director
  Childe hernia
  grooved
  Key hernia
  Kocher
  Koenig small
  Larry probe
  Lockhart Mummary fistula
  Payr
  St. Mark's fistula
Director biliary guidewire
direct pressure
direct tissue destruction
direct virtual control of biopsy
direct vision
direct-vision liver biopsy
direct visualization
DirectRay imaging device
disaccharidase deficiency
disaccharide intolerance I
disaccharide tripeptic glycerol dipalmitoyl
disaccharide tripeptide glycerol tripalmitoyl (ImmTher)
Disanthrol (casanthranol)
DISC (disabled infectious single cycle) vaccine
discharge
  blood-tinged
  bloody
  bloody nipple
  milky nipple
  mucopurulent
  mucosanguineous
  mucus
  spontaneous nipple
  suppurative
discharge diagnosis
discission blade
discission knife
discoloration of the flank
discolored mucosa
discomfort
  postprandial
  referred epigastric
discordant cellular xenograft
discordant organ xenograft
Discrene breast prosthesis
discrete bleeding source
discrete lesion
discrete mass (*not* discreet)
discrete stenosis
discrete tumor
discussion needle

disease
- Abrami
- acalculous gallbladder
- acid peptic
- acid reflux
- acute abdominal vascular
- acute idiopathic inflammatory bowel
- Addison
- adenomatous polyposis coli
- adiposis dolorosa
- adult polycystic
- AIOD (aortoiliac obstructive)
- alcoholic liver (ALD)
- alpha chain
- $alpha_1$-antitrypsin deficiency
- anal epithelial neoplasia
- Andersen
- anorectal melanoma
- atypical gallbladder
- autoimmune
- autoimmune thyroid
- autosomal dominant polycystic
- autosomal recessive
- Banti
- Barrett
- Basedow
- Behçet
- benign breast (BBD)
- Biermer
- biliary stone
- biliary tract
- black liver
- Bouchard
- Bowen
- Bradley
- brancher glycogen storage
- bronchiolitis obliterans
- bronze (Addison)
- Budd
- Byler
- calculous gallbladder
- Caroli (acute cholangitis)
- celiac (CD)
- celiac sprue

disease *(cont.)*
- Chagus
- Cherchevski
- Chiari
- cholestatic liver
- cholesterol ester storage (CESD)
- chronic granulomatous
- chronic renal
- chylopoietic
- classic triad of Rigler
- collagen vascular
- colonic mucosubmucosal elongated polyp
- colorectal
- congenital cystic liver
- connective tissue
- Cori
- Cowden
- coxsackie virus
- Crohn (CD)
- Cronkhite-Canada
- cryptosporidiosis
- cytomegalic inclusion virus
- Cushing
- cysticercus
- de Quervain thyroiditis
- debrancher glycogen storage
- Degos
- Dercum
- desmoid
- Dieulafoy
- diverticular (of the colon)
- diverticulitis
- Dubin-Sprinz
- Duncan
- duodenal ulcer
- echinococcal cyst
- end-stage liver
- erosive gastroesophageal reflux (GERD)
- esophageal reflux
- essential mixed cryoglobulinemia
- estrogen-induced liver
- extraluminal retrorectal tumor

disease *(cont.)*
extramammary Paget
Fabry
familial adenomatous polyposis (FAP)
familial visceral neuropathy
fatty liver
Fenwick
fibrocystic breast
Fiedler
fistulizing Crohn
Forbes
fulminant Wilson
functional bowel
Gamna
gastrocolic fistula
gastroesophageal reflux (GERD)
Gaucher
Gee-Herter
Gee-Herter-Heubner
Gee-Thaysen
GERD (gastroesophageal reflux)
Gierke
Gilbert
glycogen storage
gonococcal perihepatis pelvic inflammatory
Gordon
graft-versus-host (GVHD)
Graves
Grey Turner
Gross
Hartnup
Hashimoto thyroiditis
hepatic encephalopathy
hepatic Hodgkin
hepatic veno-occlusive
hepatic venous web
hepatobiliary
hepatocellular
hepatolenticular
Hers
Herter-Heubner
Hirschsprung

disease *(cont.)*
Huebner-Herter
human ehrlichial infection, Sennetsu type
Huntington
Hutinel
hydatid cyst
hyperplastic mucinous cystadenoma
IBD (inflammatory bowel)
idiopathic inflammatory bowel
ileocolic
immunologically mediated
immunoproliferative small intestinal (IPSID)
immunoproliferative small intestine
infectious
inflammatory bowel (IBD)
intercapillary glomerulosclerosis
intrahepatic
iron storage
ischemic bowel
ischemic heart
ischemic mesenteric
jejunal angiodysplasia
kinky hair
Kinnier Wilson
Klemperer
Lane
leather-bottle stomach
Leigh
Leiner
Leyden
lithiumogenic goiter
littoral cell angioma
locoregional residual
Lyme
Mediterranean lymphoma
Menetrier
Meniere
Menkes
metastatic
micrometastatic
mixed cell Hodgkin
Mondor

disease *(cont.)*
- necrotizing enterocolitis (NEC)
- necrotizing fasciitis
- neoplastic
- NERD (nonerosive reflux)
- Niemann-Pick
- nodular sclerosing Hodgkin
- nodular thyroid
- nonerosive reflux (NERD)
- nonobstructive hepatic parenchymal
- Ormond
- Osler-Weber-Rendu (OWR)
- osteitis fibrosa cystica generalisata
- Paget perianal
- parasitic
- paroxysmal motor
- Patella (pyloric stenosis)
- pathologic nipple
- pelvic inflammatory (PID)
- peptic ulcer (PUD)
- perianal Bowen
- pilonidal
- pneumatosis coli
- polycystic liver
- porphyria cutanea tarda
- primary biliary cirrhosis (PBC)
- primary sclerosing cholangitis (PSC)
- pseudomembranous colitis (PMC)
- Recklinghausen
- Rendu-Osler-Weber
- Riedel struma
- Rokitansky
- Ruysch
- Saunders
- Schaumann
- schistosomal liver
- scleroderma bowel
- sclerosing encapsulating peritonitis
- Sennetsu fever
- Siewerling-Creutzfeldt
- Simmonds
- small intestinal malignant lymphoma
- space-occupying
- Spencer

disease *(cont.)*
- stress-related mucosal (SMRD)
- struma lymphomatosis
- systemic mast cell
- systemic scleroderma
- Tangier
- terminal ileal
- triad of Rigler
- tuberculous Addison
- ulcerative colitis
- unilateral renal parenchymal
- Van Bogaert
- vancomycin-resistant *Enterococcus faecium* (VREF) infection
- veno-occlusive liver
- venous outflow obstructive
- von Hippel-Lindau
- von Recklinghausen
- von Rokitansky
- Von Gierke
- Waldmann
- Weber-Christian
- Weil
- Westphal-Strümpell
- Whipple
- Wilson
- winter vomiting
- Wolman

disease burden
disease flare
disease-free interval
disease-free survival
Disetronic diabetes management tools and instruments
Disetronic insulin pen
Disetronic insulin pump
DISH (diffuse idiopathic skeletal hyperostosis)
DISIDA scan
disinfectant
disinsertion of the papilla
disk, anal
disk forceps
disk kidney

disk punch
disk rongeur
dismal prognosis
disodium cromoglycate (DSC; DSCG)
Disolan (phenolphthalein; docusate sodium)
Disolan Forte (casanthranol; carboxymethylcellulose sodium; docusate sodium)
Disonate (docusate sodium)
Disoplex (carboxymethylcellulose sodium; docusate sodium)
disorder
  acid-peptic
  acid-related (ARD)
  bowel elimination
  deglutition
  esophageal motility
  evacuation
  exocrine pancreas
  extrapyramidal movement
  fat storage
  functional
  functional gastrointestinal (FGID)
  gastric motor
  gastric NK-like T cell lymphoproliferative
  helminthic
  iatrogenic pituitary
  immunologic deficiency
  infiltrative
  lymphoproliferative
  malignant gastrointestinal
  myeloproliferative
  neoplastic
  nonspecific esophageal motility (NEMD)
  peripheral neurologic
  post-transplant lymphoproliferative
  rectal evacuatory
  smooth-muscle motility
  underlying hematologic
disordered preoperative peristalsis
disordered vasculature
disorders of intestinal motility
Di-Spaz (dicyclomine)
dispersive electrodes
disposable airway
disposable biopsy punch
disposable proctoscope
Dispos-a-Ject plunger
disrupt impacted stone
disruption of blood supply
disruption of diaphragm
DISS air
DISS body adapter
Disse space
dissecting abdominal aneurysm
dissecting and grasping forceps
dissecting aorta
dissecting aortic aneurysm
dissecting blood from the retroperitoneal cavity
dissecting forceps
dissecting hook
dissecting probe
dissecting scissors
dissecting sponge
dissection
  axillary
  blunt
  cervical node
  diathermy (of the esophagus)
  elective lymph node
  en bloc
  extensive lymph node
  finger
  finger fracture
  fingertip
  Freer
  groin
  laparoscopic
  lateral cervical node
  lymph node
  modified neck
  node
  radical mediastinal
  radical neck

dissection *(cont.)*
  scissor
  scissors
  sharp
  sharp and blunt
  sponge
  submucosal
  VasoView balloon dissection system
dissection injury
dissection of esophagus, diathermy
dissection of gallbladder from the liver
  bed
dissection of peritoneum overlying
  the cystic duct
dissection of terminal esophagus
  and fundus of stomach
dissector (also see *cutter, scissors,*
    shears)
  Agris-Dingman submammary
  articulating
  Circon continuous flow resectoscope
  ClearCut 2 electrosurgical handpiece
  Core laparoscopic Kittner
  CPC
  Crabtree
  Crile
  curved Maryland
  CUSA (Cavitron ultrasonic Surgical
    aspirator)
  dolphin-nose dissector
  Durham
  Endo Dissect
  Endopath ETS-FLEX endoscopic
    articulating linear cutter
  Endopath EZ45 endoscopic linear
    cutter
  Endo Shears cutter
  EZ45 thoracic linear cutter
  FD-43 micro dissector
  Freer
  Fukushima-Giannotta
  grooved
  GSI balloon dissector
  hernia

dissector *(cont.)*
  Howarth
  Hurd tonsil
  Jimmy
  Kittner blunt
  Kittner dissecting scissors
  Kocher thyroid
  Maryland
  McCabe flap knife
  McCormick
  McDonald
  micro
  monopolar
  Olivecrona
  orbital rim
  oval
  Penfield
  Pivotal
  right angle
  SaphFinder surgical balloon
  SAPHtrak balloon
  short right-angle
  Spacemaker balloon
  Spacemaker VBD-300
  sponge
  spud dissector
  straight
  Swedish pattern
  tapered Maryland
  tapered right-angle
  ultrasonic
  VaporTrode
  Watson-Cheyne
Dissectron ultrasonic aspirator
disseminated gonococcal infection
disseminated intravascular coagulation
  (DIC)
disseminated intravascular coagulopathy
  (DIC)
disseminated pheochromocytoma
dissociated anesthesia
dissociative anesthesia
dissolution of gallstone
dissolution, percutaneous stone

DISS suction bottle
Distaflo bypass graft
distal bile duct
distal bile duct obstruction
distal biliary atresia
distal blind stomach
distal clot
distal colon
distal cremasteric stump
distal duodenum
distal end of transected colon
distal esophageal ring
distal esophagus
distal flow
distal gastrectomy with excision of ulcer
distal ileitis
distal lymph node metastasis
distal near-total pancreatectomy
distal nephron
distal pancreatectomy (body/tail fistula)
distal pancreatic resection
distal pulses
distal resection
distal Roux-en-Y gastric procedure
distal spatula
distal splenorenal shunt (DSR)
distal stump of artery
distal subtotal pancreatectomy
distal transection of pancreas
distance from the anal verge
distant metastasis
distant skin recurrence
distend
distended abdomen
distended afferent loop
distended gallbladder
distended loop of sigmoid colon
distended loop of small bowel
distensibility
distention
  abdominal
  bladder
  colonic
  gallbladder
distention *(cont.)*
  gaseous
  gastric
  liver
  postprandial
  progressive abdominal
  rectal
distortion of normal parenchyma
distraction hook
distraction rod
distractor pin
disturbance of self-esteem
diuresis
diuretic therapy
Diva laparoscopic morcellator
diversion, biliopancreatic
diversion proctitis
diversionary ileostomy
diverticula (see *diverticulum*)
diverticular disease of the colon
diverticulectomy
  Harrington esophageal
  Meckel
  open
diverticulectomy of hypopharynx
diverticulitis
  acute
  cecal
  chronic
  recurrent episodes of
  sigmoid
diverticulization of duodenum
diverticuloscope
diverticulosis
diverticulum (pl. diverticula)
  colonic
  congenital
  cricopharyngeal
  end-stage
  epiphrenic
  esophageal
  false
  Ganser
  Graser

diverticulum *(cont.)*
- hepatic
- hyperplastic mucosal
- hypopharyngeal
- intestinal
- intraluminal duodenal (IDD)
- intramural
- juxtapapillary
- Kirchner
- large pharyngeal
- lateral
- Meckel
- midesophageal
- perforated
- perforation of
- periampullary
- pharyngoesophageal
- pulsion
- Rokitansky
- subdiaphragmatic
- traction
- true
- volvulated Meckel diverticulum
- wide-mouthed mucosal
- Zenker

diverticulum of Nuck
diverting colostomy
diverting ileostomy
diverting loop ileostomy
diverting proximal colostomy
diverting stoma
divided-stoma colostomy
Divine colostomy appliance
diving goiter
division of cystic duct between clips
division of short gastric vessels
division of stricture
di-wing anoscope
Dix foreign body device
Dixon-Thomas-Smith clamp
Dizmiss (meclizine HCl)
DJJ (duodenojejunal junction)
DKA (diabetic ketoacidosis)
DLP cardioplegic needle
DME (drug metabolizing enzyme)
D-Modem and insulin pump therapy
DMP 504
DMSO (dimethyl sulphoxide)
DNA flow cytometry
DNA ploidy abnormality
DNA repair gene
DNA tumor virus
Doane knee retractor
Dobbhoff biliary stent
Dobbhoff feeding tube
Dobbhoff gastrectomy feeding tube
DOBI (Dynamic Optical Breast Imaging System)
dobutamine
docetaxel
Docucal-P (phenolphthalein; docusate calcium)
documented loss of blood elements
docusate calcium
docusate potassium
docusate sodium
Döderlein (Doederlein) bacillus
dog-bite infection
Dohn-Carton brain retractor
Dohrmann-Rubin cannula
DOK (docusate sodium)
DoLi S extracorporeal shock-wave
dolichocolon
dolorosa (painful) anesthesia
dolphin-nose dissector
dolphin-nose grasper
dolphin-nose grasping forceps, tissue well, double-action
Domeboro powder, tablets (aluminum sulfate; calcium acetate)
dome of diaphragm
dome of liver
Dome-Paste (zinc oxide; calamine; gelatin)
dominant breast mass
domperidone
domperidone maleate
Donaghy angled suture needle holder

donation, organ
Donati suture
Don Congreve trocar set
Don Duralap scissors
Donnagel (attapulgite)
Donnagel-PG
Donnamar (hyoscyamine sulfate)
Donna-Sed (atropine sulfate; scopolamine hydrobromide; hyoscyamine hydrobromide; phenobarbital)
Donnatal (atropine sulfate; scopolamine hydrobromide; hyoscyamine sulfate; phenobarbital)
Donnazyme (pancreatic lipase; protease; amylase)
donor
 cadaveric
 CMV-positive
 living related
 non-heart-beating
 organ
donor blood
donor kidney
donor hepatectomy
donor pancreatectomy
donor-specific bone marrow augmentation
donor-specific transfusion (DST)
Don peritoneal scissors
Donphen
donut mastopexy
Dooley nail
dopa agonist
dopamine
dopamine agonist
Doppler-guided hemorrhoid artery ligation (DGHAL)
Doppler, Nicolet Elite obstetrical
Doppler sonography
Doppler ultrasonography
Doppler ultrasound intestinal blood flow measurement
Dorbane (danthron)
Dorbantyl Forte (danthron)
Dor fundoplasty
Dormia basket catheter
Dormia noose
Dornier gallstone lithotriptor
Dornier HM3 waterbath lithotriptor
Dorros infusion/probing catheter
dorsal linear incision
dorsal lithotomy (*not* dorsolithotomy) position
dorsal mesogastrium
dorsal pancreas
dorsal pancreatic artery
dorsal plate
dorsal point
dorsal position
dorsal recumbent position
dorsal supine position
dorsal surface of the thyroid gland
dorsal vein complex
Dorsey ventricular cannula
dorsiflexion view
dorsomedial incision
dorsoplantar view
dorsosacral position
dorsosupine position
Dosalax (senna concentrate; alcohol)
Dos Santos needle
DOS Softgels (docusate sodium)
Dostinex (cabergoline)
Dott retractor
Doubilet sphincterotomy
double-action jaws
double-action parallel pliers and wire cutter
double-action rongeur
double-action wire cutter
double-action wire extraction pliers
double-armed (DAS) suture
double barrel colostomy
double barrel ileostomy
double barrel reservoir
double binocular operating microscope
double-bladed knife
double bubble duodenal sign

double buttress laparoscopic hernioplasty
double channel
double channel endoscope
double clamp
double clamping
double contrast barium enema (DCBE)
double contrast barium meal
double drape
doubled semitendinosus and gracilis autograft (DST&G)
double duct sign
double-edged razor blade
double-ended curette
double-ended nail
double-ended right-angle retractor
double gallbladder
double-head ceiling mount reflector
double-headed P190 stapler
double hernia
double hook
double hollow nail
double hook Lovejoy retractor
double-H plate
double incision
Double J indwelling catheter
double J-shaped reservoir
Double J ureteral catheter
double lumen endobronchial tube
double lumen endoprosthesis
double lumen papillotome
double lumen tube
double mesh graft
double-occluding clamp
double pedicle flap
double pedicle TRAM flap
double pigtail endoprosthesis
double pigtail stent
double-pointed needle
double-post Mayo stand
double prong fork
double puncture laparoscope
double pyloroplasty
double reverse alpha sigmoid loop
double seton modified surgical approach to transsphincteric anal fistula repair
double-spoon forceps
double S-shaped curvature
DoubleStent biliary endoprosthesis
double tertian malaria
double tracking of barium
double-wrap graciloplasty
doubly ligated
doubly ligated and divided
doubly ligated suture
doughnut kidney
doughy abdomen
Douglas cannula
Douglas, cul-de-sac of
Douglas fold
Douglas forceps
Douglas pouch
Douglas procedure (suture of tongue for micrognathia)
Douglas rectal snare
Douglas rectouterine pouch
Douglas skin graft
Dow Corning breast prosthesis
Dow Corning ileal pouch catheter
dowel graft
Dowen forceps
downbiting rongeur
Down epiphyseal knife
Downey hemilaminectomy retractor
downhill esophageal varices
Downing cartilage knife
Downing retractor
Downing staple
Down syndrome
Doxidan (phenolphthalein; docusate calcium)
Doxil (doxorubicin hydrochloride liposome injection)
Doxinate
doxorubicin hydrochloride liposome injection
Doyen abdominal retractor

Doyen abdominal scissors
Doyen bone mallet
Doyen clamp
Doyen costal elevator
Doyen costal rasp
Doyen forceps
Doyen intestinal forceps
Doyen myoma screw
Doyen retractor
Doyen rib elevator
Doyen rib rasp
Doyen scissors
Doyen vaginal retractor blade
D-penicillamine
DPL (diagnostic peritoneal lavage)
DPT-1 (diabetes prevention trial type 1)
Dr. Caldwell Senna Laxative (senna concentrate)
Dr. Dermi-Heal (allantoin; zinc oxide; Peruvian balsam)
Draffin bipod suspension apparatus
drag, instrument
Dragstedt skin graft
drain
- Becker external
- Blair silicone
- Blake
- Blake wound
- Chaffin-Pratt
- Charnley suction
- cigarette
- closed suction
- Davol
- Davol sump
- external ventricular (EVD)
- flat Silastic suction
- fluted J-Vac
- four-wing Malecot
- Hemovac
- Hemovac Hydrocoat
- Heyer-Schulte wound
- Jackson-Pratt (JP)
- Jackson-Pratt gold branch Hemaduct
- J-Vac

drain *(cont.)*
- large-bore silicone
- lumbar
- Mikulicz
- monofilament nylon
- nasobiliary
- Nélaton rubber tube
- nylon threads as
- Penrose
- percutaneous
- percutaneous closed-catheter
- peripancreatic
- peritoneal
- Pezzer
- placement of intraperitoneal
- prophylactic
- Quad-Lumen
- Relia-Vac
- rubber
- Shirley wound
- Silastic drip
- spinal
- stab-wound
- suction
- sump
- sump-Penrose
- Surgivac
- transpapillary
- T-tube
- two-wing Malecot
- van Sonnenberg sump
- ventriculoperitoneal
- ventriculostomy
- Wangensteen
- wound
- Wound-Evac

drainable ostomy pouch
drainage
- catheter
- dependent
- endoscopic
- endoscopic biliary
- enteric
- gravity

drainage *(cont.)*
- green-brown
- internal biliary
- J-Vac closed wound
- mucopurulent
- nasobiliary
- nasogastric
- nasopancreatic
- needle
- percutaneous abscess and fluid drainage (PAFD)
- percutaneous antegrade biliary
- percutaneous transhepatic (PTD)
- perianal
- preoperative endoscopic
- presacral
- regional lymphatic
- retroperitoneal
- sanguineous
- Seroma-Cath wound drainage system
- serosanguineous
- suction
- surgical
- transduodenal
- transgastric
- transpapillary
- transrectal
- Tru-Close wound drainage system
- T-tube
- wound

drainage gastrostomy
drainage of palate abscess
drainage of pancreatic exocrine secretions
drainage of pus
drainage procedure
drainage tube
draining abscess
drain site evisceration
Drake-Willock peritoneal dialysis system
Dramamine (dimenhydrinate)
Dramamine II (meclizine HCl)
Dramanate (dimenhydrinate)
Dramilin (dimenhydrinate)
Drapanas shunt
drape
- adhesive
- adhesive plastic
- beach chair shoulder
- Bedel
- Convertor
- double
- Emerald
- fenestrated
- foot
- head
- impervious
- Incise
- Ioban antimicrobial incise
- Ioban Vi-Drape
- isolation
- Iso-Seal
- Kaycel towel
- lint-free
- Microban
- NeuroDrape surgical
- Opmi microscope
- Opraflex incise
- paper
- plastic
- povidone-iodine impregnated
- Sensability lubricated plastic sheet for breast self-examination
- shoulder
- Steri-Drape plastic incise
- sterile
- sterile paper
- 3M skin
- U-drape
- Vi-Drape

draped out
drawing pin
drawtape
Dreiling tube
drenching sweat

Dressinet netting bandage
dressing (see also *bandage*; *packing*)
ABD
ABD pad
absorbent gauze
Accuzyme
AcryDerm absorbent wound
AcryDerm advanced wound
AcryDerm border island
AcryDerm hydrogel sheet
AcryDerm Sheet
AcryDerm Strands
Acticoat burn
ACU-derm wound
Adaptic
Adaptic X Xeroform gauze nonadhering
Adcon-L
Adcon-P
adhesive
adhesive tape
Aeroplast
AlgiDERM calcium alginate gel
AlgiDERM alginate wound
alginate wound
AlgiSite alginate wound
Algosteril alginate wound
Alldress composite wound
Allevyn hydrocellular foam
Allevyn nonadherent
Aloe Vesta protective ointment
Alogsteril
antiseptic
Aquacel Hydrofiber
Aquaphor
Aquasorb hydrogel
Aquasorb transparent hydrogel
Arglaes antimicrobial barrier film
ArtAssist compression
Avitene "flour"
Band-Aid
Betadine
Betadine-soaked Owen
Bioclusive

dressing *(cont.)*
Bioclusive transparent
Biolex wound gel
Biopatch foam wound
BioPatch antimicrobial
BlisterFilm transparent
Blue Goo
bolus
BreakAway absorptive wound
breast support
bulky
Bunnell
Buro-Sol
calcium alginate
CaraKlenz
carbohydrate polymer gel
Cariel
CarraFilm transparent film
CarraGauze wound strips
CarraSmart foam
CarraSmart self-adhesive foam
Carra Sorb H wound
Carra Sorb M freeze-dried gel
Carrasyn hydrogel wound
Carrasyn V
CicaCare topical gel sheeting
cidofovir gel
CircPlus compression
Circulon
Clean Seals
ClearSite absorbent hydrogel wound
ClearSite borderless
ClearSite Hydro Gauze
Coban
cold compressive
collagen-alginate wound
collodion
CombiDerm absorbent cover
CombiDerm ACD
Comfeel Plus
Comfeel Purilon
Comfeel Ulcus occlusive
compression wrap
compressive

dressing *(cont.)*
Conform
Conformant contact-layer wound
corrective soft
cotton
Covaderm composite wound
Covaderm Plus adhesive barrier
Coverlet adhesive surgical
Cover-Roll adhesive gauze
Cryo/Cuff ankle
Curaderm hydrocolloid
Curafil hydrogel
Curafoam foam wound
Curagel hydrogel
Curasol
Curasorb calcium alginate
Curity Oil emulsion
Curity saline
Dermabond
Dermagran wound
DermaMend foam wound
DermaMend hydrogel
DermaNet contact-layer wound
DermaSorb
DermAssist hydrocolloid
DermAssist wound filling
Dermatell hydrocolloid
DiabGel hydrogel
Domeboro powder
Dome-Paste
dry
dry sterile
DuoDerm CGF
DuoDerm hydroactive gel
DuoDerm SCB
Dyna-Flex compression
elastic salve
elasticized gauze
Elastikon
Elastomull double-woven stretch
Elastoplast
Elta Dermal hydrogel
ENTaxis nasal
Epigard compositive wound

dressing *(cont.)*
Epi-Lock wound
epistaxis
Esmarch
Excilon sponge
ExuDerm hydrocolloid
Exu-Dry absorptive
Fabco gauze bandage
Fellonet ointment gauze
felt
Fibracol collagen-alginate
Fibracol Plus collagen
figure-of-8 (or figure-8)
First Aid
Flexinet
Flexzan foam wound
fluff
foam gauze
Forvade
4 x 4 gauze
4 x 8 gauze
Fuller shield
Furacin gauze
FyBron alginate wound
gauze
Gentell alginate wound
Gentell foam wound
GeriMend
Glasscock ear
Greer goo
Handages
Hepafix
hyCURE collagen hemostatic wound
hyCURE G hydrogel
HydraGran absorbent
Hydrasorb foam wound
Hydrofiber
hydrogel
hydrophilic powder
hydrophilic semipermeable
absorbent polyurethane foam
HyFil hydrogel
Hypafix
Hypergel hydrogel

dressing *(cont.)*
Iamin
Iamin gel wound
iLEX skin
Inerpan flexible burn
Intelligent dressing
Interceed
Interceed TC7
IntraSite (graft T starch copolymer)
IntraSite gel
Iodoflex absorptive
iodoform gauze
Iodosorb absorptive
Irrijet DS
island
Jelonet (paraffin-soaked tulle)
Jobst breast support
Jones
Kalginate alginate wound
Kalginate calcium alginate
Kaltostat Fortex
Kaltostat wound packing material
Kerlix
Kling adhesive
Koch-Mason
LYOfoam A
LYOfoam C
LYOfoam T
LYOfoam tracheostomy
Maxorb alginate wound
Medifil collagen hemostatic wound
Medipore Dress-it surgical
Mepilex self-adherent foam
Mepitel contact-layer wound
Mepore absorptive
Merogel
Mesalt ribbon
Microfoam
Mills
Mitraflex
Mitraflex Plus
modified Robert Jones
moleskin strips
Montgomery strap

dressing *(cont.)*
Mother Jones (modified Robert Jones)
MPM hydrogel
Multidex hydrophilic powder
Multidex wound-filling material
No Sting Barrier Film
nonadherent gauze
nonadhesive
nonocclusive
Normigel hydrogel
Nu-Brede
NuDerm hydrocolloid
Nu Gauze sponge
Nu-Gel clear hydrogel wound
NUVO barrier film
Oasis wound
occlusive
O'Donoghue
Omiderm mesh
Omiderm plain
Omiderm transparent adhesive film
OpSite
OpSite Flexigrid transparent adhesive film
Optipore sponge
OsmoCyte PCA pillow wound
Owen gauze
palm-to-axilla
PanoPlex hydrogel
patch
Pedi-Boro Soak Packs
Peri-Strips Dry
Piliel hair
Pillo Pro
pledget
Polyderm foam wound
Polyderm hydrophilic polyurethane foam
Poly Mem
Polyskin II
pressure
Primaderm semipermeable foam
Primapore absorptive wound

dressing *(cont.)*
Primer compression
Pro-Clude transparent film wound
ProCyte transparent adhesive film
Proderm Topical
Profore wound
PSD Gel
RepliCare hydrocolloid
Repliderm collagen-based
Repliderm wound
Reston foam wound
Reston hydrocolloid
Restore
rigid
Robert Jones
Robert Jones bulky soft
Royl-Derm nonadherent wound
SAF-Clens
Saf-Gel hydrogel
Scar Care
Scarlet Red ointment
SCB
Schanz
SeaSorb alginate wound
2nd Skin wound
Seprafilm bioresorbable membrane
Shur-Clens
SignaDress hydrocolloid
Silastic
silk mesh gauze
Silon wound
Silvadene (silver sulfadiazine)
Silverlon wound packing strips
SIS wound
SiteGuard MVP transparent adhesive film
SkinTegrity hydrogel
Snugs
Sof-Band bulky bandage
Sof-Kling
Sof-Rol
SofSorb absorptive
soft bulky
SoftCloth absorptive

dressing *(cont.)*
Sof-Wick sponge
Solosite
SoloSite wound gel
SorbaView composite wound
Sorbsan topical wound
Spand-Gel
Spyrogel hydrogel wound
stent
Stericare
Steri-Strips
sterile
Stimson
StrataSorb composite wound
SurePress compression
SureSite transparent adhesive film
Surgicel
Suture-Self
Sween Prep skin
Synthaderm occlusive wound
SyringeAvitene
TAB (tumescent absorbent bandage) wound
Tegaderm
Tegaderm HP
Tegaderm transparent
Tegagel hydrogel dressing and sheet
Tegagen HG alginate wound
Tegagen HI alginate wound
Tegapore contact-layer wound
Tegasorb
Telfa
Telfa gauze
Telfa Plus
Thera-Boot compression dressing or wrap
THINSite with BioFilm hydrogel topical wound
Tielle Plus absorbent adhesive dressing with multilayer structure
tie-over
toe-to-groin modified Jones
Transeal transparent adhesive
Transorbent multilayer

dressing *(cont.)*
- transparent
- transparent adhesive film
- transparent polyethylene
- Tubegauz
- Tubex gauze
- Tubigrip
- tumescent absorbent bandage (TAB)
- Ultec hydrocolloid
- UltraKlenz
- Ultrafera wound
- Ultrex
- Uniflex polyurethane adhesive surgical
- Uni-Site
- Unna-Flex compression
- Unna-Pak compression
- Vari/Moist wound
- Vaseline gauze
- Vaseline petrolatum
- Veingard transparent
- Velpeau
- Veni-Gard I.V. Stabilization
- Ventex wound
- Versalon
- Viasorb wound
- Vigilon occlusive
- Vitacuff
- Webril
- wet-to-dry
- wide-mesh petroleum gauze
- Wound Stick
- WoundSpan Bridge II
- Woun'Dres hydrogel
- Xeroflo
- Xeroflogauze
- Xeroform gauze
- Zipzoc stocking compression

dressing forceps
dressing scissors
DRG Sherlock threaded suture anchor
dried-out material
Driessen hinged plate
drifting spleen
Drilac dressing
drill
- Acra-Cut wire pass
- Adson twist
- air
- air-powered cutting
- Anspach power
- archimedean hand
- battery-driven hand
- biflanged
- Black and Decker
- bone
- Bosworth
- brace
- Bunnell hand
- cannulated
- Cebotome
- Cement Eater
- centering
- cervical
- Championnière bone
- Charnley centering
- Charnley femoral condyle
- Cherry-Austin
- Children's Hospital hand
- chuck
- Cloward
- Coballoy twist
- Codman wire pass
- Collison
- cortex
- cortical
- cranial
- Crutchfield hand
- Cushing flat
- Cushing perforator
- dental
- D'Errico perforating
- Elan-E power
- femoral condyle
- fingernail
- flat
- flex
- Gray bone

drill *(cont.)*
- Hall air
- Hall large-bore
- Hall Micro E
- Hall Surgairtome
- Hall Versipower
- hand
- hand-operated
- high-speed twist
- hip fracture compaction
- Hudson brace
- Hudson cranial
- Kirschner hand
- Kirschner wire
- Küntscher (Kuentscher)
- Mam
- Mathews hand
- McKenzie perforating twist
- MicroAire
- microsurgery
- Mira Mark III cranial
- Moore hand
- Osteone air
- otologic
- patellar
- Pease bone
- penetrating
- Penn fingernail
- perforating twist
- Phoenix cranial
- Pilot
- pneumatic
- Ralk hand
- Raney cranial
- Raney perforator
- right-angle dental
- Shea
- Smedberg hand
- Smedberg twist
- Smith automatic perforator
- Smith cranial
- spiral
- step
- Stille bone
- Stille cranial

drill *(cont.)*
- Stille hand
- Stille-Sherman bone
- Stryker microsurgery
- subchondral
- Synthes
- Toti trephine
- Treace
- trephine
- Trinkle
- twist
- wire
- wire pass
- Xomed
- Zimmer hand

drill bit
- cannulated
- hip fracture compaction
- Howmedica Microfixation System
- Leibinger Micro System
- Luhr Microfixation System
- Storz Microsystems
- Synthes Microsystems

drill blade

drill bushing

drill flat

drill guide
- ACL (anterior cruciate ligament)
- Adson
- neutral and load

drill hole

drill pin

drill point
- cannulated
- carbon steel
- Crutchfield
- Raney-Crutchfield
- Stille

drill/reamer, MicroAire

drill set, Hudson cranial

drill trephine

drinker
- binge
- social
- weekend

drinking habits
drip infusion cholangiography (DIC)
Drisite brand fabric reinforcement
driver
  blade plate
  bullet
  Flatt
  Hall
  Harrington hook
  Jewett
  Küntscher (Kuentscher) nail
  K-wire
  Linvatec
  Lloyd nail
  Massie
  Micro Series wire
  nail
  Orthoairtome wire
  Paramax angled
  plate
  power
  prosthesis
  staple
  supine position
  Sven-Johansson
  Teflon-coated
driver-bender-extractor, Rush
driver-extractor
  Hansen-Street
  Ken
  McReynolds
  Sage
  Schneider
  Zimmer
driving the camera
droloxifene
dromedary kidney
dronabinol
drop test
droperidol
droplet infection
drotaverine
drowned lung
drug antagonism
drug cessation
drug class
  aminosterol
  antacid
  anthelmintic
  anticholinergic
  antiemetic
  antihyperglycemic
  antihypertensive
  antinauseant
  antineoplastic
  antisecretory
  antispasmodic
  aperient
  aperitive
  ATPase (adenosine triphosphatase) inhibitors
  bacteriostatic
  benzodiazepine
  bile acid sequestrant
  bowel evacuant
  carminative
  cathartic
  cholagogue
  counterirritant
  COX-2 inhibitor
  digestant
  digestive enzyme
  discutient
  emetic
  5-hydroxytryptamine (5-HT) receptor antagonist
  fluoropyrimidine
  general anesthetic
  H_2 blocker
  hemorroidal agent
  hemostatic
  hepatics
  hydragogue
  hydrocholeretic
  immunizing agent
  immunosuppressant
  laxative
  local anesthetic

drug class *(cont.)*
plasma expander
proliferation signal inhibitor
proton pump inhibitor
purgative
SSRI (selective serotonin reuptake inhibitor)
substituted benzimidazole
sulfonylurea
taeniacide
taxane, taxoid
theraccine
thiazolidinedione
vaccine
vermicide; vermifuge
vulnerary
drug fever
drug-induced cholestasis
drug-induced constipation
drug-induced gastritis
drug-induced hepatitis
drug-induced steatosis
drug metabolism
drug-metabolizing enzyme (DME)
drug toxicity
Drummond hook
Drummond, marginal artery of
Drummond syndrome
DRx (Digital Response)
dry colostomy
dry dressing
dry heaves (retching)
dry necrosis
dry sterile dressing
dry swallow on esophageal manometry
dry vomiting
DSC; DSCG (disodium cromoglycate)
DSMC Plus (casanthranol; docusate potassium)
DSRS (distal splenorenal shunt)
D-S-S (docusate sodium)
DST (donor-specific transfusion)
DST&G (doubled semitendinosus and gracilis) autograft
DTAFA (descending thoracic aorta-to-femoral artery) bypass graft
D-thyroxine
D-TRON insulin delivery pump
DTRs (deep tendon reflexes)
DTT (dynamic transverse traction) hook
dual-cup grasping forceps, double-action
dual irrigation adapter
DualMesh biomaterial graft
dual onlay bone graft
dual phase spiral CT scan
dual plate
dual tracer imaging
Dubecq-Princeteau angulating needle holder
Dubin and Amelar classification of varicoceles
Dubin-Johnson syndrome
Dubin-Sprinz disease
Dubin-Sprinz syndrome
Dubois scissors
duckbill forceps
duckbill elevator
duckbill forceps
duckbill rongeur
duck nose micrograsper
duct
accessory pancreatic
beaded hepatic
common bile (CBD)
common hepatic
cystic
distal bile
ductal
extrahepatic bile
extrahepatic biliary
fusiform widening of
gall
hepatic (right and left)
Hering
interlobular bile
intrahepatic
intrahepatic bile

duct *(cont.)*
  intrahepatic biliary
  lactiferous
  main pancreatic (MPD)
  middle extrahepatic bile
  normal caliber
  omphalomesenteric
  pancreatic
  perilobular
  preampullary portion of bile
  prepapillary bile
  subvesical
  terminal bile
  thyroglossal
  vitelline
  vitellointestinal
ductal calculus
ductal carcinoma
ductal carcinoma in situ (DCIS)
ductal carcinoma of prostate
ductal dilatation
ductal dilation
ductal duct
ductal ectasia of breast
ductal epithelium
ductal irregularities with dilation and stenosis
ductal obstruction
ductal proliferation
duct cell carcinoma
duct ectasia
duct lesion
ductless gland
duct lumen
duct of Luschka
duct of Santorini
duct of Wirsung
ductogram, mammary
ductography, direct contrast
duct papilloma
duct-to-duct anastomosis
ductus arteriosum
Duecollement hemicolectomy
Duecollement maneuver
Duet glucose monitor
Duette catheter
Duffield scissors
Duhamel colon operation
Duhamel laparoscopic pull-through procedure
Duke bleeding time (BT)
Duke cannula
Dukes Astler-Coller modified staging system
Duke trocar
Dulcagen (bisacodyl)
Dulcolax (bisacodyl)
Dulcolax Bowel Prep Kit (bisacodyl)
dullness
  hepatic
  liver
  shifting
  splenic
  tympanitic
dullness to percussion
dull pain
dull purple lung
dull right upper quadrant pain
dumbbell-shaped shadow
dummy seed catheter
Dumon-Gilliard prosthesis introducer
Dumon-Gilliard prosthesis pushing tube
Dumont dissecting forceps
Dumont microdissecting forceps
dumping stomach
dumping syndrome
Duncan disease
Dunhill artery forceps
Dunlop-Shands view
Dunn biopsy
duodenal aspirate
duodenal atresia
duodenal bubble
duodenal bulb
duodenal bulb apex
duodenal bulb deformity
duodenal cap
duodenal C-loop

duodenal contents examination
duodenal decompression
duodenal diversion
duodenal end of dorsal pancreatic duct
duodenal end of main pancreatic duct
duodenal erosion
duodenal fistula
duodenal fold
duodenal fossa
duodenal gland
duodenal ileus
duodenal impression on liver
duodenal ligament
duodenal loop
duodenal lumen
duodenal mucosal cells
duodenal papilla
duodenal perforation
duodenal polyp
duodenal recess
duodenal rupture
duodenal scarring
duodenal seromyectomy
duodenal sphincter
duodenal string test
duodenal stump
duodenal sweep
duodenal switch
duodenal terminus
duodenal ulcer
duodenal ulcer disease
duodenal ulcer perforation (DUP)
duodenal ulceration
duodenal vein
duodenal villi
duodenal wall hamartoma
duodenal web
duodenitis
  chronic atrophic
  erosive
duodenobiliary pressure gradient
duodenobiliary reflux
duodenocolic fistula
duodenoenterostomy
duodenogastric reflux (DGR)
duodenogastroscopy, retrograde (RDG)
duodenoileal bypass
duodenoileitis
duodenojejunal angle
duodenojejunal flexure
duodenojejunal fold
duodenojejunal fossa
duodenojejunal junction (DJJ)
duodenojejunal recess
duodenojejunal sphincter
duodenojejunostomy
duodenomesocolic fold
duodenopancreatic reflux
duodenorenal ligament
duodenoscope (see also *endoscope*)
  Fujinon EVD-XL video
  master
  MIS Source
  Olympus
  Olympus JF-1T20 flexible
    therapeutic
  Olympus JF-1T30 flexible
    therapeutic
  Olympus JF-V10 video
  Olympus JTI-T10
  Olympus PJF-7.5 pediatric duodeno-
    fiberscope
  Olympus TJF-160F video
  Olympus TJF-V10
  Pentax ED-3430T video
  Pentax ED-3440T video
  Pentax FD-34V fiberoptic
  two-channel
  transverse
duodenum
  C-loop of
  curve of
  descending
  distal
  scarified
  supravaterian
  suspensory muscle of
duodenum deformed by scarring

DuoDerm CGF (control gel formula) dressing
DuoDerm dressing
DuoDerm SCB (sustained compression bandage) dressing
Duopress guide
Duopress plate
DUP (duodenal ulcer perforation)
Du Pen epidural catheter
Du Pen long-term epidural catheter
Duphalac (lactulose)
duplex kidney
duplication cyst
DuPont Cronex x-ray film
Duraclon (clonidine hydrochloride injection)
Duraclose clip applier
DuraGen graft
Duragesic-25 (fentanyl) transdermal patches
DURAglide stone removal balloon
DURAglide3 stone removal balloon
Duralap J-hook
Duralap Metzenbaum scissors
dural elevator
dural graft
dural hook
dural knife
dural needle
Duralone-40 (methylprednisolone acetate)
Duralon occlusion balloon
dural punch
dural retractor
dural scissors
dural tack-up suture
dural tenting suture
dural traction suture
Duramorph (morphine sulfate)
Duranest MPF (etidocaine; epinephrine)
Durapatite graft
Duraprep kit
dura-protecting forceps
duration of loop formation
Duray-Read gouge
Durelast bandage
Duret lesion
Durham dissector
Durham retractor
Durmarker
Durmont-style dissecting forceps
Duros implant
duskiness, stomal
dusky cyanosis
dusky medulla
dusky stoma
dust-borne infection
duToit staple
Duval clamp
Duval distal (caudal) pancreatico-jejunostomy
Duval elevator
Duval-Scheie hemorrhoidal forceps
Duval tissue-grasping forceps
Duverney gland
DuVries incision
DVP flush shunt
DVT (deep vein [venous] thrombosis)
dwarfism
  achondroplastic
  cretin
  diastrophic
  Lorain-Levi
  pituitary
Dwyer-Hall plate
D-xylose absorption test
Dyclone (dyclonine HCl)
dyclonine HCl (Dyclone)
dye (see also *stain*)
  Congo red
  Evans blue
  indigo carmine
  Lymphazurin
  methylene blue
  radiopaque
  rapid emptying of
dye laser
dye spraying

dye worker's cancer
dymanthine HCl
dimantine HCl
Dymelor (acetohexamide)
Dymenate (dimenhydrinate)
Dyna-Flex compression dressing
Dyna-Flex compression wrap
Dynalink self-expanding biliary stent
  system
  lipolytic
  liver
  liver phosphorylase
  medium chain acyl-CoA
    dehydrogenase
  pancreatic
  protease digestive
  proteinase
  proteolytic
  serum liver
dynamic compression (DCP) plate
DynamicDeca steerable catheter
dynamic graciloplasty
dynamic ileus
dynamic locking nail
Dynamic Optical Breast Imaging
  System (DOBI)
Dynamic PACSPlus
dynamic pharyngeal radiography
dynamic/spastic ileus
dynamic stress x-ray view
dynamometer, Collin
Dynarex
DynaStat surgical hemostatic
DynaWell
dynograph
Dyonics arthroscopic blade
Dyonics cannula
Dyonics cystoscope
Dyonics laparoscope system
Dyonics rod-lens endoscope
Dyonics Vision 325z endoscope camera
Dyonics 0° 10 mm rigid laparoscope
Dyonics 7208130 rigid laparoscope
Dyonics 8007 rigid laparoscope
DyoVac suction punch
dysarthria
dyschezia
dysenteric algid malaria
dysenteric diarrhea
dysentery, bacillary
dysentery bacillus
dysfunction
  bone marrow
  endocrine
  gastrointestinal
  hepatocyte
  multiorgan
  neuroimmune
  peristaltic
  polyglandular
  sphincter of Oddi
  stress-induced organ
dysfunctional uterine bleeding (DUB)
dysgenesis, anorectal
dysimmunity
dyskinesia
  bile duct
  biliary
  esophageal
dysmotility
  esophageal
  generalized gut
  gut
  small intestinal
dyspepsia
  acid
  biliary cholelithic
  flatulent
  functional
  gastric
  nonorganic
  nonulcer
  postcholecystectomy flatulent
  ulcer-like
dyspeptic symptoms
dysphagia
  contractile ring
  esophageal

dysphagia *(cont.)*
  intermittent
  liquid food
  oropharyngeal
  postfundoplication
  postoperative
  postvagotomy
  pre-esophageal
  progressive
  sideropenic
  soft food
  solid food
  vallecular
dysphagia lusoria
dysphagia nervosa
dysphagic
dyspituitarism
dysplasia
  anal squamous
  arteriohepatic
  bilateral nodular
  caudal
  epithelial
  focus of hepatocyte
  high-grade
  mammary
  polypoid
dysplasia with associated lesion or mass (DALM)
dysplastic lesion
dysproteinemia, familial
dysrrhythmia, gastric
dyssynergia
dyssynergic esophagus
dystrophy, adiposogenital

E, e

EAC (expandable access catheter)
EAEC (enteroadherent *E. coli*)
Eagle-Barrett syndrome (prune-belly syndrome)
eagle's beak bone-cutting forceps
ear and endaural instruments
ear blade
ear forceps
Earle hemorrhoid clamp
Earle rectal probe
ear loop
early appendicitis
early gastric cancer (EGC)
early ligation of venous drainage
early menarche
early menopause
early postoperative complication
early recurrence
early satiety
Early Treatment Diabetic Retinopathy Study
early zoster
ear packing sponge
ear wick sponge
Easi-Lav
easily reducible hernia
EASL (European Association for the Study of the Liver)
Eastern Cooperative Oncology Group (ECOG)
East-West retractor
Easy $A1_c$ test
easy bruisability
easy fatigability
EasySafe disposable syringe
Eating Attitudes Test
eating habits
Eaton agent
EBA (extrahepatic biliary atresia)
EBCT (electron-beam computed tomography)
Ebner gland
EBL (endoscopic band ligation)
EBL (estimated blood loss)
Ebstein lesion
EBV (Epstein-Barr virus) infection
EBVS (EBV susceptibility)
ECA (enterobacterial common antigen)
E-CABG (endoscopic coronary artery bypass graft)
E-cadherin expression test for classification of breast carcinoma
E.CAM+ coincidence-imaging
E.CAM dual-head emission imaging system
eccentric drill guide

eccentric dynamic compression (EDCP) plate
eccentric lesion
eccentric restenosis lesion
eccentrically
ecchymosis (pl. ecchymoses)
ecchymosis of inguinal ligament
ecchymosis, perineal
ecchymotic
eccrine carcinoma
echinococcal cyst
echinococcal cyst disease
echinococciasis
Echinococcus granulosus
Echinococcus multilocularis
Echinococcus liver cyst
Echlin bone rongeur
Echlin duckbill rongeur
Echlin laminectomy rongeur
Echlin-Luer rongeur
Echlin rongeur forceps
ECHO (enterocytopathogenic human orphan) virus infection
echocolonoscope (see *colonoscope*)
echoendoscope (see *endoscope*)
echogastroscope (see *gastroscope*)
EchoGen (perflenapent)
echogenic liver
Echols retractor
EchoMark catheter
Eck fistula
Eckhoff mapping pen
Eckhout vertical gastroplasty
ECL (enterochromaffin-like) cell
Eclipse TMR laser
ECOG (Eastern Cooperative Oncology Group) performance status
E. coli 0157:H7 pathogen
E. coli serotype O157:H7
E Cotton bandage
Ecotrin
ectasia
  duct
  ductal (of breast)

ectasia *(cont.)*
  mammary ductal
  vascular
ectatic aneurysm
ecthyma, contagious
ecthyma gangrenosum
ectodermal cells of neural crest origin
ectopic ACTH syndrome
ectopic antidiuretic hormone secretion
ectopic anus
ectopic cortisol-producing tumor
ectopic gastric mucosa
ectopic hormone production
ectopic hyperinsulinism
ectopic hyperparathyroidism
ectopic midline thyroid tissue
ectopic pancreatic tissue
ectopic placement of thyroid tissue in the tongue
ectopic pregnancy
ectopic spleen
ectopic testis
ectopic thyroid nodule
edema
  ambulant
  angioneurotic
  antral
  bronchiolar
  bronze
  bullous-like
  cardiac
  cerebral
  dependent
  epithelial
  focal
  generalized (anasarca)
  gestational
  heat
  hereditary angioneurotic
  ileocecal
  inflammatory
  laryngeal
  local
  lymphatic

edema *(cont.)*
  lymphedema
  malignant
  massive pulmonary hemorrhagic
  osmotic
  patchy intercellular
  pedal
  pericholecystic
  periorbital
  peripheral
  pitting
  premenstrual
  presacral
  pretibial
  pulmonary
  Quincke
  renal
  retinal
  visceral
edema fluid
edema neonatorum
edema of parotid gland
edematous brain
edematous gallbladder
edematous hyperemic mucosa
edematous kidney
edematous tag
edentulous
Eder cotton applicator
Eder endoscope
Eder-Hufford esophagoscope
Eder 180 10 mm rigid laparoscope
Eder-Puestow dilator and shaft
Eder-Puestow metal olive dilator
edge
  ligament reflecting
  liver
  Poupart ligament shelving
Edgeahead phaco slit knife
edible vaccine
Edlich gastric lavage tube
Edmondson Grading System for hepatocellular carcinoma
Edmondson-Steiner classification
Edmondson-Steiner histologic grading of hepatocellular carcinoma
Edmonton fresh islet protocol
Edna towel clamp
Edna towel forceps
edrophonium test
Edwards hook
Edwards-Levine hook
Edwards-Levine rod
Edwards reverse ratchet rod
Edwards woven Teflon aortic bifurcation graft
EEA (end-to-end anastomosis)
EEA Auto Suture stapler
EEA stapler gun
EEA stapling of varices
EES (expandable esophageal stent)
EFAD (essential fatty acid deficiency)
effect
  angioprokinetic
  corset
  hepatotoxic
  Joule-Thompson
  pinchcock
Effer-Syllium
efferent limb
efferent loop of the jejunum
Effler-Groves forceps
Effler-Groves hook
Effner/Arthrotek endovideolaparoscope
Effner rigid laparoscope
effusion
  bloodstained
  hemorrhagic
  joint
  pancreatic pleural
  pericardial
  peritoneal
  pleural
  pleuropericardial
  pulmonary
  serous
  subdural
  unilateral pleural

eflornithine
Egan mammography
EGC (early gastric cancer)
EGD (esophagogastroduodenoscopy)
EGF (epidermal growth factor)
EGG (electrogastrogram)
Eggers bone plate
EG (esophagogastric) junction
EGS Model 100 electrogalvanic
  stimulator
EGTA (esophageal gastric tube airways)
Egyptian splenomegaly
EHEC (enterohemorrhagic *E. coli*)
EHL (electrohydraulic lithotripsy)
Ehlers-Danlos syndrome
EHM (extrahepatic metastasis)
ehrlichial infection, human, Sennetsu
  type
EHT (electrohydrothermo) electrode
EIA-2 (enzyme-linked immunoassay)
EIC (extensive intraductal carcinoma)
eicosapentaenoic acid
EIEC (enteroinvasive *E. coli*)
eight-lumen esophageal manometry
  catheter
Eikenella corrodens (formerly
  Bacteroides corrodens, HB-1)
Einhorn dilator
Einhorn string test
EIT (endoscopic injection therapy)
ELAD (extracorporeal liver assist
  device)
Elan-E power drill
Elase (fibrinolysin; desoxyribonuclease)
Elastase
elastic band ligation
elastic bandage
elastic ligature
elastic salve dressing
elastic stable intramedullary nail (ESIN)
elastic wrap bandage
Elastic Foam bandage
elasticized gauze dressing
Elastikon dressing
Elastikon elastic tape
elastomer bandage
Elastomull bandage
Elastomull double-woven stretch
  dressing
Elastoplast bandage
Elastoplast dressing
ELCA laser
Elder Helio cystoscope
Eldisine (vindesine sulfate)
elective herniorrhaphy
elective lymph node dissection
elective shunt procedure
elective sigmoid resection
elective surgical procedure
electrical impedance breast scanning
  system
electrical neutrality
electrical shock
electric anesthesia
electric cast saw
electrocautery
  bipolar
  Bovie
  Bugbee
  EndoClip
  Fine
  hook
  low-current
  monopolar
  multipolar
  needle-tip
  needlepoint
  Neoflex bendable
  Ultrashear
  Valleylab
electrocautery knife
electrocautery pencil
electrochemical glucose-monitoring
  test strip
electrocoagulating biopsy forceps
electrocoagulation
  bipolar
  monopolar
  transendoscopic
electrocoagulator (see *coagulator*)

electrode
  ACMI monopolar
  Aspen laparoscopy
  ball-tip
  BiLAP bipolar needle
  Bugfee
  button
  Cameron-Miller
  coagulation
  Coaguloop resection
  concentric-needle
  Corson needle
  EHT (electrohydrothermo)
  glass pH
  J-hook
  L-diamond
  L-wedge
  Mitek VAPRTM T thermal
  Salinetrode
  short spatula
  SingleBAR
  SilverBullet
  single-fiber EMG
  spatula
  spoon
  square-L
  StarBAR
  suction irrigation (SIE)
  surface
electrode and probe
electrode introducer
electrode pad
electrodesiccation of tumor
electrogalvanic stimulator
electrogastrogram (EGG)
electrogastrography
electrohydraulic lithotripsy (EHL)
electrohydraulic probe
Electrolase
electrolyte abnormality
electrolyte balance
electrolyte concentration
electrolyte disturbance
electrolyte imbalance
electrolyte losses
electrolyte management
electrolyte panel
  bicarbonate (bicarb) (HCO_3^-)
  calcium (Ca)
  chloride (Cl^-)
  CO_2
  potassium (K)
  sodium (Na)
electrolyte solution, polyethylene glycol
electrolyte, stool
electrolyte therapy
  Multilyte-40
  Normosol-M and 5% Dextrose
  Normosol-R and 5% Dextrose
  Normosol-R, Normosol-R pH 7.4
  Nutrilyte II
  Plasma-Lyte A pH 7.4
  Plasma-Lyte R
  Plasma-Lyte 56
  Plasma-Lyte 148
  Rehydralyte
  Resol
  Ringer injection
  Ringer injection, lactated
electrolyte-polyethylene glycol lavage solution
electrolyzed acid water
electromagnetic focusing field (EFF) probe
electromechanical coupling
electromechanical dissociation and gastroparesis
electromyogram, electromyography (EMG)
  colonic
  conventional concentric
  pelvic floor
  single-fiber
  ureteral
electron accelerator, Mobetron
electron-beam computed tomography (EBCT)
electronic microscopy

electrophoresis
  hemoglobin
  pulsed-field gel
  serum protein
ElectroProbe
Electroscope disposable laparoscopic scissors
Electrosurgery Insulation Test Set
electrosurgical cutting knife
electrosurgical desiccation
electrosurgical pencil
electrosurgical snare polypectomy
electrosurgical therapy
electrosurgical unit (see *cautery; cutter; dissector; knife*)
elemental diet
elevated alkaline phosphatase
elevated alpha-fetoprotein
elevated bilirubin
elevated BUN
elevated ESR
elevated LFTs
elevated pancreatic tumor markers
elevated plasma basal calcitonin level
elevated plasma stimulated calcitonin level
elevated portal pressure
elevated reticulocyte count
elevated serum calcitonin
elevated total serum T_4
elevated WBC
elevating spoon
elevation of anterior abdominal wall
elevation of head of the bed
elevation of right hemidiaphragm
elevator
  Adson periosteal
  angular
  Aufranc periosteal
  Bennett bone
  Bethune periosteal
  Blair
  blunt
  bone

elevator *(cont.)*
  Bowen periosteal
  Boyle uterine
  Bristow periosteal
  Brophy periosteal
  Buck
  Buck periosteal
  Cameron-Haight periosteal
  Campbell periosteal
  Carroll-Legg periosteal
  Chandler bone
  Cheyne periosteal
  chisel edge
  Cloward osteophyte
  Cloward periosteal
  Cobb periosteal
  Cobb spinal
  Cohen periosteal
  Converse periosteal
  Coryllos-Doyen periosteal
  Cottle-MacKenty
  Crawford dural
  Crego
  curved periosteal
  Cushing-Hopkins periosteal
  Cushing Little Joker
  Cushing periosteal
  Cushing pituitary
  Cushing staphylorrhaphy
  Darrach
  Davidson-Sauerbruch-Doyen periosteal
  Dawson-Yuhl-Key
  Dawson-Yuhl periosteal
  D'Errico periosteal
  Doyen costal
  Doyen rib
  duckbill
  dural
  Duval
  Endotrac
  Farabeuf periosteal
  flat narrow
  Fomon periosteal

elevator *(cont.)*
Forman nasal
fracture-reducing
Frazier dural
Freer periosteal
Freer septal
Freer septum
Gardner
Guilford-Wright duckbill
Hajek-Ballenger septal
hand
Harrington spinal
Henahan
Herczel rib
Hibbs chisel
Hoen periosteal
House endaural
House stapes
Iowa University periosteal
Jannetta duckbill
joker periosteal
Joseph periosteal
J periosteal
Kahre-Williger periosteal
Kennerdell-Maroon
Key periosteal
Kirmission periosteal
Kleinert-Kutz periosteal
Kocher
Lambotte
lamina
Lane
Lane periosteal
Langenbeck
Langenbeck periosteal
Lempert narrow
Lempert periosteal
Lewis periosteal
liberator
Locke
Love-Adson periosteal
lumbosacral fusion
M.H.G.
MacKenty periosteal

elevator *(cont.)*
Malis
Matson-Alexander
Matson rib
McGlamry
Mead periosteal
Molt periosteal
Moore bone
nasal
OSI Extremity
osteophyte
Paparella duckbill
Penfield
periosteal
Phemister
Presbyterian Hospital staphylorrhaphy
Ray-Parsons-Sunday staphylorrhaphy
Rhoton
rib
Rish periosteal
Roberts-Gill periosteal
Rochester lamina
Rochester spinal
Rosen
round-tapped periosteal
Sauerbruch rib
Sayre
Sayre periosteal
Scott-McCracken periosteal
Sebileau periosteal
Sedillot periosteal
septal
Shambaugh-Derlacki duckbill
Shambaugh narrow
Sheffield hand
Sisson fracture reducing
spinal
staphylorrhaphy
Stille
straight periosteal
Sunday staphylorrhaphy
Swanson

elevator *(cont.)*
  Tabb
  Take-Apart
  Tegtmeier
  Tenzel
  T handle
  Tronzo
  von Langenbeck periosteal
  Ward periosteal
  Wiberg periosteal
  wide periosteal
  Willauer-Gibbon periosteal
  Williger periosteal
  Woodson
  Yankauer periosteal
  Yasargil
elevator dissector
elimination diet
elimination of stool
ELISA (enzyme-linked immunosorbent assay)
ELISA buffer
ELISA IgG
ELISA titer; ELISA-3 titer
Elite Farley retractor
Ellence (epirubicin hydrochloride)
Elliot forceps
Elliott B solution
Elliott femoral condyle blade plate
Elliott gallbladder forceps
elliptical incision
ElMed rigid laparoscope
Elmor tissue morcellator
Elmore radiofrequency tissue morcellator
elongated colon
elongated mass
elongate pattern
elongated PR interval
Eloxatin (oxaliplatin)
Elsberg brain cannula
Elsberg ventricular cannula
Elta Dermal hydrogel dressing
Elta gauze dressing
Elta wound cleanser
Eltroxin (levothyroxine sodium)
Elucigene test
embalming fluid
embarrassment, circulatory
embolic mesenteric infarction
embolic necrosis
embolism
  air
  amniotic fluid
  arterial missile
  bile pulmonary
  gas
  mesenteric
  multiple
  pulmonary
  shotgun pellet
  tumor
embolization
  angiographic variceal
  transcatheter variceal
  transhepatic (THE)
embolization of bleeding vessel
embolize bleeding vessel
embolus, massive pulmonary
embryological line
embryological remnant of the third pharyngeal pouch
embryonal cell carcinoma
embryonal tumor of neural crest origin
embryonic cell transplantation
embryonic chromaffin cells
embryotomy scissors
Emdogain enamel matrix protein
Emerald drape
Emerald fabric
emergency appendectomy
emergency intubation
emergency laparotomy
emergency operation
emergency tracheostomy
emergent appendectomy
emergent endoscopic sclerotherapy
emergent herniorrhaphy

emergent operation
emergent surgery
emesis (see *vomiting*)
  coffee-grounds
  gagging without
  induction of
  retching of
  retching without
Emete-con
emetic reflex
Emetrol (fructose, dextrose, and phosphoric acid)
EMG (electromyogram) needle
Emit 2000 cyclosporine specific assay
Emitasol (metoclopramide) nasal spray
emitefur
Emmett cotton swab forceps
Emmett fistula hook
Emmett tenaculum hook
emollient laxative
emphysema, subcutaneous
emphysematous cholecystitis
emphysematous gastritis
emphysematous lung
empiric antibiotic regimen
empirical diagnosis
empirical therapy
emptying
  delayed gastric
  gallbladder
  gastric
empyema of gallbladder
EMR (endoscopic mucosal resection) suction cap method
EMT emergency medicine tube
emulsification
emulsified perflubron blood substitute
emulsion
  intravenous fat
  lipid
Emulsoil
EN (enteral nutrition)
enamel crypt
enamel matrix protein for wound healing
ENANB (enterically transmitted non-A, non-B) hepatitis (former name)
en bloc augmentation mammoplasty
en bloc axillary node dissection
en bloc distal pancreatectomy
en bloc resection
en bloc splenectomy
en bloc vein resection
Encapslon catheter
encapsulated brain abscess
encapsulated breast implant
encapsulated fluid collection
encapsulated mass
encapsulated neoplasm
encapsulated nodule
encasement of splenic vein
encephaloid gastric carcinoma
encephalomyocarditis virus
encephalomyopathy, subacute necrotizing
encephalopathy
  bilirubin
  hepatic (HE)
  portal-systemic (PSE)
  portosystemic (PSE)
  post-shunt
  Wernicke
encircled
encircling
encopresis
encroachment of tumor
endamebic abscess
endarterectomy scissors
endarterectomy shunt
endaural instrument
endaural retractor
end-biting forceps
end colostomy
end-cutting reciprocating saw
end-diastolic volume
endemic (colloid) goiter
endemic cretinism
endemic goiter
endemic nonbacterial gastroenteritis

Ender awl
Ender flexible medullary nail
Ender pin
Ender rod
end-expiratory pressure
end expiration
End-Flo laparoscopic irrigating system
end ileostomy
Endius endoscope
Endius spinal endoscopic camera endoscope
end-loop colostomy
end-loop ileocolostomy
end-loop ileostomy
Endo-AID suction irrigation
EndoALPHA integrated endosurgical system
endoanal coil
endoanal ultrasound
Endo Avitene hemostatic agent
Endo Babcock clamp
Endo Babcock surgical grasper
Endobag laparoscopic specimen retrieval system
endobiliary stent
endobiliary stenting
endobrachyesophagus
endobronchial fistula
endobronchial lesion
EndoCab ELISA
EndoCab enzyme linked immunosorbent assay (ELISA)
endocardial tumor
ENDOcare nitinol stent (urinary)
Endo Catch specimen retrieval bag
endocervical mucosa
Endocet (oxycodone/acetaminophen)
Endo Cinch laparoscopic grasper
Endo Cinch suturing system
endoclip, absorbable
Endo Clip laparoscopic clip applicator
Endo Close surgical stapler
Endocodone (oxycodone hydrochloride)
EndoCoil biliary stent
EndoCoil esophageal stent
EndoCPB (endovascular cardiopulmonary bypass) catheter
endocrine dysfunction
endocrine function
endocrine gland
endocrine pancreas hormone
endocrine pathology
endocrine therapy
endocrine tumor of the pancreas
endocrinopathy
Endocut cautery device
Endodan (oxycodone/oxycodone terephthalate/aspirin)
endodermal
Endo Dissect laparoscopic instruments
endoesophageal probe
endoesophageal tube
Endo-Flex balloon dilator
Endo-Flo irrigation system
Endo-Flo probe
end-of-treatment response
Endo-Gauge
endogenous bacteria
endogenous infection
endogenous inflammatory mediator production
endogenous insulin
endogenous obesity
endogenous parathyroid hormone
endogenous TSH stimulation
Endo GIA suture stapler
Endo GIA II stapler
Endo Grasp laparoscopic forceps
Endo Grasp roticulator
Endo Hernia clip applier
Endo Hernia surgical stapler
Endo Hernia Universal stapler
Endoknot suture needle
Endolap laparoscope
Endolap rigid laparoscope
Endolase laparoscope
Endolase rigid laparoscope
Endolav lavage pump

Endoloop disposable chromic ligature suture instrument
Endoloop ligature
Endoloop suture
Endo Lumenal gastroplication device
EndoLumina bougie
EndoLumina II transillumination system
endoluminal ultrasound (EUS)
Endo Lung device
endolymphatic sac
endolymphatic shunt
EndoMate camera
EndoMate Grab Bag endoscopic specimen retrieval bag
EndoMed laparoscopic systems
EndoMed LSS laparoscopic system
endometrial carcinoma
endometrial polyp
endometrial resection and ablation (ERA) resectoscope sheath
endometrial stromal sarcoma
endometriosis
endometritis
Endopath circular stapler
Endopath curved intraluminal stapler
Endopath EMS hernia stapler
Endopath ES reusable endoscopic stapler
Endopath ETS-FLEX endoscopic articulating linear cutter
Endopath EZ-RF linear cutter and coagulation device
Endopath EZ45 endoscopic linear cutter
Endopath EZ45 No Knife endoscopic linear stapler
Endopath EZ46 No Knife endoscopic linear stapler
Endopath laparoscopic trocar
Endopath linear cutter
Endopath multifeed stapler
Endopath no-knife stapler
Endopath Optiview optical surgical obturator
Endopath TriStar trocar
Endopath trocar
Endopath Ultra Veress needle
endopelvic fascia
endophlebitis hepatica obliterans
Endopouch Pro specimen bag
Endo-P-Probe for endorectal ultrasonography
endoprosthesis (see also *prosthesis*)
  biliary
  double-lumen
  double-pigtail
  IntraStent Double Strut biliary
  IntraStent Double Strut XS
  IntraStent LP biliary
  large-bore bile duct
  Medoc-Celestin
  Procter-Livingstone
  Wallstent enteral
  Wilson-Cook
endorectal ileal pouch
endorectal ileal pull-through
endorectal pull-through procedure
Endo Retract
end-organ response
Endosac specimen bag
endoscope (see also *endoscopy*)
  ACMI rigid laparoscope
  ACMI S3565 flexible sigmoidoscope
  Adler Eagle Vision laparoscope
  Adler P.L.U.S. laparoscope
  adult endoscope
  AESOP (Automated Endoscopic System for Optimal Positioning)
  AESOP 2000; 3000
  AngioLaz Medi-Vu endoscope
  anoscope (proctoscope)
  Arthrotek rigid laparoscope
  Baho endoscope
  Bard flexible endoscope
  borescope
  Boutin thoracoscope
  bronchoscope
  Bryan rigid laparoscope

endoscope *(cont.)*
- Buie sigmoidoscope
- Cabot cystoscope
- Cabot rigid laparoscope
- CF-200Z Olympus colonoscope
- CF-UM3 echocolonoscope
- Cho/Dyonics two-portal endoscopic system
- choledochofiberscope
- Circon rigid laparoscope
- Circon videohydrothoracoscope
- colonoscope
- Comeg rigid laparoscope
- Concept/Linvatec hysteroscope
- Concept/Linvatec laparoscope
- Concept rigid laparoscope
- Cooper Surgical cystoscope
- Cor/Tek laparoscope
- Cuda 0° 10 mm rigid laparoscope
- cystoscope
- Czaja-McCaffrey rigid laparoscope
- Demir rigid laparoscope
- Desormaux endoscope
- double-channel endoscope
- double-puncture laparoscope
- duodenoscope
- Dyonics cystoscope
- Dyonics laparoscope
- Dyonics rod-lens endoscope
- Dyonics 3625 laparoscope
- Dyonics 7208130 rigid laparoscope
- Dyonics 8007 rigid laparoscope
- Dyonics 8017 laparoscope
- Dyonics 0° 10 mm rigid laparoscope
- echocolonoscope
- echogastroscope
- Eder 180° 10 mm rigid laparoscope
- Effner/Arthrotek laparoscope
- Effner rigid laparoscope
- Elder Helio cystoscope
- ElMed rigid laparoscope
- Endius spinal endoscopic camera
- EndoALPHA integrated end surgical system

endoscope *(cont.)*
- Endolap rigid laparoscope
- Endolase rigid laparoscope
- endometrial resection and ablation (ERA) resectoscope sheath
- enteroscope
- esophagoscope
- EVII endoscopic video system
- Fansler-Ives anoscope
- FCS-ML gastroscope
- fiberoptic choledochoscope
- fiberoptic gastroscope
- fiberoptic laryngoscope
- fiberoptic sigmoidoscope
- fiberscope
- flexible sigmoidoscope
- flexible, steerable nasolaryngopharyngoscope
- Fujinon EVS-E flexible sigmoidoscope
- Fujinon FG-100FP flexible gastroscope
- Fujinon FG-100PE flexible gastroscope
- Fujinon PRO-PC flexible sigmoidoscope
- Fujinon SIG-E2 flexible sigmoidoscope
- Fujinon SIG-EK flexible sigmoidoscope
- Fujinon SIG-ET flexible sigmoidoscope
- Fujinon SIG-PC flexible sigmoidoscope
- Fujinon UGI-PE flexible gastroscope
- gastroscope
- Heine sigmoidoscope
- Henke-Sass rigid laparoscope
- Henke-Sass Wolf laparoscope
- Hirschman anoscope
- Hopkins rigid glass lens
- Iglesias fiberoptic resectoscope
- InjecTx customized cystoscope
- Inspex rigid laparoscope

endoscope *(cont.)*
InstrumentMakar laparoscope
intubating laryngoscope
InVISION to endoscope
ITI (Instrument Technology Inc.) 0.5 mm rigid borescope
Jacobscope-Palmer laparoscope
Jarit cystoscope
Jarit 0° 10 mm rigid laparoscope
Jarit 0° 5 mm rigid laparoscope
Jasan flexible fiberoptic sigmoido-scope
Jasan JFE choledochoscope
Jasan rigid proctoscope
Kantor-Berci videolaryngoscope
Karl Storz rigid laparoscope
Kelly anoscope
Kendall esophageal sonascope
Killian-Lynch laryngoscope
Kleinsasser anterior commissure laryngoscope
KLI rigid borescope
laparoscope
laser laparoscope
Linvatec 7570R 0° 10 mm rigid laparoscope
Linvatec rigid laparoscope
Lloyd Davies sigmoidoscope
MacIntosh laryngoscope
Marlow rigid laparoscope
Marlow videolaparoscope
Medi-Vu
Miller laryngoscope
MIS Source sigmoidoscope
monoscopic endoscope
"mother-baby" dual endoscope
Mueller 0° 5 mm rigid laparoscope
nasolaryngopharyngoscope
Naunton Morgan proctoscope
Navigator flexible endoscope
new variable stiffness (VS) colono-scope
Olympus A5214 0° 10 mm rigid laparoscope

endoscope *(cont.)*
Olympus A5215 rigid laparoscopic system
Olympus A5254 0° 10mm rigid laparoscope
Olympus A5255 30° 10 mm rigid laparoscope
Olympus A5257 0° 10 mm rigid laparoscope
Olympus A5258 rigid 0° 10 mm rigid laparoscope
Olympus CF-1T10L flexible gastroscope
Olympus CF-1T20L flexible gastroscope
Olympus CF-P20L flexible gastro-scope
Olympus CF-10L flexible sigmoido-scope
Olympus CF-20L flexible gastro-scope
Olympus CF-100S flexible sigmoidoscope
Olympus CF-140I videocolono-scope
Olympus CF-140L videocolono-scope
Olympus CF-140S videocolono-scope
Olympus CF-1TS2 flexible sigmoidoscope
Olympus CF-1T100L forward-viewing videocolonoscope
Olympus CF-1T10L flexible gastroscope
Olympus CF-1T10L flexible therapeutic colonoscope
Olympus CF-1T20L flexible gastroscope
Olympus CF-1T20L flexible therapeutic colonoscope
Olympus CF-1TS2 flexible sigmoidoscope
Olympus CF-200Z colonoscope

endoscope *(cont.)*
Olympus CF-20L flexible colonoscope
Olympus CF-20L flexible gastroscope
Olympus CF-30L flexible colonoscope
Olympus CF-P10S flexible sigmoidoscope
Olympus CF-P20L flexible gastroscope
Olympus CF-Q160AL/I innoflex videocolonoscope
Olympus CF-Q160L/I/S video sigmoidoscope
Olympus CF-V10S sigmoidoscope
Olympus CF-Q140I
Olympus CF-Q160L/I/S video-colonoscope
Olympus CF-Q160L/I/S video-sigmoidoscope
Olympus CHF-B20 transduodenal choledochofiberscope
Olympus CHF-BP30 transduodenal choledochofiberscope
Olympus CHF-CB30 choledocho-scope
Olympus CHF-P20 choledocho-scope
Olympus CHF-P20Q choledocho-scope
Olympus CPF-P10-S sigmoidoscope
Olympus CV-1 endoscopic system
Olympus CV-100 endoscopic system
Olympus CYF-3 OES cystofiber-scope
Olympus cystoscope
Olympus Evis Exera 160 endoscope
Olympus Evis 140 endoscope reprocessing system
Olympus Evis Q-200V video
Olympus fiberoptic sigmoidoscope
Olympus flexible sigmoidoscope
Olympus GF-UM130 ultrasound gastroscope

endoscope *(cont.)*
Olympus GF-UM3 and CF-UM20 ultrasonic
Olympus GIF-EUM2 echoendo-scope
Olympus GIF-HM gastroscope
Olympus GIF-K gastroscope
Olympus GIF-N30 gastrofibero-scope
Olympus GIF-100 videogastroscope
Olympus GIF-140
Olympus GIF-160
Olympus GIF-1T10 flexible thera-peutic gastroscope
Olympus GIF-1T10 and GIF20 echoendoscope
Olympus GIF-1T10 flexible thera-peutic gastroscope
Olympus GIF-1T140 videogastro-scope
Olympus GIF-1TV10 flexible gastroscope
Olympus GIF-2T10 flexible gastro-scope
Olympus GIF-2T20 flexible thera-peutic gastroscope
Olympus GIF-N30 gastrofibero-scope
Olympus GIF-P140 videogastro-scope
Olympus GIF-PQ20 flexible gastro-scope
Olympus GIF-PV10 pediatric video-gastroscope
Olympus GIF-Q140 videogastro-scope
Olympus GIF-Q160 gastrointestinal videoscope
Olympus GIF-XP20 flexible gastro-scope
Olympus GIF-XQ140 videogastro-scope
Olympus GIF-XQ20 flexible multi-purpose gastroscope

endoscope *(cont.)*
Olympus GIF-XQ30 flexible multipurpose gastroscope
Olympus GIF-XT30 gastrofiberoscope
Olympus GIF-XP160 SlimSIGHT gastrointestinal videoscope
Olympus GIF-XP20 flexible gastroscope
Olympus GIF-XQ140 videogastroscope
Olympus GIF-XQ20 flexible multipurpose gastroscope
Olympus GIF-XQ30 flexible multipurpose gastroscope
Olympus GIF-XT30 gastrofiberoscope
Olympus GIF-XV10 videogastroscope
Olympus HYF-XP flexible hysteroscope
Olympus hysteroscope
Olympus JF-1T20 flexible therapeutic duodenoscope
Olympus JF-1T30 flexible therapeutic duodenoscope
Olympus JF-UM20 echoendoscope
Olympus JF1T10 fiberoptic duodenoscope
Olympus OSF flexible sigmoidoscope
Olympus OSF-2 flexible sigmoidoscope
Olympus OSF-235 flexible sigmoidoscope
Olympus PCF-10 flexible pediatric colonoscope
Olympus PCF-140I pediatric video colonoscope
Olympus PCF-140L pediatric video colonoscope
Olympus PCF-160AL/I video colonoscope
Olympus PJF-7.5 pediatric duodenofiberscope

endoscope *(cont.)*
Olympus SIF-100 video push enteroscope
Olympus SIF-M magnifying enteroscope
Olympus SIF10 enteroscope
Olympus SlimSIGHT gastrointestinal videoscope
Olympus TGF-2D flexible gastroscope
Olympus TJF-100
Olympus TJF-160F videoduodenoscope
Olympus TJF-M20
Olympus URF-P2 translaparoscopic choledochofiberscope
Olympus VU-M2 and XIF-UM3 echoendoscope
Olympus XQ230 gastroscope
Optik laparoscope
Optik rigid laparoscope
ORI electronic endoscopy system
otoscope
panendoscope
Pentax EC-3430F videocolonoscope
Pentax EC-3430L videocolonscope
Pentax EC-3440F videocolonoscope
Pentax EC-3440L videocolonoscope
Pentax EC-3830 videocolonoscope
Pentax EC-3830L videocolonoscope
Pentax EC-3830TL videocolonoscope
Pentax EC-3840L videocolonoscope
Pentax EC-3840T videocolonoscope
Pentax ECN-1530 videocholedochonephroscope
Pentax ED-3430T videoduodenoscope

endoscope *(cont.)*
- Pentax ED-3440T videoduodenoscope
- Pentax EG-1840 videogastroscope
- Pentax EG-2530 gastroscope
- Pentax EG-2540 videogastroscope
- Pentax EG-2731 gastroscope
- Pentax EG-2901 flexible gastroscope
- Pentax EG-2930 gastroscope
- Pentax EG-2940 videogastroscope
- Pentax EG-3430 videogastroscope
- Pentax EG-3440 videogastroscope
- Pentax EG-3830T videogastroscope
- Pentax EG-3840T videogastroscope
- Pentax ES-3830 videosigmoidoscope
- Pentax ES-3840 videosigmoidoscope
- Pentax FC-38LX flexible gastroscope
- Pentax FG-24V fiberoptic gastroscope
- Pentax FG-29H flexible gastroscope
- Pentax FG-29V fiberoptic gastroscope
- Pentax FG-29X flexible gastroscope
- Pentax EG-1840 videogastroscope
- Pentax EG-2530 videogastroscope
- Pentax EG-2540 videogastroscope
- Pentax EG-2731 videogastroscope
- Pentax EG-2901 flexible gastroscope
- Pentax EG-2930 videogastroscope
- Pentax EG-2940 videogastroscope
- Pentax EG-3430 videogastroscope
- Pentax EG-3440 videogastroscope
- Pentax EG-3830T videogastroscope
- Pentax EG-3840T videogastroscope
- Pentax ES-3830 videosigmoidoscope
- Pentax ES-3840 videoendoscope
- Pentax EUP-EC124 ultrasound gastroscope

endoscope *(cont.)*
- Pentax FCN-15H flexible choledochoscope
- Pentax FC-38LV fiberoptic colonoscope
- Pentax FC-38LX flexible gastroscope
- Pentax FC-38MV fiberoptic colonoscope
- Pentax FD-34V fiberoptic endoscope
- Pentax fiberoptic sigmoidoscope
- Pentax flexible sigmoidoscope
- Pentax FG-24V fiberoptic gastroscope
- Pentax FG-29H flexible gastroscope
- Pentax FG-29V fiberoptic gastroscope
- Pentax FG-29X flexible gastroscope
- Pentax FG-36UX echoendoscope
- Pentax FS flexible sigmoidoscope
- Pentax FS-34A flexible sigmoidoscope
- Pentax FS-34V fiberoptic sigmoidoscope
- Pentax FS-38H flexible sigmoidoscope
- Pentax-Hitachi FG32UA endosonographic system
- Pentax SIG-E2 fiberoptic sigmoidoscope
- Pentax W fiberoptic endoscope
- PercScope percutaneous diskectomy
- pharyngoscope
- Pilling rigid laparoscope
- push enteroscope
- rectoscope (proctoscope)
- Reichert fiberoptic sigmoidoscope
- Reichert flexible sigmoidoscope
- Reichert MH-1 flexible sigmoidoscope
- Reichert SC-48 flexible sigmoidoscope
- REI rigid laparoscope

endoscope *(cont.)*
- resectoscope
- Rhinoline endoscopic system
- Riester economy otoscope
- rigid endoscope
- rigid-lens endoscope
- rigid sigmoidoscope
- semirigid sigmoidoscope
- Schindler semiflexible gastroscope
- self-retaining laryngoscope
- Semm rigid laparoscope
- Semm/Wisap laparoscope
- side-viewing
- SIF10 Olympus enteroscope
- sigmoidoscope
- SITEtrac
- Solos cystoscope
- Solos rigid laparoscope
- Sonde enteroscope
- SP-501 Sonoprobe endoscopy
- specialized tissue aspirating resectoscope (STAR)
- Spiess
- SpineScope percutaneous
- STAR (specialized tissue-aspirating resectoscope)
- StereoEndoscope
- stereotaxic
- St. Mark's sigmoidoscope
- Storz bronchoscope
- Storz cystoscope
- Storz esophagoscope
- Storz hysteroscope
- Storz resectoscope
- Storz rigid laparoscope
- Storz 26003 AP 0° 10 mm rigid laparoscope
- Storz 26033 AP 0° 10 mm rigid laparoscope
- Storz 26033 BP 0° 10 mm rigid laparoscope
- Stryker 380-10 0° 10 mm rigid laparoscope

endoscope *(cont.)*
- Stryker 380-11 0° 10 mm rigid laparoscope
- Stryker 380-12 30° 10 mm rigid laparoscope
- Surgenomic
- SurgiScope
- Syringe Avitene delivery system
- 3-Dscope laparoscope
- Toshiba video
- transparent cap-fitted
- Tuttle proctoscope
- two-channel
- URF-P2 choledochoscope
- variable stiffness
- VideoHydro laparoscope
- videoscope
- videoresectoscope
- videothoracoscope
- Visicath
- V. Mueller rigid laparoscope
- Weck-Baggish rigid laparoscope
- Weck 110405 0° 5 mm rigid laparoscope
- Weck 110800 rigid laparoscope
- Weck operating laparoscope
- Weck 0° 10 mm rigid laparoscope
- Welch Allyn flexible sigmoidoscope
- Welch Allyn videosigmoidoscope
- Wolf 8937.31 0° 10 mm rigid laser laparoscope
- Wolf Lumina rigid laparoscope
- Wolf 170° 12 mm rigid laparoscope
- Wolf 7732 rigid laparoscope
- Wolf 8934.40 rigid laparoscope
- Wolf rigid laparoscope
- Wolf 10/5 (L-angle) operative laparoscope
- Wolf videoresectoscope
- WuScope system
- Xillix LIFE-GI fluorescence endoscopy System
- XQ230 Olympus gastroscope

endoscope *(cont.)*
Zeiss Endolive endoscope
Zimmer rigid
endoscope-assisted microneurosurgery
endoscope-controlled microneurosurgery
endoscopic ablation
endoscopic antireflux procedure
endoscopic argon beam plasma coagulation
endoscopic articulating (EAS) stapler
endoscopic-assisted transumbilical augmentation mammoplasty
endoscopic balloon sphincteroplasty (EBS)
endoscopic band ligation (EBL)
endoscopic BiCAP probe
endoscopic bile duct procedure
endoscopic biliary decompression
endoscopic biliary drainage
endoscopic biliary endoprosthesis
endoscopic biliary stent
endoscopic biopsy
endoscopic biopsy forceps
endoscopic biopsy surveillance
endoscopic bougienage
endoscopic catheterization
endoscopic confocal microscopy
endoscopic cryoablation
endoscopic cryotherapy
endoscopic cystogastrostomy
endoscopic decompression
endoscopic dilation
endoscopic Doppler ultrasound
endoscopic drainage
endoscopic dual tip Kittner
endoscopic forceps
endoscopic gastroplasty
endoscopic grasping forceps
endoscopic heat probe
endoscopic injection
endoscopic injection sclerosis
endoscopic injection therapy (EIT)
endoscopic intraperitoneal perforation
endoscopic laser cautery
endoscopic laser cholecystectomy
endoscopic ligation
endoscopic light source
halogen
strobe flash
xenon flash
endoscopic mucosal ablation
endoscopic mucosal resection (EMR)
endoscopic mucosectomy
endoscopic multifeed (EMS) TA-90 stapler
endoscopic optical coherence tomography (EOCT)
endoscopic papillectomy (EP)
endoscopic papillotomy
endoscopic polypectomy
endoscopic prosthesis
endoscopic resection
endoscopic retrograde balloon dilation
endoscopic retrograde biliary drainage (ERBD)
endoscopic retrograde cholangiography (ERC)
endoscopic retrograde cholangiopancreatography (ERCP)
endoscopic retrograde cholangiopancreatography/endoscopic sphincterotomy (ERCP/ES)
endoscopic retrograde parenchymography (ERP)
endoscopic reversal technique
endoscopic sclerotherapy
endoscopic sewing machine technique
endoscopic small bowel biopsy
endoscopic snare
endoscopic sonography
endoscopic sphincterotomy (ES)
endoscopic stent placement
endoscopic suction-cap technique
endoscopic suction cup
endoscopic surveillance
endoscopic suture-cutting forceps
endoscopic suturing

endoscopic tissue sampling
endoscopic transaxillary augmentation mammoplasty
endoscopic transpapillary catheterization of the gallbladder (ETCG)
endoscopic ultrasonography (EUS)
endoscopic ultrasound (EUS)
endoscopic ultrasound-assisted band ligation
endoscopic ultrasound-guided fine-needle aspiration (EUS-FNA)
endoscopic variceal ligation (EVL)
endoscopic washing pipe
endoscopic Water Pik
endoscopic Zenker diverticulectomy with cricopharyngeal myotomy
endoscopically
endoscopist, gastrointestinal
endoscopy
  biliary
  gastrointestinal
  pancreatic
  small intestinal
  surveillance
  therapeutic
  transoral
  upper gastrointestinal
endoscopy-negative reflux disease (ENRD)
endoscopy with tumor ablation
Endo Mini Shears
Endo Shears cutter
endosonography
Endosound endoscopic ultrasound catheter
endostaple
Endostatin protein
Endo Stitch knot-tying device
Endo Stitch suture device
Endo Suture introducer
Endotak C lead catheter
endothelial cells
endothelial lining
endothelium
endotherapy, pancreatic
endotoxemia, portal and systemic
endotoxin-binding protein
endotoxin concentration
endotoxin level
Endotrac cannula
Endotrac elevator
endotracheal anesthesia
endotracheal intubation
endotracheal tube
endotracheal tube intubation
Endotrac probe
Endotrac rasp
Endotrac retractor
Endotrol tracheal tube
Endotube Rae-Flex oral
Endo Universal device
endovascular coagulation of blood vessel
endovascular glue
endovascular stent graft
Endoview endoscopy camera
end plate
end-sigmoid colostomy
end-stage cirrhosis
end-stage diverticula
end-stage liver disease (ESLD)
end-stage renal disease (ESRD)
end-to-back bowel anastomosis
end-to-end anastomosis (EEA) stapler
end-to-end invaginating anastomosis
end-to-end jejunoileal bypass
end-to-end suture
end-to-side anastomosis
end-to-side choledochojejunostomy
end-to-side jejunoileal bypass
end-to-side portocaval shunt
end-to-side splenorenal shunt
end-to-side suture
Enecat (barium sulfate)
enema (see also *bowel prep*)
  air-contrast barium
  analeptic enema
  barium (BE)

enema *(cont.)*
  blind
  Colomed
  contrast
  Cortenema retention
  double-contrast air barium
  5-ASA (5-aminosalicylic acid)
  flatus
  Fleet
  Fleet Bisacodyl
  Fleet Mineral Oil
  full-column barium
  gastrografin
  hydrocortisone
  hydrogen peroxide
  Kayexalate
  lactulose
  mesalamine
  methylene blue
  nuclear
  oil retention
  phosphosoda
  prednisolone
  prosphate
  retention
  Rowasa
  saline cleansing
  single-contrast barium
  small bowel
  soapsuds (SSE)
  steroid foam
  sulfasalazine
  tap water
  theophylline olamine
  "3H"
  water soluble contrast
enema contrast study
enemas until clear
energy-producing respiratory processes
energy, radiofrequency
en face ("ahn fahs")
enflurane
Enforcer SDS coronary stent
Engel-May nail
Engel plaster saw
Engerix-B (hepatitis B virus vaccine, recombinant)
engorgement of esophageal venous plexus (pl. plexi)
Enhancer (barium sulfate)
enhancer, video signal
Enker brain retractor
enlarged lymph node
enlarged spleen
enlarged thymus
enlarged uterus
enlargement
  gland
  lymph node
  nodular thyroid
  pituitary
  splenic
enlarging cystic lesion
en masse ("removed en masse")
Enproct disposable anoscope
enprostil
ENRD (endoscopy-negative reflux disease)
ENSI syringe
ensiform appendix
EnSite cardiac catheter
ensure hemostasis
Ensure nutritional therapy
ENT (ear, nose, and throat) scissors
entamebic abscess
Entamoeba histolytica
ENTaxis nasal packing dressing
enteral administration route
enteral alimentation
enteral diarrhea
enteral feeding
enteral nutrition (EN) therapy
  Attain
  Citrotein
  Compleat Modified Formula
  Comply
  Ensure
  Entrition

enteral *(cont.)*
Epulor
Fiberlan
Forta Shake
Glucerna
Immun-Aid
Impact
Introlan Half-Strength
Introlite
Isocal
Isocal HCN
Isocal HN
Isosource HN
Isotein HN
Jevity
Kindercal
Lipisorb
Lonalac
Magnacal
Meritene
MET-Rx
Neocate One +
Nitrolan
Nutraloric
Nutren
Nutrilan
Osmolite
Osmolite HN
Peptamen
Pre-Attain
Precision High Nitrogen
Precision LR
Profiber
Propimex-2
Reabilan
Reabilan HN
Replete
Resource
Resource Plus
Stresstein
Sustacal
Sustagen
Tolerex
TraumaCal

enteral *(cont.)*
Travasorb HN
Travasorb MCT
Travasorb SID
TwoCal HN
Tyrex-2
Ultracal
Vital High Nitrogen
enterically transmitted non-A, non-B (ENANB) hepatitis (former name)
enteric bacillus
enteric-coated aspirin
enteric-coated capsule
enteric colibacillosis
enteric contents
enteric cyst
enteric drainage
enteric fever
enteric fistula
enteric orphan virus
enterinsular axis
enteritis (see also *gastroenteritis*)
Campylobacter
chronic ischemic
Clostridium difficile
Crohn regional
graft
granulomatous
infectious
ischemic
nonspecific
radiation
regional
segmental
ulcerative
viral
enteroadherent *E. coli* (EAEC)
Enterobacter agglomerans
Enterobacter cloacae
Enterobacter freundii
Enterobacter gergoviae
Enterobacter hafnia
Enterobacter liquefaciens
Enterobacter sakazakii

enterobacterial common antigen (ECA)
enterobiasis
enterobiliary
Enterobius vermicularis (pinworm)
enterocele sac
enterocele, vaginal
enterochromaffin cell
enterocleisis, omental
enteroclysis
enterococcus (pl. enterococci)
Enterococcus avium
Enterococcus faecalis
Enterococcus faecium
enterocolic fistula
enterocolitis (see also *colitis*)
  antibiotic-induced
  bacterial
  chronic ischemic
  fulminant
  granulomatous
  hemorrhagic
  Hirschsprung-associated (HAEC)
  ischemic
  necrotizing (NEC)
  pseudomembranous
  regional
  ulcerative
enterocutaneous fistula
enterocystoplasty
enterocyte
enterocytopathogenic human orphan (ECHO) virus
Enterodophilus
enteroenteral fistula
enteroenteric fistula
enteroenterostomy
enterogastritis
enterogenous cyst
enterohemorrhagic *E. coli* (EHEC)
enterohepatic circulation
enteroinsular axis
enteroinvasive *E. coli* (EIEC)
enterokinase
enterolith
enterolithotomy
enterolysis
enteropathic organism
enteropathogenic *E. coli* (EPEC)
enteropathy
  bile salt-losing
  diabetic
  exudative
  gluten
  hypercatabolic protein-losing
  lymphangiectatic protein-losing
  protein-losing
  terminal hemorrhagic
enteroperitoneal abscess
enteroptosis
enterorrhaphy
enteroscope (see *endoscope*)
  magnifying
  Olympus SIF10
  push
  SIF10 Olympus
  Sonde
  temporary
  tube
  video push
enteroscopy
enterospasm
enterostenosis
enterostomal therapist
enterostomy, cutaneous
EnteroTest
EnteroTest Pediatric
enterotomy scissors
enterotoxigenic *E. coli* (ETEC)
enterotoxin diarrhea
enterourethral fistula
enterovaginal fistula
enterovesical fistula
Enterovirus
Entero Vu (barium sulfate for suspension)
Enterra gastric stimulation device
Enterra gastrointestinal "pacemaker"
Enteryx biopolymer material

entire bowel wall
Entocort CR (budesonide)
Entolase (lipase; protease)
Entozyme (lipase; protease)
entrapment
  bowel
  catheter
  nerve
Entree Plus
Entree II laparoscopic trocar and cannula systems
Entree thoracoscopy trocar and cannula
EntriStar PEG (percutaneous endoscopic gastrostomy) tube
Entrition nutritional therapy
Entrobar (barium sulfate [methylcellulose diluent])
enucleation of thrombosed hemorrhoid
enucleation of tumor
enucleation scissors
enucleator, gland
envelope, axillary
enveloping scar tissue
Enview camera
EnVision autoclavable 3CCD (three chip) camera head
enzyme
  brancher
  cyclophilin
  debrancher
  digestive
  DME (drug-metabolizing)
  fumarylacetoacetase parahydroxyphenylpyruvic acid (p-HPPA) oxidase
  lactase
  lipase
  lipolytic
  liver
  liver phosphorylase
  medium chain acyl-CoA dehydrogenase
  pancreatic
  protease digestive

enzyme *(cont.)*
  proteinase
  proteolytic
  serum liver
enzyme-linked immunoassay (EIA-2)
enzyme linked immunosorbent assay (ELISA)
enzyme panel
enzyme replacement therapy
EOCT (endoscopic optical coherence tomography)
EORTC (European Organization for Research and Treatment of Cancer)
eosinophil (also eosinophile)
eosinophilic esophagitis
eosinophilic gastritis
eosinophilic gastroenteritis
eosinophilic gastroenteritis syndrome
eosinophilic granuloma
eosinophilic material
eosinophil smear
eosphagogastric orifice
EOTC (endoscopic optical coherence tomography)
EP (endoscopic papillectomy)
EPC pain control
EPEC (enteropathogenic *E. coli*)
"epi" (epinephrine)
Epi-C (barium sulfate)
Epic ophthalmic 3-in-1 laser
epicritic pain
epidemic gastroenteritis
epidemic gastroenteritis virus
epidemic keratoconjunctivitis virus
epidemic nonbacterial gastroenteritis
epidemic vomiting
epidermal carcinoma
epidermal growth factor (EGF)
epidermal inclusion cyst
epidermoid carcinoma
epidermoid cyst
epidermoid skin cysts and benign craniofacial and long bone tumors (Gardner syndrome)

epidermolysis bullosa dystrophica
epidural abscess
epidural anesthesia
epidural blood patch graft
epidural catheter
epidural hematoma
epidural hemorrhage
Epigard composite wound dressing
epigastralgia
epigastric angle
epigastric discomfort
epigastric distress
epigastric fold
epigastric hernia
epigastric incision
epigastric mass
epigastric pain
epigastric reflex
epigastric region
epigastric spot
epigastric tenderness
epigastric vessel
epigastrium
epiglottis
EpiLaser laser
Epi-Lock wound dressing
epinephrine ("epi")
epinephrine and cisplatin injectable gel
epinephrine level
epinephrine/norepinephrine level
epiphrenic diverticulum
epiphyseal bar, excision of
epiphyseal cartilage plate
epiphyseal ischemic necrosis
epiphyseal knife
epiphyseal staple
epiplocele
epiploectomy
epiploic appendage
epiploic appendix
epiploon abscess
epirubicin HCl
episiotomy scissors
episodic colic
episodic vomiting
epistaxis dressing
epitendineum
epithelial cell lining
epithelial cell thymoma
epithelial component
epithelial edema
epithelial hyperplasia
epithelialization
epithelioid hemangioendothelioma
epithelium
  Barrett
  bile duct
  columnar
  crypt
  glandular
  junctional
  pseudostratified
  pyramidal
  salmon-pink
  squamous
  stratified
  surface
  transitional
  villous
epithelium crypt
epitheloid leiomyoma
epitope, alpha-Gal
EpiTouch laser
Epivir-HBV (lamivudine)
Epley maneuver
EPO (epoetin alfa)
epoetin alfa
Eppendorf biopsy forceps
Eppendorf-Tischler biopsy forceps
Epstein-Barr virus (EBV) infection
Epstein bone rasp
Epstein neurological hammer
EPT (endoscopic papillotomy)
EPTFE (expanded polytetrafluoro-ethylene) vascular suture
Epulor nutritional therapy
Equalactin (calcium polycarbophil)
Equilet (calcium carbonate)

equivocal pancreatic cytology
equivocal primary peristalsis
ER+ (estrogen-receptor positive)
ER– (estrogen-receptor negative)
ERA (endometrial resection and ablation) resectoscope sheath
ERBD (endoscopic retrograde biliary drainage)
ERBE Endocut electrocautery generator
erbium:YAG (Er:YAG) laser
Erbotom F2 electrocoagulation unit
ERC (endoscopic retrograde cholangiography)
ERCP (endoscopic retrograde cholangiopancreatography)
ERCP brush sample
ERCP cannula
ERCP catheter
ERCP/ES (endoscopic retrograde cholangiopancreatography/ endoscopic sphincterotomy)
ERCP-guided biopsy
ERCP-induced rupture
ERCP insertion of tube or stent
ERCP manometry
ErCr:YAG laser
Erdheim cystic medial necrosis
erect view
Ergamisol (levamisole HCl)
Ergoset (bromocriptine mesylate)
ergotamine tartrate
ER-ICA (estrogen receptor immunochemical assay)
Eriksson muscle biopsy cannula
Erlangen magnetic colostomy device
Erlangen-type papillotome
erosion
  duodenal
  gallstone
  gastric
  gastric antral
  salt and pepper duodenal
  linear
erosion into biliary tree
erosion into pericardial sac
erosion into pleural cavity
erosion or ulceration of surface
erosive duodenitis
erosive esophagitis
erosive gastritis
erosive gastroesophageal reflux disease (GERD)
erotic vomiting
ERP (endoscopic retrograde parenchymography)
eructation
erythema multiforme
erythema nodosum
erythema of abdominal wall
erythema, palmar
erythematous lesion
erythematous streak
erythrocyte sedimentation rate (ESR)
Erythroflex catheter
erythroid agenesis
erythromycin
erythromyin-induced cholecystitis
ES (endoscopic sphincterotomy)
Esberitox
Escherichia coli (E. coli)
Escherichia coli granuloma
Escherichia coli melanosis
Escherichia coli pneumatosis
Escherichia coli polyposis
Escherichia coli taeniae
Escherichia coli O157:H7 assay
E.S.I. Bite Block
ESI instrument adapter to AMCD cord
ESLD (end-stage liver disease)
Esmarch bandage
Esmarch dressing
Esmarch plaster knife
Esmarch plaster scissors
Esmarch plaster shears
esomeprazole magnesium
EsophaCoil self-expanding esophageal stent
esophageal A ring

esophageal achalasia
esophageal acid infusion test
esophageal adenocarcinoma
esophageal angina
esophageal aperistalsis
esophageal artery of aorta
esophageal artery of inferior thyroid
esophageal atresia
esophageal balloon
esophageal balloon technique
esophageal body
esophageal body motor function
esophageal bougie
esophageal bougienage
esophageal B ring
esophageal brushing
esophageal cancer
esophageal candidiasis
esophageal clearing
esophageal colic
esophageal contractile ring
esophageal contraction
esophageal cytomegalovirus
esophageal degeneration
esophageal dilatation
esophageal dilation
esophageal diverticulum
esophageal/duodenal decompression
  device
esophageal dyskinesia
esophageal dysmotility
esophageal dysphagia
esophageal electrocardiogram
esophageal foreign body
esophageal function test
esophageal gastric tube airways (EGTA)
esophageal gland
esophageal groove of liver
esophageal hernia
esophageal hiatal hernia
esophageal hiatus
esophageal impression
esophageal inlet
esophageal intubation
esophageal-jejunal anastomosis
esophageal lead
esophageal leiomyoma
esophageal lengthening
esophageal leukoplakia
esophageal lumen
esophageal manometry
esophageal motility disorder
esophageal motility study
esophageal mucosa
esophageal mucosal ring
esophageal muscular ring
esophageal myotomy
esophageal myotomy via thoracoscopy
esophageal obstruction
esophageal obturator airway
esophageal opening
esophageal pain
esophageal peristaltic pressure
esophageal pH
esophageal pH analysis
esophageal pH monitoring
esophageal pH test
esophageal plexus
esophageal plexus of nerves
esophageal pouch
esophageal pressure recording
esophageal reflux
esophageal reflux disease
esophageal resection
esophageal ring, distal
esophageal rupture
esophageal shunt
esophageal sling procedure
esophageal sound
esophageal spasm, diffuse
esophageal spasm mimicking angina
esophageal spasm mimicking
  myocardial infarction
esophageal sphincter
  hypertensive
  inferior
esophageal stenosis
esophageal stent

esophageal stricture
esophageal tear
esophageal temperature
esophageal temperature probe
esophageal transection with para-esophagogastric devascularization
esophageal transit time
esophageal tube
esophageal tumor
esophageal ulceration
esophageal variceal bleeding
esophageal variceal sclerosis
esophageal variceal sclerotherapy
esophageal varices, direct ligation of
esophageal varicosities
esophageal varix (pl. varices)
esophageal vein
esophageal venous plexus (pl. plexi)
esophageal web
esophageal window
esophageal Z-Stent with Dua antireflux valve
esophagectomy
  Ivor Lewis
  Ivor Lewis two-stage subtotal
  minimally invasive
  near-total
  open
  thoracoabdominal
  total
  total thoracic
  transhiatal
  transhiatal blunt
esophagitis
  acid-pepsin reflux
  alkaline
  bacterial
  Barrett
  Candida
  Candida albicans esophagitis
  candidal
  chemical
  chronic peptic
  CMV (cytomegalovirus)
esophagitis *(cont.)*
  corrosive
  eosinophilic
  erosive
  fungal
  herpetic
  infectious
  nonreflux
  peptic
  pill
  polycystic chronic
  postoperative
  radiation
  reflux (RE)
  regurgitant
  retention
  stasis
  ulcerative
esophagocele, acquired
esophagocolic anastomosis
esophagodiverticulostomy
esophagoduodenostomy
esophagoenterostomy
esophagogastrectomy
esophagogastric (EG) junction
esophagogastric anastomosis
esophagogastric complex
esophagogastric fat pad
esophagogastric fundoplasty with fundic patch (Thal-Nissen procedure)
esophagogastric intubation
esophagogastric junction
esophagogastric orifice
esophagogastric sphincter
esophagogastric tamponade
esophagogastric varices
esophagogastric vestibule
esophagogastroduodenoscopy (EGD), small-caliber
esophagogastroplasty
esophagogastroscopy
  Abbott
  Clagett Barrett

esophagogastroscopy *(cont.)*
intrathoracic
Johnson
Thal
Woodward
esophagogastrostomy
cervical
intrathoracic
esophagoglottal closure reflex
esophagogram (see *esophagram*)
esophagojejunostomy
end-to-end
end-to-side
loop
mechanical
mediastinal
Roux-en-Y
Roux-Y
stapled
transhiatal
esophagomyotomy
circumferential
Heller
laparoscopic
modified Heller
open
thoracic short
thoracoscopic
esophagoplasty
balloon
behind-sternum colon
cervical
colic patch
colonic
gastric patch
gastric tube
gastric tubular
Grondahl-Finney
intrathoracic
laparoscopic
large intestine
one-stage posterior mediastinal
patch
pectoralis myocutaneous

esophagoplasty *(cont.)*
pediatric
peptic
reverse gastric tube
single-step
subtotal
transmediastinal posterior
esophagosalivary reflex
esophagoscope (see also *endoscope*)
cine-esophagoscope
double-channel
Eder-Hufford rigid
Holinger
Jackson
Jesberg
Kelling
Kendall esophageal sonascope
large-bore rigid
Negus rigid
Olympus EF
Schindler
Storz
esophagospasm
esophagostenosis
esophagostomy
esophagotomy
cervical approach
distal
feeding
subtotal
thoracic approach
vertical
esophagotracheal (ET) junction
esophagram, barium
esophagus
achalasia of
aperistaltic
Barrett
B ring of
columnar-lined
corkscrew
curling
distal
dyssynergic

esophagus *(cont.)*
  nutcracker
  scleroderma-like
  short-segment Barrett
  spastic
  tortuous
  tubular
esophageal dilator
Espocan needle
ESR (erythrocyte sedimentation rate)
ESRD (end-stage renal disease)
essential fatty acid (EFA)
essential mixed cryoglobulinemia
essential fatty acid deficiency
Esser skin graft
esterase stain
esterified estrogen
estimated blood loss (EBL)
Estinyl (ethinyl estradiol)
Estrace (estradiol)
estradiol
Estratab (esterified estrogen)
Estridge biopsy needle
estrogen and progesterone receptors
estrogen-induced liver disease
estrogen metabolism
estrogen receptor
estrogen-receptor-negative (ER–) tumor
estrogen-receptor-positive (ER+) tumor
estrogen receptor status
estrone
Estrone Aqueous (estrone)
ESWL (extracorporeal shock-wave lithotripsy)
ESWT (extracorporeal shock-wave therapy)
ET (enterostomal therapy) nurse
ETCG (endoscopic transpapillary catheterization of the gallbladder)
ETEC (enterotoxigenic *Escherichia coli*)
Ethamolin (ethanolamine oleate)
ethanolamine oleate sclerosant
ethanol consumption
ethanolism
Ethibond Excel polyester suture
Ethibond needle
Ethibond suture
Ethicon Endo-Surgery trocar
Ethicon Excel suture
Ethicon suture
Ethicon Teflon paste
Ethiflex suture
Ethiguard blunt point
Ethilon monofilament nylon suture
ethinyl estradiol
ethmoid forceps
ethmoidolacrimal suture
ethmoidomaxillary suture
ethmovomerine plate
Ethox Corporation
Ethrane (enflurane)
ethylene oxide gas
Ethyol (amifostine)
etidocaine; epinephrine
etiology, infectious
etiology undetermined
etiology unknown
etoformin HCl
EtOH, ETOH (ethanol; ethyl alcohol)
ETOH intoxication
etomoxir
etoposide injection
e-TRAIN 110 AngioJet catheter
ET tube
Eubacterium lentum
Eubacterium limosum
Eucestoda (cestoda) tapeworm
Euglucon (glyburide)
euglycemia
EU-M30S endoscopic ultrasonography receiver
eunuchoidism
Euro bag
Euro-Collins (EC) multiorgan perfusion kit
European Association for the Study of the Liver (EASL)

European Organization for Research
  and Treatment of Cancer (EORTC)
EUS (endoluminal ultrasound)
EUS (endoscopic ultrasonography)
EUS (endoscopic ultrasound)
EUS-FNA (endoscopic ultrasound-
  guided fine-needle aspiration)
EUS-guided cytology
EUS-guided fine-needle aspiration
  biopsy
euthymic
euthyroid goiter
euthyroid sick syndrome (ESS)
euthyroid state
Evac-Q-Kwik (bisacodyl)
Evac-Q-Mag
Evac-Q-Sert
Evac-Q-Tabs
evacuant (see *bowel prep*; *enema*)
evacuating clot
evacuation, digital rectal
evacuation disorder
evacuation proctography
Evac-U-Gen
Evac-U-Lac
Evalose (lactulose)
evanescent
Evans blue dye
Evans tissue forceps
Eve tonsil snare
evening primrose oil (EPO)
eventration of diaphragm
Everest medical bipolar instrument
everolimus
Evershears and Evershears II bipolar
  scissors
eversion, rectal
evert
Evert-O-Cath catheter
everting mattress suture
EVII endoscopic video system
evisceration
EVL (endoscopic variceal ligation)
Ewald breakfast
Ewald evacuator tube
Ewald gastric lavage tube
Ewald test meal
Ewald tube
Ewing sarcoma
Ewing tumor
Ewingella americana
ex vivo liver-directed gene therapy
Ex-Lax
Ex-Lax Extra Gentle
Ex-Lax Gentle Nature
Ex-Lax Maxium Relief
Ex-Lax Stool Softener
exacerbation of pain
ExacTech blood glucose monitor
examination
  darkfield microscopic
  digital rectal
  gross
  microscopic
  physical
eXamine cholangiography catheter
exanthematous necrosis
Excalibur Plus PC electrosurgical
  generator
excavated gastric carcinoma
excavator
  curved
  House
Excelart short-bore MRI
Excel GE electrochemical glucose
  monitoring strip
Excel irrigation system
excellent visualization
Excel polyester suture
excess fluid loss in stool
excess fluid volume
excessive bleeding
excessive cortisol production
excessive mechanical ventilation
excessive PEEP
excessive postprandial antral distension
excessive splenic sequestration of red
  cells

excess TSH stimulation
exchange
  blood
  fluid
  gas
  impaired gas
Excilon sponge dressing
excimer laser
excised scar
excision
  laser hemorrhoid
  wide
excisional biopsy
excision of branchial cleft vestige
excision of primary tumor
exclusion, wide
exclusion bypass
exclusion clamp
exclusion diet
excoriation
excreta
exemestane
exenteration
exfoliation
exfoliative gastritis
Exidine-4 chlorhexidine
exisulind
exit site of catheter
exit wound
exocrine drainage from pancreatic allograft
exocrine function
exocrine gland
exocrine pancreas
exocrine pancreas disorder
exocrine pancreatic cancer
exocrine pancreatic insufficiency
exocrine secretion
exogenous bicarbonate
exogenous calcium
exogenous infection
exogenously administered
exogenous obesity
exogenous thyroid hormone
exomphalos-macroglossia-gigantism syndrome
exophthalmic goiter
exophthalmos
exophytic adenocarcinoma
exophytic carcinoma
exophytic mass
Expand-A-Band breast binder
expandable esophageal stent (EES)
expandable metal stent
expandable olive
expanded polytetrafluoroethylene
expander, tissue
expanding reamer
expansile abdominal mass
expectoration
explantation of breast implant
exploration
  abdominal
  common bile duct (CBDE)
  surgical
exploratory celiotomy
exploratory incision
exploratory laparotomy
exploratory surgery
exploring cannula
explosive diarrhea
eXpose retractor
exposure to chemicals
Express PTCA catheter
ExpressView blood glucose monitor
exquisitely tender abdomen
exquisite pain
exquisite tenderness
exsanguinated
exsanguinating hemorrhage
exsanguination
Exserohilum rostratum
extended-field radiotherapy (EFRT)
extended right hepatectomy
extended right hepatic lobectomy
extended-survival graft
extension nail
extensive DCIS (ductal carcinoma in situ)

extensive florid transmural ganglioneuromatosis
extensive intraductal carcinoma (EIC)
extensive lymph node dissection
extensive pancreatic necrosis
extensive transmural ganglioneuromatosis
exteriorization colostomy
exteriorize the colon
external anal sphincter
external beam radiotherapy and 5-FU
chemoradiotherapy
external biliary fistula
external bleeding
external clot
external fistulization of intestine
external hemorrhoid
external inguinal ring
external ligament
external oblique aponeurosis
external oblique fascia
external oblique muscle
external pancreatic fistula
external rectal sphincter
external ring
external skin tag
external spermatic fascia
external urethral orifice
external ventricular (EVD) drain
extirpation of tissue
extirpative surgery
extra-abdominal injury
extra-adrenal pheochromocytoma
extra-articular graft
extracellular concentration
extracellular fluid
extracellular material (ECM)
extracellular matrix
extracellular space
extracorporeal
extracorporeal anastomosis
extracorporeal knot
extracorporeal shock-wave lithotripsy
(ESWL)
extracorporeal shock-wave therapy
(ESWT)
eXtract specimen bag
extracting forceps
extraction balloon technique
extraction, stone
extractor
Austin Moore
bone
bone plug
break screw
Cherry
cloverleaf pin
corkscrew femoral head
endoscopic magnetic
femoral head
FIN
Fox
Glassman stone
Jewett
Kalish Duredge wire
Küntscher (Kuentscher)
Massie
metatarsal head
Moore prosthesis
Murless fetal head
Nicoll
Rousek
Schneider
staple
Sven-Johansson
Extractor three-lumen retrieval balloon
extractor-driver, Schneider
extractor-impactor, Fox
extradural abscess
extradural anesthesia
extradural hemorrhage
extrahepatic abdominal carcinoma
extrahepatic bile
extrahepatic bile duct
extrahepatic bile duct carcinoma
extrahepatic biliary atresia
extrahepatic biliary cystic dilation
extrahepatic biliary duct

extrahepatic biliary system
extrahepatic cholangiolitis
extrahepatic cholestasis
extrahepatic cirrhosis
extrahepatic duct involvement
extrahepatic malignancy
extrahepatic obstruction
extrahepatic portal venous hypertension
extrahepatic spread
extraintestinal
extraluminal retrorectal tumor
extramucosal myotomy
extramucosal stitch
extranodal extension of lymph node metastasis
extranodal growth
extranodal T cell lymphoma
extraparathyroidal tumor
extraperitoneal abscess
extraperitoneal approach
extraperitoneal fascia
extraperitoneal fat
extraperitoneal lymphocele
extraperitoneal organ
extraperitoneal space
extraperitoneal tissue
extrapyramidal movement disorder
extrasphincteric anal fistula
Extra Sport coronary guidewire
extrathyroidal invasion
extravasate
extravasated blood
extravasated contrast media
extravasation of contrast
extravasation of dye
extravasation of erythrocytes
extravascular fluid
Extra View balloon
ExtreSafe catheter
ExtreSafe needle
extrinsic lesion
extrinsic obstruction
extrinsic sphincter
extrude
extruding
extubate
extubation
exudate
exudation, peritoneal
exudative ascites
exudative colitis
exudative enteropathy
exudative peritonitis
ExuDerm hydrocolloid dressing material
Exu-Dry absorptive dressing
exulceratio simplex
eyelid edema
eye magnet
eye needle
eyepiece
eye spear sponge
eye wick sponge
EZ Detect colorectal screening test kit
E-Z Flap cranial bone plate
EZ45 thoracic linear cutter/stapler
Ez-HBT test
E-Z Tac soft tissue reattachment system
eZY WRAP abdominal binder

F, f

Fabco gauze bandage dressing
FABRase (alpha-galactosidase)
Fabrazyme (agalsidase beta)
Fabry disease
FAC (ferric ammonium citrate)
face-lift scissors
face, moon
faceplate (of ostomy appliance)
  Marlen Neoprene All-Flexible
  Torbot
  United Surgical Hypalon
faceted gallstone
facial cannula brush
facial muscle weakness
facies (surface)
  cushingoid
  moon
facies abdominalis
facies anterior corporis pancreatis
facies anterior glandulae suprarenalis
facies anterior prostatae
facies anterior renis
facies anteroinferior corporis pancreatis
facies anterosuperior corporis pancreatis
facies articularis capitis costae
facies articularis ossium
facies articularis tuberculi costae
facies colica lienis
facies colica splenis
facies costalis pulmonis
facies diaphragmatica cordis
facies diaphragmatica hepatis
facies diaphragmatica lienis
facies diaphragmatica pulmonis
facies diaphragmatica splenis
facies gastrica lienis
facies gastrica splenis
facies hepatica
facies hippocratica
facies inferior hepatis
facies inferior linguae
facies inferior pancreatis
facies inferolateralis prostatae
facies interlobaris pulmonis
facies intestinalis uteri
facies lateralis ovarii
facies lateralis testis
facies medialis ovarii
facies medialis pulmonis
facies medialis testis
facies mediastinalis pulmonis
facies posterior corporis pancreatica
facies posterior glandular suprarenalis
facies posterior hepatis
facies posterior prostatae
facies posterior renis

facies pulmonalis cordis
facies pulmonalis dextra cordis
facies pulmonalis sinistra cordis
facies renalis glandulare suprarenalis
facies renalis lienis
facies renalis splenis
facies sternocostalis cordis
facies superior hepatis
facies urethralis penis
facies vesicalis uteri
facies visceralis hepatis
facies visceralis lienis
facies visceralis splenis
FACT (Focal Angioplasty Catheter Technology)
FACT (focused appendix computed tomography)
factitial proctitis
factitious thyrotoxicosis
factor
  clotting
  coagulating
  coagulation
  growth
  intrinsic
  precipitating
  predisposing
  tissue growth (TGF)
  tumor necrosis (TNF)
factor V Leiden as a cause of Budd-Chiari syndrome
factor V Leiden heterozygote
factor VIII R:WF (von Willebrand factor)
factor VIII SQ, recombinant (ReFacto)
Factor One Medical
Fahey-Compere pin
Fahey retractor
failed nipple valve
failed shunt surgery
failing bone marrow
failure
  fulminant hepatic
  fulminant hepatocellular

failure *(cont.)*
  left-sided congestive heart
  organ
  right-sided congestive heart
failure of child to mature
failure of pancreatic ducts to fuse
failure to thrive
fair skin
falciform ligament
falciform retinal fold
falciparum malaria
Falcon coronary catheter
falling hematocrit
fallopian hiatus
false colonic obstruction
false diverticula
false-positive result
familial adenomatous polyposis (FAP)
familial adenomatous polyposis coli
familial amyloid polyneuropathy
familial chloride diarrhea
familial cholemia
familial cholestasis
familial chronic idiopathic jaundice
familial colorectal polyposis
familial dysproteinemia
familial gastrointestinal polyposis
familial hepatitis
familial hypercalcemia with nephrocalcinosis and indicanuria (blue-diaper syndrome)
familial hyperparathyroidism
familial hypocalciuric hypercalcemia
familial hypoproteinemia with lymphangiectatic enteropathy
familial intestinal polyposis
familial intestinal pseudo-obstruction
familial intrahepatic cholestasis
familial Mediterranean fever
familial nonhemolytic jaundice
familial pancreatic cancer
familial pancreatitis
familial patent ductus venosus
familial polyposis coli (FPC)

familial polyposis syndrome
familial ulcerative colitis
familial visceral neuropathy
family history of breast cancer
family history, positive
FAMMM (familial atypical multiple
  mole melanoma) syndrome
famotidine
fan retractor
Fanelli guide
Fansler-Ives anoscope
Fansler proctoscope
Fansler speculum
FAP (familial adenomatous polyposis)
Farabeau-Lambotte rasp
Farabeuf bone rasp
Farabeuf bone-holding forceps
Farabeuf-Collin rasp
Farabeuf-Lambotte bone-holding
  forceps
Farabeuf periosteal elevator
Farabeuf rasp
Farabeuf raspatory
Farabeuf retractor
far-away metastasis
Fareston (toremifene citrate)
farmer's lung
Farrell cotton applicator
Farrior-Dworacek canal chisel
Farrior wire-crimping forceps
Farr spring-wire retractor
Farr wire retractor
fascia
  anterior rectus
  autologous rectus abdominis
  clavipectoral
  cribiform
  dartos
  deep
  deltopectoral
  Denonvillier
  endoabdominal
  external oblique
  external spermatic

fascia *(cont.)*
  Gerota
  internal oblique
  lateral oblique
  pectineus
  pectoral
  pectoralis
  posterior rectus
  preperitoneal
  rectus
  Scarpa
  spigelian
  transversalis
  Waldeyer
fascia anchor
fascial absorbable suture
fascia lata graft
fascia layer
fascial band
fascial bridge
fascial closure
fascial closure of trocar site
fascial defect
fascial graft
fascial layer
fascial plane
fascial-splitting incision
fascial stranding
fascia of abdomen
fascia/peritoneum funnel
fascia reapproximated
fascicular sarcoma
fasciitis, necrotizing
Fasciola gigantica
Fasciola hepatica
fasciolopsiasis
Fasciolopsis buski
Faslodex
fast-absorbing surgical gut (plain)
Fast-Cath introducer catheter
fast Fourier transform (FFT) technique
  for EGG analysis
fasting
fast smear

FASTak suture anchor
fastener
  ROC suture
  ROC XS suture
  Suture Clinch
Fastin anchor
fasting
fasting blood glucose
fasting chemistry panel
fasting diet
fasting gastric bile acid test
fasting gastrin level
fasting hyperinsulinemia
fasting hypoglycemia
fasting insulin and glucose levels
fasting serum gastrin
F.A.S.T. 1 (First Access for Shock and Trauma) System
FastPack test
Fastrac gastrostomy access port
FasTrac guidewire
FasTracker catheter
FastTake blood glucose monitoring system
fat
  abdominal
  blurred pericecal (on CT scan)
  dietary
  interposed omental
  intramuscular
  mesenteric
  omental
  paucity of
  perinephric
  perirenal
  preperitoneal
  protruding
  subcutaneous
fatal anaphylaxis
fatal hereditary tyrosinemia
fat cell
fat creeping
fat emulsion, intravenous
fatigability
fat metabolism
fat necrosis
fat necrosis of breast
fat pad, abdominal
fat pad retractor
fat plane
fat saponification
fat-soluble bilirubin
fat-soluble vitamin
fat storage disorder
fat-storing liver cell
fat towel
fatty acid bile acid conjugate (FABAC)
fatty acid metabolism
fatty acid
fatty ascites
fatty cirrhosis
fatty food intolerance
fatty foods
fatty infiltration of liver
fatty kidney
fatty liver
fatty liver disease
fatty liver hepatitis
fatty liver of pregnancy (obstetric yellow atrophy)
fatty liver relation to HAART
fatty meal
fatty meal sonogram (FMS)
fatty micromedionodular cirrhosis
fatty necrosis
fatty stools
fatty tissue
faucial thermal-tactile stimulation
Faure forceps
Favaloro-Morse rib spreader
Favaloro sternal retractor
favorable prognosis
Fazier modified suction tube
FBA (fecal bile acid)
FCIS (Flint Colon Injury Scale)
FCPA2 ultrafast laser
FCS-ML II colonoscope

FCS-ML II endoscope
FCS-ML II gastroscope
FCS (full cervical spine) view
FDA (Food and Drug Administration)
FD-43 microdissector
FDL (fluorescein dilaurate) test
FeatherTouch CO_2 laser
feathery degeneration
feathery pattern of barium in small
  bowel
febrile agglutinin panel
febrile illness
fecal alpha$_1$-antitrypsin test
fecal analysis
fecal bile acid (FBA)
fecal contamination of food or water
fecal continence
fecal fat analysis
fecal fat excretion, 24-hour
fecal fat study
fecal fistula
fecal flora
fecal impaction
fecal incontinence
fecal incontinence score
fecalith, appendiceal
fecal mass
fecal material
fecal obstruction
fecal occult blood
fecal occult blood test (FEOT)
fecal-oral route of virus transmission
fecal-oral transmission
fecal osmolarity
fecal peritonitis
fecal reservoir
fecal residue
fecal stasis
fecal stream
fecal stream diversion
fecal transmission
fecaluria
fecal urobilinogen
fecal vomitus

Fecatest
feces (see *stool*)
  impacted
  inspissated
feces smear
feculence
feculent
feculent drainage
feculent vomitus
Federici sign
fedotozine
feedback mechanism
feeding (see also *formula*)
  Amin-Aid powdered
  bolus
  Build Up enteral
  Citrotein liquid
  Clinifeed Iso enteral
  Compleat-B liquid
  continuous drip
  Criticare HN elemental liquid
  Enrich
  Ensure Plus liquid
  enteral
  Entrition Entri-Pak
  Finkelstein
  Flexical enteral
  forced
  Fortison enteral
  gastrostomy
  gavage
  half-strength
  Hepatic-Aid powdered
  HN (high nitrogen)
  hyperosmotic
  intermittent drip
  intravenous (I.V., IV)
  Isocal HCN (high calorie and
    nitrogen) liquid
  Isotein HN
  isotonic
  Jevity isotonic liquid nutrition
  lactose-free
  Lonalac

feeding *(cont.)*
  low-residue
  Magnacal
  Meritene liquid
  NJ (nasojejunal)
  Osmolite HN liquid
  parenteral
  Portagen
  Precision Isotein HN powdered
  Precision Isotonic powdered
  Precision LR powdered
  Renu
  Resource
  Stresstein
  Sustacal HC (high calorie) liquid
  Sustacal HN liquid
  TraumaCal enteral liquid
  Traum-Aid HBC
  Travasorb HN powdered
  Travasorb MCT liquid
  Travasorb STD
  tube
  Vital
  Vitaneed
  Vivonex HN powdered
  Vivonex T.E.N.
feeding gastrostomy tube
feeding jejunostomy
feeding tube
Feen-A-Mint
Fehland colon resection clamp
Fehland intestinal clamp
Feilchenfeld splinter forceps
Feild (*not* Field) blade
Feild-Lee brain biopsy needle
Felig insulin pump
FELL suction tube
Fellonet ointment gauze dressing
felt dressing
Felty syndrome
female catheter
female reamer
feminizing tumor
femoral artery
femoral canal
femoral condyle drill
femoral-cutaneous nerve
femoral guide pin
femoral head extractor
femoral head necrosis
femoral hernia repair
femoral intermedullary guide
femoral ligament
femoral lymphadenopathy
femoral neck nail
femoral plate
femoral pulse
femoral shaft reamer
femoral sheath
femoral vein
femorocrural graft
femorocutaneous nerve
femorodistal PTFE graft
FemRx Soprano cryotherapy system
Femtosecond laser keratome
FEN (fluids, electrolytes, nutrition)
FENa (fractional excretion of sodium)
fenestrated bowel grasper
fenestrated cup biopsy forceps
fenestrated drape
fenestrated grasper
fenestrated reamer
fenestrated tube
fenestration saw
fenfluramine
Fenger gallbladder probe
fenoctimine; fenoctimine sulfate
fentanyl citrate
Fentanyl Oralet (fentanyl)
Fenwick disease
FEOT (fecal occult blood test)
FEP polymer
Ferguson bone-holding forceps
Ferguson brain suction tube
Ferguson forceps
Ferguson-Frazier suction tube
Ferguson gallstone scoop
Ferguson hemorrhoidectomy

Ferguson-Moon rectal speculum
Ferguson view
Fergusson dressing scissors
Fergusson forceps
Fergusson gallstone scoops
Fergusson hemorrhoidal clamp
Fergusson speculum
Fergusson suction tube
Feridex (ferumoxides)
Feridex I.V. (ferumoxides injectable solution)
feritin concentration
ferric ammonium citrate (FAC)
Ferris biliary duct dilator
FerriSeltz (ferric ammonium citrate [FAC])
Ferris Smith intervertebral disk rongeur
Ferris Smith-Kerrison forceps
Ferris Smith-Kerrison laminectomy rongeur
Ferris Smith laminectomy rongeur
Ferris Smith pituitary jaw rongeur
Ferris Smith rongeur forceps
Ferris Smith-Spurling disk rongeur
Ferris Smith tissue forceps
ferrite filter
ferritin, serum
ferromagnetic tamponade
Festalan
Festal II
fetal cortical tissue graft
fetal (early, intermediate, late) death
fetal diagnosis
fetal goiter
fetal substantia nigra graft
Feth-R-Kath epidural catheter
fetor hepaticus
fever
  acute rheumatic
  aseptic
  bullous
  cat-bite
  cat-scratch
  Colorado tick

fever *(cont.)*
  dehydration
  dengue
  drug
  enteric
  familial Mediterranean
  hepatic
  herpetic
  high-grade
  intermittent
  low-grade
  Mediterranean
  parenteric
  puerperal
  rat-bite
  relapsing
  rheumatic
  San Joaquin Valley
  scarlet
  Sennetsu
  septic
  steroid
  syphilitic
  yellow
  valley
fever of unknown or undetermined origin (FUO)
fever spike
Festal II
FFP (fresh frozen plasma)
FFT line
FGS and FCS endoscope
FGS-ML II endoscope
FGS-ML II gastroscope
FHF (fulminant hepatic failure)
FHIT (fragile histidine triad)
FHP (familial hypofibrinogenemia)
Fiberall (calcium polycarbophil)
FiberCon (calcium polycarbophil)
fiber, dietary
Fiberlan (lactose-free formula)
Fiberlase laser
Fiber-Lax (calcium polycarbophil)
Fiber-Norm (calcium polycarbophil)

Fiber One bran cereal
fiberoptic choledochoscope
fiberoptic endoscope
fiberoptic gastroscope
fiberoptic injection sclerotherapy (FIS)
fiberoptic light cable
fiberoptic panendoscopy
fibers, circular muscle
fiberscope (see *endoscope*)
fiber-splitting incision
Fibracol collagen-alginate dressing
Fibracol Plus collagen wound dressing
Fibrijet adhesive
fibrillary bacteria
Fibrillex (NC-503)
fibrin glue
fibrin glue adhesive
fibrinogen
fibrinoid lung
fibrinoid necrosis
fibrinolysin and desoxyribonuclease
fibrinolysis
fibrinous adhesions
fibrinous polyp
fibrin sealant
fibrin sponge
fibroadenoma of breast
fibroadipose tissue
fibroblastic ingrowth
fibroblastic tissue response
fibrocartilaginous pad
fibrocartilaginous plate
fibrocongestive splenomegaly
fibrocystic breast
fibrocystic breast syndrome
fibrocystic disease of breast
fibrocystic disorder of breast
fibroepithelial papilloma
fibroepithelial polyp
fibrofatty infiltration of pancreas
fibrofatty tissue
fibrogenesis
fibroglandular tissue
fibroid degeneration
fibrolamellar carcinoma
fibrolamellar hepatocarcinoma
fibrolamellar hepatocellular carcinoma (HCC)
fibrolamellar hepatoma
fibroma
fibromyoma
fibromyxoma
fibronectin-repeat domains
fibroplasia
fibrosarcoma
fibrosing piecemeal necrosis
fibrosis
  alcoholic
  arachnoid
  bridging
  chronic sclerosing hyaline
  congenital hepatic (CHF)
  cystic
  diffuse lobular
  inflammatory
  lung
  noncirrhotic portal (NCPF)
  pancreatic
  periductal
  periportal
  perisinusoidal
  perivenular
  portal
  portal-to-portal
  progressive perivenular alcoholic (PPAF)
  retroperitoneal
  secondary biliary
  sinusoidal
  transmural
fibrosis of liver
fibrosis of lung
fibrosis of thyroid
fibrotic liver
fibrotic pattern
fibrous adhesion
fibrous capsule of kidney

fibrous change
fibrous fullness
fibrous goiter
fibrous obliterative cholangitis
fibrous septum
fibrous sheath
fibrous stroma
fibrous stromal tissue
fibrous thyroiditis
fibrous tissue
fibrous tuberosity
fibrous tumor (desmoid)
fibrovascular polyp
fiducial plate
Fiedler disease
field
  bloodless
  operative
  surgical
field block anesthesia
fifth vital sign (pain)
figure-of-8 (or figure-8) dressing
figure-of-8 interscapular bandage
figure-of-4 (or figure-4) position
filament-forming bacillus
filariasis
file, Bayonet bone
filiform bougie
filiform guide for Lefort sound
filiform papilla
filiform polyposis
filiforms and followers
filler tube
fillet local flap graft
filleted the tract open
filling defect, radiolucent
filling of gallbladder with fluid
film (see also *position, projection, view)*
  absorbable gelatin
  Accu-Flo dura
  AP (anteroposterior)
  chiropractic
  comparison

film *(cont.)*
  cross-table lateral
  decubitus
  digital subtraction
  DuPont Cronex x-ray
  Knuttsen bending
  lateral decubitus
  low-contrast
  NUVO barrier
  oblique
  overhead
  PA (posteroanterior)
  plain
  portable
  postevacuation
  preliminary
  prone
  Repel abdominal
  Repel-CV abdominal
  scout
  skull
  spot
  stress
  suboptimal
  subtraction
  supine
  upright
film-based viewing
filmless imaging
filmy adhesion
Filshie clip applier
Filshie female sterilization clip
filter
  CO_2 gas
  OmniFilter
  PFR95
Filtzer interbody rasp
fimbriated fold
final diagnosis
Fine cross-action retractor
FIN extractor
Fine-Kerrison cervical rongeurs
finely fatty foamy liver
fine needle

fine-needle aspirate
fine-needle aspiration (FNA)
fine-needle aspiration biopsy
fine-needle aspiration cytology
fine-needle biopsy
fine-needle percutaneous cholangiogram
fine-needle transhepatic cholangiogram
fine-tip forceps
fine tissue forceps
fine-toothed forceps
fine-tooth fenestrated grasper
fingerbreadth
finger dissection
finger fracture dissection
finger fracture of liver
finger fracture technique
fingernail drill
finger retractor
finger ring cutter
fingerstick (see *lancet*)
fingertip dissection
fingertip lesion
Finney pyloroplasty
Finochietto forceps
Finochietto laminectomy retractor
Finochietto-Metzenbaum scissors
Finochietto needle
Finochietto retractor
Finochietto rib spreader
Finochietto thoracic scissors
FIN pin guide
FiO_2
Firlit drip stent
firm and rubbery gland
firm mass
firm neoplasm
First Access for Shock and Trauma
(F.A.S.T.) system
First Aid Bandage Company
First Aid triple-antibiotic bandage
first branch of the external carotid
artery
First Choice reagent strips
first-degree hemorrhoid
first-degree history
first-degree relative
first duodenal sphincter
first-pass effect
first rib rongeur
first rib shears
First Warning breast cancer screening
device
FIS (fiberoptic injection sclerotherapy)
Fisch bone rongeur
Fisch dural hook
Fischer cone biopsy excisor
Fischer transfixing pin
Fischer ventricular cannula
Fisch micro hook
Fisch rectal probe
Fisch retractor
FISH (fluorescence in situ hybridization)
Fisher and Paykel humidifier
Fisher exact test
Fisher guide
Fisher half pin
fisherman's knot
Fisher rasp
fishhook hook
fish insulin
Fishman-Doubilet test
fishmouth incision
fishmouth suture
fish-odor syndrome (trimethylaminuria)
fish-scale gallbladder
Fiskars Softouch scissors
fissure
anal
azygos
chronic fissure refractory to
conservative treatment
portal
rectal
umbilical
fissurectomy
fissure in ano

fissure of lung
fistula (pl. fistulae, fistulas)
  abdominal
  abdominal wall
  anal
  anoperineal
  anorectal
  anovestibular
  aortoduodenal
  aortoenteric
  aortoesophageal
  aortosigmoid
  appendiceal
  arteriovenous (AV)
  biliary
  biliary-cutaneous
  biliary-duodenal
  biliary-enteric (bilioenteric)
  bladder
  Blom-Singer tracheoesophageal
  brachioaxillary bridge graft (BAGF)
  brachiosubclavian bridge graft
    (BSGF)
  branchial
  Brescia-Cimino AV
  bronchobiliary
  bronchocavitary
  bronchoesophageal
  bronchopleural
  cholecystenteric
  cholecystocholedochal
  cholecystocolonic
  cholecystoduodenal
  cholecystoduodenocolic
  cholecystoenteric
  choledochocolonic
  choledochoduodenal
  colocutaneous
  coloenteric
  colonic
  colovaginal
  colovesical
  complex anorectal
  congenital pulmonary arteriovenous

fistula *(cont.)*
  cystic
  duodenal
  duodenocolic
  Eck
  enteric
  enterocolic
  enterocutaneous
  enteroenteral; enteroenteric
  enterourethral
  enterovaginal
  enterovesical
  external biliary
  external pancreatic
  extrasphincteric anal
  fecal
  gallbladder
  gastric
  gastrocolic
  gastrocutaneous
  gastroduodenal
  gastrointestinal
  gastrojejunal-colic
  gastrojejunocolic
  genitourinary
  graft-enteric
  hepatic
  hepatopleural
  high-output
  horseshoe
  H-type
  ileorectal
  ileosigmoid
  intersphincteric anal
  intrahepatic AV
  ischiorectal
  jejunocolic
  lactiferous duct
  Mann-Bollman
  mesenteric
  mucous
  nasolabial
  orofacial
  pancreatic cutaneous

fistula *(cont.)*
- pancreatic enteric
- pancreaticocutaneous
- pancreaticopleural
- parietal
- perineovaginal
- pilonidal
- rectal
- rectourethral
- rectovaginal
- rectovesical
- refractory pancreatic
- respiratory-esophageal
- retroperitoneal
- sigmoidovesical
- small bowel
- splanchnic AV
- splenic AV
- suprasphincteric
- thyroglossal
- tracheoesophageal (TE, TEF)
- transsphincteric anal
- urethrovaginal
- vesical
- vesicoenteric
- vesicouterine
- vesicovaginal
- vitelline

fistula formation
fistula hook
fistula in ano
fistula needle
fistula probe
fistula scissors
fistulation, spreading
fistulectomy
fistulization, cholecystobiliary
fistulization of esophagus
fistulization of sublingual salivary cyst
fistulizing Crohn disease
fistulogram
fistulography
fistulotomy, Parks staged
fistulous tract
Fitbox
Fitz-Hugh–Curtis syndrome
Fitzgerald aortic aneurysm forceps
five-hole (5-hole) plate
Fixateur Interne rod
fixation of breast mass to chest wall
fixation of breast mass to overlying skin
fixation pin
fixator-augmented nail
fixed-angle blade plate
fixed axillary lymph node
fixed segment of bowel
flabby abdomen
flagellate diarrhea
Flagyl (metronidazole)
flail chest
flail segment
Flanagan-Burem apposing hemicylindric graft
Flanagan spinal fusion gouge
flank
flank bruit
flank incision
flank pain
flank scar
flap
- abdominal
- advancement
- advancement of rectal
- anconeus muscle
- artery island
- Atasoy-Kleinert
- Atasoy palmar
- Atasoy triangular advancement
- axial flag
- axial pattern
- Bakamjian
- bilobed
- bipedicle
- bone
- bursal
- butterfly
- Chinese
- cross-finger

flap *(cont.)*
- cross-leg
- cross-lip
- cross-lip pedicle
- Dandy myocutaneous scalp
- deep circumflex iliac artery-iliac crest
- deltopectoral
- digital
- dorsal rotation
- dorsal transposition
- dorsalis pedis fasciocutaneous
- dorsalis pedis myofascial
- double pedicle
- double pedicle TRAM
- DRAM (de-epithelialized rectus abdominis) muscle
- entry
- extended
- extensor carpi radialis longus
- fascial
- fasciocutaneous island
- finger-fillet
- free
- free fasciocutaneous
- free fibular harvest
- free latissimus dorsi
- free temporal
- galeal
- gastrocnemius sliding
- gracilis muscle
- groin
- hemipulp
- horseshoe-shaped
- iliac osteocutaneous free
- iliofemoral pedicle
- interdigitating skin
- island
- island pedicle
- Karydakis
- Kutler digital
- lateral transverse thigh
- latissimus dorsi
- latissimus dorsi island

flap *(cont.)*
- latissimus dorsi musculocutaneous free
- latissimus dorsi myocutaneous
- liver
- lumbrical muscle
- maple leaf
- Martius flap and fascial sling
- Martius labial fat pad
- McCraw gracilis myocutaneous
- microsurgical free
- Moberg
- modified dorsalis pedis myofascial
- muscle
- musculocutaneous free
- musculotendinous
- myocutaneous
- myofascial
- necrotic
- neurocutaneous island
- neurovascular island pedicle
- nutrient
- omental
- Oriental V-Y
- osteocutaneous free
- osteoplastic
- palmar advancement
- parascapular
- pectoralis major
- pedicle
- pedicled muscle-tendon
- pericranial
- peritoneal
- peroneal island
- pulp
- radial-based
- radial forearm
- rectus abdominis
- rectus abdominis musculocutaneous free
- rectus muscle
- remote pedicle
- rotational
- rotator

flap *(cont.)*
- Rubens
- scalp
- scapular
- segmented
- single pedicle
- single pedicle TRAM
- skin
- subscapularis muscle
- Tait
- tensor fasciae latae
- thenar
- three-square
- TRAM (transverse rectus abdominis myocutaneous)
- transposition
- transverse rectus abdominis myocutaneous (TRAM)
- triangular
- triceps
- tumbler
- tummy tuck
- turned-down tendon
- vascularized
- V-Y advancement
- wraparound

flap graft, Kutler V-Y
flap knife
flapping tremor sign
flap tear
flap-valve mechanism
flap viability
flareup
flashlamp-pulsed dye laser
flashlamp-pulsed Nd:YAG laser
flashlamp-pumped pulsed dye laser
flask-shaped ulcer
flat condyloma
flat drill
flatfooted
flat grasping forceps, fenestrated, double-action
flat lesion
flat narrow elevator
flat-nose pliers
flat plate
flat plate of abdomen
flat Silastic suction drain
flat stick sponge
flat suture
Flatt driver
flattened duodenal fold
flattened T wave
flattened stool
flattening of ileal epithelium
flatulence
flatulent
flatulent colic
flatulent dyspepsia
Flatulex (simethicone)
flatus
flatus enema
flavin-containing mono-oxygenase (FMO) 2
flea-bitten kidney
fleecy mass
Fleet Babylax (glycerin)
Fleet bowel prep
Fleet Bisacodyl enema
Fleet enema
Fleet Laxative (bisacodyl)
Fleet Mineral Oil enema
Fleet Phospho-Soda (monobasic sodium phosphate; dibasic sodium phosphate)
"flesh-eating" bacteria
Fletcher's Castoria (senna concentrate)
Fletcher polypectomy forceps
fleur de lis breast reconstruction pattern
Flex Advantage kit
Flexbar Machine Corp video camera system
flex drill
Flex-EZ balloon dilator
Flex-Foam bandage
Flexguard Tip catheter
Flexiblade laryngoscope
flexible arm (Leyla) retractors

flexible dental suction
flexible endoscope
flexible endoscopic surgery
flexible esophagoscopy
flexible gastrointestinal cryotherapy
flexible medullary reamer
flexible operating instruments
flexible optical biopsy forceps
flexible retractor
flexible sigmoidoscope
flexible, steerable nasolaryngo-pharyngoscope
flexible stent
flexible ureteroscope
Flexiflo Lap G laparoscopic gastrostomy kit
Flexiflo Lap J laparoscopic jejunostomy kit
Flexiflo Stomate low-profile gastrostomy tube
Flexilite conforming elastic bandage
Flexima biliary stent system
Flexinet dressing
flexion view
Flexlase 600 laser
Flex-Master bandage
Flexon steel suture
flexor palmar plate
flexor tendon graft
FlexPack HP test
FlexPosure endoscopic retractor
Flex-T cannister
FlexTip intervertebral rongeur
FlexTube bandage
flexure
  duodenojejunal
  hepatic
  left colonic
  right colonic
  sigmoid
  splenic
Flexxicon Blue dialysis catheter
Flexzan foam wound dressing
F. L. Fischer microsurgical neurectomy bayonet scissors
FL-HCC (fibrolamellar hepatocellular carcinoma)
FLIC (Functional Living Index-Cancer)
Flint Colon Injury Scale (FCIS)
floating gallbladder
floating gallstone
floating kidney
floating liver
floating spleen
floating stool
flocculation on barium enema
Flo-Coat (barium sulfate)
FloCoil shunt
Flocor (poloxamer 188)`
Flood syndrome
floor of canal
floor of foregut
floor of inguinal region
floor, pelvic
floorstand reflector
floppy guidewire
floppy Nissen fundoplication
floppy-type Nissen fundoplication
flora
  colonic
  fecal
  intestinal
  normal
florid cirrhosis
florid duct lesion
Florinef Acetate (fludrocortisone acetate)
FloSeal Matrix hemostatic sealant
flow-compromising lesion
flower-shaped polypropylene mesh plug with multiple petal
FlowGun suction/irrigation
flow-limiting lesion
flow/pressure/resistance formula
Floxin (ofloxacin)
floxuridine (FUDR; FUdR)
flu-like syndrome
fluctuance, rectal submuscular
fluctuant abscess

fluctuant mass
fludrocortisone acetate
fluence (measurement)
fluffs dressing
Fluhrer rectal probe
fluid
  amniotic
  articular
  ascitic
  bile-stained
  bile-tinged
  bloody
  bloody peritoneal
  body
  Bouin
  cavitary
  cerebrospinal
  chylous
  clear
  cloudy
  crystalloid
  cystic
  Delafield
  dentinal
  Dialyflex dialysis
  digestive
  edema
  embalming
  extracellular
  extravascular
  free
  frothy
  gelatinous
  intercellular
  interstitial
  intracellular
  intravascular
  intravenous
  joint
  LDH level of ascitic
  loculated
  low-viscosity
  lymphatic
  meconium-stained amniotic
fluid *(cont.)*
  milky
  motor oil peritoneal
  natural body
  periappendiceal
  pericardial
  pericardial effusion
  pericholecystic
  peritoneal
  peritoneal effusion
  pleural
  pleural effusion
  prostatic
  protein-rich
  prune juice peritoneal
  sanguineous
  seminal
  serosanguineous
  serous
  spinal
  straw-colored
  subhepatic space
  synovial
  testing
  thoracentesis
  transcellular
  turbid
  turbid peritoneal
  viscous
  Zenker
fluid accumulation (from aneurysm or perforation)
fluid and electrolyte absorption
Fluid Alarm System (FAS) glove integrity system
fluid collection in pericholecystic area
fluid collection pouch
fluid-filled cleft
fluid-filled cyst
fluid-filled mass
fluid-filled papule
fluid-filled sac
fluid-filled vacuole within lens
fluid loss, gastrointestinal

fluid material
fluid overload
fluid protein
fluid resuscitation
fluid sequestration
fluid specimen, filtration of
fluid volume deficit
fluid volume excess
fluid warmer
fluid wave
fluke (trematode)
fluke, liver
flu-like syndrome
flumecino
FluMist vaccine
FLU OIA assay
fluorescein
fluorescence in situ hybridization (FISH)
fluorescence spectroscopy
FluoroNav virtual fluoroscopy system
Fluoropassiv thin-wall carotid patch
fluoropyrimidine
fluoroscopic control
fluoroscopic resolution
fluoroscopic stress x-ray view
fluoroscopy
fluorouracil (5-FU)
fluorouracil and leucovorin
Fluothane (halothane)
fluoxymesterone
flush port cap
flush-with-skin stoma
flushing
fluted J-Vac drain
fluted medullary rod
fluted titanium nail
FMO (flavin-containing mono-oxygenase) 2
FMS (fatty meal sonogram)
FNAC (fine-needle aspiration cytology)
FNH (focal nodular hyperplasia)
foam cell
foam dressing
foam gauze dressing
Foamicon (aluminum hydroxide; magnesium trisilicate)
foam roll bandage
foam sheet bandage
foam wound dressing
foamy esophagus
foamy liver
foamy material
foamy stool
Fobi pouch
focal biliary cirrhosis
focal calcification
focal colitis
focal colonic mucosal ulcer
focal dilation of the splenic vein
focal edema
focal goiter
focal hemorrhage
focal hepatocellular necrosis with hemorrhagic cyst
focal infection
focal lesion
focal necrosis
focal neurologic deficit
focal nodular hyperplasia (FNH)
focal pancreatitis
FocalSeal sealant
FocalSeal-L sealant
FocalSeal-S surgical sealant
focal small bowel obstruction
focal tenderness
focal tumor
focal ulceration and hemorrhage
foci (plural of focus)
  hypotensive
  hepatocyte dysplasia
  metastasis
  tumor
focused appendix computed tomography (FACT)
Foerster abdominal ring retractor
Foerster capsulotomy knife
Foerster sponge-holding forceps

Fogarty adherent clot catheter
Fogarty balloon
Fogarty balloon biliary catheter
Fogarty biliary probe
Fogarty-Chin clamp
Fogarty clamp
Fogarty embolectomy catheter
Fogarty forceps
Fogarty graft thrombectomy catheter
Fogarty Hydrogrip clamp
Fogarty irrigation catheter
Fogarty-type jaw
fogging of laparoscope
fog reduction elimination device (FRED)
fold
  adipose
  alar
  amniotic
  aryepiglottic
  axillary
  caval
  cecal
  cholecystoduodenocolic
  ciliary
  circular
  circulator
  costocolic
  Douglas
  duodenojejunal
  duodenomesocolic
  epigastric
  falciform retinal
  fimbriated
  flattened duodenal
  gastric
  gastropancreatic
  genital
  glossopalatine
  gluteal
  Guérin
  haustral
  hepatopancreatic
  ileocecal

fold *(cont.)*
  ileocolic
  inferior duodenal
  inferior transverse rectal
  inguinal
  interureteric
  Kerckring
  labioscrotal
  lateral umbilical
  medial umbilical
  mucosal
  Nélaton
  palatopharyngeal
  paraduodenal
  peritoneal
  rectal
  rectouterine
  sacrogenital
  semilunar
  sentinel
  sigmoid
  spiral
  superior duodenal
  superior transverse rectal
  vestigial
folded fundus gallbladder
folded gallbladder
fold pattern
Folergot-DF (belladonna alkaloids; phenobarbital; ergotamine tartrate)
Foley catheter
Foley catheter bladder decompression
Foley catheter gastrostomy tube
foliate papilla
F/O light carrier
F of follicular cancer (far-away metastasis, female, FNA-not, favorable prognosis)
folinic acid
follicle associated epithelium
follicular carcinoma
follicular cells of the thyroid
follicular cholecystitis
follicular gastritis

follicular goiter
follicular mucinosis
follow-up examination
Foloxatine (oxaliplatin)
Foltz catheter
Fomon chisel
Fomon periosteal elevator
Fomon rasp
Fonar Stand-Up MRI
Fonar-360 MRI Scanner
food
  bland
  blenderized
  cholecystokinetic
  fatty
  fried
  gas-producing
  greasy
  liquid
  spicy
Food and Drug Administration (FDA)
food bolus obstruction
food-borne gastroenteritis
food pipe
food poisoning, staphylococcal
food supplement
foot drape
foot plate
forage core biopsy
foramen cecum at the base
  of the tongue
foramen of Bochdalek
foramen of Winslow
Forane (isoflurane)
Forbes-Albright syndrome
Forbes disease
Force balloon dilatation catheter
forced alimentation
forced feeding
forceful retching
forceps (see also *hemostat*)
  Acland clamp-applying
  ACMI Martin endoscopy
  Acufex curved basket

forceps *(cont.)*
  Acufex rotary biting basket
  Adair-Allis
  Adson
  Adson bayonet dressing
  Adson bipolar
  Adson-Brown tissue
  Adson clip-introducing
  Adson dressing
  Adson dura protecting
  Adson hemostatic
  Adson hypophyseal
  Adson lightweight plain
  Adson lightweight toothed
  Adson microforceps
  Adson micro tissue
  Adson-Mixter neurosurgical
  Adson rongeur
  Adson tissue
  adventitial
  Aesculap bipolar cautery
  Alderkreutz
  Alexander biopsy
  Allen intestinal
  alligator
  alligator grasping
  alligator jaws
  alligator-type grasping
  Allis
  Allis atraumatic tissue
  Allis-TC tissue
  Allis-Willauer
  Anderson
  Angell James hypophysectomy
  Angell James reverse-action
    hypophysectomy
  angled-down
  angled-up
  anterior
  AO reduction
  approximating
  Arruga-Nicetic
  artery
  arthroscopy basket

forceps *(cont.)*
- arthroscopy grasping
- Asch
- AtrauGrip
- atraumatic
- Babcock
- Babcock atraumatic tissue
- Babcock grasping, double-action
- Babcock intestinal
- Babcock-TC
- baby Allis
- baby Babcock tissue
- baby Doyen intestinal
- baby Tischler biopsy
- Backhaus
- Backhaus towel
- Bacher flexible biopsy
- Bacon rongeur
- Baer bone cutting
- Baggish
- Bailey aortic valve cutting
- Bainbridge
- Baird
- ball-and-socket towel
- Ballantine
- Ballenger
- Ballenger sponge-holding
- Bane rongeur
- Bangerter muscle
- Bardeleben bone-holding
- Barnes-Neville
- Barraquer cilia
- Barraquer Colibri
- Barraquer suture-removing
- Barrett intestinal
- Barrett placenta
- Barrett tenaculum
- Barton obstetrical
- basket
- basket-type crushing
- Bauer
- bayonet
- bayonet bipolar
- bayonet-shaped

forceps *(cont.)*
- bayonet-type
- Beasley-Babcock
- Beer cilia
- Behrend cystic duct
- Bellucci alligator
- Bengolea artery
- Berens muscle
- Berry-TC wire-twisting
- Best gallstone
- Bevan gallbladder
- Beyer rongeur
- biarticular bone-cutting
- BiCOAG bipolar
- Billingham hemorrhoidal grasping
- Billroth
- Billroth tumor
- biopsy
- biopsy cup
- bipolar
- bipolar cautery
- Bircher-Ganske cartilage
- Bishop-Harmon
- BiSure laparoscopic
- Blake gallstone
- Blakesley suction flow
- Bloodwell
- blunt
- blunt grasping, double-action
- Boettcher artery
- Boies
- bone-biting
- bone-breaking
- bone-cutting
- bone-grasping
- bone-holding
- bone punch
- bone-splitting
- Bonney
- bottle and specimen
- bottle nose
- Bozeman sponge-holding
- brain
- brain clip

forceps *(cont.)*
- brain spatula
- brain tumor
- Brand tendon-holding
- Brand tendon-passing
- Brand tendon-tunneling
- Braun tenaculum
- Bridge
- Brigham brain tumor
- bronchoesophageal
- bronchus
- Brown-Adson
- Brown-Adson tissue
- Brown-Cushing
- Brown tissue
- Brunner intestinal
- Brunschwig artery
- Buie pile
- bulldog
- bulldog clamp-applying
- bullet-nose, tissue-well, double-action
- Burke biopsy
- Butler bayonet
- Cairns
- Cairns hemostatic
- Caparosa wire-crimping
- capsular release
- Carmalt
- Carmalt artery
- Carroll bone-holding
- Carroll dressing
- Carroll tendon-pulling
- Carroll tissue
- cartilage
- Caspar alligator
- Castroviejo-Colibri
- catheter-introducing
- cervical punch
- Chandler spinal perforating
- Charnley
- Charnley suture
- Charnley wire-holding
- Cheatle sterilizing
- Cheron polypus and dressing

forceps *(cont.)*
- Cherry-Kerrison laminectomy
- Childe approximating
- Children's Hospital intestinal
- Childs intestinal
- cholecystectomy
- Citelli punch
- clamp-applying
- claw
- claw-grasping, 2 x 3 teeth, double-action
- Cleveland bone-cutting
- clip-applying
- clip-bending
- clip-cutting
- clip-inserting
- clip-introducing
- clip-removing
- Cloward punch
- Cloward rongeur
- coagulating
- coaptation bipolar
- cobra-grasping, double-action
- Cobra rat-tooth grasping
- Colibri
- Collin-Duval lung grasping
- Collin tissue-grasping
- Collingwood Stewart hernia ring
- Collins intestinal
- Collison
- Colver tonsil-seizing
- cone-nose
- cone skull punch
- cone wire-twisting
- Cooley-Baumgarten aortic
- Cooley vascular
- Crafoord
- cranial rongeur
- Crile artery
- Crile curved
- Crile gall duct
- Crile hemostatic
- Crile-Rankin
- cup

forceps *(cont.)*
- cupped-jaw
- curved
- curved Crile
- curved Kelly
- curved mosquito
- Cushing bayonet
- Cushing bipolar
- Cushing-Brown
- Cushing delicate
- Cushing dressing
- Cushing monopolar
- Cushing rongeur
- Cushing tissue
- cutting
- CV
- cystic duct
- Dale
- Dandy scalp hemostatic
- Davis
- Davis coagulating
- Davis monopolar
- Dawson-Yuhl-Kerrison rongeur
- Dawson-Yuhl-Leksell rongeur
- DeBakey-Adson tissue
- DeBakey arterial
- DeBakey AtrauGrip
- DeBakey-Bainbridge atraumatic intestinal
- DeBakey-Bainbridge intestinal
- DeBakey-Cooley dissecting
- DeBakey-Diethrich atraumatic tissue
- DeBakey-Diethrich vascular
- DeBakey dissecting
- DeBakey double-action grasping
- DeBakey-Mixter artery
- DeBakey-Semb
- DeBakey tissue
- DeBakey vascular
- Decker alligator
- Decker microsurgical
- Deddish-Potts intestinal
- DeLee
- DeMartel appendix

forceps *(cont.)*
- DeMartel scalp flap
- Demel wire-tightening
- Demel wire-twisting
- Denis Browne intestinal holding
- depilatory
- D'Errico bayonet pituitary
- D'Errico hypophyseal
- D'Errico pituitary
- D'Errico tissue
- Desjardins gall duct
- Desjardins gallstone
- DeTakats-McKenzie brain clip
- DeVilbiss rongeur
- Dewey obstetrical
- diathermy
- dilating
- Dingman bone-holding
- DirectBite coated disposable biopsy
- disk
- dissecting
- dissecting and grasping
- dolphin nose-grasping
- double-spoon
- Doughty
- Doyen intestinal
- dressing
- dual-cup grasping
- duckbill
- Dumont dissecting
- Dumont micro-dissecting
- Dunhill artery
- dura protecting
- Durmont-style dissecting
- Duval-Crile lung
- Duval-Scheie hemorrhoidal
- Duval tissue-grasping
- eagle's beak bone-cutting
- ear
- Echlin rongeur
- Edna towel
- Effler-Groves
- electrocoagulating biopsy
- Elliot

forceps *(cont.)*
Elliott gallbladder
Emmett cotton swab
end-biting
Endo Dissect
endoscopic
endoscopic biopsy
endoscopic grasping
endoscopic suture-cutting
Eppendorf biopsy
Eppendorf-Tischler biopsy
ethmoid
Evans tissue
extracting
Farabeuf bone-holding
Farabeuf-Lambotte bone-holding
Farrior wire-crimping
Faure
Feilchenfeld splinter
fenestrated cup biopsy
Ferguson bone-holding
Fergusson
Ferris-Smith rongeur
Ferris-Smith tissue
fine-tip
fine tissue
fine-toothed
Finochietto
Fitzgerald aortic aneurysm
flat grasping, fenestrated
Fletcher polypectomy
flexible optical biopsy
Foerster sponge-holding
Fogarty
foreign body
Foss
Fox bipolar
Fraser artery
Friedman rongeur
Fujinon biopsy
gall duct
gallstone
Gardner bone
Gavin-Miller intestinal

forceps *(cont.)*
Gemini Finochietto artery
Gemini gall duct
Gemini thoracic
George
Gerald bipolar
Gerald-Brown tissue
Gerald dissecting
Gerald dressing
Gerald tissue
Gerbode
Gilbert cystic duct
Gildenberg biopsy
Gillies diathermy
Gillies lightweight
Gillies tissue
gland
Glassman-Allis intestinal
Glenn diverticulum
glenoid-reaming
Gomel micro tying
Graefe dissecting
grasping
Gray cystic duct
Green-Armytage hemostasis
Greene
Greenwood bayonet
Greenwood bipolar and suction
Greven
Gruenwald ear
Gruppe wire-crimping
Gunderson bone
Gunderson muscle
Gunnar-Hey roller
Haberer intestinal
Hajek-Koffler bone punch
Halsted artery
Halsted hemostatic mosquito
(straight/curved)
Halsted mosquito
Hardy bipolar
Hardy dressing
Hardy microbipolar
Hardy sella punch

forceps *(cont.)*
Harrington-Mixter thoracic
Harrington thoracic
Harrison bone-holding
Harrison Cripp
Harrison sterilizing
Hartmann hemostatic mosquito
Hartmann nasal dressing
Haugh
Hayes Martin
Hayton Williams wire-twisting
Healy intestinal
Heaney
Heath-Richter clip-removing
Heermann alligator
Heiss artery
Heiss Finochietto
hemoclip-applying
hemostatic
Henahan extracting
Hendrin
Herget rectal biopsy
hernia ring
Herrmann alligator
Heywood-Smith hemorrhoidal
Hibbs bone-cutting
Hildebrandt uterine hemostatic
Hinderer cartilage
Hirsch hypophysis punch
Hoen angular
Hoen scalp hemostatic
Hopkins aortic
Horsley bone-cutting
Horsley-Stille bone-cutting
Hosemann
hot biopsy
hot flexible
Hot Sampler disposable hot
House cup
Housepan clip-applying
Howard Kelly
Howmedica Microfixation System
Hudson
Hulka tenaculum

forceps *(cont.)*
Hunt tumor
Hunt-Yasargil pituitary
Hunter
Hunter splinter
Hurd bone-cutting
hypophyseal
hypophysectomy
hypophysis punch
Ingraham skull punch
intervertebral disk
intestinal-grasping
Iowa
Iowa membrane
Iselin
Jackson grasping polyp
Jackson tendon-seizing
Jacobson-Adson artery
Jacobson dressing
Jacobson hemostatic
Jacobson micro mosquito
Jacobson mosquito
Jaffee capsulorrhexis
Jannetta alligator
Jannetta bayonet
Jansen-Middleton septal
Jansen monopolar
jar
Jarell
Jarit brain
Jarit tendon-pulling
Jarvis hemorrhoid
Jawz biopsy
Jawz endomyocardial biopsy
jeweler's bipolar
Johns Hopkins
Johns Hopkins gallbladder
Johnson brain tumor
Johnson thoracic
Johnson tumor
Jones IMA
Judd-Allis intestinal
Judd-DeMartel gallbladder
Juers-Lempert rongeur

forceps *(cont.)*
Julian splenorenal
Julian thoracic
jumbo biopsy
Kalman-Mixter
Kantrowitz
Karp aortic punch
Kelly hemostatic
Kelly placenta
Kelly artery
Kern bone-holding
Kern-Lane bone
Kevorkian-Tischler biopsy
Kevorkian-Younge biopsy
kidney stone
Kielland
Kleinert-Kutz bone-cutting
Kleinert-Kutz rongeur
Kleinert-Kutz tendon
Knight bone-cutting
Knight septum-cutting
knotting
Kocher
Kocher artery
Kocher intestinal
Koeberlé
Koehne cover glass
Koerte gallstone
Kraff-Utrata tear capsulotomy
Kuehne cover glass
Lahey dissecting
Lahey Finochietto dissecting
Lahey gall duct
Lahey thyroid traction
Lalonde delicate hook
Lambotte bone-holding
laminectomy punch
lancet-shaped biopsy
Landolt spreading
Lane bone-holding
Lane intestinal
Lane screw-holding
Lane self-retaining bone-holding
Lane tissue

forceps *(cont.)*
Lange approximation
Langenbeck bone-holding
Larsen tendon-holding
laser tenaculum
laser vulsellum
Laufe
Laurer
Lees artery
Leibinger Micro System
plate-holding
Lejeune thoracic
Leksell rongeur
Lempert rongeur
LeRoy scalp clip-applying
Lester muscle
Lewin bone-holding
Lewin spinal-perforating
ligamentum flavum
ligature-holding
Lillehei valve
Lillie intestinal
lion
lion-jaw
Lister sinus
Liston
Liston bone-cutting
Liston-Key bone-cutting
Liston-Littauer bone-cutting
Liston-Stille bone-cutting
Littauer-Liston bone-cutting
Littlewood tissue
Livernois lens-holding
Livernois-McDonald
Llorente dissecting
Lloyd Davies rectal biopsy
Lloyd Davies rectal occlusion
Lockwood-Allis intestinal
Lockwood tissue
London College
long grasping
Long
loop
loop-type snare

forceps *(cont.)*
- loop-type stone-crushing
- Lore suction tube and tip-holding
- Lorna towel
- Love-Gruenwald alligator
- Love-Gruenwald intervertebral disk
- Love-Gruenwald pituitary
- Love-Kerrison rongeur
- Lovelace lung grasping
- Lovelace thyroid traction
- Lowman bone-holding
- Lucae dressing
- Lucae ear
- Luer hemorrhoid
- Luer rongeur
- Luer-Whiting rongeur
- Luhr Microfixation System plate-holding
- Magill catheter introducing
- Malis angled-up bipolar
- Malis bipolar cautery
- Malis bipolar coagulation
- Malis irrigation
- Malis-Jensen microbipolar
- Malis jeweler bipolar
- Markwalder rib
- Martin
- Martin cartilage
- Martin tissue
- Maryland dissecting
- Mathieu
- Max Fine tying
- Mayfield
- Mayo-Blake gallstone
- Mayo-Péan
- Mayo-Robson intestinal
- Mayo-Russian tissue
- Mayo towel
- Mazzariello-Caprini
- McCain TMJ
- McClintock
- McGee
- McGee-Priest wire
- McGee wire-crimping

forceps *(cont.)*
- McGill
- McGivney
- McGivney hemorrhoidal-seizing
- McIndoe diathermy
- McIndoe dressing
- McIndoe rongeur
- McKenzie brain clip
- McKenzie clip-applying
- McKenzie clip-bending
- McKenzie clip-introducing
- McKernan-Adson
- McKernan-Potts
- McLean-Tucker obstetrical
- McNealey-Glassman-Mixter
- McPherson
- Medco
- Medco Adson tissue
- Medco Allis tissue
- Medco Babcock
- Medco Bozeman uterine
- Medco Brown Adson
- Medco Carmalt splinter
- Medco Crile
- Medco eye dressing
- Medco Foerster sponge
- Medco Halsted mosquito
- Medco Schroder tenaculum
- Medco splinter
- Medco thumb dressing
- Medco tissue thumb
- Medicon-Jackson rectal
- Meeker
- membrane-puncturing
- meniscus
- Meriam dissecting
- Michel applying and removing
- Michel clip-applying and clip-removing
- micro
- microartery
- microbipolar
- Micro dissecting
- micro Halsted mosquito

forceps *(cont.)*
Micro Jaw rotatable Kelly
Micro-One dissecting
Micro-optical
microsurgery
Micro-Two
microvascular
MIC Thermal Option disposable biopsy
Mikulicz peritoneal
Miller rectal
Millin ligature-holding
Miltex tendon-pulling
Mixter artery
Mixter dissecting
Mixter gallstone
Mixter-O'Shaughnessy artery
Mixter thoracic
modified Allis grasping
MOLLY bipolar
monopolar grasping
Moolgaoker
Moorfield stitch
Morrison tissue
Moynihan artery
Moynihan gall duct
Muir hemorrhoid
Multibite biopsy
Mya hook
Nadler coaptation bipolar
nail-pulling
needle-nose dissecting
needle-pulling
Nelson tissue
Neville-Barnes
Nicola
NIH mitral valve
Niro bone-cutting
Niro wire-twisting
Nissen gall duct
Noyes alligator
Nussbaum intestinal
Ochsner
Oehler tissue and needle-pulling

forceps *(cont.)*
Officer sigmoidoscope biopsy
Officer tissue
Ogura tissue and cartilage
Oldberg pituitary
Olivecrona clip-applying and removing
Olivecrona-Toennis clip-applying
Olympus alligator-jaw endoscopic
Olympus basket-type endoscopic
Olympus FBK-13 endoscopic biopsy
Olympus hot biopsy
Olympus magnetic extractor
Olympus mini-snare
Olympus pelican-type endoscopic
Olympus rat-tooth endoscopic
Olympus reusable biopsy
Olympus reusable hot biopsy
Olympus rubber-tip endoscopic
Olympus shark-tooth endoscopic
Olympus tripod-type endoscopic
Olympus W-shape endoscopic
Ombredanne
optical
optical biopsy
Orr gall duct
Oschner artery
Overholt artery
Overholt clip-applying
Overholt thoracic
O'Shaughnessy artery
paddle
Paterson biopsy
Payr pylorus
Péan
peapod intervertebral disk
Peers towel
Peet
Peet splinter
Pennington grasping
Pennington tissue
Percy intestinal
perforating
Perman cartilage

forceps *(cont.)*
Phaneuf artery
pickup
Pierce
Pierse micro dissecting
Pierse tip
Pilling Weck Y-stent
pinch
pinch-band
Piper OB
pituitary
plain splinter
plain tissue
plate-holding
polyp-grasping
Poppen
Porter duodenal
Potts bronchus
Potts bulldog
Potts-Smith
Potts-Smith dressing
Potts-Smith tissue
Potts thumb
Potts vascular
Pratt rectal
Pratt tumor
Preston ligamentum flavum
Price-Thomas bronchial
Providence Hospital artery
pulpiform nucleus
punch
Quadripolar cutting
Radial Jaw single-use biopsy
Radolf
Raimondi hemostatic
Raimondi scalp
Rampley sponge-holding
Ramsay tissue
Randall stone
Raney clip-applying
Raney coagulating
Raney rongeur
Raney scalp clip-applying
ratchet-on-demand grasping

forceps *(cont.)*
rat-tooth or rat-toothed
Ratliff-Blake gallstone
Ratliff-Mayo
Re-New
rectal biopsy
Reddick Olsen
Rees-Martel flap
Reich-Nechtow
Remington Hobbs diathermy
retrograde grasping, double-action
Rhoton bipolar
Rhoton cup
Rhoton-Cushing
Rhoton dissecting
Rhoton-Tew bipolar
rib
Riches artery
Riches diathermy artery
Richter-Heath clip-removing
Richter laminectomy punch
ring
Ritebite biopsy
Robbers
Roberts artery
Robson intestinal
Rochester-Carmalt artery
Rochester gallstone
Rochester-Mixter artery
Rochester-Ochsner
Rochester-Péan artery
Rochester-Péan hemostatic
roller
rongeur
rotary
round cup
Rowe disimpaction
Rowe glenoid-reaming
Rowe-Harrison bone-holding
Rowe modified-Harrison
Rudd Clinic hemorrhoidal
Ruel
Rumel artery
Rumel thoracic

forceps *(cont.)*
- Ruskin bone-cutting
- Ruskin bone-splitting
- Ruskin-Liston bone-cutting
- Ruskin rongeur
- Ruskin-Rowland bone-cutting
- Russian tissue
- Rutherford-Morrison tissue
- Samuels
- Sarot artery
- Sauerbruch rib
- Sawtell artery
- Sawtell tonsil hemostatic
- scalp clip
- scalp flap
- Scharff microbipolar and suction
- Scheicker laminectomy punch
- Schindler peritoneal
- Schlesinger cervical punch
- Schlesinger rongeur
- Schnidt artery
- Schnidt gall duct
- Schnidt thoracic
- Schoenberg intestinal
- Schroeder tenaculum
- Schubert biopsy
- Schumacher biopsy
- Schwartz clip-applying
- Schwartz temporary clamp-applying
- Scoville brain clip-applying
- Scoville brain spatula
- screw-holding
- Scudder intestinal
- Seitzinger tripolar cutting
- seizing
- self-centering bone-holding
- sella punch
- Selman vessel
- Selverstone rongeur
- Semb bone
- Semb rib
- Semken (also Semkin)
- Semken bipolar
- Semken delicate

forceps *(cont.)*
- Semken tissue
- septal
- sequestrum
- serrated
- Sewall brain clip
- Sewall clip-applying
- Shea alligator
- Shutt Mantis retrograde
- Simpson A6635
- Simpson-Luikart
- Singley intestinal
- Singley-Tuttle tissue
- Skene tenaculum
- skull punch
- Smithwick clip-applying
- smooth-tipped jeweler's
- smooth tissue
- Snowden-Pencer
- Somer
- spatula
- SpectraScience reusable biopsy
- Spence rongeur
- Spencer Wells artery
- spinal perforating
- spiral basket
- splinter
- sponge
- sponge-holding
- spoon
- spoon-grasping
- spreading
- Spurling-Kerrison rongeur
- standard Allis grasping
- standard endoscopic
- Steinmann intestinal
- Steinmann tendon
- sterilizing
- Stevenson alligator
- Stevenson grasping
- St. George hemorrhoid-seizing
- Stieglitz splinter
- Stiles seizing
- Stille-Barraya intestinal

forceps *(cont.)*
Stille gallstone
Stille-Horsley bone
Stille-Liston bone-cutting
Stille-Luer rongeur
Stiwer bone-holding
St. Mark's dissecting
Stolte
stone-grasping
stone-holding basket
Storz Microsystems plate-holding
straight
straight biopsy cup
straight Crile
straight-end cup
straight Kelly
SureBite biopsy
suture
Sweet clip-applying
Swiss jeweler's
Synthes Microsystems plate-holding
Takahashi
Take-Apart
Taylor dressing
taper-jaw
Taylor delicate
Teale
TeleMed reusable biopsy
tenaculum-reducing
tendon
tendon-holding
tendon-passing
tendon-pulling
tendon-retrieving
tendon-seizing
tendon-tunneling
termite
Thatcher
Therma-Jaw (or Thermajaw) hot urologic
Thomas Allis
Thorek gallbladder
Thorek-Mixter gallbladder
three-armed basket

forceps *(cont.)*
three-edge cutting
three-nail
three-pronged grasping
thumb
Tilley dressing and packing
Tischler biopsy
Tischler cervical biopsy punch
Tischler-Morgan biopsy
tissue
titanium microsurgical bipolar
Toennis tumor
tonsil
tonsillar
toothed Adson tissue
toothed tissue
torsion
transsphenoidal bipolar
Troeltsch dressing
Troutman rectus
tubing
Tudor-Edwards bone-cutting
tumor-grasping
Turner Warwick
Turrell biopsy
Turrell-Wittner rectal
Tuttle thoracic
Twisk
tying
Ulrich bone-holding
Ulrich-St. Gallen
up-biting biopsy cup
Van Buren sequestrum
Van Doren biopsy
Varco gallbladder
vascular
Verbrugge bone-holding
Vickers ring tip
Walter-Carmalt splinter
Walter-Liston
Walton biopsy
Walton-Ruskin
Walton wire-pulling
Wangensteen tissue

forceps *(cont.)*
- Ward approximating
- Waugh diathermy
- Waugh dissecting
- Weller cartilage
- Westphal
- Westphal gall duct
- Wiet cup
- Wikstroem artery
- Wilde dressing
- Wilde ethmoid
- Wilde rongeur
- Wilfred Adams diathermy artery
- Williams intestinal
- Wilson-Cook
- wire
- wire-crimping
- wire-cutting
- wire-extracting
- wire-holding
- wire-pulling
- wire-tightening
- wire-twisting
- Wittner biopsy
- Wrigley
- W-shaped
- Yankauer
- Yasargil artery
- Yasargil bayonet
- Yasargil clip-applying
- Yasargil hypophyseal
- Yasargil knotting
- Yasargil micro
- Yasargil tumor
- Yeoman biopsy
- Yeoman rectal biopsy
- Yeoman-Turrell rectal biopsy
- Yeoman-Wittner rectal
- Young
- Young intestinal
- Z-Clamp
- Zenker artery

forceps speculum
forceps with needle bayonet/stylet
Ford-Dixon hemorrhoid ligator
Ford Hospital ventricular cannula
foregut
foreign body forceps
foreign body infiltrate
foreign body sensation
foreign body trauma
foreign material
forensic pathology
foreshortening of mesentery
forestomach
fork
- carotid
- double-prong
- Gardiner-Brown tuning
- Hardy three-prong
- implant application
- Jannetta
- Rhoton
- three-prong
- tuning

Formad kidney
formal laparotomy
Forman nasal elevator
Forman nasal rasp
Forman rhinoplasty scissors
formation
- bezoar
- gallstone
- gas
- gastric pouch
- Gothic arch
- hernia
- intestinal pouch
- pouch
- stone

formed stool
formula (see also *feeding*)
- Advance
- Deliver 2.0
- Enfamil with iron
- Ensure Plus
- flow/pressure/resistance
- Harris-Benedict mathematical

formula *(cont.)*
- I-Soyalac
- Impact enteral
- infant
- Isomil SF (sucrose-free)
- Lofenalac
- Lonalac
- Nursoy
- Nutramigen
- Peptamen liquid diet
- Perative
- Portagen
- PreCare Conceive nutritional supplement
- predigested protein
- Pregestimil
- Prosobee
- RCF (Ross carbohydrate-free)
- Similac PM 60/40 low iron
- Similac with iron
- SMA
- soy-based
- Soyalac
- Travasorb MCT (medium chain triglyceride) food supplement.

Foroblique lens (in cystoscope)
Forrest classification of gastroduodenal ulcer
Forta Shake nutritional therapy
Forte distal radius plate
fortification
fortisan fabric (cellulose) graft
Fortison enteral feeding
Forvade (cidofovir) gel dressing
forward-cutting knife
forwarding probe
forward oblique telescope
forward-viewing endoscope
Foscan (temoporfin, mTHPC) mediated photodynamic therapy
fossa (pl. fossae)
- adipose (of breast)
- axillary
- Broesike

fossa *(cont.)*
- duodenal
- epigastric
- gallbladder
- Gruber-Landzert
- hypogastric
- ileocecal
- infraduodenal
- inguinal
- Jobert
- Jonnesco
- Landzert
- mesentericoparietal
- mesogastric
- paraduodenal
- parajejunal (Broesike)
- retroduodenal
- Scarpa
- sigmoid
- subsigmoid
- Treitz
- umbilical
- Waldeyer

Foss bifid gallbladder retractor
Foss biliary duct retractor
Foss forceps
Foss intestinal clamp
Foster needle holder
Foster-TC needle holder
fotemustine
Fouchet test
foul-smelling stools
four-channel water-perfused system
four Fs (female, fat, forty, fertile)
four-flanged nail
four-gland hyperplasia
four-hole (4-hole) plate
four-hour glucose tolerance test
four-lumen tube
Fourneau 309 (suramin sodium)
Fournier gangrene after hemorrhoidectomy
Fournier One-Piece cannula
Fournier Toomey syringe cannula

four-quadrant hemorrhoidectomy
four-strand Savage suture
four-strand suture
fourth bronchial pouch
fourth intercostal space
fourth pharyngeal pouch
four-wire basket
foveal gastric mucosa
foveolar gastric mucosa
foveolar hyperplasia
foveolosulciolar gastric mucosa
Fowler position
Fox bipolar forceps
Fox curette
Fox sign
Foxy Pouch Cover
FPC (familial polyposis coli)
fractional epidural anesthesia
fractional spinal anesthesia
fractionated diet
fractionation of bilirubin
fraction, plasma protein
Fractura Flex bandage
fracture, basilar skull
fracture-reducing elevator
fragile histidine triad (FHIT)
fragmented tissue
fragment of tissue
Fragmin (dalteparin sodium injection)
fraise, DFDR diamond
Framer tendon-passing needle
Francis test
Francisella tularensis (formerly *Pasteurella tularensis*)
frank blood
frank blood in stool
frank cirrhosis
Frankenfeldt cotton applicator
Frankfeldt rectal diathermy snare
Frankfeldt rectal swab holder
frank gangrene of bowel
frank hemorrhage
Franklin-Silverman biopsy cannula
Franklin-Silverman biopsy needle
frank necrosis
frank perforation
frank pulmonary edema
frank pus
frank rigors
Frank-Starling curve
Frank-Starling mechanism
frank ulceration
Franseen needle
Franz abdominal retractor
Fraser artery forceps
Frater suture guide
Frazier Baron-style
Frazier brain-exploring cannula
Frazier Britetrac suction tube
Frazier cordotomy knife
Frazier dural elevator
Frazier dural hook
Frazier dural scissors
Frazier dural separator
Frazier hook
Frazier laminectomy retractor
Frazier lighted brain retractor
Frazier nerve hook
Frazier-Paparella suction tube
Frazier pituitary knife
Frazier scissors
Frazier suction tip
Frazier suction tube
Frazier suction tube obturator
Frazier ventricular cannula
Frazier ventricular needle
FreAmine amino acid solution
FreAmine HBC 6.9%
FreAmine III 3% (8.5%) with Electrolytes
freckle-like lesion
Fredet-Ramstedt pyloromyotomy
FRED (fog reduction/elimination device)
FRED Lite alcohol-free solution
free air
free air in abdomen
free air in colon

free air in GI tract
free band of colon
Freedom knife
free fat graft
free flap
free flap breast reconstruction (gluteus maximus to internal mammary vessels)
free flap transfer
free-floating testis
free fluid
freeform prosthetic mesh
free graft
freehand CT-guided biopsy
free hepatic venous pressure
free hormone
freeing up of adhesion
free intestinal graft
free intraperitoneal air
free jejunal graft
free jejunum transfer
free jejunum transfer with microvascular anastomosis
freely movable nodule
Freeman cookie cutter areola marker
free muscle graft
free nipple graft
free nipple transposition technique reduction mammoplasty
free perforation
free radical
Freer chisel
Freer dissector
free reflux
Freer periosteal elevator
Freer septal elevator
Freer septum elevator
Freer skin hook
Freer-Swanson ganglion knife
free skin graft
FreeStyle glucose monitoring device
free thyroxine (T_4)
free thyroxine index (FT_4I or FTI)
free tie (individual ligature)
free/total PSA (prostate-specific antigen) index
free transplanted graft
free water
free water infusion
freeze-dried bone graft
Freezor cryocatheter catheter
Freiberg biopsy set
Freiberg cartilage knife
Freiberg meniscectomy knife
French bougie
French dilator
French eye needle
French mushroom-tip catheter
French stent
French T-tube
frenectomy
frenoplasty
frenulectomy
frenum, lingual
frequency of stools
fresh blood clot
fresh frozen graft
fresh frozen plasma (FFP)
fresh frozen section
Fresh Start breast support
fresh whole blood
friability
friable bowel
friable clot
friable lesion
friable mass
friable mucosa
friable papilloma
friable tissue
friction knot
friction rub
fried food
Friedland scissors
Friedländer bacillus
Friedman bone rongeur
Friedman perineal retractor
Friedman rongeur forceps
Friedman rongeur

FRIEND (foreign body, radiation, infection, epithelialization, neoplasm, distal obstruction)
Frigitronics probe
Fritsch abdominal retractor
frog-leg (adj.)
frog-leg lateral view
frog-leg position
Fröhlich (Froehlich) syndrome
frondlike filling defect
frondlike pattern
frontal abscess abscess
frontal plate
frontal region
frontal suture
frontal view
front and side wire cutter
front lifting hood rectoscope tube
frontoethmoidal suture
frontolacrimal suture
frontomaxillary suture
frontonasal suture
frontoparietal suture
frontosphenoid suture
frontozygomatic suture
frosted liver
Frost stitch
frothy fluid
frown incision
frozen section
frozen section diagnosis
Frykholm bone rongeur
FTI (free thyroxine index)
FTSG (full-thickness skin graft)
fucosylated alpha-fetoprotein (AFP)
fucosylation index of alpha-fetoprotein (AFP)
FUDR; FUdR (5-fluorouracil deoxyribonucleoside) (floxuridine)
Fujinon biopsy forceps
Fujinon colonoscope
Fujinon duodenoscope
Fujinon endoscope
Fujinon EVC-M videocolonoscope
Fujinon EVD-XL videoduodenoscope
Fujinon EVE videoendoscope
Fujinon EVG-F upper GI videoendoscope
Fujinon EVS-E flexible sigmoidoscope
Fujinon FG-100FP flexible gastroscope
Fujinon FG-100PE flexible gastroscope
Fujinon flexible sigmoidoscope
Fujinon PRO-PC flexible sigmoidoscope
Fujinon SIG-E2 flexible sigmoidoscope
Fujinon SIG-EK flexible sigmoidoscope
Fujinon SIG-ET flexible sigmoidoscope
Fujinon SIG-PC flexible sigmoidoscope
Fujinon sigmoidoscope
Fujinon UGI-FP endoscope
Fujinon UGI-PE flexible gastroscope
Fujita snake retractor
Fujita suction retractor
Fukushima C-clamp
Fukushima-Giannotta curette
Fukushima-Giannotta dissector
Fukushima-Giannotta needle holder
Fukushima-Giannotta scissors
Fukushima retractor
Fukushima teardrop suction
fulgurate
fulguration, electrosurgical
fulguration of tumor
fulguration of ulcerative lesion
full activity
full backboard
full-blown bacterial peritonitis
full-blown syndrome
full-column barium enema
full-curve blade
Fuller rectal shield
Fuller shield
Fuller shield dressing
full lateral position
full length view
full-liquid diet
full Magill curve
fullness, abdominal

full-radius resector knife
full-thickness involvement
full-thickness reconstruction
full-thickness rectal biopsy
full-thickness skin graft (FTSG)
fulminant bacteremia
fulminant colitis
fulminant enterocolitis
fulminant hepatic failure (FHF)
fulminant hepatitis
fulminant liver failure or end-stage chronic liver disease
fulminant viral hepatitis (FVH)
fulminant Wilson disease
fulminating appendicitis
fulminating pancreatitis
fulminating ulcerative colitis
Fulton laminectomy rongeur
fumarylacetoacetase parahydroxyphenylpyruvic acid (p-HPPA) oxidase
FUMIR (5-fluorouracil, Mitomycin C, radiation)
functional anatomical mapping
functional bowel disease
  irritable bowel disease (IBD)
  irritable colon
functional bowel obstruction
functional bowel syndrome
functional colitis
functional constipation
functional cystic duct obstruction
functional death
functional diarrhea
functional disorder
functional dyspepsia
functional gastrointestinal disorder (FGID)
functional hyperinsulinism
functional hypoglycemia
functional intestinal obstruction
Functional Living Index–Cancer (FLIC)
functional material
functional pain
functional shrunken colon
functional spleen
functioning adrenocortical tumor
functioning allograft
functioning neoplasm
functioning thyroid tissue
fundal plication
fundal varices
fundic-antral junction
fundic gland gastritis
fundic mobilization in Nissen fundoplication
fundic mucosa
fundic patch
fundoplasty (see also *operation*)
  anterior
  Belsey IV
  Dor
  esophagogastric
  Gomez
  Hill
  laparoscopic esophagogastric
  Nissen
  posterior
  Thal-Nissen
  Toupet
fundoplasty with fundic patch
fundoplication (see also *operation*)
  Belsey Mark IV
  Belsey partial
  Belsey two-thirds wrap
  Collis-Nissen
  endoscopic
  floppy-type of Nissen
  herniated
  high-resistance
  Hill gastropexy
  intrathoracic Nissen
  laparoscopic
  laparoscopic anterior partial
  laparoscopic Nissen and Toupet
  ligamentum teres cardiopexy
  low-resistance

fundoplication *(cont.)*
  Nissen
  Nissen 360° wrap
  re-do
  Rossetti modification of Nissen
  slipped Nissen
  Toupet hemifundoplication
  transthoracic Nissen
  twisted
  videoscopic
fundus
  bald gastric
  gallbladder
  gastric
  stomach
  uterine
fungal abscess
fungal esophagitis
fungal infection
fungal smear
fungating mass
fungiform papilla
fungus
fungus-like bacteria
funicular inguinal hernia
funicular suture
funisitis
funnel, fascia/peritoneum
FUO (fever of unknown or undetermined origin)
Furacin gauze dressing
Furamide (diloxanide furoate)
furazolidone
Furniss anastomosis clamp
Furniss-Clute clamp
furodazole
furosemide
furrier suture
fused kidney
fusiform bacillus
fusiform widening of duct
fusion graft
fusion plate
fusion protein
FVH (fulminant viral hepatitis)
FyBron alginate wound dressing

G, g

Gabriel hemorrhoidal needle
Gabriel proctoscope
Gabriel rectal speculum
GAD (glutamic acid decarboxylase)
gadodiamide
Gadolite oral suspension
gadopentetate dimeglumine
Gaenslen split-heel incision
gag (see *mouth gag*)
gagging without emesis
gag reflex
gag response
Gail breast cancer model
gait plate
galactocele
galactogram
galactorrhea
galactose-1-phosphate uridyltransferase
galactosemia
Galeati gland
Galencia disposable anoscope
Gallagher rasp
Gallannaugh bone plate
gallbladder
  bilobed
  body of
  calcified
  chronically inflamed
  Courvoisier

gallbladder *(cont.)*
  dilated
  distended
  double
  edematous
  fish-scale
  floating
  folded fundus
  fundus of
  hourglass
  inflamed
  mobile
  multiseptate
  neck of
  painful palpable
  partially intrahepatic
  perforated
  porcelain
  robin's egg–blue
  sandpaper
  stasis
  strawberry
  thick-walled
  thin-walled
  totally intrahepatic
  wandering
gallbladder adenoma
gallbladder bag positioner
gallbladder bed

gallbladder bile
gallbladder calculus (pl. calculi)
gallbladder carcinoma
gallbladder colic
gallbladder contractility, impaired
gallbladder contraction
gallbladder-cystic duct junction
gallbladder disuse
gallbladder emptying
gallbladder empyema
gallbladder fistula
gallbladder fossa
gallbladder fundus
gallbladder hydrops
gallbladder ileus
gallbladder inflammation
gallbladder infundibulum
gallbladder lift
gallbladder mucosa
gallbladder polyp
gallbladder scan
gallbladder scoop
gallbladder sludge
gallbladder stasis
gallbladder stone
gallbladder trocar
gallbladder villi
gallbladder wall abscess
gallbladder wall thickening
gall duct
gall duct forceps
gall duct spoon
Gallego method
Gallie needle
gallium-arsenide (GaA) laser
gallium 67 (^{67}Ga)
gallium scan
gallows-type retractor
gallstone (see also *stone*)
  asymptomatic
  bilirubin pigment
  black pigment
  brown pigment
  cholesterol

gallstone *(cont.)*
  common bile duct
  dissolution of
  faceted
  floating
  impacted
  innocent
  large
  mixed-cholesterol
  mulberry
  opacifying
  pigmented
  radiolucent
  radiopaque
  retained
  silent
  spilled
  symptomatic
gallstone erosion
gallstone forceps
gallstone formation
gallstone ileus
gallstone ileus syndrome
gallstone in common bile duct
gallstone migration
gallstone obstruction of main pancreatic duct
gallstone pancreatitis
gallstone probe
GALT (gut-associated lymphoid tissue)
Galt cranial trephine
galvanic probe
Galzin (zinc acetate)
Gambee suture
gamma alcoholism
gamma brachytherapy
gamma globulin
gamma-glutamyl transferase (GGT)
gamma-glutamyl transpeptidase (GGTP)
gamma locking nail
Gamma radiosurgical knife
gamma transverse colon loop
Gamna disease

Gandhi knife
ganglion hook
ganglion knife
ganglionated plexus
ganglioneuroma
ganglioneuromatosis
  diffuse transmural
  diffuse transmural intestinal
  extensive florid transmural
  extensive transmural
gangrene
  appendiceal
  arteriosclerotic
  cold
  cutaneous
  decubital
  diabetic
  dry
  embolic
  emphysematous
  Fournier
  gas
  hemorrhagic
  hospital
  hot
  Meleney
  moist
  nosocomial
  Pott
  pressure
  primary
  progressive bacterial synergistic
  secondary
  static
  thrombotic
  traumatic
  venous
  wet
  white
gangrenous appendicitis
gangrenous appendix
gangrenous bowel
gangrenous cholangiolitis
gangrenous cholecystitis
gangrenous colitis
gangrenous hernia
gangrenous necrosis
gangrenous pulp necrosis
Ganser diverticulum
Gant clamp
Gantrisin
gaping wound
Garcia aorta clamp
Gardiner-Brown tuning fork
Gardner forceps
Gardner elevator
Gardner neurosurgical skull clamp
Gardner skull clamp pin
Gardner syndrome
Gardner-Wells tongs
Gardnerella vaginitis (formerly *Haemophilus vaginalis* or *Corynebacterium vaginale*)
garment hook
Garren-Edwards balloon
Garren-Edwards gastric (GEG) bubble
Garren gastric bubble
Garrett dilator
Garrett retractor
gas
  colonic
  compressed carbon dioxide
  free subphrenic
  paucity of colon
  periappendiceal
  subcutaneous
Gas-Ban (calcium carbonate; simethicone)
gas bloating
gas-bloat syndrome
gas cupula
gas density line (on x-ray)
gas embolism
gaseous cholecystitis
gaseous distention
gas exchange
gas formation
gas-forming bacteria

gas-forming liver abscess
gas-forming organism in bowel wall
GasFree Omni-Lift retractor
gas insufflation
gasless laparoscopic-assisted colostomy
gasless laparoscopy
gas pattern
gas-producing food
Gas Relief (simethicone)
gassiness
gassy
gastrectomized patient
gastrectomy
  Billroth I
  Billroth II
  distal
  distal with excision of ulcer
  hand-assisted laparoscopic
  high subtotal
  Horsley
  limited
  Maki pylorus-preserving
  near-total
  palliative
  pancreatic-preserving total
  partial
  partial, distal
  Polya
  proximal
  segmental
  subtotal
  total
  video-assisted total
gastric achlorhydria
gastric acid
gastric acid hypersecretion
gastric acid production
gastric acid secretion, decreased
gastric acid test
gastric adenocarcinoma
gastric air bubble (on x-ray)
gastric algid malaria
gastric analysis
gastric antral erosion
gastric antral mucosa
gastric antral vascular ectasia (GAVE)
gastric antrum
gastric antrum G cell
gastric artery
gastric aspirate
gastric aspiration tube
gastric atony
gastric atrophy
gastric balloon (see *balloon*)
gastric band
gastric banding, laparoscopic
gastric baseline
gastric B cell lymphoma
gastric bile acid test
gastric bubble
gastric bypass
gastric calculus
gastric calibration tube
gastric canal
gastric capacity
gastric carcinoma (linitis plastica)
gastric cardia
gastric channel
gastric colic
gastric content test
gastric contents
gastric cuff
gastric cytology
gastric decompression
gastric diet
gastric dilatation
gastric dilatation/volvulus (GDV)
gastric distention
gastric-duodenal coordination
gastric duplication cyst
gastric dyspepsia
gastric dysrrhythmia
gastric emptying
  decreased
  delayed
gastric emptying scan
gastric emptying test
gastric erosion

gastric fistula
gastric fold
gastric follicle
gastric function test
gastric fundus
gastric fundus wrap
gastric gland
gastric groove
gastric hemorrhage
gastric hypersecretion
gastric hypersecretion of hydrochloric acid
gastric hypersensitivity
gastric hypoacidity
gastric impression on liver
gastric inhibitory polypeptide (GIP)
gastric integrity
gastric juice
gastric Kaposi sarcoma
gastric lavage
gastric lavage tube
gastric leiomyoma
gastric leiomyosarcoma
gastric loop-type bypass
gastric lymph node
gastric lymphatic follicle
gastric membrane vesicle
gastric motility disorder
gastric motility study
gastric motor disorder
gastric mucin
gastric mucosa
gastric mucosa atrophy
gastric mucosa ischemia
gastric mucosal barrier
gastric mucosal fold
gastric mucosal hypertrophy
gastric mucosal pattern classification: A, AB, B, BC, C, etc.
gastric myoelectrical activity
gastric neobladder procedure
gastric NK-like T cell lympho-proliferative disorder
gastric obstruction
gastric omentum
gastric outflow obstruction
gastric outlet, dilation of
gastric outlet obstruction (GOO)
gastric outlet stricture
gastric outline (on x-ray)
gastric pacemaker
gastric pacemaker cell
gastric pacemaker region
gastric parietal cell
gastric partition
gastric partitioning
gastric perforation
gastric phase of acid secretion
gastric pit
gastric plexus
gastric polyp
gastric polyposis
gastric pool
gastric pouch
gastric protection
gastric reconstruction
  Longmire-Gutgemann
  Roux
  Turbinger
gastric remnant
gastric resection
gastric reservoir
gastric restrictive procedure
gastric retention (GR)
gastric rupture
gastric sclerosis
gastric secretion
gastric secretion rate
gastric secretory test
gastric stapling
gastric stasis and postprandial fullness
gastric stump
gastric stump cancer
gastric surface
gastric T-cell lymphoma
gastric tear
gastric tissue patch, vascularized
gastric transit time

gastric ulcer
gastric ulceration
gastric variceal bleeding
gastric varices
gastric vein
gastric venacaval shunt
gastric volvulus
gastric washing
gastric window
Gastrimmune (gemcitabine) vaccine
gastrin cell hyperfunction
gastrin, fasting serum
gastrin hormone
gastrin-induced excessive gastric acid
  production
gastrin inhibition
gastrinoma
  duodenal
  metastatic
  pancreatic
  primary
  recurrent
gastrinoma triangle
gastrin-producing tumor
gastrin-secretin stimulation
gastrin-secretin stimulation test
gastrin-secreting cell
gastrin-secreting non-beta islet cell
  tumor
gastrin-secreting tumor (gastrinoma)
gastrin-stimulated intestinal motility
gastrin stimulation test
gastrin test
gastritis
  acute
  acute erosive (AEG)
  acute hemorrhagic
  alcoholic
  alkaline reflux
  allergic
  antral
  aspirin-induced
  atrophic
  autoimmune chronic

gastritis *(cont.)*
  bile-induced
  bile reflux
  catarrhal
  chemical
  chronic
  chronic atrophic
  chronic cystic
  chronic erosive
  chronic follicular
  chronic (type B)
  cirrhotic
  corrosive
  cystica polyposa
  diffuse varioliform
  drug-induced
  emphysematous
  eosinophilic
  erosive
  exfoliative
  follicular
  fundic gland
  giant hypertrophic
  granulomatous
  Helicobacter pylori-associated
    (HPAG)
  hemorrhagic
  hypersecretory chronic
  hypertrophic
  idiopathic chronic erosive
  interstitial
  irritant
  necrotizing
  nonerosive nonspecific
  phlegmonous
  polypous
  proliferative hypertrophic
  pseudomembranous radiation
  radiation
  reflux bile
  stress
  stress-induced
  superficial
  toxic

gastritis *(cont.)*
  type A (autoimmune chronic)
  type B (hypersecretory chronic)
  type AB (idiopathic chronic [environmental])
  ulcerative
  varioliform
  viral
  zonal
gastritis varioliformis
gastroadenitis
gastroalbumorrhea
gastroanastomosis
gastroatonia
gastroblennorrhea
gastrocamera, Olympus GTF-A
gastrocardiac syndrome
Gastroccult test
gastrocele
gastrochronorrhea
gastrocolic fistula
gastrocolic ligament
gastrocolic omentum
gastrocolic reflex
gastrocolic ulcer
gastrocolitis
gastrocolonic response
gastrocoloptosis
gastrocolostomy
gastrocutaneous fistula
gastrodialysis
gastrodiaphragmatic ligament
Gastrodiscoides hominis
Gastrodiscus hominis
gastroduodenal anastomosis
gastroduodenal artery
gastroduodenal artery complex
gastroduodenal fistula
gastroduodenal lumen
gastroduodenal lymph node
gastroduodenal orifice
gastroduodenal ulcer
gastroduodenitis
gastroduodenopancreatectomy
gastroduodenoscopy
gastroduodenostomy
  Billroth I
  Jaboulay
  laparoscopic
  tube
gastrodynia
gastroenteric
gastroenteritis (see also *enteritis*)
  acute (AGE)
  acute infectious
  astrovirus
  bacterial
  calicivirus
  Campylobacter
  coronavirus
  endemic nonbacterial
  eosinophilic
  epidemic
  epidemic nonbacterial
  food-borne
  infantile
  infectious
  nonbacterial
  Norwalk
  porcine transmissible
  rotavirus
  toxic
  viral
  water-borne
  winter
gastroenteritis virus type A
gastroenteritis virus type B
gastroenteroanastomosis
gastroenterocolitis
gastroenterocolostomy
gastroenterologist
gastroenterology
gastroenteropathy
gastroenteroplasty
gastroenteroptosis
gastroenterostomy
  anterior gastric
  Balfour

gastroenterostomy *(cont.)*
  Billroth I
  Billroth II
  Braun-Jaboulay
  Courvoisier
  Finney
  Heineke-Mikulicz
  Hofmeister
  laparoscopic
  Polya
  prophylactic
  Roux
  Roux-en-Y
  Schoemaker
  short-limb Roux-en-Y
  side-to-side
  transomental posterior
  Von Haberer
  Wolfler
gastroepiploic arcade
gastroepiploic artery
gastroepiploic gland
gastroepiploic vein
gastroepiploic vessel
gastroesophageal (GE)
gastroesophageal hernia
gastroesophageal incompetence
gastroesophageal junction
gastroesophageal laceration
gastroesophageal laceration-hemorrhage syndrome
gastroesophageal reflux (GER)
gastroesophageal reflux disease (GERD)
gastroesophageal scintiscan
gastroesophageal sphincter
gastroesophageal variceal bleed
gastroesophageal variceal plexus
gastroesophageal vestibule
gastroesophageal window
gastroesophagitis
gastroesophagostomy
gastrogastrostomy
gastrogavage
gastrogenic
gastrogenous diarrhea
Gastrografin contrast medium
Gastrografin enema
Gastrografin swallow
gastrograph
gastrohepatic bare area
gastrohepatic ligament
gastrohepatic omentum
gastrohydrorrhea
gastroileac reflex
gastroileal reflex
gastroileitis
gastroileostomy
gastroinoma triangle
gastrointestinal (GI)
gastrointestinal bleeding
gastrointestinal cross
gastrointestinal cross artifact
gastrointestinal decompression
gastrointestinal dysmotility syndrome
gastrointestinal electrolytes
gastrointestinal endoscopist
gastrointestinal fistula
gastrointestinal fluid loss
gastrointestinal hemorrhage
gastrointestinal hormone
gastrointestinal hyperacidity
gastrointestinal inhibitory hormone
gastrointestinal losses
gastrointestinal manifestations of Zollinger-Ellison syndrome
gastrointestinal motility
gastrointestinal mucosa
gastrointestinal mucosal hemorrhage
gastrointestinal needle
gastrointestinal peptide
gastrointestinal perforation
gastrointestinal peristalsis
gastrointestinal plaque
gastrointestinal polyposis
gastrointestinal polyp
gastrointestinal quality of life index (GIQLI)

gastrointestinal regularity peptide
gastrointestinal series
gastrointestinal stasis
gastrointestinal stoma
gastrointestinal telangiectasia
gastrointestinal therapeutic system (GITS)
gastrointestinal toxicity
gastrointestinal tract
gastrointestinal tract bleeding
gastrointestinal tract perforation
gastrointestinal tumor
gastrointestinal ulcer
gastrointestinal ulceration
gastrojejunal anastomosis
gastrojejunal constipation
gastrojejunal loop obstruction syndrome
gastrojejunal ulcer
gastrojejunocolic fistula
gastrojejunostomy
 antecolic long-loop isoperistaltic
 Billroth II
 loop
 percutaneous endoscopic
 prophylactic
 Roux-en-Y
 Roux-Y
 stapled
gastrokinesograph
gastrolavage
gastrolienal ligament
gastrolith
gastrolithiasis
gastrologist
gastrology
gastrolysis
Gastrolyte oral solution
gastromalacia
GastroMARK (ferumoxsil) imaging agent
gastromegaly
gastromyxorrhea
gastronesteostomy
gastro-omental artery
gastropancreatic fold
gastropancreatic ligament
gastropancreatic reflex
gastroparalysis
gastroparesis
 diabetic
 idiopathic
 nondiabetic
 postvagotomy
 transient
gastroparesis diabeticorum
gastropathic
gastropathy
 benign hyperplastic
 chemical
 diabetic
 drug-induced
 hemorrhagic erosive
 hyperplastic
 hypersecretory
 hypertrophic
 idiopathic hypertrophic
 NSAID-induced
 portal hypertensive
 prolapse
 protein-losing
gastropexy
 anterior
 Belsey-Mark IV
 belt loop
 Boerema anterior
 circumcostal
 Hill posterior
 incisional
 laparoscopic-assisted
 laparoscopic-assisted percutaneous anterior
 percutaneous anterior
 posterior
 posterior diaphragmatic
 prophylactic
 T-fastener
 T-tack
gastropexy to diaphragm

gastrophrenic ligament
gastroplasty (GP)
  adjustable ring
  Albert-Lembert
  Collis
  Collis-Nissen
  Eckhout vertical
  endoscopic
  fundoplication
  fundus rotation
  Gomez horizontal
  greater curvature banded
  horizontal
  Kuzmak gastric banding
  laparoscopic
  laparoscopic horizontal
  Laws
  layer-to-layer
  Mason vertical banded
  mini
  O'Leary lesser curvature
  silicone elastomer ring vertical (SRVG)
  Stamm
  tubular vertical
  unbanded
  V-banded
  vertical banded (VBG)
  vertical ring (VRG)
  vertical Silastic ring
gastroplication
gastropneumonic
Gastroport
gastroptosis
gastroptyxis
gastropulmonary
gastropylorectomy
gastropyloric
gastrorrhagia
gastrorrhaphy
gastrorrhea
gastrorrhexis
gastroschisis, Silastic silo reduction
gastroscope (see also *endoscope*)
  FCS-ML
  Fujinon FG-100FP flexible
  Fujinon FG-100PE flexible
  Fujinon UGI-PE flexible
  MIS Source
  Olympus CF-1T10L flexible
  Olympus CF-1T20L flexible
  Olympus CF-20L flexible
  Olympus CF-P20L flexible
  Olympus GF-UM130 ultrasound
  Olympus GIF-100 video
  Olympus GIF-1T10 flexible
  Olympus GIF-1T10 flexible therapeutic
  Olympus GIF-1T140 video
  Olympus GIF-1TV10 flexible
  Olympus GIF-2T10 flexible
  Olympus GIF-2T20 flexible therapeutic
  Olympus GIF-HM
  Olympus GIF-K
  Olympus GIF-N30 gastrofibroscope
  Olympus GIF-P140 video
  Olympus GIF-PQ20 flexible
  Olympus GIF-PV10 pediatric video
  Olympus GIF-Q140 video
  Olympus GIF-XP20 flexible
  Olympus GIF-XQ140 video
  Olympus GIF-XQ20 flexible multipurpose
  Olympus GIF-XQ30 flexible multipurpose
  Olympus GIF-XT30 gastrofibroscope
  Olympus TGF-2D flexible
  Pentax EG-1840 video
  Pentax EG-2530
  Pentax EG-2540 video
  Pentax EG-2731
  Pentax EG-2901 flexible
  Pentax EG-2930
  Pentax EG-2940 video
  Pentax EG-3430 video

gastroscope *(cont.)*
  Pentax EG-3440 video
  Pentax EG-3830T video
  Pentax EG-3840T video
  Pentax FC-38LX flexible
  Pentax FG-24V fiberoptic
  Pentax FG-29H flexible
  Pentax FG-29V fiberoptic
  Pentax FG-29X flexible
  Schindler semiflexible
gastroscopy
Gastrosed (hyoscyamine sulfate)
gastrospasm
gastrosphincteric pressure gradient
gastrosplenic ligament
gastrosplenic omentum
gastrostaxis
gastrostenosis
gastrostolavage
gastrostomy
  Beck
  Depage-Janeway
  drainage
  feeding
  Gauderer-Ponsky PEG
  Gauderer-Ponsky-Izant PEG
  Glassman
  Kader
  laparoscopic
  Partipilo
  PEG (percutaneous endoscopic)
  percutaneous
  Russell PEG
  Ssabanejew-Frank
  Stamm
  Witzel
gastrostomy feeding
gastrostomy tube
gastrostomy tube placement
Gastro-Test
gastrotome
gastrotomy
gastrotonometer
gastrotonometer electronic sensor
gastrotonometry
gastrotoxic
gastrotoxin
gastrotropic
Gastrovist contrast medium
gastroxia
Gastrozepine (pirenzepine HCl)
Gas-X (simethicone)
Gaucher cell
Gaucher disease (types 1 to 3)
Gaucher splenomegaly
Gauderer Genie feeding device
Gauderer-Ponsky PEG operation
Gauderer-Ponsky-Izant PEG (percutaneous endoscopic gastrostomy)
Gau gastric balloon
gauge
  pressure
  Statham P23 strain
gauntlet bandage
gauze (see also *dressing*)
  absorbent
  Aquaphor
  elasticized
  foam
  iodoform
  Nu Gauze
  Owen
  PanoGauze hydrogel-impregnated
  Sofrature
  Surgicel
  tantalum
  Teletrast absorbable surgical gauze
  TransiGel hydrogel-impregnated gauze
  Vaseline
  Xeroform
gauze dressing
gauze packing
gauze sponge
gavage
gavage feeding
GAVE (gastric antral vascular ectasia)
Gavin-Miller intestinal forceps

Gaviscon (aluminum hydroxide;
  magnesium carbonate)
Gaviscon-2
gay bowel syndrome
Gay gland
Gaymar blanket
Gaymar Industries
Gaynor-Hart position
Gazayerli endoscopic retractor
Gazayerli knot tier
GBP (gastric bypass procedure)
GBS (group B streptococcus)
G cell
GCS (Glasgow Coma Scale)
GCT (giant cell transformation)
GD DTPA compound for MRI scan
GDM (gestational diabetes mellitus)
GDV (gastric dilatation volvulus)
GEA (gastroepiploic artery) graft
GE (gastroesophageal)
Gee-Herter disease
Gee-Herter-Heubner disease
Gee-Herter-Heubner syndrome
Geenan Endotorque guidewire
Gee-Thaysen disease
GEG (Garren-Edwards gastric) bubble
Geiger rongeur
GE junction
gel (see *dressing*; *medication*)
gelatin-resorcin-formalin glue
gelatin sponge
gelatinous carcinoma
gelatinous fluid
gelatinous material
gelatinous polyp
gelbe cell
gel-filled breast implant
Gelfilm (absorbable gelatin film)
Gelfoam (absorbable gelatin sponge)
Gelfoam cookie (pad)
Gelfoam soaked in sodium tetradecyl
  sulfate
gel-like material
Gelpi pediatric retractor
Gelpi perineal retractor
Gelpi self-retaining retractor
Gelusil (aluminum hydroxide; magnesium hydroxide; simethicone)
Gelusil-M
Gelusil-II
Gely suture
gemcitabine HCl
Gemella morbillorum
Gemini artery forceps
Gemini Finochietto artery forceps
Gemini gall duct forceps
Gemini thoracic forceps
Gemzar (gemcitabine HCl)
Genasense
Genasoft Plus (casanthranol; docusate
  sodium)
Genaton; Genaton Extra Strength
  (aluminum hydroxide; magnesium
  carbonate)
gene
  adenomatous polyposis coli (APC)
  adenoviral p53
  APC (adenomatous polyposis coli)
  beta
  beta-globin
  BRCA1
  BRCA2
  DNA repair
  HER-2/neu
  IFN-alpha 2
  MCC (mutated in colon cancer)
  MDR3
  multidrug resistance (MDR) 3
  mutant
  p53 adenoviral
  RhoC
  RhoC CTPase
  tumor suppressor
gene amplification
gene mutation
gene promoter methylation
general endotracheal anesthesia
general mask

general pathology
generalized edema (anasarca)
generalized glycogenosis
generalized gut dysmotility
generalized inflammatory state
generalized peritonitis
General Surgical Innovations (GSI)
generation, islet cell
generator
Genesis container
Genesis 2000 laser
Genestone 190 lithotriptor
gene therapy program
genetic counseling
genetic death
genetic diagnosis
genetic disorders, major causes of
  complex
  cytogenic
  environmental
  polygenic/multifactorial
  single gene (mendelian)
genetic engineering
genetic evaluation
genetic hemochromatosis
genetic heterogenicity
genetic marker
genetic material
genetic screening
genetic trait
  autosomal dominant
  autosomal recessive
Gengraf (cyclosporine)
geniculum
genital branch of genitofemoral nerve
genital carcinoma
genital fold
genital infection
genital nerve
genital ridge
genital ulcer
genitofemoral cutaneous nerve
genitofemoral nerve
genitourinary fistula
Genotropin (somatropin lyophilized powder)
Genotropin MiniQuick
Genotropin Pen 12
genotype, HCV (1-6)
Gentell wound dressing
Gentlax (senna concentrate)
GentleLASE Plus laser
gentle sump action
Gentle Touch postoperative colostomy appliance
genu of pancreatic duct
Genz-Arm pneumatic retractor
Genzyme Surgical Products
George artery forceps
Georgia (GA) law (glucose, age, LDH, AST, WBC)
Gerald bipolar forceps
Gerald-Brown tissue forceps
Gerald dissecting forceps
Gerald dressing forceps
Gerald tissue forceps
Gerbode forceps
Gerbode patent ductus clamp
GERD (gastroesophageal reflux disease)
Geref (sermorelin acetate)
GE (gastroesophageal) reflux
GE RT 3200 ADV II ultrasound system
GE Senographe 20001 digital mammography system
geriatric constipation
GeriMend dressing
Geriplex-FS
Germanin (suramin sodium)
germinal infection
germinating basal cell layer
germline RET proto-oncogene point mutations
Gerota fascia
Gerson therapy protocol
Gerzog bone mallet
gestational diabetes
gestational edema

gestational sac
GFX 2 coronary stent
GGT (gamma-glutamyl transferase)
GGTP (gamma-glutamyl transpeptidase)
Ghajar guide
Gherini-Kauffman endo-otoprobe laser
Ghon primary lesion
GI (see *gastrointestinal*)
GIA (gastrointestinal anastomosis)
GIA Auto Suture apparatus
Giampapa suturing technique
Gianotti-Crosti syndrome
giant anorectal condyloma acuminatum
giant cell
giant cell adenocarcinoma
giant cell carcinoma
giant cell hepatitis
giant cell monstrocellular sarcoma
giant cell sarcoma
giant cell thyroiditis
giant cell tumor
giant colon
giant congenital nevus (pl. nevi)
giant hypertrophic gastritis
giant peptic ulcer
Gianturco expandable (self-expanding) metallic biliary stent
Gianturco prosthesis
Gianturco-Rösch Z-stent
Gianturco-Roubin flexible coil stent
Gianturco wool-tufted wire coil
Giardia intestinalis
Giardia lamblia
giardial colitis
giardiasis
GIA stapler
Gibberella fujikuroi
gibbous deformity
Gibney bandage
Gibson-Balfour abdominal retractor
Gibson bandage
Giebel blade plate
Gierke disease
Giertz rongeur
Giertz-Shoemaker rib shears
Giertz-Stille scissors
Gifford mastoid retractor
gift-wrap suture technique
gigantism
Gigli saw
Gigli saw blade
Gigli saw guide
Gigli wire saw
Gilbert cholemia
Gilbert classification of groin hernias (types 1–5)
Gilbert cystic duct forceps
Gilbert disease
Gilbert free-formed umbrella-shaped plug
Gilbert-Rutkow-Robbins classification of groin hernias (types 1–7)
Gilbert sign
Gilbert syndrome
Gilchrist ileocecal bladder
Gildenberg biopsy forceps
Gillette joint
Gillies bone graft
Gillies bone hook
Gillies diathermy forceps
Gillies-Dingman hook
Gillies-Finochietto needle holder
Gillies hook
Gillies horizontal dermal suture
Gillies lightweight forceps
Gillies needle
Gillies needle holder
Gillies skin hook
Gillies suture
Gillies-TC needle holder
Gillies tissue forceps
Gilliland etching cannula
Gilvernet retractor
gingival gland
gingival mucosa
gingivectomy
Gingrass and Messer pin

Giordano sphincter
GIP (gastric inhibitory polypeptide)
GIP (glucose-dependent insulinotropic polypeptide)
girdle anesthesia
girth, increased abdominal
GITS (gastrointestinal therapeutic system)
Given Diagnostic Imaging System
glabellar rasp
glabrous cirrhosis
glancing wound
gland
  absorbent (lymph)
  accessory thyroid
  accessory parotid
  accessory suprarenal
  acid
  adrenal
  anal
  apocrine
  areolar
  arytenoid
  Aselli
  Bartholin
  Bauhin
  bile duct
  biliary
  Blandin
  Brunner
  buccal
  bulbocavernous
  bulbourethral
  cardiac (stomach)
  celiac
  cervical
  Ciaccio
  circumanal
  Cloquet
  Clobelli
  coil
  compound
  Cowper
  ductless

gland *(cont.)*
  duodenal
  Duverney
  Ebner
  endocrine
  esophageal
  exocrine
  fundic
  Galeati
  gastric
  Gay
  gingival
  Gley
  gustatory
  hepatic
  hyperplastic
  hypothalamus
  intermediate
  interstitial
  intestinal
  lacrimal
  lactiferous
  lenticular
  Lieberkühn (Lieberkuehn)
  lymph
  mandibular
  mesenteric
  mesocolic
  Montgomery
  Morgagni
  mucus-secreting
  multinodular
  nabothian
  oxyntic
  parathyroid
  paraurethral
  parotid
  peptic
  Peyer
  pharyngeal
  pineal
  pituitary
  Poirier
  pregnancy

gland *(cont.)*
- prehyoid
- prostate
- pyloric
- salivary
- Sand
- Sandström
- sentinel
- solitary (of large intestine)
- splenoid
- substernal thyroid
- suprarenal
- Suzanne
- sweat
- Theile
- thymus
- thyroid
- urethral
- Virchow
- Weber
- Wölfler (Woelfler)

gland atrophy
gland enlargement
gland enucleator
gland forceps
gland scissors
glandular carcinoma
glandular organ
glandular swelling
glans intraepidermal
Glaser automatic laminectomy retractor
Glasgow classification of choledocholithiasis
glass pH electrode
Glasscock ear dressing
Glasser gastrostomy tube
Glasser gastrotomy
Glassman-Allis intestinal forceps
Glassman atraumatic bowel clamp
Glassman clamp
Glassman dissecting scissors
Glassman gastrostomy
Glassman grasper
Glassman stone extractor
Gleason score
Glenn diverticulum forceps
glenoid-reaming forceps
Gley gland
gliadin, wheat
GliaSite implantable radiation therapy system
Glidewire
glimepiride tablets
glioblastoma multiforme
glipizide
Glisson capsule
Glisson cirrhosis
glistening mass
glitazone classification of diabetes drugs
global inhibition of GI function
globoid material
globular tumor
globulin
- $alpha_1$-antitrypsin
- cortisol-binding globulin
- hepatitis B hyperimmune
- thyroid-binding

globus hystericus
globus sensation
glomerular filtration rate (GFR)
glomerulopathy associated with infectious hepatitis (HB_sAg-positive)
glomerulopathy associated with visceral abscess
glomerulus (pl. glomeruli)
glossectomy
glossitis
glossopalatine fold
glossopharyngeal afferent
glottic adduction
glottic closure during deglutition
glottic thyroid
glove
- antivibratory
- Bio-Form
- Biobrane
- carpal tunnel
- Handeze fingerless

glove *(cont.)*
  Isotoner
  Jobst
  SoftFlex computer
  Tubigrip
  Valeo lifting
glove-and-stocking anesthesia distribution
glove anesthesia
glovelike distribution
Glover bulldog clamp
Glover coarctation clamp
Glover patent ductus clamp
Glover vascular clamp
GLS suture anchor
GlucaGen (glucagon)
glucagon-secreting tumor (glucagonoma)
glucagonoma syndrome
Glucerna
Gluck rib shears
Gluco-Pro nutritional supplement
Gluco-Protein OTC self-test
Glucochek Pocketlab II blood glucose system
glucocorticoid production
glucocorticosteroid-induced side effects
Glucofilm reagent strips
Glucometer DEX blood glucose monitor
Glucometer Elite R blood glucose monitor
Glucometer Encore reagent strips
Glucometer II blood glucose monitor
Gluconate skin prep tray
gluconeogenesis
Glucophage (metformin HCl)
Glucophage XR (metformin HCl extended-release)
glucose
  blood
  intravenous (I.V., IV)
  liquid
  plasma

glucose *(cont.)*
  serum
  urine
glucose administration, I.V., IV (intravenous)
glucose-dependent insulinotropic polypeptide (GIP)
glucose-galactose malabsorption
glucose intolerance
glucose metabolism
glucose meter
glucose monitor (see *blood glucose monitor*)
glucose-6-phosphatase deficiency
glucose-6-phosphate dehydrogenase (G6PD) deficiency
glucose tolerance, impaired
glucose tolerance test (GTT)
Glucostix reagent strips
glucosuria
glucosylceramide lipids
Glucotrol XL (glipizide)
Glucovance (glyburide; metformin HCl)
GlucoWatch blood glucose monitor
glucuronide
glucuronosyltransferase (liver enzyme)
glue (see also *adhesive*)
  biomedical
  cyanoacrylate
  endovascular
  fibrin
  HemaMyst aerosol adhesive
  Hemaseel APR fibrin adhesive
  Hemaseel HMN biological tissue glue
  HemaSyst sealant
  Krazy Glue
  LiquiBand topical wound closure
  percutaneous fibrin
  skin
  Superglue
  Tissucol fibrin
glutamic acid

glutamic acid decarboxylase (GAD)
  antibody
glutamine and somatropin
glutamine test
glutaraldehyde-tanned bovine collagen
  tubes
glutaraldehyde-tanned porcine heart
  valve
Glutasorb diet
gluteal fold
gluteal region
gluten, dietary
gluten enteropathy
gluten-free diet
gluten intolerance
Glutose
Gluzinski test
glyburide
glyburide/metformin hydrochloride
Glycacor assay
glycemic control
glycemic index
glycerin (Fleet Babylax)
glycerol
glycerol monoctanoate (GMOC)
  solution
glycine extended gastrin
glycocalix
glycogen infiltration of liver
glycogen storage disease
glycogen store
glycogenic acanthosis
glycogenolysis
glycogenosis
  brancher deficiency
  generalized
  hepatophosphorylase deficiency
  hepatorenal
glycopyrrolate
glycopyrronium bromide
Glycosal diabetes monitoring device
glycosuria
glycosylated hemoglobin
glycyltryptophan test
Glynase Pres Tab (glyburide)
Glypressin (terlipressin)
Glyset (miglitol)
Gmelin test
GMOC (glycerol monoctanoate)
  solution
gnawing pain
Go-Evac (polyethylene glycol-
  electrolyte solution electrolytes)
goblet cell
goblet cell hyperplasia
Godina double hook
Goelet retractor
goiter
  aberrant
  adenomatous
  Basedow
  colloid
  congenital
  cystic
  diffuse
  diffuse colloid
  diffuse multinodular
  diffuse toxic non-nodular
  diving
  dyshormonogenic
  endemic (colloid)
  euthyroid
  exophthalmic
  fetal
  fibrous
  focal
  follicular
  hyperplastic
  intrathoracic
  iodide
  iodine deficiency
  lingual
  lithiumogenic
  lymphadenoid
  multinodular
  multiple colloid adenomatous
  nodular
  nontoxic

goiter *(cont.)*
- nontoxic diffuse
- nontoxic nodular
- parenchymatous
- perivascular
- plunging
- retrovascular
- simple
- smooth
- soft
- sporadic
- substernal
- suffocative
- thyroid
- toxic
- toxic diffuse
- toxic multinodular
- toxic nodular
- toxic uninodular
- uninodular
- vascular
- wandering

goitrogen
goitrous cretinism
Golaski graft
gold (Au); gold-198 (^{198}Au)
Goldberg Anorectic Attitude Scale
Goldberg-Maxwell syndrome
Goldblatt clamp
Goldblatt kidney
Goldman-Fox dissecting scissors
Gold Probe bipolar hemostasis catheter
Gold Series
Goldstein Microspike approximator clamp
Goldstein Microspike clamp
golf-hole ureteral orifice
Goligher abdominal scissors
Goligher extraperitoneal ileostomy
Goligher retractor
GoLYTELY (polyethylene glycol-electrolyte solution) bowel prep
Gomco suction
Gomco suction tube
Gomel blade
Gomel micro tying forceps
gomer (acronym for pejorative, "get out of my emergency room")
Gomez fundoplasty
Gomez gastroplasty
Gomez horizontal gastroplasty with reinforced stoma
gonadal neoplasm
Gonadimmune
gonococcal perihepatis pelvic inflammatory disease
gonococcal perihepatitis
gonococcal peritonitis
gonorrheal proctitis
Gonzalez, meandering artery of
GOO (gastric outlet obstruction)
good prognosis
good renal function
Good rasp
Goodsall rule
Good Sam adult breathing circuit
gooseneck gouge
gooseneck rongeur
Gopalan syndrome
GORD (British/European spelling of GERD)
Gordon disease
Gore cast liner
Gore 1.5-T Torso Array
Gore-Tex banding of sigmoid colon to abdominal wall
Gore-Tex DualMesh Plus
Gore-Tex FEP-Ringed vascular graft
Gore-Tex graft
Gore-Tex MycroMesh Plus
Gore-Tex nonabsorbable surgical suture
Gore-Tex SAM (subcutaneous augmentation material) facial implant
Gore-Tex shunt
Gore-Tex soft tissue patch
Gore-Tex stretch vascular graft
Gore-Tex strips
Gore-Tex surgical membrane

Gore-Tex surgical mesh
Gore-Tex tapered vascular graft
Gore-Tex vascular graft
gorge
gorging
Gorney scissors
goserelin acetate
Gosset appendectomy retractor
Gosset retractor
gossypiboma (cotton)
Gothic arch formation
Gottron papule
Gott shunt
Gott tube
Gottschalk Nasostat
Gouffon hip pin
gouge (see also *chisel*)
  Abbott
  Acufex
  Alexander
  Andrews
  Army bone
  arthroplasty
  Aufranc
  Bishop
  bone
  Buck-Gramcko
  Campbell
  Capner
  Cobb spinal
  curved
  Dawson-Yuhl
  Duray-Read
  Flanagan spinal fusion
  gooseneck
  Guy
  Hibbs spinal fusion
  Hoen
  Hoen lamina
  Jewett
  Killian
  Lexer
  Lucas
  Metzenbaum
gouge *(cont.)*
  Meyerding curved
  mini-Lexer
  Moe
  motorized
  Murphy
  oscillating
  Partsch
  Read
  Ruben
  Sheehan
  Smith-Petersen curved
  Smith-Petersen straight
  Smith-Peterson gooseneck
  spinal fusion
  Stille bone
  straight
  swan-neck
  tendon
  USA pattern
  U.S. Army
  Watson-Jones bone
  West
  West bone
  Zielke
  Zimmer
Gould polygraph
Goulet retractor
Goulian mammoplasty
gourmand syndrome
GP (gastroplasty)
GR (gastric retention)
GR II coronary stent
gracilis muscle graft
gracilis muscle transposition
graciloplasty
grade, grading (see *classification*)
graded compression ultrasonography
graded esophageal balloon distention test
gradient
  biliary-duodenal pressure
  duodenobiliary pressure
  gastrosphincteric pressure
  hepatic venous pressure

grading neoplasm
grading of malignancy
grading tumor
Gradle scissors
gradual volume loss
graduated metal cup
Graefe dissecting forceps
Graefe dissecting hook
Graefe skin hook
Grafco all-nylon Y connector
graft
  ACL
  adipose
  adrenal medulla
  advancement flap
  Albee bone
  AlloDerm processed tissue
  allogenic (allogeneic) bone
  allogenous bone
  allograft
  AlloMatrix injectable putty bone graft substitute
  AneuRx stent
  anterior iliac crest
  anterior sliding tibial
  aortofemoral bypass (AFBG)
  aortohepatic arterial
  Apligraf (graftskin)
  Aria coronary artery bypass
  articular cartilage autograft
  autochthonous
  autogenous bone
  autogenous dermal
  autogenous fascial heterograft
  autogenous inlay
  autogenous soft tissue graft
  autologous crest bone
  autologous fat
  autologous reverse
  BAGF (brachioaxillary bridge graft fistula)
  Banks bone
  Bard Composix mesh
  Bard Sperma-Tex preshaped mesh

graft *(cont.)*
  Bard Visilex mesh
  batten
  bicortical iliac bone
  bicortical ilial strip
  bifurcated vascular graft
  Biobrane/HF skin substitute
  Biograft bovine heterograft
  BioPolyMeric
  bone chip
  bone graft substitute
  bone peg
  BonePlast
  bone-retinaculum-bone autograft
  bone-tendon-bone
  Bonfiglio bone
  bovine heterograft
  bovine pericardium
  Boyd dual-onlay bone
  BPB (bone-patellar ligament-bone) autologous
  BPB (bone-patellar tendon-bone) autologous
  brachiosubclavian bridge
  Braun skin
  Brennen biosynthetic surgical mesh
  bridge
  BSGF (brachiosubclavian bridge graft fistula)
  C
  CABG (coronary artery bypass)
  cable
  Calcitite
  calvarial free bone
  Campbell onlay
  cancellous and cortical bone
  cancellous chip bone
  Capset (calcium sulfate) bone graft barrier
  Carbo-Seal
  carbon fiber
  carbon fiber synthetic ligament
  cardiovascular patch
  cartilage

graft *(cont.)*
cavum conchal cartilage
CHAG (coralline hydroxyapatite Goniopora)
chip
Chuinard autogenous bone
clothespin spinal fusion
Codivilla bone
Collagraft bone graft matrix
composite
Composite Cultured Skin (CCS)
Composix mesh
consolidated
cortical strut
corticocancellous bone
corticocancellous chip
Cotton cartilage
Cragg endoluminal
cranial bone
cultured epithelial autograft
cutaneous
cymba conchal cartilage
Cymetra tissue replacement material
Dacron
Dacron synthetic ligament material
Daniel iliac bone
Dardik Biograft
Davis muscle-pedicle
delayed xenograft rejection (DXR)
demineralized bone
denatured homograft
Dermagraft human-based dermal replacement
Dermagraft-TC (transitional covering)
dermal collagen
devitalized bone
diamond inlay
Diastat vascular access
discordant cellular xenograft
discordant organ xenograft
Distaflo bypass
double mesh
doubled semitendinosus and gracilis autograft (DST&G)

graft *(cont.)*
Douglas skin
dowel
Dragstedt skin
DST&G (doubled semitendinosus and gracilis) autograft
DTAFA (descending thoracic aorta-to-femoral artery) bypass
dual onlay bone
DualMesh biomaterial
DuraGen
dural
Durapatite
E-CABG (endoscopic coronary artery bypass graft)
Edwards woven Teflon aortic bifurcation
endovascular stent
epidural blood patch
Esser skin
extended survival
extra-articular
fascia lata
fascial
femorocrural
femorodistal PTFE
fetal cortical tissue
fetal substantia nigra
fillet local flap
Flanagan-Burem apposing hemicylindric
flap
flexor tendon
Fluoropassiv thin-wall carotid patch
fortisan fabric (cellulose)
free
free fat
free intestinal
free jejunal
free muscle
free nipple
free skin
free transplanted
freeze-dried

graft *(cont.)*
- freeze-dried bone
- fresh frozen
- full-thickness skin
- fusion
- GEA (gastroepiploic artery)
- Gillies bone
- glutaraldehyde-tanned bovine collagen tubes
- glutaraldehyde-tanned porcine heart valve
- Golaski
- Gore-Tex
- Gore-Tex DualMesh Plus
- Gore-Tex FEP-Ringed vascular
- Gore-Tex MycroMesh Plus
- Gore-Tex stretch vascular
- Gore-Tex tapered vascular
- Gore-Tex vascular
- gracilis muscle
- Grafton DBM (demineralized bone matrix) bone
- Graftpatch
- Haldeman bone
- Hapset bone graft plaster
- Harris superior acetabular
- harvesting of
- Healos synthetic bone-grafting material
- Hedrocel bone substitute material
- Hemashield
- Hemashield enhanced
- hemicylindrical bone
- Henderson onlay bone
- Henry bone
- Herniamesh surgical mesh
- heterogeneous (heterogenous)
- heterograft
- Hey-Groves-Kirk bone
- Hoaglund bone
- homogeneous (homogenous)
- homologous
- H-shaped
- human meniscal allograft

graft *(cont.)*
- Huntington bone
- hydroxyapatitite
- IEA (inferior epigastric artery)
- iliac crest bone
- iliotibial band
- IMA (inferior mammary artery)
- impaction
- in situ vein
- Inclan bone
- infrarenal aortobifemoral bypass
- inlay
- inlay bone
- intercalary
- interfascicular nerve
- InterGard Knitted collagen coated
- Interpore
- interposition bone
- interposition Dacron
- interposition saphenous vein
- intramedullary
- Ionescu-Shiley pericardial xenograft
- irradiated
- Isotec patellar tendon
- ITA (internal thoracic artery)
- Judet
- jump
- keystone
- Kimura cartilage
- Krause-Wolfe skin
- Kutler V-Y flap
- Langenskiöld bone
- Lee bone
- Leibinger Micro Dynamic mesh
- LIMA (left internal mammary artery)
- lyophilized bone
- Marlex
- Marlex mesh
- Marlex PerFix plug
- Marlex synthetic
- Martius
- Massie sliding
- matchstick

graft *(cont.)*
- McFarland bone
- McMaster bone
- MD-111 bone allograft
- Meadox Microvel arterial
- medullary bone
- Microknit vascular
- mitral valve homograft
- morselized (morcellized) bone
- MycroMesh biomaterial
- myocutaneous
- Ne-Osteo bone morphogenic protein (BMP)
- nerve
- neuroplasty fat
- neurovascular island
- Nicoll
- Nicoll cancellous bone
- nontubed closed distant flap
- nontubed open distant flap
- nylon mesh
- Ollier thick split free
- Ollier-Thiersch skin
- onlay
- onlay cancellous iliac
- onlay mesh
- OP-1 implant
- open weave mesh
- Opteform 100HT bone
- osteoarticular
- osteocartilaginous
- osteochondral
- osteoperiosteal
- Osteoset bone graft substitute
- Overton dowel
- pancreatic allograft
- Papineau
- Parietex composite mesh
- Paritene mesh
- particulate
- patellar tendon
- pedicle
- pedicle bone
- peg

graft *(cont.)*
- PepGen P-15 (peptide-enhanced)
- percutaneous autogenous dowel bone
- PerioGlas bone graft material
- Perma-Flow coronary bypass
- PermaMesh
- Perma-Seal dialysis access
- peroneus brevis
- PFTE (polyfluorotetraethylene)
- Phemister onlay bone
- pigskin
- polyester tripled hamstring
- polyfluorotetraethylene (PTFE)
- polyglactin mesh dural
- polytetrafluoroethylene mesh
- polyvinyl sponge
- porcine dermal collagen
- porcine xenograft
- porous polyethylene
- portacaval H
- portocaval synthetic H-graft
- postage stamp
- postage-stamp type skin
- powdered bone
- PowerLink endoluminal
- ProOsteon 500 bone implant
- Proplast
- prosthetic femorodistal
- proud
- PTFE (polytetrafluoroethylene)
- pulmonary autograft (PA)
- Pyrost
- Rapidgraft arterial vessel substitute
- Repliform
- Reverdin epidermal free
- Russe bone
- Ryerson bone
- sandwiched iliac bone
- saphenous vein extracranial-intracranial bypass
- Sauvage
- segmental
- semitendinosus
- sentinel skin paddle

graft *(cont.)*
Sepramesh biosurgical composite mesh
seromuscular intestinal patch
short vessel
silicon-velvet composite
single onlay cortical bone
skin
skull bone
sliding inlay
slit-cut mesh
Solvang
Soto-Hall bone
Sperma-Tex preshaped mesh
split calvarial bone
split-thickness skin
spreader
stem cell autograft
strut bone
subclavian-external carotid artery
Sure-Closure skin-stretching system
Surgipro Prolene mesh
SurgiSis sling/mesh
Synergraft
Tait
temporal fascia
Thiersch
Thiersch medium split free
Thiersch thin split free
Thomas extrapolated bar
Thoralon biomaterial
three-strand semintendinosus tendon
TransCyte skin substitute
transplanted stamp
Trelex mesh
tricortical bone
tricortical ilial strip
tube flap
tumbler
Unigraft bone
Unilab Surgibone
Vascu-Guard bovine pericardial surgical patch
vascularized fibula

graft *(cont.)*
Vascutek
Vectra vascular access (VAG)
vein
Venaflow vascular
Visilex mesh
Weaveknit vascular
Wesolowski vascular
Wilson bone
Wolfe
Wolfe full-thickness free
Wolfe hand surgery
Wolfe-Kawamoto bone
wraparound flap bone
XenoDerm
xenograft
Y-shaped graft
Zenith AAA (abdominal aortic aneurysm) endovascular
Zenotech
Z-plasty local flap

GraftAssist vein and graft holder
graft copolymer
GraftCyte gauze wound dressing
graft delamination
graft elongation
graft enhanced with collagen
graft-enteric fistula
graft enteritis
graft fracture
grafting
grafting suction tube
graft irradiation
graft loading pattern
graft loosening
graft morselizer
graft necrosis
Graftpatch
graft rejection
graft survival
Grafton DBM (demineralized bone matrix) bone graft
Graftskin human skin product
graft-versus-host disease (GVHD)

graft-versus-host reaction
graft-versus-tumor activity
Graham closure with omental pouch
Graham-Cole cholecystography
Graham dural hook
Graham muscle hook
Graham nerve hook
Graham omental pouch
Graham patch
Graham plication
Graham scale for drug-induced gastric damage
Graham test
Graham-Field Inc.
grain handler's lung
gram-negative bacillus
gram-negative bacteria
gram-negative diplococci
gram-negative organism
gram-negative rod
gram-negative sepsis
gram positive
gram-positive bacillus
gram-positive bacteria
gram-positive organism
Gram stain
Gram stain and culture
Gram stain of stool
granddaughter cyst
GraNee grasper needle
granisetron HCl
granny knot
Granocyte (lenograstim)
Grant aneurysm clamp
Grant gallbladder retractor
granular appearance
granular-cell tumor
granular kidney
granularity
granulation tissue
Granulderm (trypsin; Peruvian balsam)
granule
  DiPAS-positive
  hemosiderin
  Weibel-Palade
Granulex (trypsin; Peruvian balsam)
granulocyte colony stimulating factor (G-CSF)
granulocyte-macrophage colony stimulating factor
granulocytic sarcoma
granulocytopenia
granuloma (pl. granulomas, granulomata)
  amebic
  calcified
  ceroid-like histiocytic granuloma
  eosinophilic
  hepatic
  inflammatory
  noncaseating tubercle-like
  portal zone
  rectal
granuloma inguinale
granulomatosis, intestinal lipophagic
granulomatous cholangitis
granulomatous colitis
granulomatous disease
granulomatous enteritis
granulomatous enterocolitis
granulomatous gastritis
granulomatous hepatitis
granulomatous ileitis
granulomatous infection
granulomatous mastitis
granulomatous thyroiditis
granulomatous transmural colitis
granulomatous ulcer
granulosa cell carcinoma
granulosa cell tumor
GranuMed (trypsin; Peruvian balsam)
grapefruit diet
Graser diverticulum
grasper
  alligator grasper/forceps
  atraumatic
  blunt-nose
  bottle-nose
  bowel
  bullet-nose

grasper *(cont.)*
dolphin-nose
duck-nose micrograsper
Endo Babcock
Endo Cinch
Endo Grasp
fenestrated
fenestrated bowel
fine-tooth fenestrated
four-pronged polyp
Glassman
Hasson
Hunter style double-action bowel
laparoscopic
long dolphin nose
MetraGrasp
Pivotal
pointed-nose
Pollock
Questus Leading Edge
Reddick
Reddick-Saye suture
reusable
Riza-Ribe
round-nose
stationary
Storz dolphin-nose
grasper needle
grasping forceps (see *forceps*)
grasping loop
Grassi test
grater reamer
Graves disease
Graves speculum
gravity drainage
gravity, specific
gray tumor
Gray bone drill
Gray cystic duct forceps
gray foam bandage
Gray reamer
gray-scale ultrasonography
gray-scale ultrasound
Grayson ligament in hand
greasy food
great imitator
Great Smokies intestinal permeability test kit
greater curvature banded gastroplasty
greater curvature of stomach
greater curvature ulcer
greater omentum (omentum majus)
greater peritoneal sac
greater trochanter
great vessel injury
Green-Armytage hemostasis forceps
Greenberg clamp
Greenberg Universal retractor
green-brown drainage
Greene biopsy needle
Greene forceps
Greene retractor
green liver
Green muscle hook
green stools
Green thyroid retractor
Greenville gastric bypass
Greenwald cutting loop
Greenwald flexible endoscopic electrode
Greenwich catheter
Greenwood bayonet forceps
Greenwood bipolar and suction forceps
Greer EZ Access drainage pouch
Greer's goo dressing (hydrocortisone, nystatin, zinc oxide)
Gregory baby profunda clamp
Gregory carotid bulldog clamp
Gregory DeBakey bulldog clamp
Gregory external clamp
Gregory stay suture
Grenoble-Paris-Rennes (GPR) robot microscope
Greven forceps
Grey Turner sign of retroperitoneal hemorrhage
GRFoma pancreatic endocrine tumor
gridiron incision

Griffen Roux-en-Y bypass
Grinfeld cannula
Gripper needle
gritty material
gritty tumor
Grocco sign
groin dissection
groin flap
groin hernia
groin incision
groin mass
Grollman catheter
Grondahl-Finney esophagogastroplasty
groove
  esophageal (on liver)
  gastric
  Liebermeister
  oval-form colonic
  radial
  spindle colonic
grooved dissector
grooved titanium rod
groove pancreatitis
grooving reamer
Groshong PICC catheter
gross blood
gross blood in stool
gross blood with small clots
Gross coarctation occlusion clamp
Gross disease
gross diagnosis
Grosse and Kempf locking nail system
Grosse-Kempf interlocking medullary nail
gross lesion
Gross operation
Gross test
gross tumor
gross tumor involvement
grounded patient
ground-glass appearance (on x-ray)
ground-glass body of Hadziyannis
ground-glass cell
ground-glass pattern
group B streptococcus (GBS)
Grover clamp
Grover meniscus knife
growth, extranodal
growth plate
growth plate abscess
growth retardation
Gruber-Landzert fossa
Gruber suture
Gruentzig balloon catheter
Gruenwald ear forceps
Gruenwald neurosurgical rongeur
grumous material
Grüntzig (Gruentzig)
Grüntzig balloon
Grüntzig balloon catheter
Gruppe wire-crimping forceps
Grynfeltt hernia
Grynfeltt triangle
GS (Gardner syndrome)
GSI (General Surgical Innovations)
GSI balloon dissector
GSI Spacemaker II
GSRS (gastrointestinal symptom rating scale)
GSW (gunshot wound)
G6PD deficiency
G-suit external counterpressure device
G-34 ("big gastrin")
GII EasyAnchor
GII Snap-Pak anchor
G tube
guaiac-negative stool
guaiac-positive nipple discharge
guaiac-positive stool
guaiac test of occult blood in stool
Guardian ring bracket
Guardian suction cannister
guarding
  involuntary
  muscle
  voluntary
guarding of abdomen
guarding sign

Guardsman femoral screw
gubernaculum
Gudebrod, Inc., instruments
Guedel disposable airway
Guedel plastic airway
Guedel rubber airway
Guenzberg test
Guérin fold
Guibor Silastic tube
guidance
  sonographic
  ultrasound
Guidant Origin system
guide
  Accu-Line
  acetabular
  ACL drill
  Acufex tibial
  adjustable angle
  Adson drill
  Adson dural protector
  Adson saw
  alignment
  Arthrex femoral
  Arthrex tibial
  Bailey-Gigli saw
  ball-tipped Küntscher (Kuentscher)
  barrel
  Blair saw
  bone wire
  Bullseye
  calibrated pin
  Cloward drill
  Cushing-Gigli saw
  Cushing saw
  Davis saw
  DePuy femoral acetabular overlay
  drill
  Duopress
  eccentric drill
  Fanelli
  femoral intramedullary
  FIN pin
  Fisher

guide *(cont.)*
  Ghajar
  Gigli saw
  Guyon catheter
  Hall-Dundar drill
  Hewson cruciate
  Hewson drill
  Hoffmann pin
  Howell tibial
  intercondylar drill
  intramedullary
  Iowa trumpet needle
  Lebsche saw
  ligature
  long axial alignment
  Lunderquist-Ring torque
  nail rotational
  needle
  neutral and load drill
  neutral drill
  patellar drill
  PCA cutting
  PCA medullary
  picket fence
  Pilot suture
  Pinn.ACL
  Poppen Gigli saw
  Raney saw
  Reese osteotomy
  Richards angle
  saw
  stationary angle
  Synthes wire
  T-bar
  telescopic wire
  tibial cutter
  tibial cutting
  tibial drill
  Todd-Wells
  trocar
  Trumpet needle
  tube
  tunnel drill
  wire

guide *(cont.)*
XMB tibial reaming
Yasargil ligature
guide bushing
guide catheter
guided imagery
guided microsurgery
guided-needle aspiration cytology
guided-needle biopsy
guided transcutaneous biopsy
guideline
Böhler (Boehler)
Hartel
Letournel
guide pin
ball-point
ball-tip
calibrated
guide sleeve
guide tube
guidewire
ACS (Advanced Catheter Systems)
ACS Hi-Torque Balance Middleweight
Amplatz Super Stiff
angiographic
atherolytic
atherolytic reperfusion
Athlete coronary
Bentson floppy-tip
Critikon
Director biliary
Extra Sport coronary
FasTrac
Flex
flexible
flexible J
floppy
floppy-tipped
Geenan Endotorque
Glidewire
high-torque floppy
Hi-Per Flex
Hi-Torque Flex-T

guidewire *(cont.)*
Hi-Torque Floppy (HTF)
Hi-Torque Intermediate
Hi-Torque Standard
HPC
hydrophilic
Hyperflex
Iguana
J
J-tip
J-tipped exchange
J-tipped hydrophilic
J-tipped spring
Linx exchange
long taper/stiff shaft Glidewire
Lumina
Lunderquist
Magnum
Medrad
Microvasive Glidewire
Microvasive stiff piano wire
Mustang steerable
PDT
preformed
QuickSilver hydrophilic-coated
Radiofocus Glidewire
Redifocus
Rosen
ROTACS
Schwarten LP
shapeable
Silk
Sof-T
soft-tipped
Sones
SOS
steerable
straight
TAD
Teflon-coated
Terumo
TherOx 0.014 infusion
Tracer hybrid
transluminal angioplasty

guidewire *(cont.)*
  USCI
  VeriFlex
  WaveWire
  Wholey Hi-Torque Floppy
  Wholey Hi-Torque Modified J
  Wholey Hi-Torque Standard
  Zebra exchange
guidewire exchanged
guidewire exchange technique
guidewire for needle localization
guidewire introducer
guiding catheter
Guidor barrier
Guidor surgical mesh
Guilford-Wiet foot plate pick
Guilford-Wright double-edged sickle knife
Guilford-Wright duckbill elevator
Guilford-Wright flap knife
Guilford-Wright micro bone curette
Guilford-Wright stapes pick
Guilford-Wright suction tube
Guillain-Barré syndrome
guillotine blade
Guleke bone rongeur
gullet
gull-wing incision
gum, karaya
gum rubber Martin bandage
gun (see *stapler*)
Gunderson bone forceps
Gunderson muscle forceps
Gunnar-Hey roller forceps
gunshot wound (GSW)
GunSlinger shoulder orthosis
gurgle (bowel sound)
gurgling bowel sounds
Gusberg hysterectomy clamp
Gussenbauer suture
gusseted arm board
gustatory anesthesia
gustatory gland
gut
  artificial
  caffeine
  catgut
  nervous
  plain
Gutaform
gut-associated lymphoid tissue (GALT)
gut dysmotility
Gutgemann clamp
Gutgemann-Longmire gastric reconstruction
gut-hormone profile
Guthrie fixation hook
gut suture
gutter
  lateral
  left
  paracolic
  right
gutter wound
Guy gouge
Guyon catheter guide
Guyon catheter introducer
Guyon-Péan kidney clamp
guy suture
GVAX pancreatic vaccine
GVHD (graft-versus-host disease)
Gwilliam clamp
gynecologic pain
gynecologic tumor
gynecomastia
Gynex angle hook
Gynex Emmett tenaculum
Gynex extended-reach needle

H, h

H_2 (histamine 2)
HAART (highly active antiretroviral therapy)
Haberer abdominal spatula
Haberer forceps
Haberer intestinal clamp
habit (pl. habits)
 bowel
 change in bowel
 dietary
 drinking
 drug
 eating
 smoking
habitus
 asthenic
 body
 gracile
 large
HACA (human antichimeric antibody)
Hadefield-Clarke syndrome
Hadziyannis, ground-glass body of
HAEC (Hirschsprung-associated enterocolitis)
Haemonetics Cell Saver 5
Haemonetics red blood cell collection protocol
Haemophilus ducreyi
Haemophilus haemolyticus
Haemophilus influenzae
Haemophilus influenzae type B
Haemophilus parahaemolyticus
Haemophilus parainfluenzae
Haemophilus vaginalis
Hafnia alvei (formerly *Enterobacter hafniae*)
Hafter diet trick
Hagedorn needle
Hagie hip pin
Hagie pin nail
Hagie sliding nail plate
Hahn bone nail
HAI (histologic activity index)
Haid cervical plate
Haight-Finochietto rib retractor
Haimovici arteriotomy scissors
hairy cell leukemia
Hajek antrum rongeur
Hajek-Ballenger septal elevator
Hajek chisel
Hajek-Koffler bone punch forceps
Hajek-Koffler laminectomy rongeur
Hajek-Koffler punch
Hajek laminectomy punch
Hajek mallet
Hakansson bone rongeur

Hakim-Cortis ventriculoperitoneal
shunt
HAL (hemorrhoid arterial ligation)
Haldane-Priestley tube
Haldeman bone graft
Haley's M-O (magnesium hydroxide; mineral oil) (now Phillips' M-O)
half-and-half nail
half-circle microplate
half-circle plate
half-hitch knot
halflife of circulating thyroid hormone
half pin
half-strength feeding
Halifax clamp
Halifax interlaminar clamp
Hall air drill
Hall air-driven oscillating saw
Hallberg biliointestinal bypass
Hall driver
Hall-Dundar drill guide
Halle dura knife
Halle infant speculum
Hall large bore drill
Hall Micro E drill
Hall Micro E oscillating saw
Hall Micro E reciprocating saw
Hall Micro E sagittal saw
Hall rod
Hall sternal saw
Hall Surgairtome drill
Hall Versipower drill
Hall Versipower oscillating saw
Hall Versipower reamer
Hall Versipower reciprocating saw
hallux nail
halo effect (on x-ray)
halofuginone
halogen endoscopic light source
halogen exam lamp
halo melanoma
halo pin
Halotestin (fluoxymesterone)
halothane
halothane-induced hepatitis
halothane poisoning
HALS (hand-assisted laparoscopic surgery)
Halsey nail scissors
Halsey needle holder with tungsten carbide inlay
Halsey-TC needle holder
Halsted artery forceps
Halsted-Bassini herniorrhaphy
Halsted hemostat
Halsted mosquito forceps
Halsted hemostatic mosquito forceps (straight/curved)
Halsted inguinal herniorrhaphy
Halsted mosquito forceps
Halsted operation
Halsted radical mastectomy
Halsted suture
HALT-C (hepatitis C antiviral long-term treatment to prevent cirrhosis) study
Halverson classification of groin hernias (types 1–4)
Halverson-McVay classification of groin hernias (class 1–4)
hamartoma
  benign
  bile duct
  duodenal wall
  pancreatic
hamartomas throughout the GI tract
hamartomatous gastric polyp
hamartomatous intestinal polyposis
hamartomatous lesion
hamartomatous polyp
hamartomatous polyposis
hamburger sign
Hamel test
Hamilton bandage
Hamman sign
hammer
  Berliner percussion
  Buck neurological

hammer *(cont.)*
  Buck percussion
  Cloward
  Davis percussion
  Dejerine-Davis percussion
  Dejerine percussion
  Epstein neurological
  Küntscher (Kuentscher)
  neurological
  percussion
  Rabiner neurological
  slotted
  Taylor percussion
  Traube neurological percussion
  Trömner (Troemner) percussion
Hampton air
Hampton line (on x-ray)
Hancke/Vilmann biopsy handle
  instrument
Handages dressing
hand-assisted laparoscopic colectomy
hand-assisted laparoscopic gastrectomy
hand-assisted laparoscopic hemicolec-
  tomy
hand-assisted laparoscopic surgery
  (HALS)
hand-assisted laparoscopy
hand-assisted sigmoidectomy
hand drill
hand elevator
H&H (hemoglobin and hematocrit)
handheld retractor
handheld ultrasonic nebulizer
handheld UV light
hand instrument
handle
  Bill axis traction
  Bill traction
  blade
  DeBakey ring
  elevator, T
  E-Z off reusable plastic knife
  Gigli saw
  Gigli-Strully saw

handle *(cont.)*
  Hancke-Vilmann biopsy
  Hunstad infiltration
  knife
  Kollman dilator
  laryngeal mirror
  Lysonics
  Medi-Vac Flexi-Clear suction
  Medi-Vac Yankauer suction
  octagon-threaded
  pistol-grip spring
  reinsulate "U" style
  ring
  scalpel
  Siegel knife
  standard laparoscopic
  Strully Gigli saw
  Take-Apart
  T, elevator
  thumb
  Tip-Trol
  Townsend
  Turner
  Turner Warwick diathermy scalpel
  type reamer
  U
  universal
  universal chuck
handle-type reamer
hand-operated drill
hand piece bandage
HandPort hand-assist device
hand retractor
hand roller
hand-sewn anastomosis
Hands Free knee retractor
Hanger test
hanging panniculus (also see *apron*)
Hanks Balanced Salt Solution (HBSS)
Hanot-Chauffard syndrome
Hanot cirrhosis
Hansen-Street nail
Hansen-Street pin
Hansen-Street plate

H_2 antagonist
Ha1A human monoclonal antibody
Hapset bone graft plaster
haptoglobin, serum
HAR (hyperacute rejection)
Hara classification of gallbladder inflammation
hard adhesion
hard fixed mass
hard stool passage
hard stools
Hardy bipolar forceps
Hardy dressing forceps
Hardy microbipolar forceps
Hardy sella punch
Hardy sella punch forceps
Hardy spinal retractor
Hardy suction tube
Hardy three-prong fork
Hare pin
Hariri-Heifetz needle
Harken auricle clamp
Harlow plate
Harm posterior cervical plate
Harmonic hemorrhoidectomy
Harmonic Scalpel Ultracision
Harpenden caliper
Harpoon suture anchor
Harrell Y stent (airway)
Harrington compression rod
Harrington distraction rod
Harrington esophageal diverticulectomy
Harrington hook
Harrington hook clamp
Harrington hook driver
Harrington-Mayo thoracic scissors
Harrington-Mixter thoracic forceps
Harrington retractor
Harrington rod
Harrington rod clamp
Harrington scissors
Harrington spinal elevator
Harrington splanchnic retractor
Harrington thoracic forceps
Harris band
Harris-Beath axial hindfoot view
Harris-Benedict energy requirement equation
Harris center-cutting acetabular reamer
Harris condylocephalic nail
Harris condylocephalic rod
Harris hip nail
Harris medullary nail
Harrison bone-holding forceps
Harrison Cripp artery forceps
Harrison knife
Harrison-Nicolle polypropylene peg
Harrison spot test
Harrison sterilizing forceps
Harris plate
Harris superior acetabular graft
Harris tube
Harris view
Hartley breast prosthesis
Hartmann bone rongeur
Hartmann closure of rectum
Hartmann hemostatic mosquito forceps
Hartmann mosquito forceps
Hartmann nasal dressing forceps
Hartmann nasal speculum
Hartmann point
Hartmann pouch
Hartmann procedure
Hartmann resection of bowel
Hartmann tonsil punch
Hartnup disease
Hartshill rectangle rod
Hartzler ACX-II or RX-014 balloon catheter
Hartzler angioplasty balloon
Hartzler Micro II balloon
Hartzler rib retractor
Harvard infusion pump
Harvard 2 dual syringe pump
harvesting of graft
harvesting of organ
Harvey hospital prognostic nutritional index

Harvey Stone clamp
Harvey suture scissors
Harvey wire-cutting scissors
Hashimoto struma
Hashimoto thyroiditis
Hassall corpuscles
Hasson blunt-end cannula
Hasson grasper
Hasson laparoscopy cannula
Hasson open laparoscopy cannula
Hasson SAC (stable access cannula)
Hasson technique
Hasson trocar
Hastings frame
HAT (hepatic artery thrombosis)
Hatcher pin
hatching test
Haugh forceps
haustra (pl. of haustrum)
haustral blunting
haustral fold
haustral indentation
haustral markings
haustral pattern
haustral pouch
haustrum (pl. haustra)
HAV (hepatitis A virus)
Haverfield-Scoville hemilaminectomy retractor
Havrix (hepatitis A vaccine, inactivated)
Hawkeye suture
Hawkeye suture needle
Hawkins breast localization needle
Hayes anterior resection clamp
Hayes Martin forceps
Haynes brain cannula
Haynes pin
Haynes retractor
Haynes scissors
Hays hand retractor
Hay test
Hayton Williams wire-twisting forceps
Hb (hemoglobin)
HB (hepatitis B)
HbAg, HBAg ("H-bag") (hepatitis B antigen)
HB_cAb (hepatitis B core antibody)
HB_cAg (hepatitis B core antigen)
HB_eAb (hepatitis B "e" antibody)
HB_eAg (soluble "e" antigen in hepatitis B)
HB_eAg-negative wild-type precore HBV
HBIG (hepatitis B immune globulin)
HB_sAb (hepatitis B surface antibody)
HB_sAg (hepatitis B surface antigen)
HB_sAg carrier
H_2 blocker
H_2 breath test
HBSS (Hanks Balanced Salt Solution)
HBV (hepatitis B virus)
HCA (hepatocellular adenoma)
HCC (hepatocellular carcinoma) nodule
HCl (hydrochloride)
HCO_3^- (bicarbonate)
hCS (human chorionic somato-mammotrophin)
HCS (hematocystic spot)
Hct (hematocrit)
HCV (hepatitis C virus)
HCV co-infection
HCV RNA
HDAg (delta antigen)
HD5 (human defensin 5)
HD5 immunoreactivity
HD 85 (barium sulfate)
HDI 3000 ultrasound system
HDL (high-density lipoprotein)
HDL cholesterol
HD 200 Plus (barium sulfate)
HD II (or 2) total hip prosthesis
HDV (hepatitis D virus)
HE (hepatic encephalopathy)
headache
head CT
head drape

headlight
  Burton
  Clar 55
head of pancreas
headrest, Malcolm-Rand radiolucent
head trauma
healed erosive GERD (gastroesophageal reflux disease)
healed per primam
healed yellow atrophy
Healey revision acetabular component
healing (or healed) by primary intention
healing (or healed) by secondary intention
healing ulcer
Healos synthetic bone-grafting material
Health Buddy monitoring device
HealthCheck monitor
health-related quality of life (HRQOL)
HealthShield antimicrobial mediastinal wound drainage catheter
Healy intestinal forceps
Heaney biopsy curette
Heaney clamp
Heaney forceps
Heaney hysterectomy retractor
Heaney needle
Heaney needle holder
Heaney needle holder with tungsten carbide inlays
Heaney retractor
Heaney-TC needle holder
heart block
heartburn (pyrosis)
Heart Laser (for transmyocardial revascularization)
heat edema
heater probe
heater probe ablation
heater probe coagulation
Heath-Richter clip-removing forceps
Heath ligature scissors
Heath mallet
Heath suture scissors
heaves, dry
heavy alcohol use
heavy-duty femur plate
heavy-duty two-tooth retractor
heavy side plate
heavy silk suture
heavy wire suture
Hebra blade
Hectorol (doxercalciferol)
Hedblom rib retractor
Hedrocel bone substitute material
heel ulcer
Heerfordt-Waldenstrom syndrome
Heermann alligator forceps
Heffington lumbar seat
Hegar-Baumgartner needle
Hegar bougie
Hegar rectal dilator
Hegemann-Diethrich vascular scissors
Hegenbarth clip forceps
Heidenhain cell
Heidenhain pouch
Heifitz clamp
Heimlich maneuver for choking
Heine G series loupe
Heineke-Mikulicz gastroenterostomy
Heineke-Mikulicz pyloroplasty
Heine K series loupe
Heine sigmoidoscope
Hein rongeur
Heinz bodies
Heiss artery forceps
Heiss Finochietto artery forceps
Heiss soft tissue retractor
Heister valve
helical bacteria
helical computed tomography (CT)
helical suture
Helicide (bismuth subnitrate; metronidazole; tetracycline)
Helicobacter hepaticus
Helicobacter pylori-associated gastritis (HPAG)
Helicobacter pylori bacteria in vitro

Helicobacter pylori breath test
Helicobacter pylori gastritis
Helicosol (synthetic ^{13}C-urea)
  lyophilized powder
Helidac (bismuth subsalicylate,
  metronidazole, and tetracycline)
Heliodorus bandage
Helisal rapid blood test
Helistat absorbable collagen hemostatic
  sponge
Helitene absorbable hemostatic agent
Helivax vaccine
HeliX knot pusher
helle cell
Heller-Belsey operation for achalasia of
  esophagus
Heller cardiomyotomy
Heller-Dor operation for achalasia of
  esophagus
Heller esophagomyotomy
Heller myotomy
HELLP (hemolysis, elevated liver
  enzymes, and low platelets)
  syndrome
HELLP (hemolysis with a microangio-
  pathic blood smear, elevated liver
  enzymes, and low platelet count)
  syndrome
helminth
helminthic appendicitis
helminthic disorder
helper T cell
Hema-Check test
hemagglutination inhibition/inhibiting
  (HI)
hemagglutination titer for MSA
HemaMyst aerosol adhesive
hemangioendothelial sarcoma
hemangioendothelioma, epithelioid
hemangioma
  capillary
  cavernous
  congenital
  hepatic
hemangioma *(cont.)*
  sclerosing
  strawberry
  vascular
  venous
hemangioma angioma
hemangioma of liver
hemangiomatosis, splenic capillary
hemangiopericytoma
Hemaquet catheter introducer
Hemaquet sheath introducer
Hemarrest patch
Hemaseel APR fibrin adhesive
Hemaseel HMN biological tissue glue
Hemashield enhanced graft
HemAssist blood substitute
Hemasure r/LS red blood cell filtration
  system
HemaSyst sealant
hematemesis, post-retching
Hematest
hematocellular jaundice
hematochezia
hematochezia PR (per rectum)
hematocrit (Hct)
hematocystic spot (HCS)
hematogenous dissemination of tumor
hematogenous dissemination of virus
hematogenous dissemination to distant
  organs
hematogenous route
hematogenous seeding
hematogenous spread of microorganisms
hematologic dyscrasia
hematologic malignancy
hematoma
  bowel-wall
  intramural
  nasal septal
  pelvic
  perianal
  postoperative
  rectus sheath

hematoma *(cont.)*
  subcapsular
  subdural
  subfascial
  submucosal
  vestibule of mouth
hematoma aspiration
hematoma evacuation
hematopoiesis
hematopoietic disorder
hematopoietic malignancy
hematoxylin and eosin (H&E) stain
HemDetect three-field occult blood test
heme-negative stool
hemeostatic balance
heme-positive NG aspirate
heme-positive stool
HemeSelect reagent and collection kit
hemiaxial view
hemicolectomy (also see *operation*)
  Duecollement
  extended right
  hand-assisted laparoscopic
  laparoscopic
  laparoscopic left
  left
  standard right
hemicolon
hemicylindrical bone graft
hemidiaphragm
hemigastrectomy
hemiglossectomy
hemilaminectomy knife
hemilaminectomy retractor
Hemi Sling
hemispherical contact probe
hemispherical reamer
Hemobahn endovascular stent/graft
hemobilia
Hemoccult SENSA test
Hemoccult II test
hemochromatosis, precirrhotic
hemochromatotic cirrhosis
Hemochron high-dose thrombin time (HiTT)
Hemoclip-applying forceps
Hemoclip ligating clip
hemoconcentration
Hemocor HPH
HemoCue photometer
hemodialyzer
Hemo-Drain needle
Hemo-Drain wound tube
hemodynamically significant lesion
hemodynamically stable
hemodynamically unstable
hemodynamic monitoring
hemodynamic status
hemofiltration, continuous arterio-venous (CAVH)
hemoglobin (Hb, Hgb)
hemoglobin concentration
hemoglobin crosfumaril blood substitute
hemoglobin electrophoresis
hemoglobin, glycosylated
hemoglobinopathy
Hemolink blood substitute
Hem-o-lok clamp
Hem-o-lok ligating clip
hemolysis
  chronic
  intravascular
hemolytic jaundice
hemolytic malaria
hemolytic splenomegaly
hemolytic strep (streptococcus)
hemolytic uremic syndrome (HUS)
hemolyzed blood
HemoMatic monitor
Hemopad absorbable collagen hemostat
Hemopad microfibrillar collagen hemostat
hemoperitoneal
hemoperitoneum
hemoporphyrin derivative, photo-sensitizing
hemoptysis
Hemopump
Hemopure blood substitute

Hemopure (hemoglobin glutamer-250 [bovine]) oxygen therapy system
HemoQuant fecal occult blood test
Hemorid for Women (pramoxine HCl; phenylephrine HCl)
hemorrhage
  bilateral adrenal
  concealed
  epidural
  exsanguinating
  external
  extradural
  focal
  frank
  gastric
  gastrointestinal (GI)
  internal
  interstitial
  intestinal
  intra-abdominal
  intra-alveolar
  intracranial
  intratumoral
  massive
  nasopharyngeal
  oropharyngeal
  postoperative
  punctate
  retroperitoneal
  salmon-patch
  severe
  stromal
  subarachnoid
  subdural
  submucosal
  subserosal
hemorrhagic ascites
hemorrhagic colitis
hemorrhagic consolidation of lung
hemorrhagic cyst
hemorrhagic cystitis
hemorrhagic dengue
hemorrhagic diarrhea
hemorrhagic effusion
hemorrhagic encephalitis
hemorrhagic enterocolitis
hemorrhagic fever
hemorrhagic gastritis
hemorrhagic infarct
hemorrhagic intestinal infarction
hemorrhagic malaria
hemorrhagic material
hemorrhagic mucosa
hemorrhagic myelitis
hemorrhagic necrosis of alveolar septum)
hemorrhagic necrosis of intestine
hemorrhagic necrotizing pancreatitis
hemorrhagic nephritis
hemorrhagic pancreatitis
hemorrhagic pericarditis
hemorrhagic plague
hemorrhagic pleurisy
hemorrhagic salpingitis
hemorrhagic shock
hemorrhagic speck
hemorrhagic telangiectasia
hemorrhagic tendency
hemorrhoid (pl. hemorrhoids)
  arterial ligation (HAL)
  combined
  external
  first-degree
  fourth-degree
  internal
  large refractory
  mixed
  mucocutaneous
  necrotic
  prolapsed
  prolapsing internal
  second-degree
  strangulated
  third-degree
  thrombosed
  thrombosed external
hemorrhoid arterial ligation (HAL), Doppler-guided
hemorrhoid artery

hemorrhoidal banding
hemorrhoidal clamp
Hemorrhoidal HC (hydrocortisone acetate)
hemorrhoidal O ring
hemorrhoidal plexus
hemorrhoidal prolapse
hemorrhoidal sclerotherapy
hemorrhoidal tag
hemorrhoidal vessel
hemorrhoid cryotherapy
hemorrhoidectomy
  anoderm-preserving
  closed
  contact laser
  Doppler-guided artery ligation (DHGAL)
  Ferguson
  four-quadrant
  Harmonic
  laser
  ligation
  limited
  Longo
  Lord
  Milligan-Morgan
  modified Whitehead
  Morinaga
  nonmucosal
  open diathermy-excision
  one-quadrant
  Parks
  rubber band
  scissors-excision
  stapled
  three-quadrant
  two-quadrant
hemorrhoid classification by degree (1–4)
hemorrhoid infrared photocoagulation
hemorrhoid laser excision
hemorrhoid laser vaporization
hemorrhoid quadrants
hemorrhoid sclerotherapy
Hemo-Seal
hemosiderin deposits
hemosiderin granule
HemoSleeve device
hemostasis
  complete
  meticulous
hemostasis clip
hemostasis maintained with electrocautery
hemostasis obtained with electrocautery
hemostasis of liver bed
hemostasis was achieved
hemostat (see also *clamp*; *forceps*)
  Adson
  Carmalt
  collagen
  CoStasis
  Crile
  Dandy scalp
  Halstead
  Hemopad absorbable collagen
  Hemotene absorbable collagen
  InStat MCH (microfibrillar hemostat)
  Jackson trachea
  Jacobson
  Kelly
  Kocher
  Lovelace
  Mayo
  microfibrillar
  Miculicz
  Mixter
  mosquito
  Ochsner
  Pennington
  Rochester-Péan
  Sawtell
  Schnidt tonsil
  Westphal
  Woodward

hemostatic agent
  acetylhydrolase
  Amicar
  Aquamephyton
  argatroban
  Avitene
  calcium alginate
  cellulose, oxidized
  collagen sponge, absorbable
  Collastat
  CoStasis
  DynaStat
  EndoAvitene
  Ethamolin
  ethanolamine oleate
  gelatin film
  gelatin powder
  gelatin sponge
  Gelfilm
  Gelfoam
  Helistat sponge
  Helitene absorbable
  Hemaseel HMN
  Hemopad
  Hemotene
  InStat
  InStat MCH
  MCH (microfibrillar collagen hemostat)
  Myphyton
  Novastan
  Oxycel
  phytonadione (vitamin K_1)
  Sorbsan
  Surgicel
  Surgicel Nu-Knit
  Surgifoam
  thrombin
  Thrombin-JMI
  Thrombogen topical thrombin
  Thrombostat
  Tissucol
  Trasylol
hemostatic clamp
hemostatic forceps
hemostatic sponge (see *hemostatic agent*)
hemostatic suture
Hemotene absorbable collagen hemostat
Hemotherapies Liver Dialysis Unit
hemothorax, massive
hemotympanum
Hemovac drain
Hemovac Hydrocoat drain
Hemovac suction tube
Hem-Prep (phenylephrine HCl; zinc oxide)
Hemril Uniserts (bismuth subgallate; bismuth resorcin compound; benzyl benzoate; peruvian balsam; zinc oxide)
Henahan elevator
Henahan extracting forceps
Henderson onlay bone graft
Henderson skin incision
Hendrin ductus clamp
Hendrin ductus forceps
Hendrin forceps
Henke-Sass rigid laparoscope
Henke-Sass Wolf laparoscope
Henke triangle
Henle, jejunal interposition of
Henle loop
Henley carotid retractor
Henley vascular clamp
Henner T-model endaural retractor
Hennig plaster cast spreader
Henning mallet
Henning meniscal retractor
Henning sign
Henoch-Schönlein (Schoenlein) purpura
Henry bone graft
Henry incision
hepadna virus (hepatitis B-like DNA)
Hepafix low-allergy adhesive tape dressing
Hepagene (hepatitis B vaccine)

Hepamed-coated Wiktor stent
heparin
  beef lung
  pyrogen-free
heparin anticoagulant
heparin calcium
heparin-induced thrombocytopenia (HIT)
heparin infusion prior to stentint (HIPS)
heparinize
heparinized solution
heparin lock (hep lock)
Heparin Lock Flush solution (heparin sodium)
heparin lock introducer
heparin/protamine infusion
heparin sodium & sodium chloride
heparin sulfate
heparin therapy, monitoring of
heparin whole blood
HepatAmine nutrient solution
HepatAssist bioartificial liver
hepatectomy
  cadaveric donor
  donor
  extended right
  hemi-
  laparoscopic
  left
  limited
  local
  partial
  recipient
  regional
  right
  right lobe
  segmental
  simultaneous segmental
  subsegmental
  total left
  wedge
hepatic abscess
hepatic adenoma
Hepatic-Aid powdered feeding
Hepatic-Aid II Instant Drink (multiple branched-chain amino acids)
hepatic amyloid
hepatic architecture
hepatic arterial infusion (HAI)
hepatic arterial infusion chemotherapy
hepatic arterial supply
hepatic arteriogram
hepatic artery ligation
hepatic artery portal vein fistula
hepatic artery system
hepatic artery thrombosis (HAT)
hepatic atrophy
hepatic bed
hepatic bifurcation
hepatic calculus
hepatic capsular vasculitis
hepatic capsule
hepatic carcinoma
hepatic cell carcinoma
hepatic cirrhosis
hepatic colic
hepatic coma
hepatic cord
hepatic degeneration
hepatic duct
hepatic duct calculus
hepatic dullness
hepatic encephalopathy (HE)
hepatic failure
hepatic fever
hepatic fibrosis
hepatic fistula
hepatic flexure of colon
hepatic function test
hepatic gland
hepatic glycogen
hepatic glycogen storage
hepatic glycogen stores
hepatic granuloma
hepatic hemangioma
hepatic hilum
hepatic Hodgkin disease

hepatic hydrothorax
hepatic infarction
hepatic insufficiency
hepatic iron stores
hepatic ligament
hepatic lithiasis
hepatic lobectomy
hepatic lobular parenchyma
hepatic lobule
hepatic lymph node
hepatic necrosis
hepatic nerve plexus
hepatico- (see *hepato-* entries)
hepaticoenterostomy (also hepato-enterostomy)
hepaticojejunostomy (see *hepato-jejunostomy*)
hepatic obstruction
hepaticoportoenterostomy
hepatic osteomalacia
hepaticostomy
hepaticotomy
hepatic outflow tract
hepatic parasitic cyst
hepatic parenchyma
hepatic parenchymal cell
hepatic perfusion index (HPI)
hepatic phosphorylase deficiency
hepatic plexus
hepatic porphyria
hepatic-renal angle
hepatic resection
hepatic reserve
hepatic rupture
hepatic sclerosis
hepatic segmentectomy
hepatic segment of liver
hepatic sinusoid
hepatic stem cell
hepatic tenderness
hepatic transaminase
hepatic triad
hepatic vein
hepatic vein occlusion
hepatic vein thrombosis
hepatic vein outflow
hepatic vein stent
hepatic vein thrombosis
hepatic vein vena cava thrombosis
hepatic veno-occlusive disease
hepatic venous drainage
hepatic venous isolation by direct hemo-perfusion (HVI-DHP)
hepatic venous outflow
hepatic venous outflow block
hepatic venous outflow obstruction (HVOO)
hepatic venous pressure gradient
hepatic venous web disease
hepatic web
hepatic web dilation
hepatic wedge pressure
hepatitis (pl. hepatitides)
  acute mononucleosis-like
  acute parenchymatous
  acute viral (AVH)
  alcoholic
  amebic
  anesthetic
  anicteric
  anti-HBe-positive
  autoimmune
  cholestatic viral
  chronic
  chronic active (CAH)
  chronic active viral (CAVH)
  chronic active viral, non-A, non-B (CAVH-NAB)
  chronic active viral, type B (CAVH-B)
  chronic aggressive
  chronic fibrosing
  chronic interstitial
  chronic lobular (CLH)
  chronic persistent (CPH)
  chronic persisting
  chronic progressive
  coinfection with

hepatitis *(cont.)*
- concomitant acute alcoholic
- delta
- drug-induced
- ENANB (enterically transmitted non-A, non-B) (now C)
- enterically transmitted, non-A, non-B (ET-NANB) (now C)
- familial
- fatty liver
- fulminant
- fulminant viral (FVH)
- giant cell
- granulomatous
- halothane-induced
- hepatobiliary
- herpetic
- hyperglobulinemic
- infectious (type A)
- INH-induced
- intrahepatic, of pregnancy
- ischemic
- isoniazid-induced
- lobular
- lupoid
- malarial
- MS-1
- MS-2
- mumps
- NANB (non-A, non-B) (now C)
- neonatal
- newborn
- non-A, non-B (NANB) (now C)
- noninfectious
- normal carrier
- occult
- persistent viral (PVH)
- persistent viral, non-A, non-B (PVH-NAB) (now C)
- persistent viral, type B (PVH-B)
- plasma cell
- post-transfusion
- quiescent
- recurrent

hepatitis *(cont.)*
- serum
- subacute
- subclinical
- testing
- toxic
- toxoplasmosis
- transfusion
- viral
- yellow fever

Hepatitis Activity Index
hepatitis-associated antigen (HAA)
hepatitis A vaccine, inactivated
hepatitis A virus (HAV)
hepatitis B vaccine (HBV)
hepatitis B (serum hepatitis)
hepatitis B antigen (HbAg)
hepatitis B core antibody (HBcAb)
hepatitis B core antigen (HB_cAg)
hepatitis B “e” antibody (HB_eAb)
hepatitis B “e” antigen (HB_eAg)
hepatitis B hyperimmune globulin
hepatitis B immune globulin (HBIg)
hepatitis B immunoglobulin (HBIg)
hepatitis B surface antibody (HB_sAb)
hepatitis B surface antigen (HB_sAg)
hepatitis B vaccine
hepatitis B virus (HBV)
hepatitis B virus surface antigen (HB_sAg)
hepatitis B virus vaccine, inactivated
hepatitis C, noncirrhotic
hepatitis C vaccine
hepatitis C virus (HCV) (formerly non-A, non-B)
hepatitis D (delta hepatitis)
hepatitis D (delta) virus (HDV)
hepatitis D virus antigen (HDV Ag)
hepatitis delta (type D)
hepatitis delta virus (HDV)
hepatitis E (type E)
hepatitis E virus (HEV)
Hepatitis Resource Network (HRN)
hepatitis F

hepatitis G virus (HGV)
hepatitis serologic marker
hepatization
hepatobiliary disease
hepatobiliary hepatitis
hepatobiliary scan
hepatobiliary scintigraphy
hepatobiliary tree
hepatoblastoma
hepato- (also *hepatico-*)
hepatocarcinogenic pesticide
hepatocarcinoma, fibrolamellar
hepatocellular adenoma (HCA)
hepatocellular ballooning
hepatocellular carcinoma (HCC)
hepatocellular cholestasis
hepatocellular disease
hepatocellular iron storage
hepatocellular jaundice
hepatocellular necrosis
hepatocerebral intoxication
hepatocholangiolitic carcinoma
hepatoclavicular view
hepatocolic ligament
hepatocystic
hepatocystocolic ligament
hepatocyte
 ballooning degeneration of
 cobblestone pattern of
 lipid-laden
 periportal
hepatocyte dysfunction
hepatocyte nuclear factor-1 alpha (HNF-1 alpha)
hepatodiaphragmatic interposition of colon (Chilaiditi syndrome)
hepatoduodenal ligament compression
hepatoduodenal-peritoneal reflection
hepatoduodenal reflection
hepatoduodenoperitoneal reflection
hepatoenteric anastomosis
hepatoerythropoietic porphyria (HEP)
hepatoesophageal ligament
hepatofugal flow
hepatogastric duodenal ligament
hepatogastric ligament
hepatogenous jaundice
hepatogenous pigment
hepatoiminodiacetic acid (HIDA)
hepatojejunostomy (also hepaticojejunostomy)
 complex
 high
 hilar
 intracystic
 laparoscopic
 left
 palliative
 pediatric
 peripheral
 right
 right and left
 Roux-en-Y
 side-to-side
 simple
hepatojejunostomy with cutaneous stoma
hepatojugular reflux (HJR)
hepatolenticular degeneration
hepatolenticular disease
hepatolienal cirrhosis
hepatolithiasis with biliary stricture, complicated residual
hepatologist
hepatology
hepatoma, fibrolamellar
hepatomegaly
 congestive
 painful
hepatopancreatic ampulla sphincter
hepatopancreatic fold
hepatopancreatoduodenectomy
hepatopathy, radiation
hepatopetal flow
hepatophosphorylase deficiency glycogenosis
hepatophrenic ligament
hepatopleural fistula
hepatoportal sclerosis

hepatoportoenterostomy, Kasai-type
hepatoptosis
hepatopulmonary syndrome
hepatorenal angle
hepatorenal ligament
hepatorenal pouch
hepatorenal recess
hepatorenal syndrome (HRS)
hepatorrhaphy
hepatosplenic infestation
hepatosplenomegaly
hepatotomy
hepatotoxic effect
hepatotoxicity
hepatotoxic range
hepatoumbilical ligament
Hep-B-Gammagee
hep lock catheter
Hep-Lock (heparin sodium) flush
Hep-Lock U/P (heparin sodium) flush
Heprofile ELISA (enzyme-linked immunosorbent assay)
heptadecapeptide
Heptalac lactulose solution
Heptavax-B vaccine
Heptazyme
Heptodin (lamivudine)
Heptovir (lamivudine)
herald bleed
herbal therapy
Herbert bone screw
Herbert saw
Herbert-Whipple bone screw
HercepTest
Herceptin (trastuzumab) monoclonal antibody
Hercules Nd:YAG laser system
Hercules plaster and bandage scissors
Hercules plaster shears
Hercules 7000 mobile x-ray unit
Herculink biliary stent
Herculink 14 biliary stent system
Herculon suture
Herczel rasp
Herczel rib elevator
hereditary angioedema
hereditary angioneurotic edema
hereditary cancer
hereditary carcinoma
hereditary elliptocytosis
hereditary hemorrhagic telangiectasia (HHT)
hereditary MEA (multiple endocrine adenomatosis) syndrome
hereditary MTC (MEN 2A and MEN 2B, and familial non-MEN MTC)
hereditary nonpolyposis colorectal cancer (HNPCC)
hereditary pancreatitis
hereditary tyrosinemia
heredofamilial disease
Herget rectal biopsy forceps
Hering canal
Hering duct
Hermansky-Pudlak syndrome
HERMES surgery monitoring unit
Hermesh-3 polypropylene mesh
hermetic external shunt
Hermitage Hospital Products
Hernandez-Ros bone staple
hernia (pl. hernias, herniae)
  abdominal wall
  acquired
  axial hiatal
  Barth
  Béclard
  bilateral
  bilateral incarcerated scrotal
  bilateral inguinal
  bilocular femoral
  Bochdalek
  cecal
  Cheatle-Henry
  Cloquet
  combined hernia
  complete
  concealed

hernia *(cont.)*
concentric hiatal
congenital
contralateral
Cooper
crural
diaphragmatic
direct inguinal
double
double-loop
dry
duodenal jejunal
easily reducible
epigastric
esophageal
extrasaccular
fascial
fat
fatty
femoral
funicular inguinal
gangrenous
gastroesophageal
gluteal
groin
Grynfeltt
Hesselbach
Hey
hiatal
Holthouse
iliacosubfascial
incarcerated
incisional
incomplete
indirect inguinal
infantile
inguinal
inguinal with scrotal extension
inguinocrural
inguinofemoral
inguinolabial
inguinoscrotal
inguinosuperficial
internal

hernia *(cont.)*
intersigmoid
interstitial
intestinal
intra-abdominal
intraepiploic
intrailiac
intraparietal
intrapelvic
irreducible
ischiatic
ischiorectal
Krönlein (Kroenlein)
Larrey
Laugier
Lesgaft
levator
Littré
lumbar
Malgaigne
Maydl
mesenteric
mixed hiatal
Morgagni
nontraumatic
oblique
obturator
obturator hernia
pannicular
pantaloon
paracolostomy
paraesophageal
paraesophageal hiatal
paraesophageal hiatus
parahiatal
paraileostomal
paraperitoneal
parasaccular
parasternal
parastomal
paraumbilical
parietal
pediatric
perineal

hernia *(cont.)*
- peritoneal
- Petit
- postoperative
- postoperative paraesophageal hiatus
- properitoneal inguinal
- pudendal
- recurrent
- recurring
- reducible
- retrograde
- retroperitoneal
- retropubic
- retrosternal
- Richter
- Rieux
- Rokitansky
- rolling hiatal
- sciatic
- scrotal
- sliding esophageal
- sliding hiatal
- slipped
- spigelian
- spontaneous lateral ventral
- spontaneous ventrolateral
- stoma
- strangulated
- strangulated paraesophageal
- strangulation
- transthoracic diaphragmatic
- traumatic
- Treitz
- trocar
- type I hiatal
- type II hiatal
- umbilical
- unilateral
- uterine broad ligament
- Velpeau
- ventral
- ventrolateral
- vesical
- "W"

hernia defect
hernia dissector
hernia en bissac
hernia knife
hernial lipoma
hernial orifice
hernial sac
Herniamesh surgical mesh graft
hernia pouch
hernia repair
hernia ring forceps
hernia rupture
hernia sac does not traverse the internal ring
hernia spoon
herniated preperitoneal fat
herniation of bowel
herniation, physiological gut-loop
hernioplasty (also see *herniorrhaphy; operation*)
- double-buttress laparoscopic
- LAP-TAPP (laparoscopic transabdominal preperitoneal)
- laparoscopic
- mesh plug
- modified Shouldice
- modified TAPP
- open mesh-plug
- preperitoneal
- TAPP (transabdominal preperitoneal) laparoscopic
- tension-free
- TEP (totally extraperitoneal) laparoscopic
- totally (or total) extraperitoneal laparoscopic
- transabdominal preperitoneal laparoscopic

herniorrhaphy (see also *hernioplasty*; *operation*)
- Bassini inguinal
- elective
- emergent
- Halsted-Bassini

herniorrhaphy *(cont.)*
- Halsted inguinal
- Hill-type hiatus
- Lichtenstein
- Macewen
- Madden incisional
- McVay
- open
- pants-over-vest
- Ponka
- Shouldice inguinal
- umbilical
- ventral
- vest-over-pants

Herp-Check
herpes mucositis
herpes simplex virus (HSV)
herpes type 5 virus (cytomegalovirus)
herpes ulcer
herpesvirus
herpes whitlow infection
herpes zoster virus (HZV)
herpetic esophagitis
herpetic hepatitis
herpetic vesicle
Herplex Liquifilm (idoxuridine)
Herrick kidney pedicle clamp
Hers disease
Herter-Gee disease
Herter-Heubner disease
Hertra-2 polypropylene mesh
HER-2/neu gene
Hertzler rib retractor
Herzberg test
Herzyme
Hespan (hetastarch) plasma volume expander
Hesselbach hernia
Hesselbach ligament
Hesselbach triangle
Hessel-Nystrom pin
Hessert triangle
hetastarch plasma volume expander
heterogeneous (heterogenous) graft
heterogeneous parenchyma
heterograft
- arterial
- bone
- bovine
- porcine
- stentless

heteroplasmy
heterotopia, gastric
heterotopic pancreas
heterotopic pancreatic tissue
heterotopic tissue
heterotopic transplantation
Hetrazan (diethylcarbamazine citrate)
HEV (hepatitis E virus)
Hewlett-Packard ultrasound system
Hewson cruciate guide
Hewson drill guide
Hexabrix (ioxaglate meglumine; ioxaglate sodium)
hexafluoropropylene-VDF suture
hexocyclium
Hextend blood substitute
Hextend plasma volume expander
Heyer-Schulte neurosurgical shunt
Heyer-Schulte Pour-Safe bag
Heyer-Schulte tissue expander
Heyer-Schulte wound drain
Hey hernia
Hey-Groves-Kirk bone graft
Heywood-Smith hemorrhoidal forceps
HF infrared laser
"H. flu" (slang for *Haemophilus influenzae*)
Hgb (hemoglobin)
HGD (high-grade dysplasia)
HGH (human growth hormone)
HGV (hepatitis G virus)
HHT (hereditary hemorrhagic telangiectasia)
HHV-8 (human herpesvirus-8)
hiatal hernia
hiatal stenosis
hiatus
- aortic

hiatus *(cont.)*
  diaphragmatic
  esophageal
  fallopian
  semilunar
  sternocostal
hiatus hernia
Hibbs blade
Hibbs bone-cutting forceps
Hibbs chisel
Hibbs chisel elevator
Hibbs mallet
Hibbs retractor
Hibbs spinal fusion gouge
Hibbs-Spratt curette
Hibiclens (chlorhexidine gluconate; alcohol)
HIB polysaccharide vaccine
Hib (*Haemophilus influenzae* type b) vaccine
hiccup (pl. hiccups)
hiccuping
Hickman catheter
Hicks lugged plate
HIC wire guide
HIDA (hepato-iminodiacetic acid)
HIDA Kinevac
HIDA/PRIDA scan
HIDA scan
HIDA sincalide
hidradenitis suppurativa
Hieshima coaxial catheter
HIFU (high-intensity focused ultrasound)
Higgins technique for ureterointestinal anastomosis
high-bulk, low-fat diet
high-calcium bath dialysis
high-carbohydrate diet
High Definition Imaging (HDI) 3000 ultrasound system
high-density lipoprotein (HDL)
high-dose dexamethasone suppression test
high-energy gunshot wound
high-energy laser
high failure rate
high fever, shock, and death
high-fiber diet
high-flow cannula
high-flow electronic insufflator
high-frequency cutting loop
high-frequency miniprobe
high-frequency probe
high-grade angioinvasive follicular carcinoma
high-grade dysplasia (HGD)
high-grade fever
high-grade lesion
high-grade malignancy
high-grade obstruction
high-grade obstructive lesion
high imperforate anus
high index of suspicion
high-intensity focused ultrasound (HIFU)
high intracellular concentration
high ligation
high ligation of hernia sac
high lipase
highly active antiretroviral therapy (HAART)
highly selective vagotomy
highly vascular tumor
Highmore abscess
high-output fistula
high-pitched bowel sounds
high-protein diet
high-pressure catheter
high-pressure shunt
high-pressure zone
high recurrence rate
high-residue diet
high-resistance fundoplication
high-resolution computed tomography
high-resolution ultrasound
high-resolution video monitor
high-riding ballotable prostate

high-riding prostate
high-risk population
high-roughage diet
high small bowel obstruction
high-speed twist drill
high spinal anesthesia
high sphincter pressure
high subtotal gastrectomy
high torque dermabrader
high-velocity gunshot wound
high-volume/low-pressure cuff
high volume reflux
hilar involvement
hilar lesion
hilar obstruction
hilar plate
hilar stricture
hila of kidney
Hildebrandt uterine hemostatic forceps
Hill antireflux operation
Hill cluster harvest technique
Hill-Ferguson rectal retractor
Hill fundoplasty
Hill gastropexy
Hill gastropexy fundoplication
Hill hiatus hernia repair
Hill median arcuate repair
Hill operation
Hill posterior gastropexy
Hill procedure
Hill rectal retractor
Hill repair for esophageal reflux
Hill-Sachs lesion
Hi-Lo Evac endotracheal tube
Hi-Lo Jet tracheal tube
Hi-Lo tracheal tube
hilum (pl. hila)
    hepatic
    kidney
    lung
    pulmonary
    renal
    splenic
hilus, kidney
Himmelstein sternal retractor
Hinchey diverticulitis grading system
Hinderer cartilage forceps
hindgut (distal colon and rectum)
hindgut dysfunction
hinge rod
Hinkle-James rectal speculum
hip fracture compaction drill
hip pin
Hippocrates bandage
Hippuran
HIPS (heparin infusion prior to stenting)
hip spica cast
hip-to-ankle view
Hirsch hypophyseal punch
Hirsch hypophysis punch forceps
Hirschman anoscope
Hirschman pile clamp
Hirschman proctoscope
Hirschman rectal speculum
Hirschsprung-associated enterocolitis (HAEC)
Hirschsprung disease
Hirschsprung enterocolitis
hirsutism
Hirulog (bivalirudin)
His, angle of
Histalog stimulation test
histamine blocker
histamine-resistant achlorhydria
histamine test
histamine-2 (H_2) receptor agonist
histamine-2 (H_2) receptor antagonist
Histerone 100 (testosterone)
Histoacryl Blue (HAB) tissue adhesive
Histoacryl glue (cyanoacrylate) tissue adhesive
Histoacryl glue adhesive
histologic activity index (HAI)
histologic diagnosis
histologic grading
histologic involvement of axillary lymph node

histologic lesion
histologic type
histology
histopathological diagnosis
histopathologic examination
histopathologic preparation
histopathology
Histoplasma capsulatum polysaccharide antigen (HPA)
history of radiation therapy to the neck
HIT (heparin-induced thrombocytopenia
Hitachi Model 737 multichannel analyzer
Hitachi 2.0 diagnostic ultrasound system
HI VAC tubing
Hi-Vegi-Lip (pancreatase; lipase; protease; amylase)
HLA (human lymphocyte antigen)
HLA crossmatch
HLA haplotype
HME Intertech
HM4 lithotriptor
HMTV (human mammary tumor virus)
HNB angiographic catheter
HNF-1 alpha (hepatocyte nuclear factor-1 alpha)
HNKC (hyperosmolar nonketotic coma)
HNPCC (hereditary nonpolyposis colorectal carcinoma)
H_2O absorption
Hoaglund bone graft
hoarseness
hoarse voice
Hobbs balloon dilator
Hobb view
hobnail cirrhosis
hobnailed appearance of liver surface
hobnail liver
hockey-stick appearance of catheter tip
hockey-stick incision
Hodge intestinal decompression tube
Hodgkin disease
Hodgkin lymphoma
hoe, Joe (retractor)
Hoen angular forceps
Hoen clamp
Hoen gouge
Hoen hemilaminectomy retractor
Hoen intervertebral disk rongeur
Hoen lamina gouge
Hoen laminectomy rongeur
Hoen nerve hook
Hoen periosteal elevator
Hoen scalp hemostatic forceps
Hoen scalp retractor
Hoen skull plate
Hoen ventricular needle
Hoffmann pin guide
Hofmeister anastomosis
Hofmeister gastroenterostomy
Hofmeister technique
Hohmann bone retractor
Hohn central venous catheter
Hoke osteotome
Holihesive Skin Barrier (for ostomy skin)
Holinger esophagoscope
Holinger open-end aspirating tube
Hollander test
Hollister Convex Insert
Hollister First Choice pouch
Hollister gastrostomy tube
Hollister Guardian F Skin Barrier
Hollister Holligard pouch
Hollister Karaya 5 ostomy pouch
Hollister Karaya Seal pouch
Hollister Premium paste
Hollister Premium pouch
hollow chisel
hollow mill reamer
hollow needle
hollow viscus
holmium (Ho) laser
holmium laser resection of the prostate (HoLRP)
holmium:YAG (yttrium-argon-garnet) laser

HoLRP (holmium laser resection of the prostate)
Holscher knee retractor
Holscher nerve root retractor
Holt nail
Holt nail plate
Holter tube
Holter valve
Holthouse hernia
Holzheimer retractor
Homans sign
home parenteral nutrition (HPN)
Home Access Hepatitis C Check kit
homeostasis, glucose
HomMed Sentry/Observer monitor
homogeneous graft
homogeneous material
homologous graft
homosexual rectal trauma
homovanillic acid (HVA)
homozygotes
honeycombed appearance
honeycomb lung
honeycomb mucosa
honeycomb pattern
hood forceps
Hood stoma stent
hook
 Acufex nerve
 Adson
 Adson dissecting
 Adson dural
 Adson nerve
 André
 APRL (Army Prosthetics Research Laboratory)
 Austin Moore
 Barr
 Barr crypt
 Barr fistula
 Barsky skin
 bayonet-shaped
 bifid
 Blair palate

hook *(cont.)*
 blunt
 blunt nerve
 Bobechko
 bone
 Boyes-Goodfellow
 Braun
 button
 buttressed
 Cairns-Oliver
 Carroll skin
 caudal
 cautery
 C-D (Cotrel-Dubousset)
 clawed pedicle
 Cloward cautery
 Cloward dural
 compression
 cordotomy
 corkscrew dural
 Cotrel-Dubousset (C-D)
 Crile
 Crile nerve
 crypt
 Culler
 Cushing angular
 Cushing dural
 Cushing gasserian ganglion
 Cushing nerve
 Dandy nerve
 DePuy nerve
 dissecting
 distraction
 double
 Drummond
 DTT (dynamic transverse traction)
 dura
 dural
 Edwards
 Edwards-Levine
 Effler-Groves
 Emmett fistula
 Emmett tenaculum
 Fisch dural

hook *(cont.)*
Fisch dural
Fisch micro
fishhook
fistula
Frazier dural
Frazier nerve
Freer skin
ganglion
garment
Gillies bone
Gillies-Dingman
Gillies skin
Godina double
Graefe dissecting
Graefe skin
Graham muscle
Graham nerve
Green muscle
Guthrie fixation
Gynex angle
Harrington
Hoen nerve
House crura
House foot plate
House oval window
House strut
Isola
Iterson trachea
Jackson trachea
Jameson muscle
Jannetta
jig
Jordan
Joseph skin
Keene compression
Kennerdell-Maroon
Kilner skin
Kirby muscle
Kleinert-Kutz skin
Knodt
Kocher
Krayenbuehl (Krayenbühl) vessel
Küntscher nail extracting

hook *(cont.)*
Lahey Clinic dural
Lahey Clinic nerve
Lambotte bone
laminar
laser
Leatherman
Love nerve root
Lucae nerve
Malis nerve
malleable
Marino transsphenoidal
Martin rectal
meniscus
micro
micro dural
micro nerve
Micro-One
Miltex tissue twist
Moe spinal
Moe square-ended
Moss
muscle
Mya
nail-extracting
Neivert polyp
nerve
O'Brien rib
pedicle
Pratt
Pratt crypt
Pratt rectal
prosthetic
Rhoton
rib
right-angle
Rogozinski
Rosser crypt
Sachs dural
Saunders-Paparella stapes
Scoville nerve
Selby II
Selverstone cordotomy
Shambaugh fistula

hook *(cont.)*
  Shambaugh microscopic
  sharp
  shoe of the
  side-opening
  skin
  sliding barrel
  Smillie
  Smithwick button
  Smithwick nerve
  Smithwick sympathectomy
  Speare dural
  spring
  Starion thermal cautery
  Stewart crypt
  straight dural
  Strully dural
  suture
  sympathectomy
  Take-Apart nerve
  tendon
  T-handled
  Toennis dural
  tracheal
  traction
  transsphenoidal
  transverse
  transverse process
  Trautman Locktite prosthetic
  TSRH (Texas Scottish Rite Hospital)
  twist
  Tyrell
  Valleylab electrocautery interchangeable
  valve
  vessel
  Volkmann bone
  Weary nerve
  Yankauer
  Yasargil spring
  Zielke
  Zimmer caudal
  Zuelzer
hook clamp
hooked intramedullary nail
hooked medullary nail
hook electrocautery
hook-end intramedullary pin
hook knife
hook-lying position
hook pin
hook scissors, single-action
hook wire localization, CT-directed
hookworm
Hopkins aortic forceps
Hopkins clamp
Hopkins lens system
Hopkins plaster knife
Hopkins rigid glass lens endoscope
Hopkins rod-lens system for rigid choledochoscope
Hopkins II forward oblique telescope
Hopkins II telescope
Hopmann papilloma
Hopmann polyp
Horizon stent (temporary/urinary)
Horizons C-13 urea breath test for *H. pylori*
horizontal gastroplasty
horizontal incision
horizontal mattress suture
horizontal position
horizontal retractor
horizontal suture
horizontal transmission
hormonally active
hormonal therapy
hormone
  counter-regulatory
  endocrine pancreas
  endogenous parathyroid
  exogenous thyroid
  free
  gastrointestinal
  GI inhibitory
  HGH (human growth)
  human growth (HGH)
  inhibiting
  long-acting thyroid-stimulating (LATS)

hormone *(cont.)*
  parathyroid (parathormone)
  recombinant human thyroid-stimulating
  thyroglobulin thyroid
  thyroid (TH)
  thyrotrophic
  thyrotropin-releasing (TRH)
  TSH (thyroid-stimulating)
hormone-dependent
hormone-induced hypopituitarism
hormone-induced pancreatitis
hormone receptor site
hormone-refractory disease
hormone-sensitive breast cancer
Horn endo-otoprobe laser
Horn sign
horseshoe abscess
horseshoe fistula
horseshoe kidney
horseshoe-shaped incision
Horsley anastomosis
Horsley bone-cutting forceps
Horsley bone rongeur
Horsley gastrectomy
Horsley-Stille bone-cutting forceps
Horsley-Stille rib shears
Horsley suture
hose-pipe appearance of terminal ileum
Hosemann forceps
host cell membrane
host constituent
host defense mechanism
host immune mechanism
host immune responsiveness
hot appendix
hot biopsy
hot biopsy forceps
hot defect
hot flexible forceps
hot knife
hot laser
hot nodule
Hot Sampler disposable hot biopsy forceps
hot-shot PCR (polymerase chain reaction) test
hot spot
Hotsy Cautery
Houget maneuver
Hough ("huff") hoe
Hounsfield unit
hourglass constriction of gallbladder
hourglass contraction of the stomach
hourglass deformity
hourglass gallbladder
hourglass pattern
hourglass-shaped lesion
hourglass stomach
House-Barbara shattering needle
House crura hook
House cup forceps
House endaural elevator
House excavator
House-Fisch dural retractor
House foot plate hook
House knife
House needle
House oval window hook
Housepan clip-applying forceps
House-Paparella stapes curette
House-Radpour suction-irrigator
House-Rosen needle
House separator
House stapes curette
House stapes elevator
House stapes speculum
House strut hook
House suction-irrigation tube
Houston, valve of
Howard Kelly artery forceps
Howarth dissector
Howel-Evans syndrome
Howell coronary scissors
Howell-Jolly body
Howell tibial guide
Howmedica Microfixation cranial plate
Howmedica Microfixation System forceps

Howmedica Microfixation System pliers
Howmedica Universal compression screw
Howmedica Vitallium staple
Howship-Romberg sign
Ho:YAG (holmium:yttrium-argon-garnet) laser
Ho:YAG LTK (holmium: YAG laser thermal keratoplasty), noncontact
HPAG (*Helicobacter pylori*-associated gastritis)
HPC guidewire
hpf (high-power field)
HPI (hepatic perfusion index)
HPN (home parenteral nutrition)
HR (heart rate)
H_2 receptor agonist
H_2 receptor antagonist
H_2 receptor-blocker
H_2 receptor-blocking drug
HRN (Hepatitis Resource Network)
HRQOL (health-related qualify of life)
HRS (hepatorenal syndrome)
HRT (hormone replacement therapy) patch
H-shaped capsular incision
H-shaped configuration
H-shaped graft
H-shaped ileal pouch
H-shaped microplate
H-shaped plate
HSP (heat shock protein) antigen
H-TRON plus V100/V40 insulin infusion pump
H-type fistula
Hubbard plate
hubbed needle
Huber needle
Huckstep nail
Hudson brace drill
Hudson cranial drill
Hudson cranial rongeur
Hudson forceps
Huebner-Herter disease
Hueter bandage
Hufnagel clamp
huge stools
Hughston view
huHMFG1
Huibregtse-Katon papillotome
Hulka clip applicator
Hulka tenaculum forceps
Humalog insulin
Humalog Mix 75/25
Humalog Pen (insulin delivery device)
human antichimeric antibody (HACA)
human cell transplantation
human chorionic gonadotropin
human defensin 5 (HD-5)
human growth hormone (HGH)
human hemoglobin cross-linked with glutaral
human herpesvirus 1 (HHV-1)
human herpesvirus 2 (HHV-2)
human herpesvirus 3 (HHV-3)
human herpesvirus 4 (HHV-4)
human herpesvirus 5 (HHV-5)
human herpesvirus 6 (HHV-6)
human herpesvirus 7 (HHV-7)
human immunodeficiency virus (HIV)
human insulin
human islet allograft
human islets
human lymphocyte antigen (HLA)
human mammary tumor virus (HMTV)
human meniscal allograft
human papillomavirus (HPV) infection
human T-cell leukemia virus
human T-cell lymphoma virus (HTLV I and II)
human T-cell lymphotropic virus type I (HTLV-I)
Humatrix Microclysmic gel
Humatrope (somatropin)
Humatro-Pen (growth hormone delivery device)
humeral head retractor
humeral mechanism

humeral rod
Humicade
humidifier lung
Hummingbird wand
humoral host defense mechanism
humpback Weitlaner retractor
hump, buffalo
Humphries clamp
Humulin L (human insulin zinc [rDNA])
Humulin R (human insulin [recombinant])
Humulin R pen (insulin delivery device)
Humulin 30/70 (insulin; isophane insulin)
Humulin 50/50 (isophane human insulin [rDNA]; human insulin [rDNA])
Humulin 70/30 (isophane human insulin [rDNA]; human insulin [rDNA])
Humulin-U (extended insulin zinc)
Humulin U Ultralente (extended insulin human zinc [rDNA])
hum, venous
hunger pain
Hunner ulcer
Hunstad infiltration handle
Hunstad punch
Hunter forceps
Hunter-Sessions balloon
Hunter Silastic rod
Hunter splinter forceps
Hunter-style double-action bowel grasper
Hunter tendon rod
Huntington bone graft
Huntington disease
Hunt-Lawrence pouch
Hunt-Reich trocar
Hunt tumor forceps
Hunt-Yasargil pituitary forceps
Huppert test
Hupp trachea retractor
Hurd bone-cutting forceps
Hurd tonsil dissector and pillar retractor
Hurst bullet-tip dilator
Hurst mercury bougie
Hurst-Tucker pneumatic dilator
Hürthle (Huerthle)
Hürthle cell carcinoma
Hürthle cell neoplasm
Hürthle cell tumor
Hurwitz dialysis catheter
Hurwitz esophageal clamp
Hurwitz thoracic trocar
HUS (hemolytic uremic syndrome)
Huschke ligament
Husk bone rongeur
Hutchinson freckle
Hutchinson-Weber-Peutz syndrome
Hutinel disease
HVA (homovanillic acid)
HVI-DHP (hepatic venous isolation by direct hemoperfusion)
HVOO (hepatic venous outflow obstruction)
HVS (herpesvirus simplex)
hyalin
  alcoholic
  Mallory
hyaline necrosis
hyaluronidase
Hybrid Capture CMV DNA test
Hybrid Capture cytomegalovirus DNA test
Hybrid Capture HPV DNA test
hybrid sphincterotome
Hybritech Tandem PSA ratio (free PSA/total PSA) (PSA, prostate-specific antigen)
Hycamtin (topotecan hydrochloride)
hyCURE collagen hemostatic wound dressing
hyCURE G hydrogel dressing
hyCURE protein powder wound-filler dressing
hydatid cyst

hydatid cyst disease
hydatidiform mole (molar pregnancy)
hydatid liver cyst
hydatid, Morgagni
hydatid polyp
hydatid sand
Hyde shunt
hydragogue
HydraGran absorbent dressing
hydralazine
Hydrapak
Hydrasorb foam wound dressing
Hydrate (dimenhydrinate)
hydrated
hydration
hydration status
hydrazine sulfate
hydremic ascites
Hydrocel bone substitute
hydrocelectomy
hydrocele of the cord
hydrocele, postoperative
hydrocele trocar
hydrochloretic drug
hydrochloric acid test
hydrochloride (HCl)
hydrocholeretic
Hydrocil Instant (psyllium hydrophilic
  mucilloid)
Hydrocol (hydrocolloid dressing)
Hydrocollator heating unit
hydrocolloid dressing
hydrocortisone
hydrocortisone acetate
hydrocortisone enema
hydrocortisone foam
Hydrofiber dressing
hydrogel dressing
hydrogel sheet
hydrogen breath test
hydrogen ion
hydrogen peroxide enema
Hydrolyser microcatheter
Hydromer Aquatrix II
Hydromer coated bipolar coagulation
  probe
Hydron burn bandage
hydrophilic guidewire
  J-tipped
  straight
hydrophilic powder dressing
hydrophilic semipermeable absorbent
  polyurethane foam dressing
hydrops of gallbladder
hydrostatic balloon
hydrostatic balloon catheter
hydrostatic decompression
HydroSurg laparoscopic irrigator
Hydro-Temp probe
hydrothorax
  chylous
  hepatic
hydroxyapatite adhesive
hydroxyapatite-coated pin
hydroxyapatitite graft
hydroxylation
hydroxymethylacyfulvene (HMAF)
hydroxyurea tablet
HyFil hydrogel dressing
Hyfrecator 2000
Hyfrecator pencil sheath
Hyfre-Fav
hygroscopic condensor
Hylaform (hylan polymer) viscoelastic
  gel
Hylagel-Nuro viscoelastic gel
Hylasine viscoelastic gel
Hylin rasp
hyoid bone
hyoscyamine sulfate
Hyosophen (atropine sulfate; scopolamine hydrobromide; hyoscyamine
  hydrobromide; phenobarbital)
Hypafix dressing
Hypafix nonwoven tape
Hypaque contrast medium
Hypaque-Cysto contrast medium
Hypaque Meglumine (diatrozoate
  meglumine iodine)

Hypaque Sodium (diatrozate
 sodium iodine)
Hypaque-76 (diatrozate meglumine;
 diatrozate sodium)
Hypaque swallow
hyperacidity
 gastric
 gastrointestinal
hyperactive bone marrow
hyperactive bowel sounds
hyperactive sphincter
hyperacute rejection (HAR)
hyperacute rejection of porcine
 xenograft
hyperadrenocorticalism
hyperal (hyperalimentation)
hyperaldosteronism
hyperalimentation
 central
 intravenous (I.V., IV)
 parenteral
 peripheral
hyperamylasemia
hyperbaric anesthesia
hyperbaric spinal anesthesia
hyperbilirubinemia
 conjugated
 idiopathic unconjugated
 neonatal
 unconjugated (UCB)
hypercalcemia, familial hypocalciuric
hypercalcemia with nephrocalcinosis
 and indicanuria
hypercalcitoninemia
hypercalciuric
hypercaloric diet
hypercapnia
hypercatabolic protein-losing
 enteropathy
hypercellular gland
hypercellularity
hyperchloremia
hyperchloremic acidosis
hyperchlorhydria
hypercholesterolemia
hypercortisolism
hyperdistention of abdomen
hyperemesis gravidarum
hyperemia
hyperemic mucosa
hyperestrogenism
hyperfunction
 adrenal cortex
 medulloadrenal
 pituitary
 thyroid
hyperfunction of adrenal medulla
hyperfunctioning adenoma
hyperfunctioning spleen
hypergastrinemia with acid
 hypersecretion
Hypergel hydrogel dressing
hyperglobulinemic hepatitis
hyperglobulinemic purpura
hyperglycemia
 diabetic
 postpancreatectomy
 symptomatic
Hyper-Had camera
HyperHep (hepatitis B immune
 globulin)
hyperinsulinar obesity
hyperinsulinemia
hyperinsulinemic-euglycemic glucose
 clamp
hyperinsulinism
 ectopic
 functional
 iatrogenic
hyperinterrenal obesity
Hyperion LTK laser
hyperkalemia
hyperkeratosis, esophageal
hyperkinetic circulatory state
hyperlipidemia
hyperlipoproteinemia
hyperlucent lung
hypermagnesemia

hypermetabolic state
hypermetabolism
hypermobile kidney
hypermotility of bowel
hypernatremia
hypernephroid carcinoma
hyperosmolar coma
hyperosmolarity
hyperosmolar nonketotic coma (HNKC)
hyperosmotic feeding
hyperoxaluria, enteric
hyperparathyroidism
  ectopic
  familial
  primary
  secondary
  tertiary
hyperparathyroid state
hyperpepsinogenemia
hyperperistalsis
hyperphosphatemia
hyperpigmentation of the skin
hyperplasia
  adrenal
  antral G cell
  appendiceal
  basal cell
  benign
  benign prostatic
  Brunner gland
  chief cell
  congenital adrenal
  congenital virilizing adrenal
  crypt
  cystic breast
  ductal
  epithelial
  focal epithelial
  focal nodular (FNH)
  four-gland
  foveolar
  gastric mucosal
  giant lymph node
  giant of gastric mucosa

hyperplasia *(cont.)*
  goblet cell
  islet cell
  lipomatous
  long-standing adenomatous
  lymphoid
  lymphonodular
  nodular lymphoid (NLH)
  nodular regenerative (NRH)
  physiologic
  primary thyroid
  refractory
  squamous
  thyroid
  transmissible murine colonic
  unilateral
  verrucous
hyperplasmic obesity
hyperplastic adenomatous polyp
hyperplastic alveolar mucosa
hyperplastic gastric polyp
hyperplastic gland
hyperplastic goiter
hyperplastic-hypertrophic obesity
hyperplastic lesion
hyperplastic mucinous cystadenoma
hyperplastic mucosal diverticula
  in gallbladder
hyperplastic obesity
hyperplastic polyp
hyperplastic polyposis of the colon
hyperprotidic diet
hyperpyrexia
hyperresonance
hyperresonant abdomen
hyperrugosity
hypersecretion
  acid
  aldosterone
  colonic
  gastric acid
  glucagon
  pituitary
  vasoactive intestinal peptide

hypersecretory gastropathy
hypersensitivity, gastric
hypersplenism
hyper-TBG-nemia (thyroid-binding globulin)
hypertension
  adrenal
  benign
  borderline
  essential
  extrahepatic portal venous
  idiopathic portal (IPH)
  labile
  malignant
  noncirrhotic portal
  portal
  presinusoidal intrahepatic portal
  primary
  renal
  renovascular
  splenoportal
  surgically correctable
  systemic venous
hypertensive crisis
hypertensive ischemic ulcer
hypertensive LES (lower esophageal sphincter)
hyperthermia catheter
hyperthyroidism
  apathetic
  classic
  Graves disease
  iodine-induced
  masked
  primary
  secondary
  silent thyroiditis
  subacute thyroiditis
  thyrotoxicosis factitia
  toxic adenoma
  toxic diffuse
  toxic multinodular goiter
  transient (Jod-Basedow phenomenon)
hypertonic plasma
hypertonic saline
hypertonic state
hypertrophic cirrhosis
hypertrophic gastritis
hypertrophic gastropathy
hypertrophic obesity
hypertrophic papilla
hypertrophic pyloric stenosis
hypertrophied mucosa
hypertrophied muscular layer
hypertrophy (see *hyperplasia*)
hyperuricemia
hyperventilation
hypervitaminosis
hypnosis anesthesia
hypoacidity, gastric
hypoactive bowel sounds
hypoalbuminemia
hypobaric anesthesia
hypobetalipoproteinemia
hypocalcemia, postoperative
hypocalcemic tetany
hypocalciuria
hypochloremia
hypochloremic metabolic acidosis
hypochlorhydria
hypochondriac fossa
hypochondriac region
hypochondriasis
hypochondrium (pl. hypochondria)
hypodermic needle
hypoechoic area (on ultrasound)
hypofibrinogenemia, familial (FHP)
hypofunction, adrenal cortex
hypofunctioning
hypogammaglobulinemia
hypoganglionosis of colon
hypogastric artery ligation
hypogastric fossa
hypogastric region
hypogastric vessel
hypogastrium

hypoglycemia
  alcoholic
  alimentary
  autoimmune
  drug-induced
  fasting
  idiopathic
  ketotic
  leucine-induced
  neonatal
  postprandial
  reactive
hypoglycemia with macroglossia
hypoglycemic crisis
hypoglycemic shock
hypoglycemic symptoms
hypoglycosylation syndrome, type 1a
hypogonad obesity
hypoinsulinemia, postsurgical
hypoinsulinism
hypokalemia
hypokalemic metabolic acidosis
hypomastia
hypomenorrhea of hyperthyroidism
hypometabolism
hypomotility, postprandial antral
hyponatremia
hypoparathyroidism
  idiopathic
  neonatal
  pseudo-
  transient
  transitory neonatal
hypopharyngeal diverticulum
hypopharyngeal or cricopharyngeal
  region
hypopharyngeal wall
hypopharynx
hypophosphatemia
hypophosphatemic
hypophyseal forceps
hypophysectomy forceps
hypophysectomy-induced
  hypopituitarism
hypophysial pouch
hypophysis punch forceps
hypopituitarism
  hormone-induced
  hypophysectomy-induced
  iatrogenic
  postablative
  radiotherapy-induced
hypoplasia
  bile duct
  organ
  syndromatic hepatic ductular
hypoplasmic obesity
hypoplastic lung
hypoproteinemia, idiopathic
hypoproteinemia with lymphangiectatic
  enteropathy
hyposalivation
hypospadias
hypotension, orthostatic
hypotensive anesthesia
hypotensive episode
hypotensive esophageal contraction
hypotensive focus (pl. foci)
hypothalamic pituitary level
hypothalamic release of CRF
hypothalamus gland
hypothermia, gastric
hypothermic anesthesia
hypothyroidism
  acquired
  congenital
  goitrus
  iatrogenic
  iodine
  juvenile
  PAS (P-aminosalicylic acid)
  phenylbutazone-induced
  postablative
  postsurgical
  post-therapeutic
  primary
  resorcinol-induced
  secondary

hypothyroid obesity
hypotonic duodenography
hypotonic fluid
hypovolemia secondary to acute hemorrhage
hypovolemia-induced metabolic acidosis
hypovolemic shock
hypoxemia
hypoxia
Hyrtl sphincter
hysterical anesthesia
hysterical colic
hysterical vomiting
hysteroscope
Hy-Tape latex-free surgical tape

I, i

Iamin (prezatide copper acetate)
Iamin gel wound dressing
Iamin hydrating gel (Blue Goo)
Iamin-IB solution (prezatide copper acetate)
I&D (incision and drainage)
I&O, I/O (intake and output)
IAP (International Association of Pancreatology)
IAS (intra-abdominal sepsis)
iatrogenic cause
iatrogenic Cushing syndrome
iatrogenic hyperinsulinism
iatrogenic hypopituitarism
iatrogenic hypothyroidism
iatrogenic infection
iatrogenic malabsorption
iatrogenic pituitary disorder
iatrogenic thyroiditis
iatrogenic trauma
IBC (inflammatory breast cancer)
IBD (inflammatory bowel disease)
IBD (irritable bowel disease)
IBS (irritable bowel syndrome)
IBW (ideal body weight)
Icar (carbonyl iron)
iced lactated Ringer solution
iced saline lavage
Ice hair trimming shears
ice water swallow
ICF (intracellular fluid)
ICHOP (intractability, cancer, hemorrhage, obstruction, perforation)
icing liver
icodextrin
ICP (intrahepatic cholestasis of pregnancy)
ICP (intracranial pressure) catheter
icteric leptospirosis
icteric phase of hepatitis
icteric sclerae
icteric skin
icterohemorrhagic leptospirosis
icterus
  conjunctival
  scleral
icterus gravidarum
icterus gravis
Idealbind bandage
IDD (intraluminal duodenal diverticulum)
IDDM (insulin-dependent diabetes mellitus)
ideal body weight (IBW)
identified, suture-ligated, clamped, and cut

identify the appendix
identify the inguinal anatomy
idiopathic anal fissures
idiopathic and diabetic gastroparesis
idiopathic autoimmune hemolytic anemia
idiopathic bile acid malabsorption
idiopathic chronic erosive gastritis
idiopathic colitis
idiopathic Cushing syndrome
idiopathic gastrointestinal bleeding
idiopathic gastroparesis
idiopathic hypertrophic gastropathy
idiopathic hypoglycemia
idiopathic hypoproteinemia
idiopathic inflammatory bowel disease
idiopathic intestinal pseudo-obstruction
idiopathic megacolon
idiopathic obstruction
idiopathic pancreatitis
idiopathic poor fixation of the right colon
idiopathic portal hypertension (IPH)
idiopathic proctocolitis
idiopathic steatorrhea
idiopathic thrombocytopenic purpura (ITP)
idiopathic unconjugated hyper-bilirubinemia
idoxifene
IDST (intraductal secretin test)
IEA (inferior epigastric artery) graft
IECRT (intraoperative endoscopic Congo red test)
I-Flow nerve block infusion kit
IFN-alpha 2 gene
IgA (immunoglobulin A)
  mesangial
  polymeric
IgA antigen complex
IgA deficiency
IgD (immunoglobulin D)
IgE (immunoglobulin E)
IgE-mediated immune reaction (type 1)
IgE-mediated injury
IgF-1 (insulin-like growth factor 1)
IgG (immunoglobulin G)
IgG-2A monoclonal antibody
Iglesias fiberoptic resectoscope
IgM anti-HAV antibody
IgM anti-HB_c antibody
IgM antibody
IgM (immunoglobulin M)
Iguana guidewire
IHA (intrahepatic atresia)
IHOP (intractability, hemorrhage, obstruction, perforation)
ILA surgical stapler
ILC (interstitial laser coagulation)
ileal conduit
ileal crypt
ileal inflow tract
ileal J pouch
ileal lesion
ileal neobladder
ileal pouch anal anastomosis (IPAA)
  H-shaped
  J-shaped
  S-shaped
  W-shaped
ileal primary tumor
ileal pull-through procedure
ileal resection
ileal reservoir
ileal secretion
ileal S pouch
ileal stasis
ileal varices
ileal villous atrophy in the absence of jejunal villous atrophy
ileal W pouch
ileectomy
ileitis
  allergic
  backwash
  Crohn
  dietetic
  distal

ileitis *(cont.)*
- granulomatous
- infectious
- obstructive dysfunctional
- prestomal
- regional
- segmental
- terminal

ileoanal anastomosis
ileoanal endorectal pull-through
ileoanal pouch
ileoanal pull-through procedure
ileoanal reservoir
ileoascending colostomy
ileocecal edema
ileocecal fat pad
ileocecal fold
ileocecal fossa
ileocecal junction
ileocecal orifice
ileocecal pouch
ileocecal recess
ileocecal valve
- competent
- incompetent

ileocecitis, infectious bacterial
ileococcygeus muscle
ileocolectomy
ileocolic arcade
ileocolic artery
ileocolic cecal artery
ileocolic disease
ileocolic fold
ileocolic plexus
ileocolic resection
ileocolic vein
ileocolic vessel
ileocolitis
- Crohn
- regional
- transmural
- ulcerative

ileocolonoscopy
ileocolostomy
- end-loop
- LeDuc-Camey

ileoconduit
ileocystoplasty
- Camey
- LeDuc-Camey

ileogastric reflex
ileogastrostomy
ileogram
ileo-ileal anastomosis
ileoproctostomy
ileorectal anastomosis (IRA)
ileorectal fistula
ileorectostomy
ileoscopy, retrograde
ileoscopy through stoma
ileosigmoid colostomy
ileosigmoid fistula
ileosigmoid knot
ileosotomy closure
ileostomate
ileostomist
ileostomogram
ileostomy
- blowhole
- Brooke
- continent
- Dennis-Brooke
- diversionary
- diverting
- diverting loop
- double-barrel
- end
- end-loop
- Goligher extraperitoneal
- incontinent
- J-loop
- Kock continent
- Kock reservoir
- loop
- loop-end
- permanent loop

ileostomy *(cont.)*
  pouched
  split
  temporary loop
  terminal
ileostomy appliance
ileostomy bag
ileostomy closure
ileostomy diarrhea
ileostomy effluent
ileostomy stoma
ileotransverse colon anastomosis
ileotransverse colostomy
ILE-SORB absorbent gel
ileum
  antimesenteric border of distal
  mesentery of
  terminal
ileus
  adhesive
  adynamic
  adynamic
  decreased
  duodenal
  dynamic
  gallbladder
  gallstone
  mechanical
  meconium
  occlusive
  paralytic
  postoperative
  spastic
ileus subparta
iLEX skin protectant paste dressing
iliac colon
iliac crest biopsy
iliac crest bone aspiration
iliac crest bone graft
iliac lymph node
iliac node
iliac vein
iliac vessel
iliofemoral triangle
iliohypogastric nerve
ilioinguinal ligament
ilioinguinal nerve
ilioinguinal ring
iliopectineal arch
iliopectineal line
iliopsoas ring
iliopsoas sign
iliopsoas test
iliopubic tract
iliotibial band graft
Ilizarov telescoping rod
illicit drug
illness, febrile
Illumen-8 guiding catheter
Illumina PROSeries laparoscopy system
Ilopan-Choline (dexpanthenol; choline bitartrate)
Ilozyme
ILS (intraluminal stapler)
ILUS (intraluminal ultrasound) catheter
IM (intramedullary) rod
IMA (inferior mammary artery) graft
IMA (inferior mesenteric artery) retractor
IMA (internal mammary artery)
ImageChecker M1000
image-guided pancreatic core biopsy
image-guided surgery
Imagent GI (perflubron)
Imager ac rectal suspension (barium sulfate)
imagery, guided
IMAGE TEC video camera system
image, video
imaging (also *image; scan; scanner; ultrasound*)
  ACAT (automated computerized axial tomography)
  acoustical shadowing
  Acuson Aspen ultrasound system
  AddOn-Bucky
  Airis II open MRI system
  Aloka 650 ultrasound system

imaging *(cont.)*
Aspen ultrasound system
Atlas 2.0 diagnostic ultrasound system
ATL UM 9 HDI Colorflow ultrasound system
AU5 Harmonic ultrasound system
Aurora MR breast imaging system
AutoSonix system
B-mode acquisition and targeting (BAT)
barium enema
barium swallow
BAT (B-mode acquisition and targeting) system
BI-RADS (Breast Imaging Reporting and Data System)
Bisound AP 3000 Colorflow ultrasound system
breast
Bruel & Kjaer 3535 ultrasound system
Bucky
computed tomography laser mammography (CTLM)
Computerized Thermal Imaging system
cross-sectional
CTLM (computed tomography laser mammography)
diffraction-enhanced
digital x-ray detector
Digitizer Director
DirectRay device
dual-phase spiral CT scan
Dynamic PACSPlus system
E.CAM+ coincidence-imaging
E.CAM dual-head emission imaging
EBCT (electron-beam computed tomography)
electron-beam computed tomography (EBCT)
endoanal ultrasound

imaging *(cont.)*
endoscopic optical coherence tomography (EOCT)
endoscopic ultrasonography
endosonography
EOCT (endoscopic optical coherence tomography)
EU-M30S endoscopic ultrasonography receiver
evacuation proctography
FACT (focused appendix computed tomography)
fluorescence spectroscopy
FluoroNav virtual fluoroscopy system
focused appendix computed tomography (FACT)
FONAR-360 MRI scanner
galactogram
GE RT 3200 ADV II ultrasound system
Given Diagnostic Imaging System
Gore 1.5-T Torso Array
graded compression ultrasonography
helical computed tomography
Hercules 7000 mobile x-ray unit
Hewlett-Packard ultrasound system
High Definition Imaging (HDI) 3000 ultrasound system
Hitachi 2.0 diagnostic ultrasound system
iiRAD DR1000C
ImageChecker M1000
IMiG-MRI
intraoperative laparoscopic cholangiography
IsoStent radioisotope stent
LAST (large-area sensing technology) imager
Longport Digital Scanner (LDS)
magnetic resonance cholangiopancreatography (MRCP)
magnetic resonance neurography (MRN)

imaging *(cont.)*
mammary ductogram
MammoSite RTS
Mammotome ultrasound system
MRCP (magnetic resonance cholangiopancreatography)
MRN (magnetic resonance neurography)
M2A Swallowable Imaging Capsule
native tissue Harmonic imaging (NTHI)
Olympus EU-M30S endoscopic ultrasonography receiver
Olympus GF-UM130 ultrasound gastroscope
omega sign
Opdima digital mammography system
Open Sky MRI
optical coherence (OCT)
Optistar MR contrast delivery system
Palpagraph mammography device
Perception 5000 PC-based ultrasound scanner
percutaneous transhepatic cholangiography (PTC)
PowerVision ultrasound system
pulse inversion Harmonic
rectal contrast medium
reflectance spectroscopy
reflectant spectral photometer
Senographe 2000D digital mammography system
SenoScan mammography
Signa Special Procedures (SP) system
Skylight system
Softscan laser scanner
SonoCT Real-Time Compound Imaging
SonoSite 180 handheld ultrasound
spectroscopy
Stratis II MRI system

imaging *(cont.)*
Synergy ultrasound system
TDMS (Trex digital mammography system)
Technos ultrasound system
terahertz wave
thyroid ultrasonography
Toshiba EccoCee ultrasound system
Toshiba 270 ultrasound system
TrakBack ultrasound catheter
transperineal ultrasonography
TransScan 2000 breast mapping device
Trex digital mammography system (TDMS)
Xillix LIFE-GI fluorescence endoscopy system
Xplorer 1000 digital x-ray system
Xplorer digital

imaging agent (also see *medications*)
Anatrast (barium sulfate)
AngioMark
Apomate
arcitumomab
Baricon
barium sulfate
Barobag
Baro-cat
Baros
Barosperse
Bear-E-Bag Pediatric
Bear-E-Yum GI
Bilopaque
Cardio-Green (CG) (indocyanine green)
CEA-Scan (arcitumomab)
Cholografin Meglumine (iodipamide meglumine)
Combidex
Conray 400 (iothalamate meglumine)
Definity (perflutren)
Digibar 190
Enecat (barium sulfate)

imaging *(cont.)*
Enhancer (barium sulfate)
Entrobar (barium sulfate [methylcellulose diluent])
Epi-C (barium sulfate)
FAC (ferric ammonium citrate)
Feridex (ferumoxides)
ferric ammonium citrate (FAC)
FerriSeltz (ferric ammonium citrate [FAC])
ferumoxsil
Flo-Coat (barium sulfate)
gadodiamide
Gadolite oral suspension
Gastrografin (diatrizoate meglumine; diatrizoate sodium)
GastroMARK (ferumoxsil)
glucagon
gold Au-198 (^{198}Au)
HD 85 (barium sulfate)
HD 200 Plus (barium sulfate)
Hexabrix (ioxaglate meglumine; ioxaglate sodium)
Hypaque-Cysto contrast medium
Hypaque Meglumine 30%; 60% (diatrozoate meglumine iodine)
Hypaque Sodium 25%; 50% (diatrozate sodium)
Hypaque Sodium; Hypaque Sodium 20% (diatrozate sodium [59.87% iodine])
Hypaque-76 (diatrozate meglumine; diatrozate sodium)
Imagent GI (perflubron)
Imager ac (barium sulfate)
ImmuRAID-AFP
^{123}I murine MAb to alpha-fetoprotein (AFP)
^{131}I murine MAb to alpha-fetoprotein (AFP)
^{131}I 6B-iodomethyl-19-norcholesterol
^{111}In altumomab pentetate (monoclonal antibody)

imaging *(cont.)*
indocyanine green
^{111}In satumomab pendetide (monoclonal antibody)
insulin ^{125}I
insulin ^{131}I
Intropaste (barium sulfate)
iobenzamic acid
iocetamic acid
iodipamide meglumine
iodixanol
Iodotope (sodium iodide ^{131}I)
ioglycamic acid
iohexol
iopanoic acid
iothalamate meglumine
iothalamate sodium
Iotrex
ioversal
ipodate calcium
ipodate sodium
Isovue-370 (iopamidol)
Kinevac (sincalide)
LeuTech
Liqui-Coat HD (barium sulfate)
LumenHance (manganese chloride tetrahydrate)
Magnevist (gadopentetate dimeglumine)
manganese chloride tetrahydrate
mangofodipir trisodium
MD-Gastroview (diatrozoate meglumine; diatrozoate sodium)
Medebar Plus (barium sulfate)
Medescan (barium sulfate)
meglumine diatrizoate
meglumine iocarmate
meglumine iothalamate
meglumine ioxaglate
methylene blue
Miraluma (technetium ^{99m}Tc sestamibi kit)
MS-325
NeoTect disease-specific

imaging *(cont.)*
- nofetumobab
- nonionic contrast media
- Novopaque (barium sulfate)
- OctreoScan 111 (^{111}In pentetreotide)
- Omnipaque (iohexol)
- Omniscan (gadodiamide)
- OncoScint CR/OV (^{111}In satumomab pendetide)
- OptiMARK (gadoversetamide injection)
- Optiray 350 (ioversal)
- Optison
- Oragrafin sodium (ipodate sodium)
- pentagastrin
- Peptavlon (pentagastrin)
- perflenapent
- perflisopent
- perflutren
- Prepcat (barium sulfate)
- Quantison
- ReVele
- sincalide
- Sitzmarks (polyvinyl chloride)
- sodium amidotrizoate
- sodium iothalamate
- sodium ioxaglate
- sodium ipodate
- sodium mitrizoate
- sodium tyropanoate
- Sonazoid ultrasound
- SonoRx (simethicone-coated cellulose suspension)
- stannous sulfur colloid
- technetium ^{99m}Tc ethylene dicysteine (EC)
- technetium ^{99m}Tc sestamibi
- Telepaque (topanoic acid)
- Teslascan (mangafodipir trisodium)
- Tomocat (barium sulfate)
- Tonopaque (barium sulfate)
- tyropanoate sodium
- Vascoray (iothalamate meglumine; iothalamate sodium)

imaging *(cont.)*
- Verluma (nofetumobab)
- Visipaque (iodixanol)

imaging workup
IMAGN 2000 cellular analysis test
Imagyn clip applier
imbibe
imbricated posterior wall closure
imbricating suture
imbrication of diaphragm
IMED infusion device
imidoacetic acid radioactive agent
imiglucerase
immature neutrophils (bands)
immediate decompression
Immergut suction coagulation tube
imminent cardiac collapse
Immix bioabsorbable implant
IMMIX CB implant
immobilize, immobilization
immobilizing bandage
ImmTher (disaccharide tripeptide glycerol tripalmitoyl)
ImmTher (disaccharide tripeptide)
Immun-Aid
immune complex
immune deficiency
immune electron microscopy
immune mechanism
immune response
immunity, cell-mediated
immunizing agent
immunoassay, PP-CAP IgA enzyme
immunoblastic lymphoma large cell
immunoblastic sarcoma
immunoblot analysis
ImmunoCard STAT! Rotavirus test
immunocompetency
immunocompromised patient
immunodeficiency, severe combined (SCID)
immunoelectrophoresis
immunogenicity
immunoglobulin A (IgA)

immunoglobulin D (IgD)
immunoglobulin E (IgE)
immunoglobulin G (IgG)
immunoglobulin I (IgI)
immunoglobulin M (IgM)
immunohistochemical detection
immunohistochemical staining
immunohistochemistry
immunoinflammatory sequelae
immunologic deficiency disorder
immunologic insulin resistance
immunologically mediated disease
immunomodulation
immunomodulator
immunomodulatory protocol
immunoproliferative small intestinal disease (IPSID)
immunoreactive parathyroid hormone (iPTH)
immunosuppressant cocktail
immunosuppression, corticosteroid-based
immunosuppressive agent
immunosuppressive drug
immunosuppressive protocol
immunosuppressive steroid weaning
ImmuRAID-AFP (technetium ^{99m}Tc murine MAb to human alpha-fetoprotein)
Immurait (IgG-2A monoclonal antibody)
Immodium, Imodium A-D (loperamide)
Impact enteral formula
impacted calculus
impacted feces
impacted gallstone
impacted stool
impaction
  basket
  fecal
  intestinal
  stone
impaction graft
impaction lesion
impactor, Browne pneumatic
impactor rod
impaired cellular defense mechanism
impaired esophageal peristalsis
impaired excretion of conjugated bilirubin
impaired fat metabolism
impaired gallbladder contractility
impaired gas exchange
impaired glucose tolerance
impaired nutritional state
impaired regeneration syndrome (IRS)
impaired skin integrity
impaired thymic development
impaired wound healing
impalement injury
  abdominal
  anorectal
  transcorpus
IMP-Capello arm support
impedance, bioelectrical
imperforate anus
impervious drape
implant (also see *breast implant*; *prosthesis*)
  carcinomatous
  Duros drug delivery
  Gore-Tex SAM (subcutaneous augmentation material) facial implant
  Gore-Tex strips
  Immix bioabsorbable
  IMMIX CB
  iridium-192 wire
  islet cell
  lumbar anterior-root stimulator (LARSI)
  Macroplastique bladder
  peritoneal
  Restore orthobiologic soft tissue
  saline
  silicone gel
implant application fork
Implast bone cement adhesive

Import vascular-access port with BioGlide
impregnated sponge
Impress instrument tracking
impression
  cardiac, on the liver
  colic
  digastric
  duodenal
  esophageal
  gastric
  liver
  renal
  suprarenal
impromidine
impromidine HCl
improved gas exchange
ImuLyme vaccine
Imuran (azathioprine)
IMV (inferior mesenteric vein)
IMV (intermittent mandatory ventilation)
Inactivin
inadequate bowel prep
inadequate cardiac output
inadequate circulating blood volume
inadequate hemostasis of the splenic pedicle
inadequate perfusion of organ
Inamed technique
inanition
Inapsine (droperidol)
inborn error in liver bilirubin uptake and glucuronyl transferase
inborn error of metabolism
incarcerated hernia
incarcerated omentum
incarcerated sepsis
incarceration of hernia
incarceration of inguinal hernia
incarceration of loop of intestine
Incel (biricodar dicitrate)
incentive spirometry, postoperative
Incert bioabsorbable implantable sponge
In Charge diabetes control system
incidence
incidental abdominal radiograph
incidental appendectomy
incised in the direction of its fibers
Incise drape
incised ulcer
incised wound
incision
  abdominal
  Amussat
  anterolateral thoracotomy
  anteromedial
  Battle
  Battle-Jalaguiere-Kammerer
  battledore (racquet-shaped)
  bayonet-type
  Bevan abdominal
  bifrontal
  bikini skin
  bilateral subcostal
  Brunner modified
  Brunner palmar
  Bruser skin (knee)
  capsular
  celiotomy
  cervical
  Charnley
  Cherney
  Chernez
  chevron
  choledochotomy
  Cincinnati
  circumareolar
  circumferential
  circumlinear
  circumscribing
  circumumbilical
  clamshell
  coronal
  cross-tunneling
  cruciate
  C-shaped
  Cubbins

incision *(cont.)*
- Curtin
- curved
- curvilinear
- Deaver
- deltoid-splitting
- diamond-shaped
- dorsal linear
- dorsomedial
- double
- DuVries
- elliptical
- epigastric
- exploratory
- fascial-splitting
- fiber-splitting
- fishmouth
- flank
- frown
- Gaenslen split heel
- gridiron
- groin
- gull-wing
- Heineke-Mikulicz
- Henderson skin
- Henry
- hernia
- hockey-stick
- horizontal
- horseshoe-shaped
- H-shaped capsular
- infraclavicular
- inframammary
- infraumbilical
- inguinal
- intercartilaginous
- intraperitoneal
- inverted-U abdominal
- J-shaped skin
- Kammerer-Battle
- Kehr
- keyhole
- Kocher
- Kocher collar (thyroidectomy)

incision *(cont.)*
- LaRoque herniorrhaphy
- lateral
- lateral utility
- lazy H
- lazy S
- lazy Z
- L-curved
- longitudinal
- low transverse
- L-shaped
- Ludloff
- Mayfield
- Maylard
- McBurney
- medial
- medial parapatellar
- median
- median parapatellar
- midabdominal transverse
- midaxillary line
- midline
- midline abdominal
- minilaparotomy
- muscle-splitting
- Nagamatsu
- oblique
- Ollier
- omega-shaped
- palmar
- paramedial
- paramedian
- parapatellar
- pararectus
- paraumbilical
- Penduloff
- periareolar
- Pfannenstiel
- posterior
- puncture
- racquet-shaped
- recently healed surgical
- rectus sheath
- relaxing

incision *(cont.)*
- relief
- relieving
- Rethi
- right subcostal
- Rockey-Davis
- S
- saber-cut
- scoring
- semilunar
- serpentine
- S-flap
- skin
- skin crease
- smile (or smiling)
- smiling
- spindle-shaped
- split
- S-shaped
- stab
- stab wound
- standard
- standard Kocher
- steri-stripped
- sternal-splitting
- sternotomy
- straight
- subcostal
- subumbilical
- tangential
- thoracoabdominal
- through-and-through
- transverse
- T-shaped
- U-shaped
- vertical
- vertical midline
- volar
- V-shaped
- Wagner skin
- Warren
- Watson-Jones
- web space
- Wilde

incision *(cont.)*
- Willy Meyer mastectomy
- xiphoid to umbilicus
- Y
- Yorke-Mason
- Y-shaped
- Z-plasty
- zigzag
- zigzag finger

incisional biopsy
incisional hernia
incisional scar
incision and drainage (I&D) of abscess
incision extended laterally
incision extended superiorly and inferiorly
incision into rectus sheath
incision line
incision made from xiphoid to umbilicus
incision of labial frenum (frenotomy)
incisive bone
incisive canal
Incisor arthroscopic blade
incisura angularis of stomach
incisura dextra of Gans
Inclan bone graft
inclusion body
incompetent ileocecal valve
incompetent sphincter
incompetent valve
incomplete colonoscopy
incomplete hernia
incomplete UES (upper esophageal sphincter) relaxation
incontinence
- bladder
- bowel
- exercise-induced
- fecal
- ischemic fecal
- rectal
- stool
- stress
- urge

incontinent ileostomy
incontinent of stool
increased abdominal girth
increased alveolar ventilation
increased BUN
increased catecholamines
increased collateral blood flow
increased colonic phasic contractions
increased concentration of liver enzymes
increased contractility
increased direct bilirubin
increased end-tide CO_2
increased estrogen
increased gastric acid and pepsin production
increased gastric pressure
increased granularity and friability of mucosa
increased heart rate
increased intra-abdominal pressure
increased intracranial pressure
increased intraluminal pressure
increased intravascular volume
increased lactic acid
increased LFTs
increased morbidity and mortality
increased PCO_2
increased PEEP
increased portal pressure
increased preload
increased pulmonary compliance
increased renin to angiotensin
increased respiratory rate
increased secretion of PTH
increased serum sodium
increased shunt fraction
increased surface lubricity
increased telomerase activity
increased thyroid hormone synthesis
increased tidal volume
increased turnover of red blood cells
increased vascularity
increased venous capacitance
increased WBCs
increase in angiotensin
increase in metabolic rate
increase in oxygen consumption
incuTemp monitoring device
independence, insulin
independent parallel circuits
Indermil topical tissue adhesive
index (pl. indexes, indices) (see also *classification*)
  biliary saturation
  body mass (BMI)
  Bouchard
  Broder
  Crohn disease activity (CDAI)
  free thyroxine
  free/total PSA (prostate-specific antigen) index
  Harvey hospital prognostic nutritional index
  hepatic perfusion (HPI)
  nutritional
  obesity
  parietal cell
  PATI (Penetrating Abdominal Trauma Index)
  Prognostic Nutritional (PNI)
  saturation (SI)
  spleen
in diameter
Indian childhood cirrhosis
Indiana pouch procedure
Indiana reamer
indicanuria
indices (see *index*)
Indiclor (^{111}In radioimaging agent)
indigestion
indigo carmine dye
indigo carmine stain
Indigo LaserOptic treatment system
indirect bilirubin
indirect hemagglutination antibody test
indirect hemagglutination titer
indirect hepatic vein wedge pressure

indirect hernia defect
indirect hernia sac
indirect inguinal hernia
indirect laryngoscopy
indirect space
indiscriminate lesion
indium
  ^{111}In altumomab pentetate (monoclonal antibody)
  ^{111}In DTPA
  ^{111}In satumomab pendetide (monoclonal antibody)
indium 64-labeled white blood cell scan
individual ligature (free tie)
indocyanine green
indolent radiation-induced rectal ulcer
indolent thrombosis
indolent ulcer
indomethacin
induced under anesthesia
induction anesthesia
induction of anesthesia
induction of emesis
induction therapy
indurated appendix
induration
  breast
  skin
  wound
indurative necrosis
indwelling arterial line
indwelling catheter
indwelling stomal device
ineffective airway clearance
ineffective breathing pattern
Inerpan flexible burn dressing
Infanrix vaccine
infant formula
infant shunt
infant skull clamp
infantile colic
infantile embryonal carcinoma
infantile gastroenteritis
infantile liver
infantile mitochondrial myopathy
infantilism
  Brissaud
  celiac
  hepatic
  Herter
  hypophysial
  intestinal
  Levi-Lorain
  Lorain
  lymphatic
  pancreatic
  partial
  pituitary
  renal
  sexual
  universal
infarct
infarcted appendix epididymidis
infarcted bowel
infarction
  agnogenic intestinal
  bowel
  diaphragmatic myocardial (DMI)
  embolic mesenteric
  hemorrhagic intestinal
  hepatic
  intestinal
  mesenteric
  myocardial
  nonocclusive intestinal
  segmental bowel
  thrombotic mesenteric
  thyroid
In-Fast bone screw system
infected necrosis
infected necrotizing pancreatitis
infected peripancreatic purulent fluid collection
infected tissue
infection
  adenovirus
  AER (acute erosive gastritis)
  agonal

infection *(cont.)*
airborne
animal bite
apical
bacterial
biliary tract
Bunyavirus
Campylobacter
candidal
cat-bite
catheter tunnel
cat-scratch
chronic
CMV (cytomegalovirus)
colonization
community-acquired
cross
cryptogenic
cytomegalovirus (CMV)
disseminated gonococcal
dog-bite
droplet
dust-borne
EBV (Epstein-Barr virus)
ECHO (enterocytopathogenic human orphan) virus
endogenous
Epstein-Barr virus
exogenous
Fasciola hepatica
focal
fungal
genital
germinal
Giardia
gram-positive bacterial
granulomatous
human ehrlichial, Sennetsu-type
human papillomavirus (HPV)
iatrogenic
latent
local
mass
mixed

infection *(cont.)*
nosocomial
ocular
opportunistic
pelvic
postoperative
preexisting
primary
protozoal
pulmonary
pyogenic
recurrent upper respiratory tract (RURTI)
regional spread of
rickettsial
Salinem
scalp
secondary
secondary bacterial
skin
subclinical
suppurative
surgical site
systemic
systemic fungal
terminal
tick-borne
TORCH (toxoplasmosis, rubella, cytomegalovirus, herpes simplex)
tunnel
upper respiratory (URI)
upper respiratory tract (URTI)
urinary tract (UTI)
vector-borne
Vincent
viral
viral respiratory (VRI)
water-borne
wound

infection due to gram-positive bacteria
infectious arthritis
infectious avian nephrosis
infectious bacterial ileocecitis
infectious colitis

infectious disease
  communicable
  contagious
  transmissible
infectious eczematous dermatitis
infectious enteritis
infectious esophagitis
infectious etiology
infectious gastroenteritis
infectious granuloma
infectious hepatitis
infectious ileitis
infectious jaundice
infectious jejunitis
infectious mononucleosis (IM)
infectious myocarditis
infectious myositis
infectious pancreatic necrosis virus
infectious pancreatitis
infectious sigmoiditis
infectious splenomegaly
infectious stomatitis
infectious wart virus
infective colitis
infective splenomegaly
Infergen (interferon alfacon-1)
inferior border of liver
inferior central pedicle reduction
  mammoplasty
inferior constrictor muscle
inferior duodenal fold
inferior duodenal recess
inferior epigastric artery
inferior epigastric vessel
inferior esophageal sphincter
inferior hemorrhoidal artery
inferior hemorrhoidal vein
inferior laryngeal nerve
inferior lumbar triangle
inferior mesenteric artery
inferior mesenteric vein
inferior MI (myocardial infarction)
inferior myocardial infarction
inferior pancreaticoduodenal artery
inferior parathyroid gland
inferior pedicle of breast
inferior pedicle technique reduction
  mammoplasty
inferior surface of diaphragm
inferior surface of pancreas
inferior thyroid artery
inferior thyroid vein
inferior transverse rectal fold
inferior vena cava
inferior vena cava obstruction
inferior venacavography
inferolateral surface of prostate
inferomedial
infestation, parasitic
infiltrate (see *infiltration*)
infiltrate lymphoma
infiltrating adenocarcinoma
infiltrating ductal carcinoma of breast
infiltrating lesion
infiltrating lobular carcinoma
infiltration (also *infiltrate*)
  cavitary
  consolidated
  diffuse
  eosinophilic
  foreign body
  glycogen
  interstitial
  leukocytic
  lymphocytic
  mesenteric
  mononuclear
  nodular
  pulmonary
  tumor
infiltration anesthesia
infiltration of nodule
infiltrative carcinoma
infiltrative disorder
Infiniti catheter
Infinity hip system
inflamed appendicitis
inflamed appendix

inflamed gallbladder
inflamed stenosis of the sigmoid colon
inflammation
  acute
  active chronic
  adhesive
  appendiceal
  appendix
  atrophic
  caseous
  catarrhal
  cavitating
  chronic
  chronic jejunal
  circumscribed
  cirrhotic
  colonic
  confluent
  diffuse
  diffuse acute
  diffuse chronic
  erosive
  esophageal
  exudative
  fibrinous
  fibrocaseous
  fibrosing
  gallbladder
  gangrenous
  granulomatous
  hemorrhagic
  hyperplastic
  hypertrophic
  interstitial
  ischemic
  localized
  metastatic
  miliary granulomatous
  mucosal
  multifocal
  necrotic
  necrotizing granulomatous
  obliterative
  pancreatic

inflammation *(cont.)*
  pelvic
  periesophageal
  perirectal
  portal
  proliferative
  pseudomembranous
  psoas
  purulent
  recurrent
  sanguineous
  serofibrinous
  splenic
  subacute
  suppurative
  thyroidal
  transmural
  transudative
  traumatic
  ulcerative
inflammation of pouch of ileoanal pull-through
inflammation of thyroid
inflammation spleen
inflammatory bowel disease (IBD)
inflammatory breast cancer (IBC)
inflammatory cancer
inflammatory carcinoma of breast
inflammatory cascade (leading to sepsis syndrome)
inflammatory cytokine
inflammatory diarrhea
inflammatory disease of small bowel
inflammatory edema
inflammatory fibroid polyp
inflammatory fibrosis
inflammatory granuloma
inflammatory intra-abdominal process
inflammatory lesion
inflammatory mediator
inflammatory myopathy
inflammatory polyp
inflammatory process
inflammatory response

inflating bellows
inflating sigmoidoscopic bellows
inflation bag
inflator, LeVeen
infliximab monoclonal antibody
inflow cannula
INFORM HER-2/neu breast cancer test
infraclavicular incision
infraclavicular lymph node
infracolic compartment
infraduodenal fossa
infragastric
infrahepatic caval anastomosis
infrahepatic vena cava
inframammary approach in augmentation mammoplasty
inframammary incision
inframammary scar
infrapatellar view
infrarenal aortobifemoral bypass graft
infraumbilical incision
infraumbilical mound
infraumbilical position
infundibular
Infusaid chemotherapy implantable pump
Infusaid hepatic pump
Infusaid implantable drug infusion pump
InfusaSleeve II catheter
infusion
  analgesic
  constant-flow
  continuous subcutaneous insulin (CSII)
  coronary
  crystalloid
  drip
  drug
  esophageal acid
  free water
  hepatic arterial (HAI)
  lipid
  multi-lumen

infusion *(cont.)*
  nerve block
  pentagastrin
  sidehole
  syringe
  triple-lumen
  valved
  volumetric
infusion cannula
infusion pump
Inge laminectomy retractor
Ingraham skull punch forceps
ingrown (onychocryptosis) nail
inguinal adenopathy
inguinal bulge
inguinal canal
inguinal crease
inguinal exploration
inguinal floor repair
inguinal fold
inguinal hernia
inguinal hernia with scrotal extension
inguinal herniorrhaphy
inguinal incision
inguinal ligament
inguinal lymphadenectomy
inguinal lymphadenopathy
inguinal nerve
inguinal node
inguinal region
inguinal ring
  external
  internal
inguinal sphincter
inguinal triangle
inguinodynia
inguinofemoral hernia
inhalation anesthesia
inhalation mask anesthesia
inhaler
  AERx
  Spiros
inherited deficiency in natural coagulation inhibitors

inhibition
  gastrin
  global (of GI function)
inhibitor
  calcineurin
  COX-2
  HMG-CoA reductase
  monoamine oxidase (MAO)
  protein pump
  proton pump
  thrombus
inhibitory syndrome
INH-induced hepatitis
initial diagnosis
initial incision retractor
Inject-Ease 100 syringe
injection
  AccuGuide
  Bard flexible endoscopic
  Botox
  Botox sphincter
  Busulfex
  Camptosar (irinotecan HCl)
  Cidecin (daptomycin)
  clonidine HCl
  Daxor quantitative
  doxorubicin HCl liposome
  endoscopic
  epinephrine for vasoconstriction
  etoposide
  field block
  Fragmin (dalteparin sodium)
  intra-arterial bolus
  local epinephrine
  Medi-Jector Choice needle-free
    insulin
  mucosal
  multiple subcutaneous insulin (MSI)
  percutaneous ethanol (PEI)
  percutaneous ethanol tumor
  perirectal
  proximal saline
  Rebetron (interferon alfa-2b)
  Ringer
injection *(cont.)*
  sclerosing agent
  secretin
  selective
  sinus tract
  submucosal saline
injection mass
injection monitor
injection needle, aspiration
injection of epinephrine for
  vasoconstriction
injection of sclerosing agent
injection of secretin into mesentery
  arteries
injection of sinus tract
injection procedure for mammary
  ductogram or galactogram
injection sclerosis of esophageal varices
injection sclerotherapy
injector
  Injex needle-free
  Med-E-Jet inoculator
  Medi-Jector Choice
  Optistat power
  PercuPump disposable
  Pulse*Spray
InjecTx customized cystoscope
Injex needle-free injector
injury
  Ajmalin liver
  bile duct
  bile duct epithelial cell
  blunt
  diaphragmatic
  dissection
  extensive irreparable duodenal and
    pancreatic head
  extra-abdominal
  great vessel
  intraparenchymal liver
  intrathoracic
  isolated splenic
  juxtahepatic venous
  liver parenchymal

injury *(cont.)*
  major organ
  mechanism of
  penetrating
  penetrating stab wound
  recurrent nerve
  retroperitoneal
  right hepatic artery
  right hepatic duct
  seatbelt neck
  spleen
  through-and-through
  unilateral
  urethral
Injury Severity Score
inlay bone graft
inlay graft
inlet
  esophageal
  pelvic
  thoracic
inner cell mass
inner crossbar
InnerDyne single-action, single-tooth biopsy punch
InnerDyne spoon biopsy punch
Innervasc device
innervate
innervation, vagal
innocent gallstone
Innofem (estradiol)
Innofluor FPIA (fluorescence-polarization immunoassay) assay
Innohep (tinzaparin sodium)
innominate artery
innominate fascia
^{131}I uptake (thyroid function) test
inoperable case
inorganic arsenic
Inoue balloon technique
INR neurological stent
INRO surgical nail
insensible water loss (sweat, respiration, stool)
in situ
in situ breast cancer
in situ carcinoma
in situ pin
in situ vein graft
inspection
Inspex rigid laparoscope
inspiratory arrest
inspiratory muscle trainer
inspired air
inspired oxygen concentration
inspissated bile
inspissated bile syndrome
inspissated feces
inspissated material
inspissated sump syndrome
instability, MSI (microsatellite)
InStat collagen absorbable hemostat
InStat MCH (microfibrillar hemostat)
InstaTrak 3000 device
InStent balloon-expandable stent
in-stent restenosis
InStent self-expanding stent
instillation of antibiotic solution
instillation of medication
instillation therapy
Institute, National Cancer (NCI)
instrument drag
instrument guide (for flexible instruments)
instrument, sponge, and needle count
instrument wipe sponge
instrumentation of bile duct
InstrumentMakar laparoscope
instrument for biopsy of lung and pleura
instruments were removed under direct vision
insufficiency
  adrenal medullary
  corticoadrenal
  hepatic
  mesenteric vascular
  pancreatic
  pituitary

insufflate the peritoneum
insufflation
  blind needle
  gas
insufflation anesthesia
insufflation gas source
  "E" tank
  "H" tank
insufflation needle
insufflation tank room
insufflator
  carbon dioxide
  high-flow electronic
  Karl Storz N_2O Endoflator
  nitrous oxide
  Storz high-speed
Insuflon indwelling insulin delivery system
insular cirrhosis
insulated cautery
insulated coagulation suction
insulated coatings: nylon, Kynar, Teflon or ceramic
insulated Foman ball retractor
insulated instrument
insulated outer tube with Luer lock
insulation on flexible, semirigid shafts
insulation-tipped (IT) diathermic knife
insulin
  AC137 analog
  biphasic
  biphasic isophane
  dalanated
  globin zinc
  exogenous
  Humalog
  human
  isophane human
  Humulin
  Humulin L (human insulin zinc [rDNA])
  Humulin R (human insulin [recombinant])
  Humulin 30/70

insulin *(cont.)*
  Humulin 50/50
  Humulin 70/30
  Humulin-U (extended insulin zinc)
  Humulin U Ultralente (extended insulin human zinc [rDNA])
  intermediate-acting
  isophane
  Lente Insulin
  long-acting
  neutral
  neutral protamine Hagedorn (NPH)
  Novolin 70/30 PenFill
  Novolin 70/30 Prefilled
  Novolin 85/15 PenFill
  Novolin L
  Novolin N
  Novolin N PenFill
  Novolin N Prefilled
  Novolin R
  Novolin R PenFill
  Novolin R Prefilled
  NovoRapid
  NPH (neutral protamine Hagedorn)
  NPH Iletin II
  NPH-N
  Oralgen oral aerosol
  protamine zinc (PZI)
  rapid-acting
  regular
  Regular Iletin II
  Regular Iletin II U-500 (concentrated)
  Regular Purified Pork
  Semilente
  short-acting
  Ultralente
  Velosulin BR
  Velosulin BR human buffered regular
  Velosulin Human BR
insulin allergy
insulin argine
insulin aspart

insulin coma
insulin defalan
insulin deficient
insulin delivery device
  ADICOL
  Dahedi Model 25 pump
  Disetronic Insulin Pen
  Disetronic pump
  D-modem and
  D-TRON pump
  Felig pump
  H-TRON plus V100/V40 pump
  Humalog Pen
  Humulin 70/30 Pen
  Humulin R Pen
  Insuflon indwelling
  Medi-Ject needle-free
  Medi-Jector Choice needle-free
  MiniMed
  Novolin Pen
  open-looped
  OptiPen
  OptiPen Pro
  OptiSet
  portable infusion
insulin-dependent diabetes mellitus (IDDM)
insulin glargine
insulin:glucose ratio
insulin human zinc, extended
insulin ^{125}I
insulin ^{131}I
insulin independence
insulin-like growth factor 1 (IGF-1)
insulin-like growth factor-1, recombinant human (rhIGF) (mecasermin)
insulin lispro
insulinoma
insulinopathy
insulinotardic
insulin-producing tumor arising from beta cells
insulinotropic polypeptide, glucose-dependent (GIP)
insulin pump (see *insulin delivery device; pump*)
Insulin Reaction gel (glucose)
insulin receptors
insulin resistance, immunologic
insulin resistance in gestational diabetes
insulin resistance in the obese
insulin resistance syndrome
insulin-resistant diabetes mellitus associated with acanthosis nigricans
insulin-secreting cells
insulin-secreting tumor (insulinoma)
insulin shock
insulin sufficient
insulin tolerance test
insulin treatment
insulin zinc
  extended
  prompt
insulin zinc [pork]
insulin zinc protamine
insulin zinc suspension
  amorphous
  crystalline
InSurg laparoscopic stone basket
Insyte AutoGuard catheter
In-Tac bone-anchoring system anchor
intact airway
intact molecule assay
intake and output (I&O, I/O)
integral tip
Integrated Wound Manager
integrity
  anastomosis
  gastric
  impaired skin
Intelligent dressing
intensified immunosuppression
intention
  delayed healing by primary
  healing by primary
  healing by secondary
intentional transoperative hemodilution
interbody rasp

intercalary graft
intercapillary glomerulosclerosis
intercartilaginous incision
Interceed surgical adhesion barrier
Interceed TC7
intercellular fluid
Intercept Platelet System
interceptive conditioning
intercondylar drill guide
intercostal anesthesia
intercostal arteries
intercostal nerve block
intercostal space
intercostal veins
intercostal vessels
intercostobrachial nerve
interfascicular nerve graft
interferometry
interferon
  lymphoblastoid
  pegylated
interferon alfacon-1
interferon alfa-n1
interferon alfa-n3
interferon alfa-2a
interferon alfa-2b
interferon alfa-2b and ribavirin
interferon alfa-2b recombinant
interferon-ribavirin therapy for hepatitis C
interferon beta (IFN-B)
interferon beta-1a
interferon gamma-1b
interferon monotherapy
interfoveolar ligament
interfragmentary plate
InterGard Knitted collagen-coated graft
InterGard patch
Intergel adhesion prevention solution
interjugular node
interlaminar clamp
interleukin-4 receptor (IL-4R)
interleukin 10 (IL-10)
interlobular artery of kidney
interlobular bile duct
interlocking intramedullary nail
interlocking ligature
interlocking nail
interloop abscess
intermediate gland
intermediate Hi-Lo tracheal tube
intermediate Hi-Lo with Brandt
intermesenteric abscess
intermittent diarrhea
intermittent drainage
intermittent drip feeding
intermittent dysphagia
intermittent malaria
intermittent melena
intermittent open system
intermittent pain
intermittent suture
internal abdominal ring
internal anal sphincter (IAS)
internal biliary drainage
internal clot
internal hemorrhage
internal hemorrhoid
internal hernia
internal inguinal ring
internal mammary artery (IMA)
internal mammary lymph node
internal mammary vein
internal oblique fascia
internal oblique muscle
internal procidentia
internal rectal sphincter
internal ring
internal spermatic fascia
internal sphincterotomy
internal urethral orifice
International Association of Pancreatology (IAP)
International Islet Transplant Registry (ITR)
International Pancreas Transplant Registry
International System of Units (SI)

International Transplant Registry
Intern Line "Boston Style"
Intern Line "Physician Style"
interosseous knife
interparietal fascia
interparietal suture
interpectoral lymph node
Interpore graft
interposed omental fat
interposition bone graft
interposition Dacron graft
interposition graft
interposition of colon between liver and diaphragm
interposition saphenous vein graft
interrupted near-far, far-near suture
interrupted pledgeted suture
interrupted suture
intersphincteric abscess
intersphincteric anal fistula
intersphincteric rectal dissection
interspinous line
interstitial catheter
interstitial cells of Cajal
interstitial fluid
interstitial gastritis
interstitial gland
interstitial hemorrhage
interstitial hernia
interstitial laser coagulation (ILC)
interstitial nephritis
interstitial pancreatitis
interstitial pattern
intertrochanteric plate
interureteric fold
interval resection of redundant sigmoid
intervention
  medical
  operative
  surgical
  therapeutic
intervertebral disk forceps
intervertebral disk punch
intervertebral disk rongeur
intestinal allograft
intestinal amebiasis
intestinal anastomosis
intestinal angiodysplasia
intestinal atony
intestinal atresia
intestinal bacteria
intestinal bag
intestinal bypass
intestinal calculus
intestinal candidiasis
intestinal clamp
intestinal cleansing
intestinal colic
intestinal concretion
intestinal contents
intestinal crushing clamp
intestinal decompression
intestinal diverticulum
intestinal dysmotility and stasis
intestinal failure due to short-bowel syndrome
intestinal flora
intestinal ganglioneuromatosis
intestinal gland
intestinal glucose transport
intestinal graft radiation
intestinal-grasping forceps
intestinal hemorrhage
intestinal hernia
intestinal impaction
intestinal intussusception
intestinal invagination
intestinal juice
intestinal lipodystrophy
intestinal lipophagic granulomatosis
intestinal loop
intestinal lumen
intestinal lymphangiectasia
intestinal lymphoma
intestinal M cells
intestinal metaplasia
intestinal motility disorder
intestinal mucosa

intestinal muscle contractions
intestinal necrosis
intestinal neuronal dysplasia (IND)
intestinal obstruction
intestinal perforation
intestinal perfusion study
intestinal permeability
intestinal phase of acid secretion
intestinal plication
intestinal polyposis
intestinal polyposis II
intestinal polyposis-cutaneous
  pigmentation syndrome
intestinal prolapse
intestinal pseudo-obstruction
intestinal secretion
intestinal sepsis
intestinal stasis
intestinal stenosis
intestinal strangulation
intestinal stricturoplasty
intestinal torsion
intestinal tract
intestinal transplant
intestinal transplantation (ITx)
intestinal trichomoniasis
intestinal ulcer
intestinal urinary conduit
intestinal villous architecture
intestinal villous atrophy
intestinal web
intestine
  blind
  empty (jejunum)
  iced
  jejunoileal
  large
  mesenteric
  segmented
  small
  straight
intestinointestinal reflex
intestinum crasum
intestinum caecum
intestinum ileum
intestinum jejunum
intestinum rectum
intestinum tenue mesenteriale
in the midaxillary line
intolerance
  gluten
  heat
  lactose
  sucrose
in toto
intoxication, hepatocerebral
intra-abdominal abscess
intra-abdominal adhesion
intra-abdominal bleeding
intra-abdominal fluid collection
intra-abdominal hemorrhage
intra-abdominal hernia
intra-abdominal ileal reservoir
intra-abdominal mass
intra-abdominal pressure
intra-abdominal sepsis (IAS)
intra-abdominal sheer stress
intra-abdominal wall
intra-abdominal wall musculature
intra-alveolar hemorrhage
intra-anal pressure
intra-anal wart
intra-aortic balloon (IAB)
intra-aortic endovascular sonography
intra-arterial bolus injection
intra-arterial chemotherapy catheter
intra-articular shaver
intracanalicular papilloma
Intracath catheter
Intracath needle
intracellular bacteria
intracellular compartment
intracellular fluid (ICF)
intracellular organism
intracellular protein
intracellular space
intracellular water
IntraCoil

intracolonic Kaposi sarcoma
Intracone intramedullary reamer
intracorporeal anastomosis
intracorporeal shock-wave lithotripsy (ISWL)
intracranial clamp
intracranial mass lesion
intracranial tumor
intracrural fiber
intractability, cancer, hemorrhage, obstruction, perforation (ICHOP)
intractable abscess
intractable diarrhea
intractable leg ulcer
intractable ulcer
intractable ulcerative colitis
intractable vomiting
intracuticular suture
intracystic papilloma
intradeglutitive phase of swallowing
intradermal suture
IntraDose (cisplatin/epinephrine) gel
intraductal carcinoma of breast
intraductal papilloma
intraductal pressure
intraductal secretin test (IDST)
intradural abscess
intraepidermal carcinoma
intraepithelial carcinoma
intraepithelial nonkeratizing carcinoma
intraesophageal acid test
intraesophageal peristaltic pressure
intraesophageal pH test
intraesophageal stent
Intraflex intramedullary pin
intragastric balloon
intragastric bubble
intragastric pH mapping
intragastric pressure
intragraft polymerase chain reaction (PCR) assay
intrahaustral contraction ring
intrahepatic abscess
intrahepatically
intrahepatic atresia
intrahepatic AV fistula
intrahepatic bile duct
intrahepatic biliary cystic dilation
intrahepatic biliary duct
intrahepatic cholangiocarcinoma
intrahepatic cholangioenterostomy
intrahepatic cholangiolitis
intrahepatic cholestasis of pregnancy (ICP)
intrahepatic cirrhosis
intrahepatic disease
intrahepatic duct
intrahepatic hepatitis of pregnancy
intrahepatic radicle
intrahepatic sclerosing cholangitis
intrahepatic stone
intrahepatic stricture
intrahepatic transjugular portosystemic shunt
intralesional therapy
Intralipid fat emulsion
intralobular biliary canal
intralobular fibrosis
intraluminal (ILS) stapler
intraluminal acid
intraluminal contents
intraluminal cyst
intraluminal esophageal pressure
intraluminal manometry
intraluminal occluding suture
intraluminal pH electrode test
intraluminal shelf (infolding of the media)
intraluminal Silastic esophageal stent
intraluminal stone
intramammary sulcus
intramedullary (IM)
intramedullary anesthesia
intramedullary graft
intramedullary guide
intramedullary nail
intramedullary pin
intramedullary rasp

intramedullary reamer
intramesenteric abscess
intramucosal development
intramural abscess
intramural bowel mass
intramural colonic air
intramural duodenal hematoma after blunt abdominal trauma
intramural edema
intramural esophageal rupture
intramural fistulous tract
intramural hematoma
intramuscular abscess
intranasal anesthesia
Intran disposable pressure measurement catheter
intraocular malignancy
intraocular melanoma
Intra–Op autotransfusion
intraoperative autologous transfusion (IOAT)
intraoperative bile spillage
intraoperative chemical splanchnicectomy
intraoperative cholangiogram
intraoperative cholangiography (IOC)
intraoperative endoscopic Congo red test (IECRT)
intraoperative laparoscopic cholangiography
intraoperative pancreatography
intraoperative trauma
intraoperative ultrasound
intraoperative view
intraoral anesthesia
intraosseous anesthesia
intraosseous abscess
intraosseous probe
intraosseous suture anchor
intrapapillary terminus
intraparenchymal liver injury
intraperitoneal abscess
intraperitoneal adhesion
intraperitoneal air
intraperitoneal blood
intraperitoneal cavity
intraperitoneal drain placement
intraperitoneal hyperthermic chemotherapy (IPHC)
intraperitoneal incision
intraperitoneal onlay mesh (IPOM) hernia repair technique
intraperitoneal viscus
intrapulmonary shunting
intrarectal ultrasound
intrarenal reflux
IntraSite (graft T starch copolymer)
IntraSite gel
IntraSite hydrogel dressing
intraspinal anesthesia
IntraStent DoubleStrut biliary endoprosthesis
IntraStent DoubleStrut XS stent
IntraStent LP biliary stent
intrathoracic esophagogastroscopy
intrathoracic goiter
intrathoracic injury
intrathoracic Nissen fundoplication
intratracheal anesthesia
intratumoral catheter
intravariceal sclerotherapy
intravascular compartment
intravascular fluid
intravascular stent
intravascular ultrasound (IVUS) catheter
intravascular volume
intravascular volume status
intravenous (I.V., IV)
intravenous alimentation
intravenous administration of fluids
intravenous administration of medications
intravenous amino acids
intravenous anesthesia (IVA)
intravenous calcium gluconate
intravenous cholangiogram (IVC)
intravenous extension of tumor

intravenous feeding (IVF)
intravenous fluid
intravenous fluid bolus
intravenous fluid therapy
intravenous glucose administration
intravenous hydration
intravenous hyperalimentation
intravenous Instant Timer
intravenous line sepsis
intravenous nutritional therapy (also see *feeding formula*)
  FreAmine HBC 6.9%
  FreAmine III 3% (8.5%) with Electrolytes
  HepatAmine (multiple branched-chain essential and nonessential amino acids; electrolytes)
  Iodo-Pak (sodium iodide)
  Iodopen (sodium iodide)
  Molypen
  MulTE-Pak-5 (multiple trace elements [metals])
  Neotrace-4
  PedTE-Pak-4
  Pedtrace-4 (multiple trace elements)
  Zinca-Pak
intravenous piggyback
intravenous pole
intravenous push
intravenous regional anesthesia
intravenous sedation anesthesia
intravenous sponge
intravenous tolbutamide
intravenous vasopressin
intraventricular cannula
intraventricular catheter
intrepid PTCA angioplasty catheter
intrinsic factor
intrinsic muscles of the larynx
intrinsic plus position
intrinsic stenotic lesion
introducer
  Bard Safety Excalibur catheter
  Becton-Dickinson

introducer *(cont.)*
  Check-Flo
  Ciaglia
  Cook
  Czaja-McCaffrey rigid stent
  Desilets-Hoffman catheter
  electrode
  Endosuture
  Fast-Cath
  guidewire
  Guyon catheter
  Hemaquet catheter
  Hemaquet sheath
  heparin lock
  Key-Med Nottingham
  laparoscopic
  Littleford-Spector
  LPS Peel-Away
  Micropuncture Peel-Away
  Moss G-tube PEG kit
  Mullins catheter
  Naviguide
  Nottingham
  Nottingham semirigid
  Oasis One Action stent
  Pacesetter
  peel-away
  percutaneous lead
  percutaneous tracheostomy
  permanent lead
  Dumon-Gilliard prosthesis
  Swartz SL Series Fast-Cath
  Tuohy-Borst
  Wilson-Cook prosthesis
introducer sheath
introduction of endoprosthesis by ERCP (endoscopic retrograde cholangio-pancreatography)
Introlan Half-Strength
Introlite (lactose-free formula)
Intron A (interferon alfa-2b, recombinant)
Intropaste (barium sulfate)
intubate

intubating laryngoscope
intubation
  endotracheal
  esophageal
  esophagogastric (EG)
  nasal
  nasogastric (NG)
  nasotracheal
  oral
  orotracheal
Intuitive system
intussuscepted bowel
intussusception
  agonic
  appendiceal
  bowel
  colic
  double
  enteric
  ileal
  ileocecal
  ileocolic
  intestinal
  jejunogastric
  postmortem
  retrograde
intussusceptum
intussuscipiens
invaginated
invagination
  intestinal
  stomal
invasion
  adjacent organ
  blood vessel
  capsular
  chest wall
  depth of
  extrathyroidal
  local
  lymphatic
  lymphocyte
  metastatic
  mucosal
invasion *(cont.)*
  tissue
  tumor
  tumorous hepatic
invasion outside the thyroid
invasive breast cancer
invasive carcinoma
invasive ductal carcinoma
invasive lesion
invasive lobular carcinoma
invasive neoplasm
invasive procedure
invasive thyroiditis
invasive tumor
inversion ankle stress view
inversion-ligation appendectomy
inversion, nipple
Inverta-PEG tube
inverted ductal papilloma
inverted loop sign
inverted nipple
inverted papilloma
inverted suture
inverted-U abdominal incision
inverted U-pouch ileal reservoir
inverted V sign (on x-ray)
inverting suture
Investa suture
InView clear leggings
in vitro
in vivo
involuntary guarding
involuntary reflex rigidity
involution
involvement, mucosal (see also invasion)
INVOS 2100 early warning test for breast cancer
INX stainless steel stent (neurovascular)
Inyo nail
IOAT (intraoperative autologous transfusion)
Ioban antimicrobial incise drape
Ioban 2 antimicrobial films

Ioban Vi-Drape
iobenzamic acid
IOC (intraoperative cholangiogram)
iocetamic acid contrast medium
iodide goiter
iodinated contrast agent
iodinated contrast media
iodine
  ^{123}I murine MAb to alpha-fetoprotein (AFP)
  ^{125}I
  ^{131}I 6B-iodomethyl-19-norcholesterol
iodine-deficiency goiter
iodine hypothyroidism
iodixanol
iodocholesterol scanning
Iodoflex absorptive dressing
Iodoflex solid gel pad dressing
iodoform gauze dressing
iodoform gauze pack
Iodo-Pak (sodium iodide)
Iodopen (sodium iodide)
iodophor-impregnated adhesive drape
iodophor scrub
iodoquinol
Iodosorb absorptive dressing
Iodosorb wound cleansing gel dressing
Iodotope (sodium iodide ^{131}I)
IoGen
ioglycamic acid
iohexol
Ionescu-Shiley pericardial xenograft
ion-exchange resin
ion laser
IontoDex (dexamethasone sodium phosphate)
iontophoresis
IOP (intraoperative pressure)
iopamidol
iopanoic acid contrast medium
IOS immunoassay system
Iotec cannula
Iotec trocar
iothalamate sodium
Iotrex radioisotope
ioversal
Iowa membrane forceps
Iowa trumpet needle guide
Iowa University periosteal elevator
IPAA (ileal pouch-anal anastomosis)
ipecac-induced cardiotoxicity
ipecac-induced myopathy
ipecac-induced vomiting
ipecac syrup
IPH (idiopathic portal hypertension)
IPHC (intraperitoneal hyperthermic chemotherapy)
IPHP (intraperitoneal hyperthermic perfusion)
ipodate (also iopodate)
ipodate calcium
ipodate contrast medium
ipodate sodium
IPOM (intraperitoneal onlay mesh)
ipoxygenase
IPPB (intermittent positive pressure breathing)
iprofenin
IPSID (immunoproliferative small intestine disease)
ipsilateral arm lymphedema
ipsilateral brain mass
ipsilateral breast
ipsilateral internal mammary lymph node
ipsilateral lymph node
ipsilateral pneumoscrotum
ipsilateral side
ipsilateral supraclavicular node
ipsilateral thyroid lobe
ipsilateral thyroid lobectomy
ipsilateral vocal cord paralysis
iPTH (immunoreactive parathyroid hormone)
IRA (ileorectal anastomosis)
Iressa
iridium-192 (^{192}Ir)

iridium-loaded stent
iridium ribbon
iridium seed
iridium wire implant
irinotecan HCl injection
IRIS coronary stent
Irish node
Iris Medical EndoProbe
iris scissors
IRMA blood analysis system
IRMA-M test
IRMA SL test
irofulven
iron-binding capacity of blood
iron-deficiency anemia
iron liver
iron-overload syndrome
iron storage disease
iron store
irradiated graft
irradiation, graft
irradiation injury
irradiation of donor organ
Irravac irrigator
irreducible hernia
irregular amputated mucosal pattern
irregular mass
irregularity
irreversible chronic graft rejection
irrigant, Renacidin
irrigate and aspirate until clear
irrigated with warm saline
irrigating solution, physiological
irrigating syringe, Toomey
irrigation, irrigator
  Asepto
  closed-system
  Coloplast
  Conseal
  copious
  Dansac
  Endo-AID suction
  End-Flo laparoscopic
  Endo-Flo

irrigation *(cont.)*
  Excel
  FlowGun
  House suction
  HydroSurge laparoscopic
  Irravac
  IrrigaTORR
  Irrijet DS
  Lap Vacu-Irrigator
  Nibbler
  Orthotec
  Pathfinder
  pressurized pulsatile
  Ringer
  Shambaugh
  Squirt wound
  StrykeFlow suction
  suction
  Surgilav
  tissue
  United Ostomy
  Vozzle Vacu-Irrigator
irrigation instrument
irrigation of colostomy
irrigation pump
irrigation tubing
irrigator (see *irrigation*)
IrrigaTORR device
Irrijet DS debridement and irrigation system
Irrijet DS wound irrigation system
irritability
irritable bowel disease (IBD)
irritable bowel syndrome (IBS)
  constipation-predominant
  diarrhea-predominant
irritable colon
irritable stricture
irritant gastritis
irritation, peritoneal
irritative diarrhea
irritative lesion
IRS (impaired regeneration syndrome)

ischemia
  bowel loop
  chronic
  gastric mucosa
  mucosal
  myocardial
  necrotic
  nonocclusive mesenteric
ischemia/reperfusion
ischemic bowel
ischemic bowel disease
ischemic bowel loop
ischemic colitis
ischemic enteritis
ischemic enterocolitis
ischemic fecal incontinence
ischemic heart disease
ischemic hepatitis
ischemic kidney
ischemic mesenteric disease
ischemic necrosis
ischemic needle of femoral head (INFH) necrosis
ischemic skin ulcer
ischiatic hernia
ischiorectal abscess
ischiorectal fistula
ischiorectal fossa block anesthesia
ischiorectal fossa plane
ischiorectal hernia
ischiorectal pad of fat
Iselin forceps
ISG (immune serum globulin)
Ishak classification of chronic hepatitis C (0–6)
ISI laparoscopic instruments
island
  macroscopic
  squamous
  tissue
island dressing
island flap
islet allotransplant
islet amyloid polypeptide (IAPP)
islet autotransplant
islet cell
islet cell allografting
islet cell antibody
islet cell autoantibody
islet cell generation
islet cell hyperplasia
islet cell implant
islet cell neoplasm
islet cell preparation
islet cell tumor
islet cryopreservation
islet separation technology
Isletest-GAD test
Isletest-ICA kits for detection of islet cell autoantibodies
islets of Langerhans
islets, pancreatic
islet transplantation
Iso-Bac reinforcement
Isoband bandage
isobaric spinal anesthesia
isobutyl 2-cyanoacrylate (IBC) tissue adhesive
Isocaine HCl (mepivacaine HCl)
Isocal HCN (high calorie and nitrogen) enteral feeding
Isocal HN enteral feeding
isodense
isodensity
isoechoic
isoenzyme of LDH
isoenzyme, Regan
isoflurane
isofylline
isoimmunization
Isola hook
Isola rod
isolate
isolated gastric varices
isolated splenic injury
isolated thyroid-stimulating hormone deficiency
isolation

isolation drape
Isolex 300i stem cell selection system
Isolyser
IsoMed implantable drug pump
Isomil DF (soy protein formula)
Isomil SF (sucrose-free) formula
isoniazid-induced hepatitis
Isopan (magaldrate)
Isopan Plus (magaldrate; simethicone)
isoperistaltic anastomosis
isoperistaltic ileal reservoir
isoprene strap
isopropyl alcohol
isoproterenol
Iso-Seal drape
isosexual virilization
isosorbide dinitrate (ID)
isosorbide mononitrate
Isosource HN
Isospora belli
Isospora hominis
Isospora natelenis
IsoStent radioisotope stent
Isotec patellar tendon graft
Isotein HN enteral feeding
isotomic fluid secretion
Isotoner glove
isotonic feeding
isotope meal
isotope tracer
isovaleric acid
isovaleric acid CoA dehydrogenase deficiency
isovaleric acidemia (IVA)
isovaleryl CoA carboxylase deficiency
Isovue-370 (iopamidol)
I-Soyalac formula
Israel rasp
Israel retractor
ISSE optical dissecting and suction cannula
isthmectomy
isthmus
isthmus of thyroid
isthmusectomy
ISWL (intracorporeal shock-wave lithotripsy)
ITA (internal thoracic artery) graft
ITC balloon catheter
ITC radiopaque balloon catheter
itching
Iterson trachea hook
ITI (Instrument Technology, Inc.) 0.5 mm rigid endoscope
ITI rigid borescope
Ito cell
Ito cell sarcoma
ITR (International Islet Transplant Registry)
itraconazole (Sporanox)
ITx (intestinal transplantation)
I.V., IV (intravenous)
IVA (isovaleric acidemia)
IVAC Core·Check thermometer
IVAC electronic thermometer
IVAC MedSystem III multichannel infusion pump
IVAC SmartSite needleless system
IVAC Space·Saver volumetric pump
IVAC Vital·Check device
IVAC volumetric infusion pump
Ivalon rectopexy
Ivalon sponge
Ivalon sponge rectopexy
Ivalon sponge-wrap operation
IVC (intravenous cholangiogram)
IVC stenosis
IVC venous sampling for catecholamines
Ivemark syndrome
ivermectin
Ives anoscope
Ives-Fansler anoscope
IVF (intravenous feeding)
IVF (intravenous fluids)
Ivor Lewis esophagectomy

Ivor Lewis esophagogastrectomy
Ivor Lewis two-stage subtotal
esophagectomy
IVUS (intravascular ultrasound)
catheter
Ivy Biomedical Systems
Ivy bleeding time (BT)

J, j

Jaboulay gastroduodenostomy
Jaboulay pyloroplasty
jackknife position
Jackman orthogonal catheter
Jackson battery
Jackson bone extension clamp
Jackson esophageal bougie
Jackson esophagoscope
Jackson grasping polyp forceps
Jackson, inside curve
Jackson intervertebral disk rongeur
Jackson laryngeal atomizer
Jackson laryngectomy tube
Jackson Open-End aspirating tube
Jackson-Pratt (JP)
Jackson-Pratt catheter
Jackson-Pratt drain
Jackson-Pratt gold branch Hemaduct wound drain
Jackson retractor
Jackson scissors
Jackson tendon-seizing forceps
Jackson trachea hemostat
Jackson trachea hook
Jackson trachea tenaculum
Jackson trachea tube
Jackson tracheal bistoury
Jackson Velvet eye aspirating tube
jackstone calculus
Jacobs distraction rod
Jacobson-Adson artery forceps
Jacobson bulldog clamp
Jacobson dressing forceps
Jacobson hemostatic forceps
Jacobson micro mosquito forceps
Jacobson microneurosurgical scissors
Jacobson micro probe
Jacobson microvascular knife
Jacobson microvascular needle holder with tungsten carbide inlays
Jacobson mosquito forceps
Jacobson-Potts vascular clamp
Jacobson probe
Jacobson-TC needle holder
Jacobson vessel knife
Jacobs-Palmer laparoscope
Jacoby test
Jacuzzi
Jaeger lid plate
Jaffee capsulorrhexis forceps
Jahnke anastomosis clamp
Jako laryngeal suction tube
Jamaican vomiting sickness
Jameson dissecting scissors
Jameson muscle hook
Jameson scissors

Jamestown Canyon virus
Jamshidi biopsy needle
Jamshidi liver biopsy needle
J&J Medical (Johnson & Johnson)
Janeway lesion
Janeway procedure
Jannetta alligator forceps
Jannetta aneurysm neck dissector
Jannetta bayonet forceps
Jannetta dissector
Jannetta duckbill elevator
Jannetta forceps
Jannetta fork
Jannetta hook
Jannetta knife
Jannetta-Kurze dissecting scissors
Jannetta posterior fossa retractor
Jannetta probe
Jansen curette
Jansen mastoid retractor
Jansen-Middleton septal forceps
Jansen monopolar forceps
Jansen rasp
Jansen retractor
Jansen rongeur
Jansen scalp retractor
Jansen-Wagner retractor
Japanese classification of gastric
  carcinoma
jar forceps
Jarcho self-retaining uterine cannula
Jarell forceps
Jarit brain forceps
Jarit cystoscope
Jarit-Kerrison laminectomy rongeur
Jarit laparoscope
Jarit-Liston bone rongeur
Jarit P.E.E.R. retractor
Jarit rigid laparoscope
Jarit Rotator
Jarit-Ruskin bone rongeur
Jarit tendon-pulling forceps
Jarit 0° 5 mm rigid laparoscope
Jarit 0° 10 mm rigid laparoscope
Jarvis clamp
Jarvis hemorrhoid forceps
Jasan flexible fiberoptic sigmoidoscope
Jasan JFE choledochoscope
Jasan rigid proctoscope
jaundice
  acholuric
  acquired hemolytic
  anhepatic
  benign postoperative
  breast milk
  Budd
  choleric
  cholestatic
  chronic acholuric
  chronic familial
  chronic idiopathic
  congenital familial nonhemolytic
  congenital hemolytic
  familial chronic idiopathic
  familial nonhemolytic
  hematogenous
  hemolytic
  hepatocellular
  hepatogenous
  infectious
  leptospiral
  malignant
  malignant obstructive
  mechanical
  neonatal
  newborn
  nonhemolytic
  obstructive
  painless
  parenchymal
  physiologic (newborn)
  retention
  scleral
  spirochetal
  yellow
jaundiced plasma
jaundiced skin
Javid carotid artery clamp

Javid shunt
Javorski test
jaw gib
jaw thrust
Jawz biopsy forceps
Jawz endomyocardial biopsy forceps
JC DNA virus
JDM (juvenile diabetes mellitus) (now classified as type 1)
Jegher syndrome
jejunal angiodysplasia
jejunal aspirate
jejunal atresia
jejunal biopsy
jejunal feeding tube
jejunal limb
jejunal loop
jejunal loop interposition of Henle
jejunal pouch
jejunal rupture
jejunal syndrome
jejunal ulcer
jejunectomy
jejunitis
  allergic
  dietetic
  infectious
  nongranulomatous
jejunocolic fistula
jejunoileal bypass (JIB)
  Payne-DeWind
  Scott
jejunoileitis
jejunoileostomy, Roux-en-Y distal
jejunojejunostomy
jejunostomy
  afferent
  decompression
  endoscopic
  feeding
  laparoscopic
  loop
  needle catheter
  percutaneous endoscopic (PEJ)

jejunostomy *(cont.)*
  subserosal needle catheter
  Witzel
jejunostomy catheter
  Baker
  decompression
  feeding
  Flexiflo Lap J
  laparoscopic
  loop
  MIC
  needle
  Witzel
jejunostomy tube
jejunum
  arterial arcades of
  coils of
  mesentery of
  proximal
  windows of
Jelco I.V. catheter
Jelco needle
Jelco winged I.V. catheter
jelly
  Wharton
  Xylocaine
jelly-like material
Jelonet (paraffin-soaked tulle) dressing
Jenckel cholecystoduodenostomy
Jennings mouth gag
Jensen sarcoma
Jergesen I-beam plate
Jergesen tapered plate
Jergesen tube
Jesberg aspirating tube
Jesberg esophagoscope
jet lesion
jet pilot position
Jeter lag screw
Jeter position screw
Jevity isotonic liquid nutrition
jeweler's bipolar forceps
Jewett driver
Jewett extractor

Jewett gouge
Jewett nail
Jewett nail overlay plate
JFB III endoscope
J-hook cannula
J-hook electrode
J-hook ElectroProbe
JIB (jejunoileal bypass)
jig, cutting
jig hook
J ileal reservoir
Jimmy dissector
JL4 (Judkins left 4 cm curve) catheter
JL5 (Judkins left 5 cm curve) catheter
J needle
J needle technique
Jober fossa
Jobson Horne probe
Jobst glove
Jobst stockings
Jod-Basedow phenomenon (transient hyperthyroidism)
JODM (juvenile-onset diabetes mellitus) (now classified as type 1)
Joe hoe retractor
Johannesberg staple
Johannson hip nail
Johns Hopkins bulldog clamp
Johns Hopkins coarctation clamp
Johns Hopkins forceps
Johns Hopkins gallbladder forceps
Johns Hopkins gallbladder retractor
Johnson & Johnson Medical
Johnson brain tumor forceps
Johnson esophagogastrostomy
Johnson retractor
Johnson thoracic forceps
Johnson tumor forceps
joint fluid
joker (slang for instrument)
joker periosteal elevator
Joll thyroid retractor
Jolles test
Jones compression pin
Jones compression plate
Jones dressing
Jones IMA forceps
Jones position
Jones thoracic clamp
Jones towel clip
Jones view
Jonnesco fossa
Jordan-Bookwalter retractor
Jordan hook
Jordan needle
Jorgenson scissors
Joseph button-end knife
Joseph dissecting scissors
Joseph hook
Joseph nasal rasp
Joseph nasal scissors
Joseph periosteal elevator
Joseph skin hook
joule (J)
Joule-Thompson effect in endoscopic cryotherapy
Joystick
J periosteal elevator
J pouch, two-loop ileal
J-shaped ileal pouch
J-shaped reservoir
J-shaped skin incision
J-shaped tube
J-tipped hydrophilic guidewire
J tube
J-turn maneuver with endoscope
Judd-Allis intestinal forceps
Judd-DeMartel gallbladder forceps
Judd ventral hernia repair
Judet graft
Judet radius view
Judkins 4 diagnostic catheter
Juers-Lempert rongeur forceps
jugal suture
jugular line
jugular venous distention
jugular versus peripheral ACTH levels

juice
  acid-peptic
  appetite
  gastric
  intestinal
  pancreatic
Julian splenorenal forceps
Julian thoracic forceps
jumbo biopsy forceps
jump graft
jumper's knee position
junction
  anorectal
  cardioesophageal (CE)
  choledochopancreatic ductal
  cystic-choledochal
  cystocholedochal
  esophagogastric (EG)
  fundic-antral
  gastroesophageal (GE)
  ileocecal
  duodenojejunal
  mucocutaneous
  pancreaticobiliary ductal
  pyloroduodenal
  squamocolumnar
  tracheoesophageal (TE; TEF)
  ureteropelvic
junction of papillary and reticular dermis
junction of right and left hepatic ducts
junction of second and third portions of duodenum
Juven nutritional supplement
juvenile angiofibroma
juvenile cirrhosis
juvenile diabetes mellitus (JDM) (now classified as type 1)
juvenile embryonal carcinoma
juvenile hypothyroidism
juvenile melanoma
juvenile-onset diabetes mellitus (JODM) (now classified as type 1)
juvenile pattern
juvenile polyp
juvenile polyposis
juvenile polyposis coli
juxtacortical osteogenic sarcoma
juxtaglomerular cells
juxtahepatic venous injury
juxtapyloric ulcer
J-Vac closed wound drainage
J-Vac suction reservoir
J wire
J-wire guide

K, k

K (potassium)
Kader gastrostomy
Kaessmann nail
Kahn dissecting scissors
Kahn-Frazier suction tube
Kahn uterine trigger cannula
Kahre-Williger periosteal elevator
Kaletra (lopinavir/ritonavir)
Kalginate alginate wound dressing
Kalginate calcium alginate dressing
Kalish Duredge wire extractor
Kalman-Mixter forceps
Kalman needle holder with tungsten carbide inlay
Kalt needle
Kaltostat calcium alginate dressing
Kaltostat Fortex high-absorbent wound dressing
Kaltostat pad (high-absorbent) dressing
Kaltostat rope dressing
Kaltostat wound packing material
Kam Vac suction tube
Kanavel brain-exploring cannula
Kaneda plate
Kaneda rod
Kantor-Berci videolaryngoscope
Kantor sign
Kantrowitz artery forceps
Kantrowitz thoracic clamp
Kantrowitz vascular scissors
Kanulase
Kaodene Non-Narcotic (kaolin; pectin; bismuth subsalicylate)
Kao Lectrolyte
kaolin
Kaopectate
Kao-Spen (kaolin; pectin)
Kapectolin (kaolin; pectin)
Kaplan PenduLaser 115 surgical laser system
Kaposi sarcoma, intracolonic
Kapp-Beck-Thomson clamp
Kapsinow test
karaya powder
Karaya 5 paste
Karaya 5 seal
Karaya ring ileostomy appliance
Karl Storz endoscope
Karl Storz endoscopy video camera system
Karl Storz N_2O Endoflator
Karl Storz rigid laparoscope
Karl Storz Take-Apart instruments
Karmody venous scissors
Karnofsky rating scale
Karp aortic punch forceps

Kartchner carotid artery clamp
Kartush insulated retractor
Karuse nasal snare
Karydakis flap
Karydakis pilonidal cyst excision
karyotype determination
Kasai peritoneal venous shunt
Kasai portoenterostomy
Kasdan retractor
Kashiwado test
Kaslow intestinal tube
Kasof (docusate potassium)
Kasugai classification of chronic
  pancreatitis
Kato test
Kay aorta clamp
Kaycel towel
Kayer-Fleischer ring
Kaye scissors
Kaye tamponade balloon catheter
Kaye-TC scissors
Kayexalate enema
Kay-Lambert clamp
Kayser-Fleischer ring
K blade
K-C (kaolin; pectin; bismuth
  subcarbonate)
kcal (kilocalorie, calorie)
KDF-2.3 catheter
K-dissector sponge
K-Dur (potassium chloride)
Keel Cobra One-Piece cannula
Keel Cobra Toomey syringe cannula
Keene compression hook
Kefzol
Kehr incision
Kehr sign
Keith abdominal needle, straight,
  triangular point
Keith abdominal triangle
Keith needle
Kelling esophagoscope
Kelling test
Kelly abdominal retractor
Kelly anoscope
Kelly artery forceps
Kelly clamp
Kelly dissecting scissors
Kelly fistula scissors
Kelly forceps, curved
Kelly hemostat
Kelly hemostatic forceps
Kelly-Locklin scissors
Kelly-Paterson syndrome
Kelly placenta forceps
Kelly plication suture
Kelly proctoscope
Kelly rectal speculum
Kelly retractor
Kelly scissors
Kelly sphincteroscope
Kelly straight proctoscope
Kelly tapered proctoscope
keloid scar
Kelsey pile clamp
Kemerovo virus
Ken sliding nail
Kendall esophageal sonascope
Kendall Healthcare Company
Kendall sontatemp
Kennerdell-Maroon elevator
Kennerdell-Maroon hook
Kennerdell-Maroon orbital retractor
Keofeed feeding tube
ketoacidosis
keratome
keratome blade
keratosis
  actinic
  lacelike
  pharyngeal
  seborrheic
  senile
Kerckring duodenal fold
Kerlix bandage
Kerlix disposable laparotomy sponge
Kerlix dressing
Kern bone-holding clamp

Kern bone-holding forceps
Kern-Lane bone forceps
kernicterus
Kerrison down-biting rongeur
Kerrison forceps
Kerrison laminectomy rongeur
Kerrison punch
Kerrison rongeur
KESS constipation scoring system
Kessel plate
Kessler suture
Kestrone 5 (estrone)
Ketek (telithromycin)
ketoacidosis
    alcoholic
    diabetic
ketoconazole
ketone
ketonuria
ketoprofen
ketorolac tromethamine
ketosis, benign dietary
ketosis-prone diabetes mellitus
ketosis-resistant diabetes mellitus
KetoSite test for status of ketoacidosis
ketotic hypoglycemia
Kevorkian biopsy tip
Kevorkian-Tischler biopsy forceps
Kevorkian-Townsend biopsy curette
Kevorkian-Younge biopsy curette
Kevorkian-Younge biopsy forceps
Keyes cutaneous punch
Keyes dermal punch
Key hernia director
Key-Med Atkinson endoprosthesis
Key-Med Nottingham introducer
Key periosteal elevator
Key rasp
keyhole incision
keyhole surgery
keystone graft
kidney
    abdominal
    afferent vessels of

kidney *(cont.)*
    amyloid
    arcuate artery of
    Armanni-Ebstein
    arteriosclerotic
    artificial
    Ask-Upmark
    atrophic
    biopsy of
    cake
    cicatricial
    congested
    contracted
    cow
    crush
    cyanotic
    cystic
    disk
    donor
    doughnut
    dromedary
    duplex
    edematous
    fatty
    fibrous capsule of
    flea-bitten
    floating
    Formad
    fused
    Goldblatt
    granular
    hila of
    horseshoe
    hypermobile
    interlobular artery of
    ischemic
    large red
    medullary sponge
    mortar
    movable
    mural
    myelin
    myeloma
    pancake

kidney *(cont.)*
- pelvic
- polycystic
- putty
- pyelonephritic
- Rose-Bradford
- sacciform
- sclerotic
- sigmoid
- sponge
- supernumerary
- thoracic
- wandering
- waxy

kidney calculus
kidney cancer
kidney abscess
kidney colic
kidney function test
kidney laceration
kidney stone
kidney stone forceps
kidney transplant
Kidney Internal Splint/Stent (KISS) catheter
kidney-shaped placenta
kidney tubule
kidney tumor
Kielland forceps
Kiernan space
Kifa catheter
killer T cell
Killian antrum cannula
Killian gouge
Killian-Lynch laryngoscope
Killian rectal speculum
Killian septum speculum
Killian suction tube
Kilner catspaw retractor (cat's paw)
Kilner cheek retractor
Kilner dissecting scissors
Kilner hook
Kilner insulated retractor
Kilner skin hook
Kilner-TC needle holder
kilocalorie (kcal, calorie)
Kimberly Clark Ballard Medical
Kimmelstiel-Wilson syndrome
Kimura cartilage graft
Kinberg test
Kindercal nutritional therapy
Kindt carotid artery clamp
Kinesed
kinetic gallbladder study
Kinevac (sincalide)
King Systems
kinked intestine
kinked ureter
kink in bowel
kinking of CNS catheter
kink in intestine
kinky hair syndrome (Menkes disease)
Kinnier Wilson disease
Kinsella-Buie lung clamp
Kinsey atherectomy catheter
Kirby muscle hook
Kirchner diverticulum
Kiricuta breast reconstruction
Kirklin atrial retractor
Kirk mallet
Kirmission periosteal elevator
Kirmission periosteal rasp
Kirsch laser welding technique
Kirschner abdominal retractor
Kirschner hand drill
Kirschner wire drill
Kish urethral illuminated catheter
KISS (Kidney Internal Splint/Stent) catheter
kissing balloon
kissing ulcer
kit
- Adenovirus EIA test
- Alatest Latex-specific IgE allergen
- B-D Easy A1c test
- CdTOX A OIA
- Circulon System Step 2 venous ulcer dressing

kit *(cont.)*
    CloseSure procedure
    Daxor quantitative injection syringe
    Decon Mini-Plus
    Dulcolax Bowel Prep Kit (bisacodyl)
    Duraprep
    Euro-Collins (EC) multiorgan
        perfusion
    EZ Detect colorectal screening test
    Flex Advantage
    Flexiflo Lap G laparoscopic
        gastrostomy
    Flexiflo Lap J laparoscopic
        jejunostomy
    Great Smokies intestinal
        permeability
    hematopoietic progenitor assay
    HemeSelect reagent and collection
    I-Flow nerve block infusion
    Isletest and Isletest-ICA
    LeuTech radiolabeled antibody
    Matritech NMP22 test
    Moss G-tube PEG
    NeoTect
    Nerve Block Infusion
    NuMA
    NuMA test
    PainBuster infusion pain
        management
    PAK (percutaneous access kit)
    PathVysion HER-2 DNA probe
    Quick AC Enema
    Riba 3.0 SIA reagent kit for
        hepatitis C
    Russel gastrostomy
    standard bunny
    Surgi-Start Kit single basin set
    Three-Spring Reservoir Wound
        Suction Drainage
    Tridrate Bowel Evacuant
    Trinity adenovirus EIA test
    Virgo antimitochondrial antibody)
    V-scan test
Kitano knot
Kittner blunt dissector
Kittner clamp
Kittner dissecting scissors
Kittner retractor
Kittner sponge
Klatskin liver biopsy needle
Klatskin tumor
Klear-Temp probe
Klebanoff common duct sound
Klebanoff gallstone scoop
Klebsiella
KleenSpec dispenser
KleenSpec disposable anoscope
Kleihauer-Betke acid elution test
Kleinert-Kutz bone rongeur
Kleinert-Kutz bone-cutting forceps
Kleinert-Kutz periosteal elevator
Kleinert-Kutz rasp
Kleinert-Kutz rongeur forceps
Kleinert-Kutz skin hook
Kleinert-Kutz synovectomy rongeur
Kleinert-Kutz tendon forceps
Kleinert-Ragdell retractor
Klein pump
Kleinsasser anterior commissure
    laryngoscope
Kleinschmidt appendectomy clamp
Klemme laminectomy retractor
Klemm sign
Klemperer disease
Kleppinger bipolar forceps
KLI rigid borescope
Klima-Schleicher biopsy needle
Klinefelter syndrome
Kling adhesive dressing
Kling elastic bandage
Kling fluff roll and sponge
Klintmalm clamp
Klippel-Trenaunay syndrome
KLS Centre-Drive screw
Knapp scissors
knee-chest position
knee-elbow position
kneeling position

knee retractor
knife (see also *blade; scalpel*)
  A-K diamond
  A-OK ShortCut
  acetabular
  Adson dural
  Adson right-angle
  amputation
  angular
  arachnoid
  arthroscopic
  Ayre
  backward-cutting
  Bailey-Glover-O'Neill commissurotomy
  Ballenger swivel
  banana
  Bard-Parker
  bayonet
  Beaver
  Beaver-DeBakey
  beveled
  Bircher meniscus
  bladebreaker
  Blount
  Bovie
  Braithwaite
  Brock commissurotomy
  Bucy chordotomy (or cordotomy)
  cartilage
  Catlin amputating
  cautery
  chondroplasty
  chordotomy (cordotomy)
  Cobalt Knife
  cobalt-60 gamma
  Cobbett
  Collin amputating
  commissurotomy
  cordotomy (chordotomy)
  crescent
  Crile gasserian ganglion
  Culbertson canal
  Cushing dural hook

knife *(cont.)*
  deep blade
  DeMarneffe meniscotomy
  Derlacki capsule
  Derra commissurotomy
  Desmarres paracentesis
  double-bladed
  Down epiphyseal
  Downing cartilage
  dural
  Edgeahead phaco slit
  electrocautery
  electrosurgical cutting
  epiphyseal
  Esmarch plaster
  flap
  Foerster capsulotomy
  forward-cutting
  Frazier cordotomy
  Frazier pituitary
  Freedom
  Freer-Swanson ganglion
  Freiberg cartilage
  Freiberg meniscectomy
  full-radius resector
  Gamma radiosurgical
  Gandhi
  ganglion
  Grover meniscus
  Guilford-Wright double-edged sickle
  Guilford-Wright flap
  Halle dura
  Harmonic Scalpel
  Harrison
  hemilaminectomy
  hernia
  hook
  Hopkins plaster
  hot
  House
  insulation tipped diathermic
  interosseous
  intimectomy
  Jacobson microvascular

knife *(cont.)*
Jacobson vessel
Jannetta
Joseph button-end
Knifelight surgical knife and light
Koos microvascular
Krull acetabular
Langenbeck flap
Langenbeck resection
LaserSonics Nd:YAG LaserBlade scalpel
LaserSonics SurgiBlade
Lebsche sternal
left-cutting
Leksell cobalt-60 gamma
Leksell Gamma
Lempert paracentesis
L hook
Lindvall-Stille
Liston amputating
Liston amputation
Liston phalangeal
Lorenz PC/TC scissors ultra-sharp
Lowe-Breck cartilage
Lowe-Breck meniscectomy
Maltz cartilage
McCabe canal
McHugh facial nerve
McHugh flap
McKeever cartilage
meniscotomy
meniscus
MicroKnife XL triple-lumen needleknife
microvascular
Midas Rex
Mori
myelotomy
needle
Neff meniscus
Neoflex bendable
NeoKnife electrosurgical
Olivecrona trigeminal
Oretorp

knife *(cont.)*
Paparella canal
Paparella drum elevator
Paparella incudostapedial
Paparella sickle
Parasmillie double-bladed
Parker
Paufique
pituitary
plaster
Premium dissecting
Questrus Leading Edge sheathed
Rayport
Reiner plaster
resection
retrograde
Ridlon plaster
right-angle
right-cutting
roentgen
roentgen radiosurgical
Rosen incision
Salenius meniscus
SatinCrescent
SatinShortcut
semilunar cartilage
sharp
Shaw I and Shaw II
Sheehy round
ShortCut
sickle
skin
skin blade
Smart Scalpel
Smillie-Beaver
Smillie cartilage
Smillie meniscus
Smith cartilage
specimen
standard dissecting
Stecher arachnoid
Stryker cartilage
swivel
Tabb double-ended flap

knife *(cont.)*
  Tabb myringoplasty
  Take-Apart
  tenotomy
  Tiemann Meals tenolysis
  Toennis dura
  201-source cobalt-60 gamma
  Typhoon microdebrider
  UltraCision ultrasonic
  vessel
  Virchow
  Visitec circular
  Visitec crescent
  Visitec stiletto
  Watson
  Weary cordotomy
  Weck
  Yamada myelotomy
  Yankauer
  Yasargil arachnoid
  Yasargil microvascular
knife blade
Knifelight illuminated retractor
Knifelight surgical knife and light
knifelike pain
Knight bone-cutting forceps
Knight needle
Knight septum cutting forceps
knife/sleeve device
Knighton hemilaminectomy retractor
Knighton laminectomy retractor
knitted Dacron graft
knitted double velour Dacron patch graft
knitted tantalum
knobby process
Knodell classification of chronic hepatitis C
Knodell periportal inflammation score
Knodt compression rod
Knodt hook
Knodt rod
knot
  Aberdeen
  arthroscopic

knot *(cont.)*
  convertible slip
  extracorporeal
  fisherman's
  friction knot
  half-hitch
  heliX knot pusher
  ileosigmoid knot
  Kitano
  LapTie endoscopic
  lockable arthroscopic
  Nicky
  ratchet
  Roeder loop
  sailorman's
  slip
  square
  surfer's
  surgeon's
  Tennessee slider
  Topel
knot geometry
knotless suture anchor
knotless anchor suture
knot of Henry
knot pusher
  Arrequi
  heliX
  MetraTie
knot tied with throws
knot tier and ligature carrier, Retter
knot tier, Gazayerli
knot tightener, Nordt
knotting forceps
Knowles bandage scissors
Knowles nail
Knowles pin
knuckle of bowel
knuckle of colon
knurled rod
Knuttsen bending view (x-ray)
Ko-Airan maneuver
Koala pressure catheter
Koala vascular clamp
Kobak pudendal block needle

Kocher anastomosis
Kocher artery forceps
Kocher bladder spatula
Kocher bronchocele sound
Kocher clamp
Kocher collar incision (in thyroidectomy)
Kocher dilatation ulcer
Kocher director
Kocher elevator
Kocher forceps
Kocher gallbladder retractor
Kocher hemostat
Kocher hook
Kocher incision
Kocher intestinal forceps
Kocher-Langenbeck ilioinguinal approach
Kocher maneuver
Kocher pylorectomy
Kocher pyloromyotomy
Kocher retractor
Kocher thyroid dissector
Koch-Mason dressing
Koch nucleus hydrolysis needle
Kock ("coke")
Kock continent ileostomy
Kock ileal reservoir
Kock ileostomy
Kock pouch modified procedure
Kock reservoir ileostomy
Kodsi scale of Candida esophagitis
Koeberlé forceps
Koenig (König)
Koenig nail-splitting scissors
Koenig rasp
Koenig small director
Koenig syndrome
Koerte gallstone forceps
Koerte rake retractor
Kogan-Burke speculum
Kogan speculum
KOH (potassium hydroxide)
KOH colpotomizer system
KOH smear
Kolantyl
Kollman urethral dilator
kombucha (yeast/bacteria/fungus symbiont)
Komprex bandage
Komprex-Binde bandage
König (Koenig) syndrome
Konsyl (psyllium)
Konsyl-D
Konsyl Orange (psyllium hydrophilic mucilloid)
Konsyl Fiber (calcium polycarbophil)
Konton catheter
Kontron intra-aortic balloon
Koos microvascular knife
Kopans breast lesion localization needle
Kostuik rod
K-Pek (attapulgite)
Krackow suture
Kraff-Utrata tear capsulotomy forceps
Krankendonk pin
K-ras gene
Kraske jackknife position in surgery
Kraske position
Kraske transsacral proctectomy
KRAS mutation (gene implicated in cancer)
Krause biopsy tip
Krause nasal snare
Krause suture
Krause-Wolfe skin graft
Krayenbuehl (Krayenbühl) vessel hook
Krazy Glue sclerosant
Kreuscher scissors
Krimpt sponge
Kristeller specula
Krokiewicz test
Kronecker aneurysm needle
Kron gall duct dilator
Krukenberg tumor
Krull acetabular knife
krypton (red) laser
K-Sponge
K.T. Medical

KTP (potassium titanyl phosphate) laser
KTP/532 laser
KTP/YAG surgical laser system
K-Tube
Kuehne cover glass forceps
Kugel approach
Kugel hernia patch
Kugel patch repair
Kulchitsky cell
Kulchitsky cell carcinoma
Kunkel syndrome
Küntscher (Kuentscher)
Küntscher awl
Küntscher condylocephalic rod
Küntscher drill
Küntscher extractor
Küntscher hammer
Küntscher intramedullary reamer
Küntscher medullary nail
Küntscher nail driver
Küntscher nail extracting hook
Küntscher pin
Kupffer cell
Kupffer cell recovery (in obstructive jaundice)
Kupffer cell sarcoma
Kurze dissecting scissors
Kussmaul sign
Kutler V-Y flap graft
Kutrase (amylase; protease; lipase; cellulase; hyoscyamine sulfate; phenyltoloxamine citrate) digestive enzymes
Küttner (Kuettner)
Küttner blunt dissector
Kuzmak gastric banding technique
Kuz-Medics total knee retractor
Ku-Zyme HP (amylase; protease; lipase; cellulase) digestive enzymes
kwashiorkor protein-energy undernutrition
Kwik-Kits
K-wire driver
Kyasanur Forest hemorrhagic fever virus
Kynar insulated coating
Kytril (granisetron hydrochloride)

L, l

LA (left atrial)
LABA (laser-assisted balloon
angioplasty)
Labbe triangle
Laborde trachea dilator
lacelike keratosis
lacerated wound
laceration
gastroesophageal
kidney
spleen
through-and-through
V-shaped
wound
La Crosse virus
Lactaid
lactase deficiency
lactase enzyme
lactate dehydrogenase (LDH)
lactated Ringer (LR) solution
lactation
lacteal vessel
lactic acid
lactic acid bacillus
lactiferous duct
lactiferous duct fistula
lactiferous gland
Lactinex
Lactobacillus acidophilus
lactoferrin
Lactomer absorbable subcuticular skin
staple
lactose-associated diarrhea
lactose breath hydrogen test
lactose deficiency
lactose enzyme
lactose-free diet
lactose-free feeding
lactose intolerance
lactose, undigested
Lactrase
lactulose enema
lactulose-mannitol test
lactulose/rhamnose permeability
(L/R ratio)
lactulose solution
lacunar ligament
Ladd band
Ladd correction of malrotation
of the bowel
Ladd procedure
Ladd syndrome
Laënnec cirrhosis
Laënnec pearl

Lafora body
LAGB (Lap-Band adjustable gastric banding) system
lag screw
Lahey bag
Lahey clamp
Lahey Clinic dural hook
Lahey Clinic nerve hook
Lahey dissecting forceps
Lahey Finochietto dissecting forceps
Lahey gall duct forceps
Lahey gland forceps
Lahey liver transplant bag
Lahey retractor
Lahey scissors
Lahey thoracic forceps
Lahey thyroid retractor
Lahey thyroid traction forceps
Lahey tissue retractor
Laing plate
Laird-McMahon anorectoplasty
LAIS excimer laser
LAK (lymphokine activated killer) cell
lake, bile
laky blood
Lalonde delicate hook forceps
LAMA (laser-assisted microvascular anastomosis or laser-assisted microanastomosis)
Lambda Plus dye laser
Lambda Plus PDL 1 (and PDL 2) laser
lambdoid suture
lambdoidal cranial suture
Lambert aortic clamp
Lambert-Kay aorta clamp
Lambert-Kay vascular clamp
Lambert-Lowman bone clamp
Lambert-Lowman chisel
lambliasis
lambliosis
Lambotte bone-holding forceps
Lambotte bone hook
Lambotte elevator
Lambotte osteotome
Lambotte rasp
lamellated pattern
lamina elevator
lamina of the aponeurosis
lamina propria
lamina retractor
laminar hook
laminated clot
laminectomy blade
laminectomy chisel
laminectomy punch
laminectomy punch forceps
laminectomy retractor
laminectomy rongeur
Lamis adapter
Lamis patella clamp
Lamis tubing set
Lamis Y tubing
lamivudine therapy
lamp, Wood
Lancereaux-Mathieu-Weil spirochetosis
lancet
  Autoclix
  auto-Lancet
  ExacTech pen
  Laser Lancet
  Lasette
  Microlet Vaculance
  Microtainer
  Softclix
  Vaculance
lancet-shaped biopsy forceps
lancinating pain
Landau trocar
landmark
  anatomic
  anatomical
  bony
Landolt spreading forceps
Landon retractor
Landzert fossa
Lane band
Lane bone-holding clamp
Lane bone-holding forceps

Lane cleft palate, 1/2 circle, cutting edge
Lane disease
Lane elevator
Lane intestinal clamp
Lane intestinal forceps
Lane operation
Lane periosteal elevator
Lane plate
Lane point
Lane procedure
Lane screw-holding forceps
Lane self-retaining bone-holding forceps
Lane tissue forceps
Lane twin stomach clamps
Lang Stevenson intestinal clamp
Lange approximation forceps
Lange-Hohmann bone retractor
Langenbeck bone-holding forceps
Langenbeck elevator
Langenbeck flap knife
Langenbeck-Kocher retractor
Langenbeck metacarpal saw
Langenbeck periosteal elevator
Langenbeck rasp
Langenbeck resection knife
Langenbeck retractor
Lange skinfold calipers
Langenskiöld bone graft
Langerhans cell
Langer line
lansoprazole
Lantus (insulin glargine)
Lanza scale for drug-induced gastric mucosal damage
Lanz low-pressure cuff endotracheal tube
Lanz pressure-regulating valve
LAO (left anterior oblique) view
lap (brief form for laparotomy)
laparoendoscopic room
Laparofan device
LaparoLift gasless laparoscopy system
LaparoLift retractor system
LaparoSAC single-use obturator and cannula
laparoscope (see also *endoscope*)
 ACMI rigid
 Adler Eagle Vision
 Adler P.L.U.S.
 Arthrotek rigid
 Bryan rigid
 Cabot rigid
 Circon rigid
 Comeg rigid
 Concept rigid
 CorTek semirigid microlaparoscope
 Cuda 0° 10 mm rigid
 Demir rigid
 diagnostic
 Dyonics 0° 10 mm rigid
 Dyonics 3625
 Dyonics 7208130 rigid
 Dyonics 8007 rigid
 Eder 180 10 mm rigid
 Effner rigid
 ElMed rigid
 Endolap rigid
 Endolase rigid
 50° Foroblique optic
 flexible video
 Henke-Sass rigid
 Henke-Sass Wolf
 Inspex rigid laparoscope
 InstrumentMakar
 Jacobs-Palmer
 Jarit 0° 5 mm rigid
 Jarit 0° 10 mm rigid
 Jarit rigid
 Karl Storz rigid
 laser
 Linvatec
 Linvatec 7570R 0° 10 mm rigid
 Linvatec rigid
 Marlow rigid
 Marlow video
 Medilas

laparoscope *(cont.)*
MicroLap Gold microlaparoscope
MiniSite
Mueller 0° 5 mm rigid
Olympus A5214 0° 10 mm rigid
Olympus A5254 0° 10 mm rigid
Olympus A5254 0° 10mm rigid
Olympus A5255 30° 10 mm rigid
Olympus A5257 0° 10 mm rigid
Olympus A5258 rigid 30° 10 mm
operating
operative
Optik rigid
Pilling rigid
REI rigid
Schoelly
Semm rigid
Solos rigid
Storz 26033 AP 0° 10 mm rigid
Storz 26033 BP 0° 10 mm rigid
Storz AP 26003 0° 10 mm rigid
Storz Hopkins
Storz rigid
Stryker
Stryker 380-10 0° 10 mm rigid
Stryker 380-11 0° 10 mm rigid
Stryker 380-12 30° 10 mm rigid
Surgitech
Surgiview
10° operating
3Dscope
VerreScope
VideoHydro
V. Mueller rigid
Weck-Baggish rigid
Weck operating
Weck 0° 10 mm rigid
Weck 110405, 0° 5 mm rigid
Weck 110800 rigid
Wisap
Wolf Lumina rigid
Wolf rigid
Wolf 10/5 (L-angle) operative
Wolf 170 12 mm rigid

laparoscope *(cont.)*
Wolf 7732 rigid
Wolf 8934.40 rigid
Wolf 8937.31 0° 10 mm rigid
0° forward optic
Zimmer rigid
laparoscope camera
laparoscopic adrenalectomy
laparoscopically assisted colorectal resection
laparoscopically assisted sigmoid resection
laparoscopically assisted vaginal hysterectomy (LAVH)
laparoscopic anterior fundoplication
laparoscopic antireflux surgery (LARS)
laparoscopic appendectomy
laparoscopic approach
laparoscopic-assisted procedure
laparoscopic-assisted vaginal hysterectomy
laparoscopic bile duct exploration
laparoscopic biopsy of liver
laparoscopic bladder neck suture suspension procedure
Laparoscopic Bowel Registry
laparoscopic bowel resection
laparoscopic Burch procedure
laparoscopic cardiomyotomy
laparoscopic cholecystectomy ("lap chole")
laparoscopic colectomy
laparoscopic colorectal cancer surgery
laparoscopic common bile duct exploration
laparoscopic contact ultrasonography (LCU)
laparoscopic cholecystectomy
laparoscopic dissection and manipulation
laparoscopic distal pancreatectomy
laparoscopic Doppler probe
laparoscopic duct exploration

laparoscopic esophagogastroplasty with
  Nissen fundoplication
laparoscopic exploration of common
  bile duct
laparoscopic extracorporeal knot
laparoscopic extraperitoneal
  sacrospinous suspension
laparoscopic fundoplication
laparoscopic gallbladder removal
laparoscopic gastric banding
laparoscopic gastrostomy
laparoscopic grasper
laparoscopic Heller myotomy
laparoscopic hernia repair
laparoscopic hernioplasty
laparoscopic herniorrhaphy
laparoscopic intracorporeal ultrasound
  (LICU)
laparoscopic introducer
laparoscopic irrigation pump
laparoscopic jejunostomy
laparoscopic Kittner device
laparoscopic laser-assisted autoaugmentation
laparoscopic laser cholecystectomy
  (LLC)
laparoscopic liver biopsy
laparoscopic lysis of adhesions
laparoscopic micro scissors
laparoscopic myotomy
laparoscopic Nissen and Toupet fundoplication
laparoscopic Nissen fundoplication with
  esophageal lengthening
laparoscopic paraesophageal hernia
  repair (LPHR)
laparoscopic pelvic lymph node dissection and extraperitoneal pelvioscopy
laparoscopic placement of peritoneal
  dialysis catheter
laparoscopic pneumodissection
laparoscopic posterior hemi-fundoplication
laparoscopic radical prostatectomy
laparoscopic repair of paraesophageal
  hernia (LRPH)
laparoscopic retractor
laparoscopic retroperitoneal
  lymphadenectomy
laparoscopic Roux-en-Y gastric bypass
laparoscopic sleeve
laparoscopic surgeon's thumb
laparoscopic surgery for peptic ulcer
  disease
laparoscopic telescope
  30° angle
  0° straight forward
  Storz
laparoscopic Toupet fundoplication
laparoscopic transcystic duct exploration
laparoscopic transcystic lithotripsy
  (LTCL)
laparoscopic transcystic papillotomy
laparoscopic trocar
laparoscopic trocar sleeve
laparoscopic tubal ligation
laparoscopic ultrasound (LUS)
laparoscopic urinary diversion
  procedure
laparoscopic uterine nerve ablation
laparoscopy
  diagnostic
  double-puncture
  hand-assisted
  laser
  needle
  single-port
  single-port, double-puncture
  single-puncture
  THL (Transvaginal Hydro
    Laparoscopy) system
  video
laparoscopy needle (see *needle*)
  Core
  Maciol
laparoscopy under local anesthesia
  (LULA)
LaparoSonic coagulating shears
  for autograft harvesting

laparotomy
emergency
exploratory
mini-
open
second-look
staging
laparotomy (lap)
laparotomy pad cover
laparotomy pad, sponge, and needle counts
laparotomy ring
laparotomy with splenectomy
laparotomy with splenorrhaphy
Lap-Band adjustable gastric banding (LAGB) system
Lap-Band closure tool
lap Nissen (laparoscopic Nissen fundoplication)
lap pad
Lapra-Ty absorbable suture clip
Lapro-Clip ligating clip system
LaproFlator device, Storz
Laprotek
Lap Sac
lap sponge
lap, sponge, and needle counts
lap tape (pad or sponge)
LAP-TAPP (laparoscopic transabdominal preperitoneal) hernioplasty
LAP (leucine aminopeptidase) test
LapTie endoscopic knot-tying instrument
Lap Vacu-Irrigator
Lapwall laparotomy sponge
Lapwall laparotomy sponge and wound protector
LAR (low anterior resection)
LAR/CAA (low anterior resection in combination with coloanal anastomosis)
LARA analyzer
lardaceous degeneration of liver
lardaceous liver
large aperture
large benign thymus gland
large bladder rupture
large-bore bile duct prosthesis
large-bore gastric feeding lavage
large-bore inflow cannula
large-bore I.V.'s (or IVs)
large-bore needle
large-bore rigid esophagoscope
large-bore silicone drains
large-bore slotted aspirating needle
large-bore Tygon tubing
large bowel
large bowel obstruction
large bowel torsion
large bowel volvulus
large-caliber tube
large cell carcinoma
large cell, immunoblastic lymphoma
large-diameter bougie
large-droplet fatty liver
large egress cannula
large gallstone
large hernia defect
large intestine
large intestine gland
large loop excision of the transformation zone (LLETZ)
large luminal diameter
large-needle biopsy
large-particle biopsy
large, noncompressible appendix
large pharyngeal diverticulum
large red kidney
large, refractory hemorrhoids
large sharp curet
large-volume crystalloid and blood resuscitation
large-volume nebulizer
large-volume paracentesis
larger-gauge polypropylene ring
largyneal polyp
LaRoque herniorrhaphy incision
Larrey hernia

Larry probe director
Larry rectal probe
LARS (laparoscopic antireflux surgery)
Larsen tendon-holding forceps
LARSI (lumbar anterior-root stimulator implant)
laryngeal abductor
laryngeal carcinoma
laryngeal edema
laryngeal mirror
laryngeal mirror with handle
laryngoflex laryngectomy tube
laryngopharyngectomy
laryngopharynx
laryngoscope (see *endoscope*)
laryngoscope blade
laryngoscopy, direct
larynx
Las Vegas One-Piece cannula
LAS (lymphadenopathy syndrome)
LASE (laser-assisted spinal endoscopy)
laser
- AccuLase excimer
- acupuncture
- alexandrite (solid-state)
- AlexLazr or AlexLAZR
- Apex Plus excimer
- ArF (argon fluorine) excimer
- argon
- argon/krypton
- argon laser
- ArthroProbe
- Aura desktop ENT
- Aurora diode-based dental
- Aurora diode soft tissue
- biocavity
- Candela 405 nm pulsed dye
- Candela SPTL
- carbon dioxide (CO_2)
- CB erbium/2.94
- Centauri Er:YAG
- CHRYS CO_2
- ClearView CO_2
- CO_2 (carbon dioxide)

laser *(cont.)*
- Coherent CO_2 surgical
- Coherent UltraPulse 5000C
- cold
- Cooper
- copper-vapor pulsed
- CorneaSparing LTK system
- coumarin pulsed-dye
- CrTMHo:YAG crystal
- CTE:YAG (CrTmEr:YAG)
- Derma K
- DermaLase ErCr:YSGG laser system
- Derma 20
- diode
- dye
- Eclipse TMR
- ELCA
- endoscopic
- Epic ophthalmic 3-in-1
- EpiLaser
- EpiTouch
- erbium:YAG (Er:YAG)
- ErCr:YAG
- excimer
- FCPA2 ultrafast
- FeatherTouch CO_2
- Femtosecond laser keratome
- Fiberlase
- flashlamp pulsed dye
- flashlamp pulsed Nd:YAG
- flashlamp-pumped pulsed dye
- Flexlase 600
- “flying spot” excimer
- gallium-arsenid (GaA)
- Genesis 2000
- GentleLASE Plus
- Gherini-Kauffman endo-otoprobe
- Heart Laser (for transmyocardial revascularization)
- He-Ne (helium-neon)
- Hercules Nd:YAG
- HF infrared
- high-energy

laser *(cont.)*
Ho:YAG (holmium:yttrium-argon-garnet) laser
holmium (Ho)
holmium:YAG (yttrium-argon-garnet)
Horn endo-otoprobe
hot
Hyperion LTK
Indigo LaserOptic
ion
Kaplan PenduLaser 115 surgical
Kirsch laser welding technique
KPT
krypton (red)
KTP (potassium-titanyl-phosphate)
KTP/532
LAIS excimer
Lambda Plus dye
Lambda Plus PDL 1 (and PDL 2)
laparoscopic
Laser Lancet
Lasermedic Microlight 830
LaserPen
LaserSonics EndoBlade
LaserSonics Nd-YAG Laser Blade
LaserSonics SurgiBlade
Laserthermia
LaserTripter MDL 3000
Lasertrolysis
LaserTweezers
LightSheer (and LightSheer SC) diode
Lightstic 180 and Lightstic 360
low-energy (LEL)
low intensity laser therapy (LILT)
low-power
LPI (Laser Photonics, Inc.)
LTK (laser thermal keratoplasty)
LX 20
Lyra
Mainster retina
Maloney endo-otoprobe
Max FiberScan
Microlase transpupillary diode

laser *(cont.)*
Microlight 830
Microprobe
midinfrared
Multi-Operatory Dentalaser (MOD)
Nd:YAG (neodymium: yttrium-aluminum-garnet)
neodymium:YAG (Nd:YAG)
neodymium:yttrium-aluminum-garnet (Nd:YAG)
Nidek EC-5000 excimer
NovaLine Litho-S DUV excimer
NovaPulse CO_2
Nuvolase 660
OcuLight
OcuLight SL diode
OLM (ophthalmic laser micro-endoscope)
OmniPulse holmium pulsed
OmniPulse-MAX holmium
Opmilas 144 Plus
Opmilas 144 Plus Nd:YAG
Opmilas CO_2 multipurpose
OtoLam
Palomar E2000 ruby
Paragon CO_2
PDT
Pegasus Nd:YAG surgical
PenduLaser 115 surgical
PerioLase
PhotoPoint
Polaris 1.32 Nd:YAG
Prima
Prostalase
Pulsar CO_2
PulseMaster
PulseMaster Nd:YAG
Pulsolith (coumarin pulsed-dye)
Q-switched neodymium:YAG
Q-switched ruby
red light neon
RevitaLase erbium cosmetic
ScleroLaser
ScleroPlus

laser *(cont.)*
- ScleroPLUS HP
- Selecta 7000
- Sharplan SilkTouch flashscan surgical
- Silhouette
- Silk Laser aesthetic carbon dioxide
- Silk Touch laser skin resurfacing
- Skinlight erbium YAG
- Skinscan
- SLP1000 (super long-pulse) diode
- SLS (Spectranetics laser sheath)
- SLS Chromos 694 long pulse ruby
- soft
- SoftLight
- Softscan
- Spectranetics laser sheath (SLS)
- STATLase-SDL diode endoscopic
- SPTL-1b vascular lesion
- STAR excimer
- stereotaxically guided interstitial
- Surgilase 150
- Surgilase CO_2
- Surgilase Nd:YAG
- THC (thulium, holmium, chromium):YAG
- Topaz CO_2
- Topaz 30 CO_2
- TruPulse CO_2
- 2040 erbium SilkLaser
- UltraFine erbium
- UltraPulse CO_2
- Unica CO_2
- Urolase fiber
- Vbeam
- VersaLight
- VersaPulse
- VersaPulse holmium
- VersaPulse Select holmium
- Versatome
- Visulas Nd:YAG
- VISX excimer laser
- VISX Star S2 excimer
- Vitesse Cos

laser *(cont.)*
- Xanar 20 Ambulase CO_2
- XeCl (xenon-chloride)
- YAG (yttrium-aluminum-garnet)
- YagLAZR or YagLazr
- yttrium-aluminum-garnet (YAG)
- Zeiss Visulas 690s
- Zyoptix

laser ablation
laser-assisted balloon angioplasty (LABA)
laser-assisted laparoscopic cholecystectomy
laser-assisted microanastomosis (LAMA)
laser-assisted microvascular anastomosis (LAMA)
laser-assisted spinal endoscopy (LASE)
laser-assisted tissue-welding technique
laser-assisted uvulopalatoplasty (LAUP)
laser ball retractor
laser biomicroscopy
"Laser Bra" procedure (see *L.I.F.T.*)
laser coagulation instrument
laser correlational spectroscopy (LCS)
laser Doppler flowmetry (LDF)
laser Doppler probe
Laser-Flex tracheal tube
Laserflo blood perfusion monitor (BPM)
Laserflo Doppler probe
laser guard shield
laser hemorrhoidectomy
laser hook
laser image custom arthroplasty (LICA)
laser-induced thermotherapy (LITT)
laser laparoscope
laser laparoscopy
laser laryngeal suction tube
Laser Lancet
laser lithotripsy
laser mammography system
Lasermedic Microlight 830 laser
laser myringotomy

laser nucleotomy
laser photoablation
laser photocoagulation
laser plume
Laser plume filter
laser probe
LaserPen laser
laser reduction mammoplasty
laser scalpel and quartz rod
LaserScissors
laser sclerosis
Laserscope device
LaserSonics EndoBlade laser
LaserSonics Nd:YAG LaserBlade scalpel
LaserSonics Surgiblade
laser stylus profilometer
laser tenaculum
laser tenaculum forceps
laser therapy, OtoLam
laser thermal keratoplasty (LTK)
laser trabeculodissection (LTD)
laser tube
Laserthermia
LaserTripter MDL 3000
Lasertrolysis
LaserTweezers
LaserTweezers 100 (LT100)
laser uterosacral nerve ablation (LUNA)
laser vaporization
laser vulsellum forceps
laser welding
Lasette lancet
Lasette laser finger perforator
Lash hysterectomy technique
lashing suture
Lasix (furosemide)
LAST (large-area sensing technology) imager
Latarjet, nerve of
late hypercapnia
late menopause
latent cancer
latent infection
lateral anterior drawer stress view
lateral bending view
lateral border of rectus sheath
lateral cervical lymphadenectomy
lateral cervical node dissection
lateral cervical spine film
lateral collateral ligament retractor
lateral compression of the iliac crest
lateral crural steal (LCS)
lateral decubitus film
lateral decubitus position
lateral decubitus view
lateral extension of laceration
lateral film
lateral fixation of arytenoid cartilage
lateral flexion and extension C-spine film
lateral gutter
lateral hypopharyngeal pouch (LHP)
lateral incision
lateral internal pelvic reservoir
lateral internal sphincterotomy
lateralizing extremity movement
lateralizing sensory deficit
lateral-lateral pouch
lateral lobe of prostate
lateral oblique fascia
lateral oblique view
lateral park bench position
lateral pectoral nerve
lateral peritoneal reflection
lateral pharyngeal diverticula
lateral reflection of colon
lateral thoracic artery
lateral tilt stress ankle view
lateral to pectoral minor muscle
lateral transverse thigh flap
lateral umbilical fold
lateral utility incision
lateral view
late stoma closure
latex allergy
latex fixation test

latex-free
latex hood
latex O ring (for ligator)
latex sclerosant
latissimus dorsi flap
latissimus dorsi island flap
latissimus dorsi muscle
latissimus dorsi myocutaneous flap
LATS (long-acting thyroid-stimulating) hormone
Latzko vesicovaginal fistula repair
Laubry-Soulle syndrome
Laufe forceps
LAUP (laser-assisted uvulopalatoplasty)
Laurence-Moon-Bardet-Biedl syndrome
Lauren classification of gastric carcinoma
Laurer forceps
lavage
  abdominal
  colonic
  copious peritoneal
  gastric
  iced saline
  PEG (polyethylene glycol)
  peritoneal
  ThermoChem-HT
lavage and suction
LAVH (laparoscopically assisted vaginal hysterectomy)
lavoltidine succinate
law, Courvoisier
Lawrence Add-A-Cath
Laws gastroplasty with Silastic collar-reinforced stoma
Lawson Tait perineorrhaphy scissors
Lawson-Thornton plate
laxative
  anthracene-type
  bulk
  bulk-forming
  contact
  emollient
  lubricant

laxative *(cont.)*
  osmotic
  saline
  stimulant
laxative abuse
laxative abuser
layer
  anatomical
  aponeurotic
  basal
  concentric
  dermal
  fascial
  mucosal
  muscular
  seromuscular
  serosal
  subcutaneous
  subcuticular
  submucosal
layered pattern
Lazaro da Silva continent perineal colostomy creation technique
Lazarus-Nelson pneumoperitoneum technique
lazy H incision
lazy S incision
lazy Z incision
LC-DCP plate
LCAD (long-chain acyl-CoA dehydrogenase deficiency)
L-Cath peripherally inserted neonatal catheter
L cell
LCHAD (long chain 3-hydroxyacyl-coenzyme A dehydrogenase deficiency)
LCIS (lobular carcinoma in situ)
LCMV (lymphocytic choriomeningitis virus)
LCS (laser correlational spectroscopy)
LCS (lateral crural steal)
LCT (long chain triglycerides)

LCU (laparoscopic contact ultrasonography)
L-curved incision
LDF (laser-Doppler flowmetry) probe
LDH (lactate dehydrogenase)
LDH (serum lactate dehydrogenase)
LDH-isoenzyme 5
L-diamond electrode
LDL (low-density lipoprotein)
LDL cholesterol
LDL/HDL ratio
LDS digital scanner
LDS stapler
LDS surgical stapler
Le Dentu suture
LE arterial insufficiency ulcer
lead colic
lead-filled mallet
lead pipe appearance
lead pipe colon
lead poisoning
Lead hand
Leadbetter-Politano ureterovesicoplasty
leading bar
leading cord method of colonofiberoscopy
Leading Lady breast prosthesis
leaflet retractor
leak, leakage
  anastomotic
  bile
  pancreatic
  stomal
leakage of cyst
leakage of tracer
leaky gut syndrome
lean body mass
leapfrog position
leather bottle stomach
Leatherman hook
leaves of diaphragm
leaves of mesentery
LeBag ileocolic urinary reservoir
Lebsche knife
Lebsche rongeur
Lebsche saw guide
Lebsche sternum knife
Lebsche wire saw
lecithin
lecithin synthesis, impaired
Lecythophora hoffmannii
Lecythophora mutabilis
LeDuc anastomosis
LeDuc-Camey ileocolostomy
LeDuc-Camey ileocystoplasty
Lee bone graft
leeches (*Hirudo medicinalis*)
Leech Wilkinson cannula
Lee cutting biopsy needle
Lee microvascular clamp
LEEP (loop electrosurgical excision procedure)
Lees artery forceps
Lee-White clotting time
Lee-White coagulation time
Lefferts rib shears
LeFort urethral sound
LeFort uterine prolapse repair
left adrenal vein
left arm weakness
left colic artery
left colon
left colonic flexure
left-cutting knife
left decubitus position
left gastric artery
left gastroepiploic artery
left gastroepiploic vein
left gutter
left hepatic artery
left hepatic duct
left hepatic lobectomy
left hepatic vein (LHV)
left internal mammary artery (LIMA)
left lateral decubitus abdominal film
left lateral decubitus position
left lobe
left lobe of liver

left lobe of thyroid
left lower quadrant (LLQ)
left pleural effusion
left pneumothorax
left renal vein
left shift
left-sided colitis
left-sided congestive heart failure
left-sided lesion
left-sided nail
left-sided segmental portal stenosis
left-sided ulcerative colitis
left subdiaphragmatic space
left supraclavicular fossa
left-to-right subtotal pancreatectomy
left upper outer quadrant
left upper quadrant (LUQ)
leg of suture
Leibinger 3-D plate
Leibinger Micro Dynamic mesh graft
Leibinger Micro Plus plate
Leibinger Micro System cranial fixation plate
Leibinger Micro System plate-holding forceps
Leibinger Micro System pliers
Leica Aristoplan laser-scanning microscope
Leigh disease
Leiner disease
leiomyoma (pl. leiomyomata)
  epithelioid
  esophageal
  gastric
  uterine
leiomyosarcoma
  gastric
  renal
  small intestine
Leishmania brasiliensis
Leishmania donovani
Leishmania tropica
leishmaniasis
Lejeune thoracic forceps
LeJour technique of reduction mammoplasty
LeJour-type breast reduction, modified
Leksell cobalt-60 gamma knife
Leksell Gamma knife
Leksell laminectomy rongeur
Leksell rongeur
Leksell rongeur forceps
Leksell-Stille thoracic rongeur
Leland-Jones vascular clamp
LEL (low-energy laser)
LeMaitre biliary catheter
Lembert suture
Lemmon rib contractor
Lempert bone rongeur
Lempert fine curette
Lempert malleus cutter
Lempert narrow elevator
Lempert paracentesis knife
Lempert periosteal elevator
Lempert rongeur
Lempert rongeur forceps
lenercept tumor necrosis factor (TNF)
lengthening, esophageal
Lennhoff sign
Lente Iletin II (insulin zinc [pork])
Lente Insulin
Lente L (insulin zinc [pork])
lenticular carcinoma
lentigo maligna melanoma
lentigo-polypose-digestive syndrome
Leonard Arm pneumatic action support device
Leonard catheter
Leo test
LE (lupus erythematosus) panniculitis
Lepley-Ernst tube
leptomeningeal carcinoma
leptospiral jaundice
leptospirosis
  icteric
  icterohemorrhagic
LeRoy clip-applying forceps
LES (lower esophageal sphincter)
  pressure

LES incompetence
LESA (lower esophageal sphincter
  augmentation)
Leser-Trelat sign
Lesgaft hernia
Lesgaft space
Lesgaft triangle
lesion
  acanthotic
  accessible
  acquired
  aneurysmal
  angiocentric immunoproliferative
  angulated
  aortic arch
  aphthous-type
  apple-core
  areolar
  Armanni-Ebstein
  atherosclerotic
  Baehr-Lohlein
  Bankart
  benign lymphoepithelial
  benign pigmented
  bifurcation
  bird's nest
  blastic
  bleeding
  Blumenthal
  Bracht-Wachter
  bull's-eye
  calcified
  cardiac valvular
  caviar
  central
  cherry-red endobronchial lesion
    of Kaposi sarcoma
  choristoma
  circular cherry-red
  coin
  complex
  concentric
  congenital
  constrictive

lesion *(cont.)*
  coronary artery
  Councilman
  critical
  cryosurgical
  culprit
  cystic
  de novo
  depigmented
  Dieulafoy
  diffuse
  discrete
  duct
  Duret
  Ebstein
  eccentric
  eccentric restenosis
  endobronchial
  enlarging cystic
  erythematous
  extrinsic
  fingertip
  flat
  florid duct
  flow-compromising
  flow-limiting
  fluctuant
  focal
  Forrest gastroduodenal
  freckle-like
  friable
  Ghon primary
  gross
  hamartomatous
  hemodynamically significant
  high-grade
  high-grade obstructive
  hilar
  Hill-Sachs
  histologic
  hourglass-shaped
  hyperplastic
  ileal
  impaction

lesion *(cont.)*
indiscriminate
infiltrating
inflammatory
intracranial mass
intrinsic stenotic
invasive
irritative
Janeway
jet
left-sided
lichenoid
linear cutaneous
local
Löhlein-Baehr
lower motor neuron
lymphoepithelial
lytic
macroscopic multicentric
malignant
Mallory-Weiss
mesenteric vascular
microscopic multicentric
mixed
molecular
mongolian spotlike
multifocal
multiverrucous friable
napkin-ring
napkin-ring annular
necrotic
nodular
noninfective endocardial
occlusive
occult
onion scale
onionskin
organic
ostial
oval cherry-red raised
papillary
papular
papulonecrotic
partial

lesion *(cont.)*
peripheral
photon-deficient
pigmented (melanotic)
pigmented satellite
polypoid
precancerous
precursor
premalignant
preneoplastic intraductal
primary
punctate keratotic
purpuric
purulent
radial sclerosing
raised, slightly pigmented
regurgitant
rheumatic
right-sided
ring-wall
satellite
scirrhous
secondary
segmental
serial
sessile
skin
skip
solitary
space-occupying
spherical
squamous anal intraepithelial
squamous intraepithelial
stenotic
structural
subtotal
supranuclear
suspicious
systemic
tandem
target
telangiectatic
tight
tortuous

lesion *(cont.)*
- total
- traumatic
- trophic
- tuberculoid
- tubular
- type A, B, or C
- ulcerated
- ulcerative
- unstable
- upper motor neuron
- valvular regurgitant
- vascular
- vasculitic
- vegetative
- vulvar
- wire-loop

LESP (lower esophageal sphincter pressure)
lesser curvature of stomach
lesser curvature ulcer
lesser esophageal sphincter (LES)
lesser multangular bone
lesser omentum
lesser palatine artery
lesser palatine foramina
lesser palatine nerve
lesser pancreas
lesser peritoneal sac
lesser sac of peritoneal cavity
Lester Martin modification of Duhamel operation
Lester muscle forceps
lethal neoplasm
lethargy
Letournel plate
letrazuril
letrozole
leucine aminopeptidase (LAP) test
leucine-induced hypoglycemia
leucovorin and fluorouracil
leukapheresis, ALPS (autologous l., processing, and storage)
leukemia
Leukine (sargramostim)
leukocyte, fecal
leukocytic infiltrate
leukocytosis
leukopenia
leukoplakia
- esophageal
- hairy
- oral

leukotrienes
LeuTech infection imaging agent
LeuTech radiolabeled antibody kit
LeuTech radiolabeled imaging agent
leuvectin
levamisole HCl
Levaquin (levofloxacin)
levator ani muscle
levator ani syndrome
levator muscle imbrication
levator span
Levbid (hyoscyamine sulfate)
LeVeen catheter
LeVeen inflator
LeVeen peritoneal shunt
LeVeen valve
level
- air-fluid
- Albarran deflecting
- blood glucose
- CA 19-9
- metabolite
- plasma glucose
- serum complement
- serum transaminase
- suppressed thyrotropin

level I axillary lymph node (low; lateral to pectoral minor)
level II axillary lymph node (middle; deep to pectoral minor)
level III axillary lymph node (high; medial to pectoral minor)
level of cricoid cartilage
level of fluid
level of nipple

Levin tube
levobupivacaine
levofloxacin
Levo-T (levothyroxine sodium)
Levothroid (levothyroxine sodium)
levothyroxine sodium (T_4)
Levovist ultrasound contrast agent
Levoxyl (levothyroxine sodium)
Levsin PB drops (hyoscyamine sulfate; phenobarbital; alcohol)
Levsin/SL (hyoscyamine sulfate)
Levsin with Phenobarbital (hyoscyamine sulfate; phenobarbital)
Levsinex (hyoscyamine sulfate)
Levsinex Timecaps
Levulan photodynamic therapy (PDT)
levulose test
Lewin bone-holding clamp
Lewin bone-holding forceps
Lewin spinal-perforating forceps
Lewis laryngeal tube
Lewis laryngectomy tube
Lewis nail
Lewis periosteal elevator
Lewis periosteal rasp
Lewis rasp
Lewis-Tanner subtotal esophagectomy and reconstruction
Lewy-Holinger Teflon injection needle
Lewy-Rubin Teflon glycerine mixture injection needle
Lewy Teflon glycerine mixture syringe
Lexan quick connect
Lexer chisel
Lexer gouge
lexipafant
Lexirin
Leyden disease
Leyla brain retractor
LFT (liver function test)
LGT laryngectomy tube
LGV (lymphogranuloma venereum)
LHMT (low-range heparin management test)
L hook knife
LHP (lateral hypopharyngeal pouch)
LHV (left hepatic vein)
Li, Lm, Ls location of esophageal varices
liarozole fumarate
Liazal (liarozole fumarate)
liberator elevator
libido, decreased
Librax
LICA (laser image custom arthroplasty)
Lich-Gregoire kidney transplant surgery
Lich ureteral implantation in transplantation surgery
lichenoid lesion
lichenoid papule
lichen planus
Lichtenberg needle
Lichtenstein hernia repair
Lichtenstein Hernia Institute
Lichtenstein herniorrhaphy
Lichtenstein onlay patch repair
Licox monitoring device
LICU (laparoscopic intracorporeal ultrasound)
Liddle aorta clamp
lidocaine topical anesthetic
Lidoject-2 (lidocaine HCl)
LIE (latissimus dorsi, iliac crest, external oblique)
Lieberkühn (Lieberkuehn)
Lieberkühn crypt
Lieberkühn gland
lienogastric ligament
lienorenal ligament
lienteric diarrhea
lienteric stool
life expectancy, limited
lifelong constipation
lifelong obesity
lifelong suppressive therapy
LIFE OxygenPac
LifeShirt monitoring system
Lifestream coronary dilatation catheter

Lifestream Personal Cholesterol
  Monitor
life-threatening
lift-and-cut biopsy
L.I.F.T. (laser-assisted internal fabrication) of breast (see *Laser Bra*)
Ligaclip clip applier
ligament
  anterior cruciate (ACL)
  Berry
  cholecystoduodenal
  Cooper
  coronary
  Dacron synthetic
  external
  falciform
  femoral
  gastrocolic
  gastrodiaphragmatic
  gastrohepatic
  gastrolienal
  gastropancreatic
  gastrophrenic
  gastrosplenic
  Grayson
  hepatic
  hepatocolic
  hepatocystocolic
  hepatoduodenal
  hepatoesophageal
  hepatogastric
  hepatogastroduodenal
  hepatophrenic
  hepatorenal
  hepatoumbilical
  Hesselbach
  Huschke
  ilioinguinal
  iliopectineal
  inguinal
  interfoveolar
  lacunar
  lienorenal
  Mackenrodt

ligament *(cont.)*
  Meckel
  median arcuate
  mucosal suspensory
  phrenicocolic
  phrenicoesophageal
  phrenoesophageal
  phrenogastric
  Poupart
  pubocervical
  reflecting edge of
  reflected portion of
  round
  sheath
  shelving edge of
  splenic
  splenocolic
  splenorenal
  suspensory breast
  synthetic
  superior pubic
  thyrothymic
  Treitz
  triangular
  umbilical
ligament of Berry
ligament of Treitz
ligament reflecting edge
ligament shelving edge
ligament sizing tube
ligaments were clamped, cut, and
  suture-ligated
ligamentum arteriosum
ligamentum flavum forceps
ligamentum gastrocolicum
ligamentum gastrolienale
ligamentum gastrophrenicum
ligamentum gastrosplenicum
ligamentum teres
ligamentum teres cardiopexy fundoplication
ligamentum venosum
ligand adhesive
Ligapack ligating reel

LigaSure vessel sealing system
Ligat test
ligated
  circumferentially
  doubly
  staple
  suture serially
ligation
  artery
  band (of esophageal varices)
  Barron
  direct
  Doppler-guided hemorrhoid artery
    (DGHAL)
  early, of venous drainage
  elastic band (EBL)
  endoscopic
  high
  hypogastric artery
  laparoscopic artery
  rubber band, of hemorrhoid
  stump
  transesophageal
  transgastric
ligation hemorrhoidectomy
ligation of branches
ligation of coronary vein
ligation of Wharton duct
ligator
  Arrequi laparoscopic knot pusher
  Barron hemorrhoidal
  Ford-Dixon hemorrhoid
  Injection Superview Speedband
  latex O rings
  Lurz hemorrhoidal suction
  McGivney hemorrhoidal
  Olympus
  rubber band
  rubber band hemorrhoidal
  Rudd-Clinic hemorrhoidal
  Rudd hemorrhoid
  St. Mark's hemorrhoidal
  Suture Lok
ligature (see also *suture*)
  elastic
  Endoloop
  free-tie
  individual
  interlocking
  popliteal vein
  pursestring
  rubber band
  silk
  stick-tie
  suture
  tape
ligature guide (see *guide*)
ligature-holding forceps (see *forceps*)
ligature needle (see *needle*)
ligature scissors (see *scissors*)
light
  Knifelight
  Pelosi Illuminator
  xenon endoscopic
light and dark blue braided stainless
  steel
lighted instrument guide and carrier
lighted retractor
light gray stool
light microscopy
light-scattering spectroscopy
LightSheer diode laser
LightSheer SC diode laser
Lightstic 180 (and 360) fiberoptic
  medical laser diffuser
ligneous thyroiditis
lignocaine
liguid nitrogen cryotherapy
LIH (Lars Ingvar Hansson) hook pin
Lillehei valve forceps
Lillie intestinal forceps
LILT (low-intensity laser therapy)
LIMA (left internal mammary artery)
  graft
LIMA-Lift
LIMA-Loop

LIMAvator chest wall retractor
limb
  afferent
  blind
  suture
  efferent
  jejunal
  Roux
  Roux-en-Y jejunal
limb stump
limbs of the thymus
limit dextrinosis
limited hemorrhoidectomy
limited life expectancy
limited pancreatectomy
limited view
limiting plate
Limitrol-DM
Limulus amoebocyte lysate (LAL)
  chromogenic endotoxin assay
limy bile
Linatrix suture
Lincoln-Metzenbaum scissors
Lincoln scissors
Lindholm tracheal tube
Lindorf lag screw or position screw
Lindvall-Stille knife
line
  anorectal
  anterior axillary
  arcuate
  arterial
  axillary
  blood outflow
  Cantlie
  central
  central venous pressure (CVP)
  dentate
  embryological
  gas density
  Hampton
  iliopectineal
  incision
  indwelling arterial
line *(cont.)*
  interspinous
  intravenous (I.V., IV)
  jugular
  Langer
  mammary milk
  midaxillary
  milk
  mucocutaneous
  pectinate
  pubic hair
  pubococcygeal
  radiopaque
  Rex-Cantli-Serege
  Richter-Monroe
  semilunar
  skin
  Spigelian
  staple
  subclavian
  suture
  Toldt
  transpyloric
  white
  Z
linea alba
linea nigra
linear calcification
linear cutaneous lesion
linear erosion
linear stapler
linear stapling device
linear streak en face
linear ulcer
linea semilunaris
line of Toldt
linezolid
lingual frenum
lingual goiter
lingual papilla
lingual thyroid
lingual tonsil
linguine sign
lining, endothelial

linitis plastica
Linnartz intestinal clamp
lint-free drape
Linton-Nachlas tube
Linton shunt
Linvatec autoclavable camera
Linvatec driver
Linvatec laparoscope
Linvatec microdebrider
Linvatec rigid laparoscope
Linvatec 7570R 0° 10 mm rigid laparoscope
lion forceps
lion-jaw forceps
liothyronine sodium
liotrix
lip lift
lip shave
lipancreatin
lipase (also see *enzyme*)
    pancreatic
    serum
lipase enzyme
lipase test for liver function
lipemia, alimentary
lipid emulsion
lipid infusion
lipid island
lipid-laden hepatocytes
lipid panel
lipid profile
lipidosis, cerebroside
lipids, serum
lipiodol CT
Lipisorb nutritional therapy
Lipitor (atorvastatin calcium)
lipoatrophic diabetes
lipoblastic sarcoma
lipodystrophy, intestinal
lipofuscin
lipolytic enzyme
lipoma
    cord
    hernial
    pancreatic
lipoma of spermatic cord
lipomatosis of pancreas, congenital
lipomatous ileocecal valve
lipomatous-like tissue
lipomatous polyp
lipopolysaccharide binding protein (LBP)
lipopolysaccharide (LPS) receptor
lipoprotein
    high-density (HDL)
    low-density (LDL)
    very low-density (VLDL)
lipoprotein X level
liposarcoma
liposhaver
liposome encapsulated doxorubicin citrate complex
Lipostructure technique
Liposyn II fat emulsion solution
liquefaction necrosis
liquefied argon gas
LiquiBand topical wound-closure glue
Liqui-Char (activated charcoal)
Liqui-Coat HD (barium sulfate)
liquid antacid
Liquiderm liquid adhesive bandage
liquid diarrhea
liquid diet
liquid food dysphagia
liquid material
Liqui-Doss (mineral oil)
liquid stools
Lister bandage scissors
Lister bougie
Lister scissors
Lister sinus forceps
Liston amputation knife
Liston bone cutter
Liston bone-cutting forceps
Liston bone rongeur
Liston forceps
Liston-Key bone-cutting forceps
Liston-Key-Horsley rib shears
Liston-Littauer bone rongeur

Liston-Littauer bone-cutting forceps
Liston phalangeal knife
Liston-Stille bone-cutting forceps
lithiasis, hepatic
lithiumogenic goiter
lithogenic bile
lithogenicity of bile
litholysis
Lithospec intracorporeal lithotriptor
Lithostar lithotripor
Lithostar multiline lithotripsy system
Lithostar nonimmersion lithotriptor
lithotomy position
lithotripsy
  coumarin green tunable dye laser
  electrohydraulic (EHL)
  extracorporeal shock-wave (ESWL)
  intracorporeal shock-wave (ISWL)
  laser
  mechanical
  percutaneous
  percutaneous transhepatic choledo-
    choscopic electrohydraulic
  through-the-scope mechanical
  tunable dye laser
  ultrasonic
lithotripsy bath
lithotripter (see *lithotriptor*)
lithotriptor (also lithotripter)
  American Endoscopy mechanical
  Browne pneumatic impactor
  Calcutript
  Circon-ACMI electrohydraulic
  computerized
  DoLi S extracorporeal shock-wave
  Dornier gallstone
  Dornier HM3 waterbath
  Dornier HM4
  electrohydraulic
  extracorporeal piezoelectric (EPL)
  Genestone 190
  intracorporeal shock-wave
  laser
  Lithospec intracorporeal

lithotriptor *(cont.)*
  Lithostar multiline lithotripsy system
  Lithostar nonimmersion
  LT.01, LT.02 piezoelectric
  Medstone STS
  Medstone STS-T transportable
    lithotripsy system
  Modulith SL 20
  Olympus
  Piezolith-EPL (extracorporeal
    piezoelectric lithotriptor)
  Pulsalith
  Sonolith 3000
  Sonolith 4000+
  Sonolith Praktis
  Swiss lithoclast
  Technomed Sonolith 3000
  Wilson-Cook mechanical
lithotriptor gantry system
lithotrite
litmus milk test
LITT (laser-induced thermotherapy)
Littauer-Liston bone-cutting forceps
Littauer stitch scissors
Littauer-West rongeur
Littleford-Spector introducer
Littler dissecting scissors
Little retractor
Little trimmer
Littlewood tissue forceps
Littmann Cardiology III stethoscope
Littmann Classic II S.E. stethoscope
Littmann Master Cardiology stetho-
  scope
Littmann Master Classic II stethoscope
littoral cell angioma
Littré hernia
Litwak cannula
Litwak left atrial-aortic bypass
Litwak mitral valve scissors
liver
  acute fatty, of pregnancy
  albuminoid
  alcoholic cirrhotic

liver *(cont.)*
alcoholic fatty
ballotable
bare area of
biliary cirrhotic
black
blue
brimstone
bronze
cadaveric
capsule of
cardiac impression on
caudate lobe of
centrilobular region of
cholestatic
cirrhosis of
cirrhotic
degenerative
degraded
diaphragmatic surface of
dome of
duodenal impression on
echogenic
end-stage
esophageal groove of
fatty
fatty infiltration of
fibrotic
finely fatty foamy
finger fracture of
floating
foamy
frosted
gastric impression on
"golfball"
green
HepatAssist bioartificial
hobnail
icing
infantile
iron
lardaceous
large-droplet fatty
left lobe of

liver *(cont.)*
lobectomy of
metastasis to
nodular
noncirrhotic
nutmeg
pigmented
polycystic
polylobar
potato
pyogenic
quadrate lobe of
renal impression on
right lobe of
sago
shock
shrunken
small-droplet fatty
stasis
sugar-icing
SYBIOL (synthetic bio-liver)
tender
trisegmentectomy of
undersurface of
visceral surface of
wandering
waxy
wedge biopsy of

liver abscess
liver adenocarcinoma
liver allotransplantation
liver and peritoneum biopsy needle
liver and spleen were congested
liver bed, surface of
liver bile
liver biopsy
liver biopsy needle (see also *needle*)
Colapinto transjugular
Franklin-Silverman
Jamshidi
Klatskin
Menghini
Tru-Cut
Tru-Cut/Vim Silverman

liver cancer
liver capsule
liver cell
liver cell adenoma
liver cell plate
liver cirrhosis
liver clotting factor
liver colic
liver death
liver dialysis
Liver Dialysis Unit system
liver diet
liver dullness
liver edge
liver edge was palpable
liver enzyme (glucuronosyltransferase)
liver failure, fulminant
liver flap
liver-flap sign
liver fluke
liver function
liver function profile
liver function test (LFT)
liver impression
liver iron store
liver-jugular sign
liver, kidneys, and spleen (LKS)
liver laceration
liverlike lung
liver lobule, central vein of
liver malfunction
liver mass with central scar
liver meal
liver metabolism
liver metastasis
liver "mets" (metastases)
liver necrosis
Livernois lens-holding forceps
Livernois-McDonald forceps
liver palms
liver panel
liver parenchyma
liver phosphorylase
liver profile
liver regeneration
liver resection
liver reticuloendothelial system function
liver segment
liver span
liver, spleen, and kidneys (LKS)
liver-spleen scan
liver tenderness
liver transplant
liver transplantation
liver trauma
liver tumor
Livewire duo-decapolar steerable
  catheter
Livewire TC ablation catheter
livid
living donor partial hepatectomy
living-related transplant (LRT)
Livingston triangle
LKS (liver, kidneys, spleen)
LLETZ (large loop excision of the
  transformation zone)
Llorente dissecting forceps
Lloyd Davies abdominal scissors
Lloyd Davies knee and leg holder
Lloyd Davies pelvic retractor
Lloyd Davies rectal biopsy forceps
Lloyd Davies rectal occlusion forceps
Lloyd Davies sigmoidoscope set
Lloyd Davies stirrups
Lloyd nail driver
Lloyd syndrome
LLQ (left lower quadrant)
LMA-Unique airway
LMA-Unique disposable laryngeal
  mask airway
Loa loa
load, viral
loader, rubber band
loading cone for McGivney ligator
lobe
  caudate (liver)
  hepatic
  ipsilateral thyroid

lobe *(cont.)*
- lateral
- left
- lower
- median
- pyramidal
- quadrate
- Riedel
- right
- upper

lobectomy
- contralateral subtotal thyroid
- hepatic
- ipsilateral thyroid
- left liver
- partial liver
- right liver
- thyroid

lobucavir
lobular architecture of liver
lobular carcinoma
lobular carcinoma in situ (LCIS)
lobular carcinoma of breast
lobular hepatitis
lobular panniculitis
lobular pattern
lobulated mass
lobulated tumor
lobulation
lobule
local and systemic capillary leak
local anesthesia (see *anesthesia*)
local control
local death
local edema
local epinephrine injection
local infection
local infiltration technique
local invasion by primary lesion
localization-compression grid plate
localization of infection
localization, preoperative
localized abscess
localized bleeding
localized irritation
localized necrosis
localized pain
localized resection
localizing tenderness
localizing test
local lesion
locally invasive tumor
local node
local peritoneal irritation
locating pin
LoCholest Light (cholestyramine resin)
Locilex (pexiganan acetate)
Locke clamp
Locke elevator
locked intramedullary nail
locked suture
locker room syndrome
Lockhart Mummary fistula director
locking loop suture
locking nail
locking pliers
locking suture
lock-stitch suture
Lockwood-Allis intestinal forceps
Lockwood tissue forceps
Lockwood underminer
locomotor
Lo-Contour tube with Murphy tip
locoregional cancer recurrence
locoregional residual disease
loculated fluid
locus of infection
Lofgren syndrome
logroll the patient
Löhlein-Baehr lesion
loin pain hematuria syndrome (LPHS)
lollipop-tree sign (on x-ray)
Lomanate (diphenoxylate HCl; atropine sulfate)
Lonalac feeding
Lonalac powder
London College forceps
Lone Star retractor

long-acting thyroid stimulator (LATS)
long-acting thyroid-stimulating hormone (LATS) test
long axial alignment guide
long axial oblique view
long axis of spleen
long-axis parasternal view
long axis view
long chain acyl-CoA dehydrogenase deficiency (LCAD)
long chain 3-hydroxyacyl-coenzyme A dehydrogenase deficiency (LCHAD)
long chain triglycerides (LCT)
long dolphin-nose grasper
longer-acting anesthetic
longer halflife
Long forceps
long grasping forceps, aggressive teeth, single-action
long grasping forceps, wavy teeth, tissue well, single-action
long intestinal tube
longitudinal esophageal stricture
longitudinal filleting of the pancreas
longitudinal incision
longitudinal muscle contraction
longitudinal myotomy
longitudinal orientation
longitudinal suture
long-limb gastric bypass
Longmire-Gutgemann gastric reconstruction
long-nose retriever snare
Longo hemorrhoidectomy
Lonox (diphenoxylate HCl; atropine sulfate)
long Péan clamp
Longport Digital Scanner (LDS)
long-segment intrahepatic biliary stricture
long segment region
long-standing adenomatous hyperplasia
long-standing stimulation of the thyroid
long splenic pedicle
long taper/stiff shaft Glidewire
long-term duodenobiliary reflux
long-term side effects of chemotherapy
long-term thyroxine therapy
long-term treatment
long thermistor
long thoracic nerve
loop
  afferent
  air-filled
  alpha sigmoid
  bowel
  colonic
  contiguous
  Cutting LOOP
  diathermic
  double reverse alpha sigmoid
  duodenal
  efferent
  gamma transverse colon
  intestinal
  ischemic bowel
  jejunal
  N-shaped sigmoid
  puborectalis
  sentinel
  sigmoid
  smart
  Surg-I-Loop
  vessel
  V+Loop
loop choledochojejunostomy
loop colostomy
loop diuretic
looped cautery
loop electrosurgical excision procedure (LEEP)
loop-end ileostomy
loop esophagojejunostomy
loop forceps
loop gastrojejunostomy
loop ileostomy
loop jejunostomy
loop mattress suture

loop of jejunum, efferent
loop of redundant colon
loopogram
loop ostomy bridge
loop suture
loop-type snare forceps
loop-type stone-crushing forceps
loose stools
loperamide
lopinavir/ritonavir
Lo-Pro tracheal tube
Lo-Pro tube with Murphy tip
LORAD StereoGuide stereotactic
breast biopsy system
Lorain-Levi dwarfism
Lord dilatation of hemorrhoids
Lord hemorrhoidectomy
lordotic view
Lore suction tube and tip-holding
forceps
Lorenz cranial plate
Lorenz PC/TC scissors ultra-sharp
knife
Lorenz shears
Lorna towel forceps
Lortat-Jacob hepatic resection
Losec (omeprazole)
loss of acidic environment
loss of aortic contour
loss of appetite
loss of energy
loss of heterozygosity (LOH)
loss of pulmonary vascular
autoregulation
loss of sigmoid curve
loss of splenic function
loss of urethral tethering
Lotronex (alosetron HCl)
Lottes pin
Lottes triflanged medullary nail
lotus position
Louis mastopexy
Louis plate
Loumanen airway (or Luomanen)
loupe (also see *microscope*)
Berger magnifying
binocular
binocular magnifying
fiberoptic (also fibreoptic)
Heine G series
Heine K series
low-power
Miltex
optical
Scanlan
SheerVision
surgical
loupe magnification
Love-Adson periosteal elevator
Love-Gruenwald alligator forceps
Love-Gruenwald intervertebral disk
forceps
Love-Gruenwald intervertebral disk
rongeur
Love-Gruenwald pituitary forceps
Love-Gruenwald pituitary rongeur
Love-Kerrison cervical rongeur
Love-Kerrison laminectomy rongeur
Love-Kerrison rongeur forceps
Lovelace lung grasping forceps
Lovelace thyroid traction forceps
Love nerve root hook
Love nerve root retractor
Lovenox (enoxaparin)
Love uvula retractor
low amino acid level
low anterior resection (LAR)
low anterior resection in combination
with coloanal anastomosis
(LAR/CAA)
low-calorie diet
low cardiac output
low-compliance hydrostatic balloon
low-contact dynamic compression
(LC-DCP) plate
low-contrast film
low-current electrocautery
low-density lipoprotein (LDL)

low-density beta lipoprotein deficiency
low-dose dexamethasone suppression test
Lowe-Breck cartilage knife
Lowe-Breck meniscectomy knife
low-energy laser (LEL)
lower airway sounds
lower border of the pancreas
lower esophageal sphincter (LES)
lower esophageal sphincter augmentation (LESA)
lower esophageal sphincter pressure (LESP)
lower esophageal sphincter resting pressure
lower gall duct forceps
lower gastrointestinal tract
lower hand retractor
lower leg saphenous vein
lower motor neuron lesion
lower panendoscopy
lower pole of the thyroid
lower respiratory tract smear
lower soft tissue attenuation of the accordion sign
lower tract obstruction
low-fat diet
low-fiber diet
low-grade encapsulated follicular carcinoma
low-grade fever
low-grade malignancy
low intensity pulsed ultrasound
low imperforate anus
low intensity laser therapy (LILT) laser
low intermittent suction
low-level endotoxemia
low lung compliance
Lowman bone-holding clamp
Lowman bone-holding forceps
Lowman-Gerster bone clamp
Lowman hand retractor
Lowman-Hoglund bone-holding clamp
Lowman-Hoglund chisel
low pelvic anastomosis
low pH
low phosphorus
low-pitched bowel sounds
low-power diet
low-power laser
low-power loupe
low-pressure catheter
low-pressure shunt
Low Profile PMV 2001 Purple tracheostomy
low-protein diet
low-range heparin management test (LHMT)
low-residue diet
low-residue feeding
low-resistance fundoplication
low-roughage diet
Lowsium Plus (magaldrate; simethicone)
Lowsley prostatic tractor
low-sodium diet
low-stage disease
low transverse incision
low urethral pressure (LUP)
low urine calcium
low-viscosity fluid
low-voltage harness
LPHS (loin pain hematuria syndrome)
LPI (Laser Photonics, Inc.) laser
LPPS hydroxyapatite adhesive
LPS (lipopolysaccharide)
LPS balloon
LPS Peel-Away introducer
LR (lactated Ringer) solution
LRT (living related transplant)
LRYGBP (laparoscopic Roux-en-Y gastric bypass procedure)
L-shaped incision
L-shaped microplate
L-shaped plate
LSTAT (life support trauma and transport) system
LTD (laser trabeculodissection)

L-thyroxine
LTK (laser thermal keratoplasty)
LT.01 lithotriptor
LT.02 piezoelectric lithotriptor
LTS (Liquid Treatment System)
Lubri-Flex stent
Lucae bone mallet
Lucae dressing forceps
Lucae mallet
Lucae nerve hook
Lucas chisel
Lucas gouge
Lucey-Driscoll syndrome
Luck-Bishop bone saw
Lucké carcinoma
Ludloff incision
Luekosilk bandage
Luer bone rongeur
Luer-Friedman bone rongeur
Luer-Hartmann rongeur
Luer hemorrhoid forceps
Luer-Koerte gallstone scoop
Luer lock
Luer-Lok syringe
Luer retractor
Luer rongeur forceps
Luer trachea retractor
Luer-Whiting rongeur forceps
Lugol solution
Lugol stain
Luhr Microfixation cranial plate
Luhr Microfixation System plate-holding forceps
Luhr Microfixation System pliers
Luhr microplate
Luhr miniplate
Luhr pan plate
Lukens PGA synthetic absorbable suture
Lukens trachea retractor
Lukes-Collins classification of lymphoma
LULA (laparoscopy under local anesthesia)
lumbar anterior-root stimulator implant (LARSI)
lumbar appendicitis
lumbar arachnoid peritoneal shunt
lumbar drain
lumbar epidural abscess
lumbar epidural anesthesia
lumbar hernia
lumbar lamina retractor
lumbar puncture needle
lumbar region
lumbar thecoperitoneal shunt
lumbar vein
lumbocostoabdominal triangle
lumboperitoneal (LP) shunt
lumbosacral fusion elevator
lumen (pl. lumina)
  appendiceal
  bile duct
  bowel
  cystic duct
  duct
  duodenal
  esophageal
  gastroduodenal
  intestinal
  monitoring
  scalloped bowel
lumenal antigen
LumenHance (manganese chloride tetrahydrate) imaging agent
Lumina guidewire
luminal bacteria
luminal colonic pH
luminal diameter
luminal microorganisms
luminal narrowing
lumpectomy and radiation
lumpectomy of breast
lumpiness in breast
lumpy material
LUNA (laparoscopic uterine nerve ablation)

LUNA (laser uterosacral nerve
ablation)
Lund Browder burn diagram, modified
Lunderquist guidewire
Lunderquist-Ring torque guide
Lundh meal
Lundholm plate
Lundh test
lung
- airless
- atelectatic
- bird-breeder's
- black
- cardiac
- cheese handler's
- coal-miner's
- drowned
- dull purple
- emphysematous
- farmer's
- fibrinoid
- fissures of
- grain handler's
- hemorrhagic consolidation of
- hilum of
- honeycomb
- humidifier
- hyperlucent
- hypoplastic
- liverlike
- malt worker's
- mason's
- meat wrapper's
- miner's
- normal gas exchange in
- pigeon-breeder's
- rudimentary
- shock
- shrunken
- silo-filler's
- silver finisher's
- smoker's
- thresher's
- vanishing

lung *(cont.)*
- welder's
- wet
- white

lung abscess
lung adenocarcinoma
lung apex
lung base
lung cancer
lung capacity
lung flukes
lung-grasping forceps (see *forceps*)
lung mass
lung metastasis
lung parenchyma
lung plague
lung retractor
lung root
lung stone
lung tumor
lung tumor resection
lung volume reduction surgery (LVRS)
Luongo hand retractor
LUP (low urethral pressure)
lupoid hepatitis
LUQ (left upper quadrant)
Luque II plate
Luque rod
Luque rod scissors
Luque-Galveston plate
Lurz hemorrhoidal suction ligator
LUS (laparoscopic ultrasound)
Lusk instruments for pediatric
endoscopic sinus surgery
luteinizing hormone
Lu-Tex
Lutkens sphincter
Lutrin photosensitizer
Luttke test
Luxtec fiberoptic system
LVEDP (left ventricular end diastolic
pressure)
LVRS (lung volume reduction surgery)
L-wedge electrode

LX 20 laser
Lycopodium clavatum (club moss)
Lyell syndrome
Lyme disease
LYMErix vaccine
lymph gland
lymph node (pl. lymph node)
(see also *node*)
abdominal
anorectal
appendicular
axillary
celiac
central
delphian
enlarged
femoral
fixed axillary
gastric
gastroduodenal
hepatic
histologic involvement of axillary
iliac
infraclavicular
inguinal
internal mammary
interpectoral
ipsilateral
ipsilateral internal mammary
level I axillary (low; lateral to pectoral minor)
level II axillary (middle; deep to pectoral minor)
level III axillary (high; medial to pectoral minor)
matted axillary
medulla of
mesenteric
pancreaticolienal
pancreaticosplenic
para-aortic
paracolic
pelvic
lymph node *(cont.)*
pericholedochal
perirectal
periumbilical
porta hepatic
prophylactic removal of uninvolved
pyloric
regional
retrorectal
Rotter
sampling of
scapular
sentinel (SLN)
shotty
Sister Mary Joseph
solitary
splenic hilar
superficial inguinal
supraclavicular
Rotter
scapular
splenic hilar
lymph node adenopathy
lymph node dissection
lymph node enlargement
lymph node group, delphian
lymph node metastasis
lymph node resection
lymph node-revealing solution (LNRS)
lymph node survey
lymph vessels of prostate
lymphadenectomy
axillary
bilateral inguinofemoral
mediastinal
lymphadenitis
lymphadenoid goiter
lymphadenopathy
axillary
femoral
infraclavicular
inguinal
supraclavicular

lymphadenopathy syndrome (LAS)
lymphangiectasia
  intestinal
  primary intestinal
  intestinal
lymphangiectatic protein-losing
  enteropathy
lymphangioma
lymphangioma of mesentery
lymphangioma of small bowel
lymphangiomatous cyst
lymphangiosarcoma
lymphangitis
lymphapheresis
lymphatic and hematogenous distant
  metastasis
lymphatic channel
lymphatic compression
lymphatic drainage
lymphatic edema
lymphatic flow
lymphatic fluid
lymphatic invasion
lymphatic medulla
lymphatic obstruction
lymphatic sarcoma
lymphatic spread
lymphatics
  abdominal
  inguinal
  mediastinal
  perirectal
Lymphazurin (isosulfan blue) dye
Lymphedema Alert Bracelet
lymphedema edema
lymphedema, neonatal
lymphoblastoid interferon, human
  (L-IFN)
lymphocele, extraperitoneal
lymphocyte-depleted Hodgkin disease
lymphocyte immune globulin
lymphocyte invasion
lymphocyte, sinusoidal
lymphocytic choriomeningitis virus
  (LCMV)
lymphocytic colitis
lymphocytotoxic antibody
lymphoepithelial lesions
lymphogenous
lymphogranuloma inguinale
lymphogranuloma venereum (LGV)
lymphoid cell thymoma
lymphoid cholangitis
lymphoid hyperplasia
lymphoid polyp
lymphoid tumor
lymphoma
  African Burkitt
  Burkitt
  diffuse
  extranodal T-cell
  follicular
  follicular center cell
  gastric B-cell
  gastric T-cell
  GI tract
  histiocytic
  Hodgkin
  immunoblastic
  infiltrate
  infiltrative
  intestinal
  large cell
  large cleaved cell
  large noncleaved cell
  Lennert
  lymphoblastic
  lymphocytic
  malignant
  mantle cell
  Mediterranean
  mixed lymphocytic-histiocytic
  mixed small and large cell
  nodular
  non-African Burkitt
  non-Hodgkin
  plasmacytoid
  polypoid
  primary GI tract

lymphoma *(cont.)*
  Rappaport classification of gastric
  small cell
  small cleaved cell
  small intestinal malignant
  small lymphocytic
  small noncleaved cell
  stomach
  U-cell
  ulcerative
lymphomatosis, struma
lymphonodular hyperplasia
lymphoproliferative disorder
lymphoproliferative syndrome
lymphosarcoma
lymphoscintigraphy
Lynch syndrome I
Lynch syndrome II
LYOfoam A dressing
LYOfoam C dressing
LYOfoam T dressing
LYOfoam tracheostomy dressing
lyophilized aortic homograft
lyophilized bone graft
lyophilized liposomal delivery system
lypressin
Lyra laser system
Lyrelle patch
lyse, lysed ("adhesions were lysed")
lysis of adhesions
Lysonics handle tubing
Lysonix 2000 soft tissue aspirator
"lytes" (electrolytes)
lytic lesion
lytic virus
Lytren electrolyte solution

M, m

Maalox (aluminum hydroxide; magnesium hydroxide)
Maalox Plus
Maalox TC
Maalox Whip
MAAP scan
MAA shunt fraction
MAb monoclonal antibody
MAb-170 monoclonal antibody
MAC (monitored anesthesia care)
Macewen hernia operation
Macewen herniorrhaphy
Machado-Guerreiro test
Machida choledochoscope
MacIntosh laryngoscope
Maciol laparoscopic suture needle set
Mackenrodt, ligament of
MacKenty periosteal elevator
Mackenzie point
MacLean test
macroaggregated albumin (MAA) lung perfusion scan
macroamylasemia
macrogenitosomia praecox
macroglobulinemia, Waldenstrom
Macrokine (WF10)
macrolobular cirrhosis
macronodular cirrhosis
macrophage function
macrophages, ceroid-laden
Macroplastique implant
macroscopic appearance
macroscopic damage
macroscopic island
macroscopic multicentric lesions
Madayag biopsy needle
Maddacrawler
Madden herniorrhaphy
Madden repair of incisional hernia
Madigan prostatectomy
Madurella mycetomatis
mafenide acetate
magakaryocytosis
magaldrate
Magaldrate Plus (magaldrate; simethicone)
Magalox Plus (aluminum hydroxide; magnesium hydroxide; simethicone)
Magerl screw placement in lower cervical spine
maggots (*Lucilia caesar; Phaenicia sericata; Pharmia regina*)
Magill catheter-introducing forceps
Magill curve
Magill forceps
Magill insulated suction tube

Magill suction tube
Magnacal liquid feeding
Magnalox (aluminum hydroxide; magnesium hydroxide)
Magnatril
MAGneedle controller
magnesia, milk of
magnesium (Mg)
magnesium citrate
magnesium, serum
magnesium sulfate
magnesium trisilicate
magnet, eye
magnetic-controlled suturing (MCS)
magnetic endoscope imaging (MEI)
magnetic positional imaging (MPI)
magnetic resonance cholangiography (MRC)
magnetic resonance cholangiography with HASTE
magnetic resonance cholangiopancreatography (MRCP)
magnetic resonance imaging (MRI)
magnetic resonance mammography (MRM)
magnetic resonance neurography (MRN)
magnetic resonance pancreatography (MRP)
magnetic resonance splenoportography
magnetic susceptibility test
Magnevist (gadopentetate dimeglumine)
magnification, power
magnifying loupe
Magnox (aluminum hydroxide; magnesium hydroxide)
Magnum guidewire
MAGPI (meatal advancement, glanuloplasty, penoscrotal junction meatotomy) operation
Magrina-Bookwalter vaginal retractor
mahogany-colored stools
MAI (*Mycobacterium avium-intracellulare*)
Maingot clamp
main pancreatic duct (MPD)
main route of drainage
Mainstay urologic soft tissue anchor
Mainster retina laser
maintaining equilibrium
maintenance fluids
main tumor
Mainz pouch urinary reservoir
Maison retractor
major crossmatch
major duodenal papilla
major organ injury
major water loss
Maki pylorus-preserving gastrectomy
malabsorption
  congenital lactose
  congenital sucrose-isomaltose
  glucose-galactose
  sucrose-isomaltose, congenital
  tryptophan
malabsorption and weight loss
malabsorption of fats
malabsorption of vitamin B_{12}
malabsorption state
malabsorption syndrome
malabsorptive diarrhea
malaise
malaise and fever
malaria
  acute
  algid
  autochthonous
  avian
  benign tertian
  bilious remittent
  cerebral
  congenital
  double tertian
  dysenteric algid
  falciparum
  gastric algid
  hemolytic
  hemorrhagic

malaria *(cont.)*
induced
intermittent
malignant tertian
nonan
ovale
pernicious
quartan
quotidian
relapsing
remittent
tertian
therapeutic
transfusion
vivax
malarial cachexia
malarial cirrhosis
malarial granuloma
malarial hepatitis
malaria-like illness
malarial knobs
malarial necrosis
malarial pigment
malarial pneumonitis
malaria smear
Malarone (atovaquone/proguanil)
Malassezia furfur
Malassezia pachydermatis
Malcolm-Lynn C-RXF cervical retractor frame
Malcolm-Lynn rongeur
Malcolm-Rand radiolucent headrest
Malcolm-Rand retractor
maldigestive diarrhea
male breast cancer
male gynecomastia
male Luer lock
male reamer
male Undies
Malecot catheter
Malecot drain, two-wing
Malecot drain, four-wing
Malecot gastrostomy tube
malformation
anorectal
arteriovenous (AVM)
congenital cardiac
congenital cavernous of splenic vein
Dieulafoy vascular
malignancy
aggressive
borderline
colorectal
extrahepatic duct
grading of
hematologic
hematopoietic
high-grade
intrahepatic duct
intraocular
low-grade
metastatic
neuroendocrine
pancreatic
primary
prostatic
staging of
thyroid
unresectable
malignancy of extrahepatic ducts
malignancy of intrahepatic ducts
malignant atrophic papulosis
malignant B-cell syndrome
malignant biliary obstruction
malignant carcinoid syndrome
malignant cell
malignant change
malignant degeneration
malignant dysphagia
malignant edema
malignant fibrous histiocytoma
malignant gastrointestinal disorder
malignant glioma tumor
malignant hyperphenylalaninemia
malignant hypertension
malignant insulinoma

malignant jaundice
malignant lentigo
malignant lentigo melanoma
malignant lesion
malignant lymphoma
malignant melanoma
malignant melanoma in situ
malignant melanoma metastatic to heart
malignant mesenchymal tumor
malignant mesothelioma
malignant mole
malignant mucoid adenocarcinoma
malignant neoplasm
malignant nephrosclerosis
malignant neurilemmoma
malignant obstructive jaundice
malignant pheochromocytoma
malignant polyp
malignant teratoma of heart
malignant tertian malaria
malignant thymoma
malignant thyroid nodule
malignant tumor
malignant tumor of thymus gland
malignant ulcer
Malignant dysphagia
Malis angled-up bipolar forceps
Malis bipolar cautery forceps
Malis bipolar coagulation forceps
Malis brain retractor
Malis elevator
Malis irrigation forceps
Malis-Jensen microbipolar forceps
Malis jeweler bipolar forceps
Malis nerve hook
Malis neurological scissors
Malis tube
malleable aluminum shaft
malleable aluminum stylet
malleable blade
malleable hook
malleable metal finger splint bandage
malleable plate
malleable probe
malleable retractor
malleable ribbon retractor
malleable scoop
malleable stylet
mallet (see also *hammer*)
  Acufex
  Bergman
  bone
  boxwood
  cervical
  copper
  Cottle
  Crane
  Doyen bone
  Gerzog
  Gerzog bone
  Hajek
  Heath
  Henning
  Hibbs
  Kirk
  lead-filled
  Lucae
  Lucae bone
  Mead
  Meyerding
  Miltex
  Ombredanne
  Ralks
  Richards
  Rush
  slotted
  Steinbach
  Surgical No Bounce
  Swanson
  Williger bone
  Wolfe-Boehler
mallet deformity
mallet finger
mallet fracture
mallet toe
malleus nipper
Mallinckrodt Laser-Flex endotracheal tube

Mallinckrodt Medical tracheal tube
Mallory body
Mallory-Head rasp
Mallory hyaline body
Mallory-Weiss lesion
Mallory-Weiss mucosal rupture
Mallory-Weiss mucosal syndrome
Mallory-Weiss mucosal tear
Mallory-Weiss procedure
Mallory-Weiss rupture
Mallory-Weiss syndrome
Mallory-Weiss tear
Malmstrom cup
malnourished
malnourishment
malnutrition
  profound
  protein-calorie (PCM)
  protein-energy (PEM)
malodorous fluid
malodorous stools
Maloney bougie
Maloney endo-otoprobe laser
Maloney mercury-filled esophageal dilator
malpighian body
malrotation of intestine
malt worker's lung
Maltsupex (nondiastatic barley malt extract)
Maltz cartilage knife
Maltz rasp
Maly test
Mam drill
mamillary suture
mammaplasty (see *mammoplasty*)
mammary atrophy
mammary calculus
mammary duct obstruction
mammary ductal ectasia
mammary ductogram
mammary dysplasia
mammary galactogram
mammary gland
mammary milk line
mammary ptosis
mammastatin protein
Mammex TR computer-aided mammography system
mammogram, mammography
  annual
  baseline
  bilateral
  computed tomography laser
  computed tomography laser mammography (CTLM)
  contoured tilting compression
  CT laser (CTLM)
  CTLM
  ductographic
  Dynamic Optical Breast Imaging System (DOBI)
  Egan
  GE Senographe 20001 digital
  laser
  magnetic resonance mammography (MRM)
  Mammex TR
  Opdima digital
  Palpagraph
  prebiopsy
  repeat
  scintimammography
  Senographe 2000D digital
  SenoScan
  Softscan laser
  step-oblique
  TDMS (Trex digital mammography system)
  Trex digital mammography system (TDMS)
  xeromammogram
  XMG (x-ray mammogram)
mammogram-guided core biopsy
mammographer
mammographically guided needle localization
mammographic findings

mammographic view
mammography (see *mammogram*)
mammoplasty, mammaplasty
  augmentation
  axillary approach in augmentation
  axillary endoscopic reduction
  BAMBI (breast augmentation mammoplasty by injection)
  "belly button" augmentation
  central cone technique reduction
  "cleavoplasty" augmentation
  "cross-the-heart" augmentation
  en bloc augmentation
  endoscopic-assisted transumbilical augmentation
  endoscopic transaxillary augmentation
  free nipple transposition technique reduction
  Goulian
  inferior central pedicle reduction
  inferior pedicle technique reduction
  inframammary approach in augmentation
  laser reduction
  LeJour technique of reduction
  "mega-pocket" augmentation
  nonrigid technique reduction
  owl incision technique reduction
  pedicle technique reduction
  periareolar augmentation
  reconstructive
  reduction
  short-scar tumescent reduction
  subglandular augmentation
  superior pedicle technique reduction
  superwet reduction
  transaxillary subpectoral
  transumbilical augmentation
  vertical bipedicle flap technique reduction
  vertical reduction
  videoendoscopic augmentation
  wet-technique reduction

mammoplasty *(cont.)*
  Wise areola mastopexy breast augmentation (WAMBA)
  Wise pattern for reduction
MammoSite RTS (radiation therapy system) catheter
Mammotest breast biopsy system
Mammotest Plus breast biopsy system
Mammotome minimally invasive breast biopsy
Mammotome probe
Mammotome ultrasound system
management, palliative pain
Mandibular Excursiometer
mandibular fracture
mandibular gland
mandril set
maneuver
  Colanis
  Duecollement
  Epley
  Heimlich
  Hoguet
  Ko-Airan maneuver
  Kocher
  Mattox
  Mendelsohn
  Mueller
  Pringle
  Valsalva
mangofodipir trisodium
manipulation, transgenic
Mann-Bollman fistula
Mann-Whitney U test (data analysis)
Mannitol
manofluorography (MFG)
manometric assessment
manometric pattern
manometric study
manometry
  anal
  aneroid
  anorectal
  balloon reflex

manometry *(cont.)*
- biliary
- ERCP
- esophageal
- point of respiratory reversal on esophageal
- preoperative esophageal
- rectal
- rectosigmoid
- sphincter of Oddi

Mansfield balloon
M antibody
manual morcellator
manual resuscitator bag
MAO (monoamine oxidase) inhibitor
Maox 42 (magnesium oxide)
MAP (mean arterial pressure)
MAP–CVP/CO (mean arterial pressure–central venous pressure/ cardiac output = systemic vascular resistance)
maple leaf flap
mapping
- anal
- functional anatomical
- intragastric pH

mapping marker
mapping pen
Maquet endoscopy table
marantic clot
marasmus protein-energy under-nutrition
Marathon guiding catheter
Marberger hilar retractor
marble bone pin
Marblen
Marburg virus
M.A.R.C. clip
Marcaine HCl (bupivacaine HCl)
Marcus grading scale for avascular necrosis
Marechal-Rosen test
Marezine
marfanoid body habitus
margin
- clear
- negative
- right costal

marginal artery of Drummond
marginal ulcer
marginal zone of the spleen
margination of white blood cells
marijuana usage
marimastat
Marinol (dronabinol)
Marino transsphenoidal hook
Marin reamer
Marjolin ulcer
marked afterload increase
marked stridor
marked thrombocytosis
marker (see also *genetic marker, tumor marker*)
- CA 15-3 RIA (radioimmunoassay) serum tumor
- Castroviejo
- CEA (carcinoembryonic antigen)
- Freeman cookie cutter areola
- genetic
- hepatitis serologic
- mapping
- methylene blue
- preoperative placement of radiologic
- radioactive-labeled
- radiopaque
- serum
- Sitzmarks radiopaque
- Skinmate
- tumor

marker transit study
Markham-Meyerding hemilaminectomy retractor
markings
- haustral (on x-ray)
- red wale (RWM)

Markov simulation model
Mark II Chandler retractor

Mark II distal femur retractor
Mark II Kodros radiolucent awl
Mark II PCL retractor
Mark II S retractor
Mark II Z knee retractor
Mark IV Moss decompression-feeding
catheter
Markwalder bone rongeur
Markwalder rib forceps
Marlen double-faced adhesive disc
Marlen Gas Relief drainage pouch
Marlen Neoprene All-Flexible faceplate
Marlen Odor-Ban ileostomy pouch
Marlen Solo ileostomy pouch
Marlen Zip Klosed pouch
Marlex band
Marlex graft
Marlex hernia repair
Marlex mesh
Marlex mesh abdominal rectopexy
Marlex mesh rectopexy
Marlex PerFix plug
Marlex plug technique
Marlex polypropylene mesh
Marlex synthetic graft material
Marlow laparoscope
Marlow Primus instrument collection
Marlow rigid laparoscope
Marlow videolaparoscope
Marlow videoscope
Marmine (dimenhydrinate)
maroon-colored stools
Marquardt bone rongeur
marrow purging ex vivo pretransplant
Marseille classification of pancreatitis
MARSpo2 Tech pulse oximeter
Marsupial adjustable belt with
attachable pouch
marsupial pouch
marsupialization of sublingual salivary
cyst (ranula)
Martel clamp
Martin anoplasty
Martin cartilage chisel
Martin cartilage clamp
Martin cartilage forceps
Martin cartilage scissors
Martin cutting needle
Martin-Davis rectal speculum
Martin laryngectomy tube
Martin meniscus clamp
Martin muscle clamp
Martin needle
Martin nerve root retractor
Martin pelvimeter
Martin rectal hook
Martin scissors
Martin sheet rubber bandage
Martin stitch scissors
Martin tissue forceps
Martius flap and fascial sling
Martius graft
Martius labial fat pad flap
Martorell hypertensive ulcer
Maryland dissecting forceps, double-
action
Maryland dissector
MAS (minimal access surgery)
Masimo SET (signal extraction
technology) pulse oximeter
mask anesthesia
mask phenomenon
Mason abdominotranssphincteric
resection
Mason Colly Seel Disc for ostomy skin
Mason gastroplasty
Mason suction tube
Mason vascular clamp
Mason vertical-banded gastroplasty
Mason-Judd suprapubic retractor
mason's lung
mass
abdominal
abdominopelvic
appendiceal
apperceptive
apple-core configuration of
body cell

mass *(cont.)*
- breast
- brittle
- colon
- concentrically laminated
- conical
- cystic
- discrete
- dominant
- dominant breast
- elongated
- encapsulated
- epigastric
- exophytic
- expansile abdominal
- fecal
- firm
- fleecy
- fluctuant
- fluid-filled
- friable
- fungating
- glistening
- groin
- hard fixed (in the thyroid)
- injection
- inner cell
- intra-abdominal
- intramural bowel
- ipsilateral brain
- irregular
- lean body
- liver
- lobulated
- lung
- molar
- molecular
- multilocular
- multinodular
- nodular
- nonthyroidal neck
- painless breast
- palpable
- palpable epigastric

mass *(cont.)*
- palpable retroareolar
- pearly white
- periumbilical
- phlegmonous
- pituitary
- polypoid
- pulsatile abdominal
- recanalization reducible
- rectal submucosal
- red cell
- reddish-brown tumor
- relative molecular
- retroareolar
- retroperitoneal
- right-sided
- right upper quadrant
- sex chromatin
- shiny
- slow-growing skin
- slowly enlarging
- soft tissue
- solid
- spiculated
- stellate
- stonelike
- tigroid

mass effect
Masset test for bile pigment in urine
Massie driver
Massie extractor
Massie II nail
Massie nail assembly
Massie plate
Massie sliding graft
Massie sliding nail
mass infection
massive acid secretion
massive bleeding
massive blood transfusion
massive coagulation
massive deposits of glycogen in muscle
massive embolism
massive fluid resuscitation

massive genital prolapse
massive hemorrhage
massive hemothorax
massive hepatic necrosis
massive ischemic necrosis
massive lower GI bleeding
massive pneumonia
massive pulmonary embolus
massive pulmonary hemorrhagic edema
massive splenic trauma
mass lesion
mass of congealed blood
Masson needle holder
Masson needle holder with tungsten
  carbide inlays
mastalgia
mast cell
mastectomy (pl. mastectomies)
  Auchincloss modified radical
  axillary node dissection
  bilateral
  breast-sparing
  complete
  Halsted radical
  lumpectomy
  McWhirter simple
  modified radical
  partial
  Patey modified radical
  preventive
  prophylactic
  quadrantectomy
  radical
  "scarless"
  segmental
  simple
  skin-sparing
  subcutaneous
  total
  two-stage technique of
  Willy Meyer incision for
mastectomy for gynecomastia
master duodenoscope
Masters intestinal clamp
Masters-Schwartz liver clamp
masticator space
Mastin muscle clamp
mastitis
  acute
  benign
  chronic
  chronic cystic
  cystic
  Dahl-Iverson
  diffuse cystic
  granulomatous
  parenchymatous
  periductal
  plasma cell
  postpartum
  puerperal
  tuberculous
mastocytosis, systemic
mastodynia
mastoid retractor
mastopathia chronica cystica
mastopexy
  anchor
  areolar
  augmentation
  Benelli
  Benelli lollipop
  Biesenberger technique of
  breast-lift
  central technique of
  circumareolar
  concentric
  crescent
  donut, doughnut
  double skin
  endoscopic-assisted
  full
  keyhole
  Keystone
  LeJour
  lollipop
  Louis
  modified

mastopexy *(cont.)*
  periareolar
  "purse-string"
  reduction
  Regnault type B
  "round block" technique of
  SAMBA (simultaneous areolar mastopexy and breast augmentation)
  short-scar technique of
  simple
  vertical
  Wise
mastotomy with abscess drainage
MAST trousers
Masuka staging system, modified, for thymic carcinoma
matchstick graft
material
  amorphous
  "anchovy paste" (in hepatic abscess)
  base
  breadlike
  calcareous
  Cellolite patty
  coffee-grounds (CGM)
  collagen hemostatic
  colloid
  contrast
  cross-reacting (CRM)
  Curaderm hydrocolloid dressing
  Cutinova Cavity wound filling
  Cymetra tissue replacement
  cytoplasmic
  Dacron synthetic ligament
  DermAssist hydrocolloid dressing
  DermAssist wound filling
  Dermatell hydrocolloid dressing
  dried out
  Enteryx biopolymer
  eosinophilic
  extracellular (ECM)
  ExuDerm hydrocolloid dressing
  fecal

material *(cont.)*
  fluid
  foamy
  foreign
  functional
  gelatinous
  gel-like
  genetic
  globoid
  gritty
  grumous
  Healos bone-grafting
  Hedrocel bone substitute
  hemorrhagic
  hemostatic
  homogeneous
  inspissated
  jelly-like
  Kaltostat wound packing
  liquid
  lumpy
  Marlex synthetic graft
  mesh graft
  mucoid
  Multidex wound filling
  myxoid
  necrotic "anchovy paste"
  noncellular
  nonfibrous
  NuDerm hydrocolloid dressing
  polyglactin absorbable suture
  polyglyconate absorbable suture
  PolyWic wound filling
  Prolene suture
  purulent
  radiopaque contrast
  refractile
  RepliCare hydrocolloid dressing
  residual calculous
  Reston hydrocolloid dressing
  sandy
  sarcoplasmic
  semisolid
  SignaDress hydrocolloid dressing

material *(cont.)*
  suture
  thickened
  tissue equivalent
Mathews hand drill
Mathews rectal speculum
Mathieu forceps
Mathieu needle
Mathieu needle holder
Mathieu needle holder with tungsten carbide inlay
Mathieu rasp
Mathieu rectal speculum
Mathieu retractor
Mathieu-TC needle holder
Mathieu trivalve rectal speculum
Matritech NMP22 test kit
matrix, extracellular
MATRIX assay
Matson-Alexander elevator
Matson rib elevator
Matson rib stripper
matted lymph node
Matthew cross-leg clamp
Mattox aorta clamp
Mattox maneuver
mattress suture
mattress-type suture
mature T-tube tract
maturing the stoma
maturity-onset diabetes mellitus (MODM) (now classified as type 2)
maturity-onset diabetes of the young (MODY)
Maunsell-Weir operation
Max FiberScan laser
Max Fine tying forceps
Max Force balloon catheter
Max Force catheter
Maxamine (aldesleukin)
MaxCast tape
Maxidone
maxillary impression
maxillofacial tube
Maxima Forté blood oxygenator
maximal O_2
maximum anal resting pressure (MARP)
Maxolon (metoclopramide)
Maxon polyglyconate monofilament suture
Maxon suture
Maxorb alginate wound dressing
Maxxim Medical
Mayaro virus
Mayfield forceps
Mayfield incision
Mayfield miniature clip applier
Mayfield neurosurgical skull clamp
Mayfield rongeur
Mayfield skull clamp pin
Mayfield temporary aneurysm clip applier
Mayfield three-pin skull clamp
Maylard incision
Mayo abdominal clamp
Mayo abdominal retractor
Mayo-Adams abdominal retractor
Mayo-Adams appendectomy catheter
Mayo-Adams appendectomy retractor
Mayo-Adams spreader
Mayo-Blake gallstone forceps
Mayo clamp
Mayo Clinic system for primary biliary cirrhosis
Mayo-Collins retractor
Mayo common duct probe
Mayo common duct scoop
Mayo common duct spoon
Mayo curved dissecting scissors
Mayo dissecting scissors
Mayo dressing scissors
Mayo external vein stripper
Mayo gall duct probe
Mayo gallstone scoop
Mayo-Guyon kidney pedicle clamp
Mayo-Harrington scissors
Mayo-Hegar needle

Mayo-Hegar needle holder with tungsten carbide inlay
Mayo hemostat
Mayo iliac/femoral cannula
Mayo-Lexer scissors
Mayo needle
Mayo-Noble scissors
Mayo-Ochsner suction trocar cannula
Mayo-Péan forceps
Mayo-Robson clamp
Mayo-Robson forceps
Mayo-Robson intestinal forceps
Mayo-Robson position
Mayo-Russian tissue forceps
Mayo scissors
Mayo stand
Mayo sterilizing pin
Mayo-Stille scissors
Mayo straight dissecting scissors
Mayo subclavian cannula
Mayo towel forceps
Mayo trocar-point needle
Mazzariello-Caprini forceps
MB (methylene blue)
MBTS (modified Blalock-Taussig shunt)
MCAD (medium-chain acyl-CoA dehydrogenase) deficiency
MCAD deficiency
MCAG (multiple colloid adenomatous goiter)
MCAS (modular clip application system)
MCAT (modular coded aperture technology) collimator
McBride pin
McBride plate
McBurney appendectomy
McBurney incision
McBurney point
McBurney sign
MCC (mutated in colorectal carcinoma) gene
McCabe canal knife
McCabe-Farrior rasp
McCabe flap knife dissector
McCabe perforation rasp
McCain TMJ cannula
McCain TMJ forceps
McCain TMJ probe
McCain TMJ scissors
McCleery-Miller intestinal clamp
McClintock forceps
McCormick dissector
McCort sign (on x-ray)
McCraw gracilis myocutaneous flap
McCulloch long suction tube
McDonald dissector
McDougal clamp
McDougal prostatectomy clamp
M cell genesis
MCFA (medium chain fatty acids)
McFarland bone graft
McGaw volumetric pump
McGee-Priest wire forceps
McGee wire-crimping forceps
McGhan breast implant
McGhan saline-filled prosthesis
McGill forceps
McGivney grasping forceps
McGivney hemorroidal ligator
McGivney hemorrhoid forceps
McGlamry elevator
MCH (mean corpuscular hemoglobin)
MCHC (mean corpuscular hemoglobin concentration)
McHugh facial nerve knife
McHugh flap knife
McIndoe bone rongeur
McIndoe diathermy forceps
McIndoe dressing forceps
McIndoe rongeur forceps
McIndoe scissors
McIntosh laryngoscope blade
McIvor blades
McIvor mouth gag
McKee tri-fin nail
McKeever cartilage knife
McKenty rasp

McKenzie brain clip forceps
McKenzie clip-applying forceps
McKenzie clip-bending forceps
McKenzie clip-introducing forceps
McKenzie clip rack
McKenzie perforating twist drill
McKernan-Adson forceps
McKernan-Potts forceps
McKinley EpM analgesic infusion pump
McLaughlin intertrochanteric plate
McLaughlin modification of Bunnell pullout
McLaughlin nail
McLean pile clamp
McLean-Tucker obstetrical forceps
McMaster bone graft
McNealey-Glassman-Mixter forceps
McNemar test (for ascites)
McPherson forceps
MCS (Magnetic Controlled Suturing)
MCS (mesocaval shunt)
MCT (medium chain triglycerides)
MCTD (mixed connective tissue disease)
MCT oil
MCV (mean corpuscular volume)
McVay classification of groin hernias (types 1-4)
McVay herniorrhaphy
McVay inguinal hernia repair
McWhirter simple mastectomy
M.D. Anderson clamp
M.D. Paramedic Bag
MD-Gastroview (diatrozoate meglumine; diatrozoate sodium)
MDI deliver device
MD-111 bone allograft
MD-60 radiopaque contrast medium
MDR (multidrug resistance) 3 gene
MEA (multiple endocrine adenomatosis) syndrome
MEA type I (Wermer syndrome)
MEA type II or IIa (Sipple syndrome)
MEA type IIB or III (mucosal neuroma syndrome)
Mead bone rongeur
Mead mallet
Meadox Microvel arterial graft
Mead periosteal elevator
Mead rongeur
meal
  barium
  Boyden test
  butter
  double contrast barium
  Ewald test
  fatty
  isotope
  liver
  Lundh
  motor test
  opaque
  pain related to
  retention
  small bowel
  test
mean arterial pressure
mean corpuscular hemoglobin (MCH)
mean corpuscular hemoglobin concentration (MCHC)
mean corpuscular volume (MCV)
mean end-expiratory pressure
mean operative time
mean transit time
meandering artery of Gonzalez
Mears sacroiliac plate
measles virus
measurement test
meat wrapper's lung
meaty appearance
meaty texture
Mebadin (dehydroemetine)
mebendazole
mebrofenin hepatobiliary function test
mecasermin (insulin-like growth factor-1, recombinant human [rhIGF])

mechanical biliary obstruction
mechanical bowel obstruction
mechanical compression of viscera
  by tumor
mechanical dead space
mechanical diarrhea
mechanical duct obstruction
mechanical extrahepatic obstruction
mechanical ileus
mechanical intestinal obstruction
mechanical jaundice
mechanical lithotripsy for bile duct
  stone
mechanically defective sphincter
mechanical obstruction
mechanical small bowel obstruction
mechanical ventilation
mechanism
  antireflux
  deflecting
  deglutition
  feedback
  flap-valve
  Frank-Starling
  host defense
  humeral
  immune
  impaired cellular defense
  pinchcock
  sphincteric
  swallowing
mechanism of injury
mecholyl study
Meckel band
Meckel diverticulectomy
Meckel diverticulitis
Meckel diverticulum
Meckel ligament
Meckel rod
Meckel scan
Meckel space
meclizine HCl
meconium ileus
meconium plug syndrome
meconium-stained amniotic fluid
MECT (multipolar electrocoagulation
  therapy)
Mectizan (ivermectin)
Mectra Tissue Sample Retainer
medications (including pharmaceuticals,
    natural substances, imaging
    agents, and prescription and
    over-the-counter drugs)
  abarelix
  Abbokinase (urokinase)
  acarbose
  Accuprep HPF powder
  Accuzyme enzymatic debriding
    agent
  Accuzyme ointment
  Accuzyme topical enzyme
  Acephen analgesic suppositories
  Aceta (acetaminophen)
  Aceta with Codeine (codeine
    phosphate; acetaminophen)
  acetohexamide
  Acidulin (glutamic acid hydro-
    chloride)
  Aciphex (rabeprazole sodium)
  ACTH
  Actidose Aqua (activated charcoal)
  Actidose with Sorbital (activated
    charcoal; sorbital)
  Actigall (ursodiol-ursodeoxycholic
    acid)
  Actimmune (interferon gamma-1b)
  Actiprep skin preparation
  Actiq (oral transmucosal fentanyl
    citrate) ("lollipop")
  activated attapulgite
  activated charcoal
  Actos (pioglitazone hydrochloride)
  Actron (ketoprofen) pain reliever
  Acutrim
  Adcon-A
  Adcon-C
  Adcon-I
  Adcon-L gel

medications *(cont.)*
Adcon-P solution
Adcon-T/N gel
adefovir dipovoxil
ADEKs multivitamin supplement
ADEKs pediatric drops
Adept (icodextrin)
Adipex-P (phentermine HCl)
Adriamycin (doxorubicin)
Adrucil (fluorouracil)
AERx (morphine sulfate)
AERx electronic inhaler (morphine sulfate)
agalsidase beta
Agoral (mineral; phenolphthalein)
ALA (alpha lipoic acid)
Alamag (aluminum hydroxide; magnesium hydroxide)
Alamag Plus (aluminum hydroxide; magnesium hydroxide; simethicone)
albendazole
Albenza Tiltab (albendazole)
Aldactone (spironolactone)
aldesleukin
Aldurazyme
Alferon N (interferon alfa-n3)
Algicon
alglucerase
Alibra (alprostadil/prazosin HCl)
Aliminase
AlitraQ formula
alitretinoin
Alka-Mints (calcium carbonate)
Alka-Seltzer (sodium bicarbonate; citric acid; aspirin; phenyl-alanine)
Alka Seltzer Extra Strength
Alka Seltzer Gold
Alkets (calcium carbonate)
Allovectin-7 (DNA/lipid complex)
Almacone (aluminum hydroxide; magnesium hydroxide; simethicone)
Aloe Vesta protective ointment

medications *(cont.)*
Alond (zopolrestat)
alosetron HCl
alpha-D-galactosidase enzyme
alpha-galactosidase
alpha lipoic acid (ALA)
AlphaNine
alprostadil
Alprox-TD (alprostadil)
Alramucil (psyllium hydrophilic mucilloid)
ALRT1550 capsules
ALternaGEL (aluminum hydroxide gel)
Altracin (bacitracin)
Alu-Cap (aluminum hydroxide gel)
Aludrox (aluminum hydroxide; magnesium hydroxide; simethicone)
aluminum carbonate gel, basic
aluminum hydroxide gel
aluminum sulfate
Alu-Tab (aluminum hydroxide gel)
ALX-0600
Amaryl (glimepiride) tablets
amber touch-and-heal (St. John's wort)
amifostine
aminoglutethimide
aminosalicylic acid
aminosidine
aminosterol
Aminosyn
Aminosyn M
Aminosyn II
Amitone (calcium carbonate)
Amphojel (aluminum hydroxide gel)
amphotericin B
Ampligen
anakinra
Analpram-HC (hydrocortisone acetate; pramoxine)
ananain
Anaspaz (hyoscyamine sulfate)

medications *(cont.)*
anastrozole
Ancef
Andractim (dihydrotestosterone gel)
Androderm testosterone transdermal patch
Androgel (testosterone)
Androsorb
Angiocidin
AngioMark contrast agent
Angiozyme
anisotropine methylbromide
annamycin
Anogesic (nitroglycerin ointment)
antacid
anthraquinone of cascara
anti-IL-2 receptor antibody
antibiotic
anticholinergic drug
Anticort
antiemetic
Antiminth (pyrantel pamoate)
antiprostaglandin
Antispas (dicyclomine HCl)
Antivert (meclizine)
Antrenyl
Antrocol
Anucort HC (hydrocortisone acetate)
Anumed (bismuth subgallate; bismuth resorcin compound; benzyl benzoate; zinc oxide; Peruvian balsam)
Anusol (pramoxine HCl; zinc oxide)
Anusol-HC (hydrocortisone acetate)
Anvirzel
Anzemet (dolasetron mesylate)
Apo-Domperidone (domperidone maleate)
Apomate radiopharmaceutical imaging agent
apomorphine
Apra (CT-2584 mesylate)
Aptosyn (exisulind)
arbaprostil

medications *(cont.)*
Arco-Lase (amylase; protease; lipase; cellulase)
Arco-Lase Plus (amylase; protease; lipase; cellulase; hyoscyamine sulfate; atropine sulfate; phenobarbital)
Arilvax yellow fever vaccine
Arimidex (anastrozole) tablets
Aromasin (exemestane) tablets
aromatic cascara fluidextract
aromatic cascara sagrada
Aroplatin
arsenic trioxide (ATO)
Arthrotec (diclofenac sodium; misoprostol)
Asacol (mesalamine) delayed-release tablets
ASAP antimicrobial solution
Ascriptin A/D
A-Spas S/L (hyoscyamine sulfate)
Atabrine
Atgam (lymphocyte immune globulin; antithymocyte)
ATO (arsenic trioxide; As2O3)
atorvastatin calcium
atovaquone/proguanil
Atrisol aerosol
Atrocholin
atropine sulfate
attapulgite
Avakine (infliximab)
Avandia (rosiglitazone maleate)
Avelox (moxifloxacin)
Avicidin
Avicine
Avitene Hemostat (microfibrillar collagen hemostat)
Axid; Axid AR (nizatidine)
Axokine (ciliary neurotrophic factor [CNTF])
azathioprine
Azulfidine EN-tabs (sulfasalazine)
BA-EDTA (bile acid-EDTA) solution

medications *(cont.)*
bacitracin
Bactrim
BalAsa (balsalazide disodium) (now Colazal)
balm of Gilead
balmony
Balneol
balsalazide disodium
Banalg
Banthine (methantheline bromide)
barberry (*Berberis vulgaris*)
Barbidonna #2 (atropine sulfate; scopolamine hydrobromide; hyoscyamine hydrobromide; phenobarbital)
Basaljel (aluminum carbonate gel, basic)
Beano (alpha-D-galactosidase enzyme)
becaplermin
Bellacane (atropine sulfate; scopolamine hydrobromide; hyoscyamine sulfate; phenobarbital)
Bellacane SR (belladonna alkaloids; phenobarbital; ergotamine tartrate)
Belladenal
belladonna alkaloid
belladonna extract
Bellafoline
Bell/ans (sodium bicarbonate)
Bellatal (phenobarbital)
Bellergal-S (belladonna extract; phenobarbital; ergotamine tartrate)
Bel-Phen-Ergot SR (belladonna alkaloids; phenobarbital; ergotamine tartrate)
BeneFin shark cartilage powder
BeneFix (coagulation factor IX [recombinant])
bentiromide
Bentyl (dicyclomine HCl)

medications *(cont.)*
benzocaine
benzquinamide
benztropine; benztropine mesylate
Beta LT (beta-alethine)
Betadine (povidone-iodine)
Betadine gel
Betathine (beta-alethine; Beta LT)
bethanechol
Bexxar (^{131}I tositumomab)
Biaxin XL (clarithromycin) extended-release tablets
Bicarbolyte
bichloroacetid acid
bile acid sequestrants
bile salts
bimoclomal
Biofreeze with Ilex analgesic ointment
BioGlue
Bio-Hep-B
biphasic insulin
biphasic isophane insulin
biricodar dicitrate
bisacodyl tannex
Bisco-Lax (bisacodyl)
bismuth subcarbonate
bismuth subgallate
bismuth subsalicylate
bisoxatin; bisoxatin acetate
bithionol
Bitin (bithionol)
Black-Draught syrup (casanthranol; senna extract)
Black-Draught tablets (senna concentrate)
blood mononuclear cells, allogenic peripheral
Blue Goo (Iamin hydrating gel)
Bonine
botulinum toxin
Bouin solution
bovine immunoglobulin concentrate
BrachySeed iodine-125 (^{125}I)

medications *(cont.)*
BrevaRex
bromelain
Bromo-Seltzer (sodium bicarbonate; citric acid; acetaminophen)
bromocriptine mesylate
Brompton's Cocktail
Brompton's Mixture (oral narcotic alcohol solution)
broxuridine
Bucladin-S
buclizine HCl
bucrylate
budesonide
Buffets II (acetaminophen; aspirin; caffeine; aluminum hydroxide)
Bumex (bumetanide)
bupivacaine HCl
Buro-Sol (aluminum sulfate)
Burow solution
Buscopan
busulfan
Busulfanex (busulfan) for injection (now Busulfex)
Busulfex (busulfan)
butenafine
Butibel (belladonna extract; butabarbital sodium)
butyrylcholinesterase
C242-DM1
CA 72–4 gastric cancer antigen tumor marker
cA2 monoclonal antibody
cabergoline
calcifediol
Calcijex (cacitriol)
calcitriol
calcium carbonate
calcium polycarbophil
Calderol (calcifediol)
Calm-X (dimenhydrinate)
Camalox
cambendezole
Camptosar (irinotecan hydrochloride) injection

medications *(cont.)*
Campyvax vaccine
Cancidas (caspofungin acetate)
Candistat-G
Candistroy
cannabinol
canstatin
Cantil (mepenzolate bromide)
capecitabine
capsaicin
Carafate (sucralfate)
carbantel lauryl sulfate
carbonyl iron
Cariel gel
CARN 750 (now CarraVex injectable)
Caroid
CarraVex injectable (formerly CARN 750)
casanthranol
Casec
caspofungin acetate
castor oil
cathartic
Cavilon barrier ointment
CDA (chenodeoxycholic acid)
CDCA (chenodeoxycholic acid)
Cd-texaphyrin photosensitizing agent
CEA-Cide
Cedax (ceftibuten)
cefadroxil
cefazolin
cefdinir
ceftibuten
Ceftin (cefuroxime)
cefuroxime
celandine (*Chelidonium majus*)
Celebra (celecoxib) (now Celebrex)
Celebrex (celecoxib)
CellCept (mycophenolate mofetil [MMF])
CellCept (mycophenolate mofetil)
Celsior organ preservation solution
Centara (priliximab)

medications *(cont.)*
- Ceo-Two (sodium bicarbonate; potassium bitartrate)
- cephalosporin
- Cephulac
- Ceredase (alglucerase)
- Cerezyme (imiglucerase)
- Certican (everolimus)
- Certiva vaccine
- Cetacaine
- cetraxate HCl
- cetuximab
- CharcoAid 2000 (activated charcoal)
- charcoal, activated
- Charcoal Plus (activated charcoal)
- CharcoCaps (charcoal)
- Charcodote
- Chardonna-2 (belladonna extract; phenobarbital)
- Chenix (chenodiol)
- chenodeoxycholic acid (CDCA)
- chenodiol
- Chenofalk
- Chirocaine (bupivacaine; levobupivacaine)
- chitosan
- ChloraPrep One-Step
- Chloresium (chlorophyllin copper complex)
- chlormethazine
- chlorophyllin copper complex (PALS tablets)
- cholagogue
- cholecystokinin
- Cholestagel (now Welchol)
- cholestyramine resin
- Choletec (^{99m}Tc mebrofenin) imaging agent
- choline chloride
- Cholografin Meglumine (iodipamide meglumine)
- Chooz (calcium carbonate)
- chromium (Cr)
- chromium picolinate

medications *(cont.)*
- chromium polynicotinate
- Chronulac (lactulose)
- Chrysalin
- Chymex (bentiromide)
- Cidex OPA
- cilansetron
- ciliary neurotrophic factor (CNTF)
- cimetidine HCl
- Cipro (ciprofloxacin)
- ciprofloxacin
- cisplatin/epinephrine gel
- Citra pH (sodium citrate)
- Citralax (magnesium citrate; magnesium sulfate)
- citrate of magnesia
- Citrocarbonate (sodium bicarbonate; sodium citrate)
- Citrotein
- Citrucel (methylcellulose)
- Citrucel Sugar Free (methylcellulose; phenylalanine)
- CLA (conjugated linoleic acid)
- clarithromycin
- clenoliximab (IDEC-151/SB-217969)
- clidinium
- clidinium bromide
- Clinimix E (amino acid with electrolytes in dextrose with calcium)
- Clinitest
- Clinoril (sulindac)
- Clomycin (polymyxin B sulfate; bacitracin; neomycin sulfate; lidocaine)
- clonidine gel
- clonidine hydrochloride injection
- clorsulon
- clortermine HCl
- closantel
- *Clostridium* botulinum toxin
- Clysodrast (bisacodyl tannex)
- CMV-IGIV (cytomegalovirus immune globulin, intravenous)

medications *(cont.)*
CNTF (ciliary neurotrophic factor)
coagulation factor IX recombinant
Coblation technology
Colace (docusate sodium)
Co-Lav (polyethylene glycol electrolyte solution; electrolytes)
Colax (phenolphthalein; docusate sodium)
Colazal (balsalazide disodium)
Colazide (balsalazide disodium)
colesevelam HCl
Colestid (colestipol)
colestipol
colistimethate
colistin
Collins solution
colloidal bismuth subcitrate
COLO-Vax
Colocort (hydrocortisone enema)
Cologel
Colomed
Colovage (polyethylene glycol-electrolyte solution)
Coly-Mycin M
Coly-Mycin S
Colyte (polyethylene glycol-electrolyte solution)
Combidex imaging agent
combretastatin
comosain
Compazine suppositories (prochlorperazine)
Compleat Modified Formula
Comply
Compro (prochlorperazine)
Comvax (*Haemophilus* b purified capsular polysaccharide; *Neisseria meningitidis* OMPC) (hepatitis B virus vaccine)
conjugated linoleic acid (CLA)
Constilac (lactulose)
Constulose (lactulose)
ConTE-Pak-4 (multiple trace elements)

medications *(cont.)*
Converspaz
Converzyme
ConXn (recombinant human relaxin, H_2)
Cope (aspirin; caffeine; magnesium hydroxide; aluminum hydroxide)
Cordox
coriander
Correctol (bisacodyl)
Correctol Extra Gentle (docusate sodium)
Cortenema (hydrocortisone)
Cortenema retention enema
Corticaine
corticorelin ovine triflutate
corticosteroid
Cortifoam (hydrocortisone acetate)
Cotara
Cotazym; Cotazym-S (lipase; protease; amylase)
Coumadin (warfarin sodium)
counterirritant
COX-2 inhibitor
Cr (chromium)
Creon
Crestor (rosuvastatin)
Cro-Man-Zin (chromium; manganese; zinc)
Cryptosporidium parvum bovine colostrum IgG concentrate
CT-2584 mesylate
CTLA4-Ig monoclonal antibody
CTP-37 theraccine
CTP37 vaccine
CY-1899
cyclizine
cyclophilin
cyclophosphamide
cycloserine (L-cycloserine)
cyclosporin A
CyPat
Cytadren (aminoglutethimide)
cytarabine liposomal

medications *(cont.)*
- CytoGam (cytomegalovirus immune globulin)
- CytoImplant (blood mononuclear cells, allogenic peripheral)
- Cytolex (pexiganan acetate) (now Locilex)
- Cytolex cream (pexiganan acetate)
- cytomegalovirus immune globulin, human
- cytomegalovirus immune globulin, solvent/detergent treated
- Cytomel (liothyronine sodium)
- cytoprotective agent
- Cytotec (misoprostol)
- Cytovene (oral ganciclovir)
- Cytoxan (cyclophosphamide)
- dacliximab monoclonal antibody
- daclizumab
- Dairy Ease (lactase enzyme)
- DairyCare
- Dakin solution
- dalanated insulin
- dalteparin sodium
- danaparoid sodium
- danthron
- daptomycin for injection
- Darbid (isopropamide)
- Daricon PB (oxyphencyclimine)
- darifenacin
- Darvocet-N 100
- dazopride; dazopride fumarate
- DC softgels (docusate calcium)
- DDAVP (desmopressin acetate)
- DDS-Acidophilus
- Debrisan (dextranomer)
- Decholin (dehydrocholic acid)
- decitabine
- Definity (perflutren)
- Degas (simethicone)
- DEHOP (diethylhomospermine)
- dehydrocholic acid
- dehydroemetine
- dehydroepiandrosterone (DHEA)

medications *(cont.)*
- Deliver 2.0 formula
- Demerol
- DENSPM (diethylnorspermine)
- deoxyspergualin
- DepoCyt (cytarabine liposomal)
- DepoMorphine (morphine sulfate)
- Derifil (chlorophyllin)
- DermaFreeze
- Dermol HC (hydrocortisone)
- Dermoplast (benzocaine; menthol)
- Dermuspray (trypsin; Peruvian balsam)
- desmopressin acetate (DDAVP)
- Devrom (bismuth gallate)
- dexamethasone sodium phosphate
- dexanabinol
- Dexatrim
- dexfenfluramine
- dexmedetomidine
- Dexol 300
- dexpanthenol
- dextran 40
- dextranomer
- DHEA (dehydroepiandrosterone)
- DHEA sulfate (DHEAS)
- DiaBeta (or Diaßeta)
- Diacol
- Dialose (docusate sodium)
- Dialose Plus (yellow phenol phthalein; docusate sodium)
- Dialume (aluminum hydroxide gel)
- Diapid (lypressin)
- Diar-Aid (loperamide)
- Diasorb (activated attapulgite)
- diazepam
- Dibent (dicyclomine)
- dibucaine
- diclofenac sodium
- dicyclomine hydrochloride
- diethylpropion
- diethylcarbamazine; diethylcarbamazine citrate
- diethylhomospermine (DEHOP; DEHSPM)

medications *(cont.)*
diethylnorspermine (DENSPM)
difenoximide HCl
difenoxin; difenoxin HCl
DiffGAM
Diffistat-G
Di-Gel (aluminum hydroxide; magnesium hydroxide; simethicone)
Di-Gel Advanced Formula (magnesium hydroxide calcium carbonate; simethicone)
Digepepsin (pancreatin; pepsin; bile salts)
digestant
Digestozyme (pancreatin; pepsin; dehydrocholic acid)
Digibar 190 (barium sulfate for suspension)
Digibar 190 imaging agent
diloxanide furoate
dimenhydrinate
Dinate (dimenhydrinate)
Diocto-C (docusate, casanthranol)
Diocto-K (docusate potassium)
Diocto-K Plus (casanthranol; docusate potassium)
Dioctolose Plus (casanthranol; docusate potassium)
Dioeze (docusate sodium)
Dipentum (olsalazine sodium)
diphenoxylate HCl
Diprivan (propofol)
Diquinol (iodoquinol)
Dirame (propiram)
disaccharide tripeptic glycerol dipalmitoyl
disaccharide tripeptide glycerol tripalmitoyl
Disanthrol (casanthranol)
disodium cromoglycate (DSC; DSCG)
Disolan (phenolphthalein; docusate sodium)

medications *(cont.)*
Disolan Forte (casanthranol; carboxymethylcellulose sodium; docusate sodium)
Disonate (docusate sodium)
Disoplex (carboxymethylcellulose sodium; docusate sodium)
Di-Spaz (dicyclomine)
Dizmiss (meclizine HCl)
DMP 504
docetaxel
docusate calcium
docusate potassium
docusate sodium
DOK (docusate sodium)
dolasetron mesylate
Domeboro powder, tablets (aluminum sulfate; calcium acetate)
domperidone
Donna-Sed (atropine sulfate; scopolamine hydrobromide; hyoscyamine hydrobromide; phenobarbital)
Donnagel (attapulgite)
Donnagel-PG
Donnatal No. 2 (atropine sulfate; scopolamine hydrobromide; hyoscyamine sulfate; phenobarbital)
Donnazyme (pancreatic lipase; protease; amylase)
Donphen
dopamine
Dorbane
Dorbantyl Forte
DOS softgels (docusate sodium)
Dosalax (senna concentrate; alcohol)
Dostinex (cabergoline)
Doxidan (phenolphthalein; docusate calcium)
Doxil (doxorubicin hydrochloride liposome injection)
Doxinate

medications *(cont.)*
doxorubicin hydrochloride liposome injection
D-penicillamine
Dramamine II (meclizine HCl)
Dramanate (dimenhydrinate)
Dramilin (dimenhydrinate)
Dr. Caldwell Senna Laxative (senna concentrate)
Dr. Dermi-Heal (allantoin; zinc oxide; Peruvian balsam)
droloxifene
dronabinol
droperidol
DSC; DSCG (disodium cromoglycate)
DSMC Plus (casanthranol; docusate potassium)
D-S-S (docusate sodium)
D-thyroxine
D-xylose
Dulcagen (bisacodyl)
Dulcolax (bisacodyl)
Dulcolax Bowel Prep Kit (bisacodyl)
DuoDerm Hydroactive (hydrocolloid gel)
Duphalac (lactulose)
Duraclon (clonidine hydrochloride injection)
Duragesic-100 (fentanyl) transdermal patches
Duralone-80 (methylprednisolone acetate)
Duramorph (morphine sulfate)
Duranest MPF (etidocaine; epinephrine)
Dyclone (dyclonine HCl)
dyclonine HCl
dymanthine HCl
dimantine HCl
Dymelor (acetohexamide)
Dymenate (dimenhydrinate)
EchoGen (perflenapent)
Ecotrin

medications *(cont.)*
edrophonium
Effer-Syllium
eflornithine
8-methoxycarbonyloctyl oligosaccharides
Elase (fibrinolysin; desoxyribonuclease)
Eldisine (vindesine sulfate)
Ellence (epirubicin hydrochloride)
Elliott B solution
Eloxatin (oxaliplatin)
Elta wound cleanser
Eltroxin (levothyroxine sodium)
Emdogain
Emete-con
Emetrol (fructose, dextrose, and phosphoric acid)
Emitasol (metoclopramide) nasal spray
emitefur
emulsified perflubron blood substitute
Emulsoil
Endocet (oxycodone/acetaminophen)
Endocodone (oxycodone hydrochloride)
Endodan (oxycodone/oxycodone terephthalate/aspirin)
Endo-Flo irrigation
Endostatin protein
Engerix-B (hepatitis B vaccine [recombinant])
Eno
enprostil
Entero Vu (barium sulfate for suspension)
Entocort (budesonide)
Entocort CR (budesonide)
Entolase
Entozyme
EPC
epinephrine & cisplatin injectable gel

medications *(cont.)*
epirubicin hydrochloride
Epivir (lamivudine)
Epivir-HBV (lamivudine)
epoetin alfa
Equalactin (calcium polycarbophil)
Equilet (calcium carbonate)
Ergamisol (levamisole HCl)
Ergoset (bromocriptine mesylate)
ergotamine tartrate
Esberitox
esomeprazole magnesium
esterified estrogens
Estinyl (ethinyl estradiol)
Estrace (estradiol)
estradiol
Estratab (esterified estrogens)
estrone
Estrone Aqueous (estrone)
Ethamolin (ethanolamine oleate)
ethanolamine oleate
ethinyl estradiol
Ethyol (amifostine)
etidocaine
etoformin HCl
etomoxir
etoposide injection
Euglucon (glyburide)
Evac-Q-Kwik (bisacodyl)
Evac-Q-Mag (magnesium citrate; citric acid; potassium citrate)
Evac-Q-Sert (sodium bicarbonate; potassium bitartrate)
Evac-Q-Tabs (phenolphthalein)
Evac-U-Gen
Evac-U-Lac
Evalose (lactulose)
everolimus
Ex-Lax
Ex-Lax Extra Gentle
Ex-Lax Gentle Nature
Ex-Lax Maximum Relief
Ex-Lax Stool Softener
exemestane

medications *(cont.)*
exisulind
extended insulin human zinc (rDNA)
extended insulin zinc
FABRase (alpha-galactosidase)
Fabrazyme (agalsidase beta)
FAC (ferric ammonium citrate)
factor VIII SQ, recombinant
famotidine
Fareston (toremifene citrate)
Faslodex (fulvestrant)
fedotozine
Feen-A-Mint
fenfluramine
fenoctimine; fenoctimine sulfate
fentanyl citrate (Actiq "lollipop")
Fentanyl Oralet (fentanyl)
fentanyl transdermal patches
Feridex I.V. (ferumoxides injectable solution)
ferric ammonium citrate (FAC)
FerriSeltz (ferric ammonium citrate [FAC])
Festalan (atropine)
Festal II
Fiberall (calcium polycarbophil)
FiberCon (calcium polycarbophil)
Fiber-Lax (calcium polycarbophil)
Fiber-Norm (calcium polycarbophil)
Fibrillex (NC-503)
5-aminosalicylic acid
5-ASA
5-FU (fluorouracil)
50% Dextrose with Electrolyte Pattern A (or N)
Flagyl (metronidazole)
Flatulex (simethicone)
Fleet Babylax (glycerin)
Fleet enema
Fleet Bisacodyl enema
Fleet Laxative (bisacodyl)
Fleet Mineral Oil enema

medications *(cont.)*
Fleet Phospho-Soda (monobasic sodium phosphate; dibasic sodium phosphate)
Fletcher's Castoria (senna concentrate)
Flocor (poloxamer 188)
Florinef Acetate (fludrocortisone acetate)
Floxin (ofloxacin)
floxuridine (FUDR; FUdR [5-fluorouracil deoxyribonucleoside])
fludrocortisone acetate
flumecinol
FluMist vaccine
fluoropyrimidine
fluorouracil & leucovorin
fluorouracil (5-FU)
fluoxymesterone
Foamicon (aluminum hydroxide; magnesium trisilicate)
Folergot-DF (belladonna alkaloids; phenobarbital; ergotamine tartrate)
folinic acid
Foloxatine (oxaliplatin)
Foscan
fotemustine (S 10036)
Fourneau 309 (suramin sodium)
Fragmin (dalteparin sodium injection)
FRED (fog reduction elimination device) solution
FRED Lite alcohol-free solution
FUDR; FUdR (floxuridine)
Furamide (diloxanide furoate)
furazolidone
furodazole
G.B.S.
gadodiamide
Gadolite oral suspension
Galzin (zinc acetate)
gamma globulin

medications *(cont.)*
Gantrisin
Gardrin (enprostil)
Gas Relief (simethicone)
Gas-Ban (calcium carbonate; simethicone)
Gas-X (simethicone)
Gastrimmune (gemcitabine)
Gastrimmune vaccine
Gastrografin (meglumine diatrizoate)
GastroMARK imaging agent (ferumoxsil)
Gastrosed (hyoscyamine sulfate)
Gastrozepine (pirenzepine HCl)
Gaviscon (aluminum hydroxide; magnesium carbonate)
Gaviscon-2
Gelfoam soaked in sodium tetradecyl sulfate
Gelusil (aluminum hydroxide; magnesium hydroxide; simethicone)
Gelusil-M
Gelusil-II
gemcitabine HCl
Gemzar (gemcitabine HCl)
Genasense
Genasoft Plus (casanthronate; docusate sodium)
Genaton
Genaton Extra Strength (aluminum hydroxide; magnesium carbonate)
Gengraf (cyclosporine)
Genotropin (somatropin lyophilized powder)
Genotropin MiniQuick
Genotropin Pen 5
Genotropin Pen 12
Gentlax (senna concentrate)
Geref (sermorelin acetate)
Geriplex-FS
Germanin (suramin sodium)
glimepiride tablets

medications *(cont.)*
glipizide
glitazone classification of diabetes drugs
globin zinc insulin
globulin, hepatitis B hyperimmune
GlucaGen (glucagon)
glucagon
Gluco-Pro nutritional supplement
Glucophage (metformin HCl)
Glucophage XR (metformin HCl extended-release)
glucose
Glucotrol
Glucotrol XL (glipizide)
Glucovance (glyburide; metformin HCl)
glutamic acid
glutamine & somatropin
Glutose
glyburide
glyburide/metformin hydrochloride
glycerin
glycerol
glycerol monoctanoate (GMOC) solution
glycopyrrolate
glycopyrronium bromide
Glynase Pres Tab (glyburide)
Glypressin (terlipressin)
Glyset (miglitol)
GMOC (glycerol monoctanoate) solution
Go-Evac (polyethylene glycol-electrolyte solution electrolytes)
gold-198 (^{198}Au)
GoLYTELY (polyethylene glycol-electrolyte solution)
Gonadimmune
gosereline acetate
granisetron HCl
Granocyte (lenograstim)
Granulderm (trypsin; Peruvian balsam)

medications *(cont.)*
Granulex (trypsin; Peruvian balsam)
GranuMed (trypsin; Peruvian balsam)
GVAX pancreatic vaccine
Haley's M-O (magnesium hydroxide; mineral oil) (new name Phillips' M-O)
halofuginone
Halotestin (fluoxymesterone)
Hanks balanced salt solution (HBSS)
Havrix (hepatitis A vaccine, inactivated)
H-BIG (hepatitis B immunoglobulin)
H_2 blocker
H_2 receptor-blocker
Hectorol (doxercalciferol)
Helicide
Helicosol (synthetic ^{13}C-urea) lyophilized powder
Helidac (bismuth subsalicylate, metronidazole, and tetracycline)
Helidac dose-pack (bismuth subsalicylate; metronidazole; tetracycline HCl)
HemAssist blood substitute (hemoglobin crosfumaril)
Hemocor HPH
hemoglobin crosfumaril
Hemopad (microfibrillar collagen hemostat)
Hemorid for Women (pramoxine HCl; phenylephrine HCl)
Hemorrhoidal HC (hydrocortisone acetate)
Hemotene (microfibrillar collagen hemostat)
Hem-Prep (phenylephrine HCl; zinc oxide)
Hemril Uniserts (bismuth subga-l late; bismuth resorcin compound; benzyl benzoate; Peruvian balsam; zinc oxide)

medications *(cont.)*
Hep-B-Gammagee
Hep-Lock, Hep-Lock U/P (heparin sodium)
Hepagene (hepatitis B vaccine)
heparin sodium
Heparin Lock Flush (heparin sodium)
HepatAmine nutrient solution
hepatitis B immune globulin
Heptalac (lactulose)
Heptavax-B
Heptazyme
Heptodin (lamivudine)
Heptovir (lamivudine)
Herceptin (trastuzumab) monoclonal antibody
Herplex Liquifilm (idoxuridine)
Herzyme
Hespan (hetastarch)
hetastarch
Hetrazan (diethylcarbamazine citrate)
hexocyclium
Hextend
Hirulog (bivalirudin)
Histerone 100 (testosterone)
Hi-Vegi-Lip
Humalog (insulin lispro, human [rDNA])
Humalog Mix 75/25
Humalog Pen
human insulin (recombinant)
human insulin zinc
Humatrope (somatropin)
Humicade
Humulin 30/70 (insulin; isophane insulin)
Humulin 50/50 (isophane human insulin [rDNA]; human insulin [rDNA])
Humulin 70/30 (isophane human insulin [rDNA]; human insulin [rDNA])

medications *(cont.)*
Humulin L
Humulin Pen
Humulin R (human insulin [recombinant])
Humulin U (extended insulin zinc)
Humulin U Ultralente (extended insulin human zinc [rDNA])
hyaluronidase
hydralazine
Hydrate (dimenhydrinate)
hydrazine sulfate
hydrochloric acid
Hydrocil Instant (psyllium hydrophilic mucilloid)
hydrocortisone
hydrocortisone acetate
hydrocortisone enema
hydrocortisone foam
hydroxymethylacyfulvene [HMAF]
hydroxyurea tablet
HylaSine gel
hyoscyamine
hyoscyamine sulfate
Hyosophen (atropine sulfate; scopolamine hydrobromide; hyoscyamine hydrobromide; phenobarbital)
HyperHep (hepatitis B immune globulin)
I-Flow nerve block infusion kit
Iamin hydrating gel (Blue Goo)
Iamin-IB solution (prezatide copper acetate [PCA])
Icar (carbonyl iron)
icodextrin
idoxifene
Ilopan
Ilopan-Choline (dexpanthenol; choline bitartrate)
Ilozyme
imiglucerase
ImmTher (disaccharide tripeptide glycerol tripalmitoyl)

medications *(cont.)*
- Imodium A-D
- Imodium, Imodium A-D (loperamide)
- impromidine HCl
- ImuLyme vaccine
- Imuran (azathioprine)
- Inactivin
- Inapsine (droperidol)
- Incel (biricodar dicitrate)
- Indiclor (indium ^{111}In radioimaging agent)
- Infanrix vaccine
- Infergen (interferon alfacon-1)
- infliximab monoclonal antibody
- Innofem (estradiol)
- Innohep (tinzaparin sodium)
- ^{111}In satumomab pendetide
- insulin argine
- insulin aspart
- insulin defalan
- insulin glargine
- insulin human, isophane
- insulin human zinc, extended
- insulin lispro, human [rDNA])
- insulin zinc
- insulin zinc protamine
- insulin zinc suspension (amorphous)
- insulin zinc suspension (crystalline)
- insulin zinc [pork]
- Insulin Reaction (glucose)
- interferon alfa-2a
- interferon alfa-2b
- interferon alfa-2b recombinant
- interferon alfa-n1
- interferon alfa-n3
- interferon alfacon-1
- interferon beta
- interferon beta-1a
- interferon gamma-1b
- Intergel adhesion prevention solution
- interleukin-4 receptor (IL-4R)
- IntraDose (cisplatin/epinephrine) gel
- IntraSite (graft T starch copolymer)

medications *(cont.)*
- IntraSite gel
- Intron A (interferon alfa-2b, recombinant
- iodipamide meglumine
- iodixanol
- iodophor
- iodoquinol
- Iodosorb wound gel
- IoGen
- iohexol
- IontoDex (dexamethasone sodium phosphate)
- ipecac syrup
- Iressa
- irinotecan HCl injection
- irofulven
- ISG (immune serum globulin)
- ISIS 2302
- Isocaine HCl (mepivacaine HCl)
- isofylline
- Isopan (magaldrate)
- Isopan Plus (magaldrate; simethicone)
- isophane human insulin (rDNA)
- isosorbide mononitrate
- itraconazole
- ivermectin
- JTT-501
- Juven nutritional supplement
- Kaletra (lopinavir/ritonavir)
- Kanulase
- Kaodene Non-Narcotic (kaolin; pectin; bismuth subsalicylate)
- Kao Lectrolyte
- kaolin
- Kaopectate (attapulgite)
- Kao-Spen (kaolin; pectin)
- Kapectolin (kaolin; pectin)
- Kasof (docusate potassium)
- Kayexalate
- K-C (kaolin; pectin; bismuth subcarbonate)
- Kefzol (cefazolin)

medications *(cont.)*
Kestrone 5 (estrone)
Ketek (telithromycin)
ketoconazole
ketoprofen
ketorolac tromethamine
Kindercal supplement
Kinesed
Kinevac (sincalide)
Kolantyl
Konsyl (psyllium)
Konsyl-D, Konsyl Orange (psyllium hydrophilic mucilloid)
Konsyl Fiber (calcium polycarbophil)
K-Pek (attapulgite)
Kutrase (amylase; protease; lipase; cellulase; hyoscyamine sulfate; phenyltoloxamine citrate) digestive enzymes
Ku-Zyme, Ku-Zyme HP (amylase; protease; lipase; cellulase) digestive enzymes
Kytril (granisetron hydrochloride)
Lactaid
lactase enzyme
Lactinex
lactose enzyme
Lactrase
lactulose solution
lamivudine
lansoprazole
Lantus (insulin glargine)
lavoltidine, lavoltidine succinate
laxative
LDP-02
lenercept
Lente Iletin II (insulin zinc [pork])
Lente L (insulin zinc [pork])
letrazuril
letrozole
leucovorin
leucovorin & fluorouracil
Leukine (sargramostim)

medications *(cont.)*
LeuTech radiolabeled imaging agent
leuvectin
levamisole HCl
Levaquin (levofloxacin)
Levbid (hyoscyamine sulfate)
levobupivacaine
levofloxacin
Levo-T (levothyroxine sodium)
Levothroid (levothyroxine sodium)
levothyroxine sodium
levothyroxine sodium & tiratricol
Levoxyl (levothyroxine sodium)
Levsin
Levsin-PB drops (hyoscyamine sulfate; phenobarbital; alcohol)
Levsin/SL (hyoscyamine sulfate)
Levsin with Phenobarbital (hyoscyamine sulfate; phenobarbital)
Levsinex Timecaps (hyoscyamine sulfate)
lexipafant
Lexirin
liarozole fumarate
Liazal (liarozole fumarate)
Librax (clidinium; chlordiazepoxide)
lidocaine
lidocaine HCl
lidocaine topical anesthetic
Lidoject-2 (lidocaine HCl)
lignocaine
Limitrol-DM
linezolid
liothyronine sodium
liotrix
lipancreatin
Lipitor (atorvastatin calcium)
liposome encapsulated doxorubicin citrate complex
LiquiBand topical wound closure glue
Liqui-Char (activated charcoal)
Liqui-Doss (mineral oil)
lobucavir

medications *(cont.)*
LoCholest
LoCholest Light (cholestyramine resin)
Locilex (pexiganan acetate)
Lomanate (diphenoxylate HCl; atropine sulfate)
Lomotil (diphenoxylate HCl; atropine sulfate)
Lonox (diphenoxylate HCl; atropine sulfate)
loperamide
lopinavir/ritonavir
Losec (omeprazole)
Lotronex (alosetron HCl)
Lovenox (enoxaparin)
Lowsium Plus
L-thyroxine
Lu-Tex
LYMErix vaccine
lymph node-revealing solution (LNRS)
Lymphazurin dye (isosulfan blue)
lymphoblastoid interferon, human (L-IFN)
lymphocyte immune globulin, antithymocyte (rabbit)
lypressin
Maalox (aluminum hydroxide; magnesium hydroxide)
Maalox Plus
Maalox TC (therapeutic concentrate)
Maalox Whip
Macrokine (WF10)
mafenide acetate
magaldrate
Magaldrate Plus
Magalox Plus (aluminum hydroxide; magnesium hydroxide; simethicone)
Magnalox (aluminum hydroxide; magnesium hydroxide) (Canada)
magnesium citrate
magnesium oxide

medications *(cont.)*
magnesium sulfate
magnesium trisilicate
Magnox (aluminum hydroxide; magnesium hydroxide)
maladrate
Malarone (atovaquone/proguanil)
Maltsupex (nondiastatic barley malt extract)
Mannitol
Maox 42 (magnesium oxide)
Marblen
Marcaine HCl (bupivacaine HCl)
Marezine
marimastat
Marinol (dronabinol)
Maxamine (aldesleukin)
Maxidone
Maxolon (metoclopromide)
MCT (medium chain triglycerides)
MD-Gastroview (diatrozoate meglumine; diatrozoate sodium)
Mebadin (dehydroemetine)
mebendazole
meclizine HCl
Mectizan (ivermectin)
Medicone (benzocaine)
Medifil
Mefoxin
Megace (megestrol acetate)
Megnatril
Menest (esterified estrogens)
Meni-D (meclizine HCl)
mepenzolate bromide
meperidine
mepivacaine HCl
Meridia (sibutramine HCl)
meropenem
Merrem (meropenem)
mesalamine delayed-release tablets
mesalazine
Metamucil (psyllium hydrophilic mucilloid; sodium bicarbonate; potassium bicarbonate)

medications *(cont.)*
metformin extended-release
metformin HCl
methantheline bromide
methoxamine
methoxyflurane
methscopolamine bromide
methylcellulose
methylprednisolone acetate
methylprednisolone sodium succinate
methyl tertiary butyl ether (MTBE)
methyltestosterone
metoclopramide nasal spray
metocurine iodide
metrizamide
metrizoate sodium
Metro I.V. (metronidazole)
metronidazole
Metryl 500
Metubine Iodide (metocurine iodide)
MetXia
microfibrillar collagen hemostat
Micronase (glyburide)
Micronized Glyburide (glyburide)
midazolam HCl
miglitol
milk of magnesia (MOM)
Milk of Magnesia–Cascara, Concentrated
Milkinol (mineral oil)
minalrestat
mineral oil
Mintezol (thiabendazole)
Mintox (aluminum hydroxide; magnesium hydroxide)
MiraLax (polyethylene glycol 3350)
Miraluma (technetium ^{99m}Tc sestamibi)
misoprostol
MitoExtra
mitomycin
Mitrolan (calcium polycarbophil)
Mivacron (mivacurium chloride)

medications *(cont.)*
Moctanin (monoctanoin)
Modane Bulk, Plus, and Soft
Modane Plus
Modane Soft
Modane Versabran
MOM (milk of magnesia)
monooctanoin
morantel, morantel tartrate
Morphelan (oral morphine)
MorphiDex
morphine HCl
morphine sulfate
morrhuate
Motilium (domperidone maleate)
Motofen (difenoxin HCl; atropine sulfate)
moxifloxacin
MPI 5020
MTBE (methyl tertiary butyl ether)
Mucomyst
MulTE-Pak-5 (multiple trace elements [metals])
Multikine
Multilyte-40 (combined electrolyte solution)
Mutamycin (mitomycin)
mycophenolate mofetil (MMF)
Mycostatin
Mylagen, Mylagen II
Mylanta Natural Fiber Supplement (psyllium hydrophilic mucilloid)
Mylanta-II
Mylicon (simethicone)
Myocet (liposome encapsulated doxorubicin citrate complex)
Nabi-Altastaph vaccine
Nabi-HB (hepatitis B immune globulin [human])
Nabi-NicVAX vaccine
Nabi-StaphVAX vaccine
Naganol (suramin sodium)
nandrolone phenpropionate
Naphuride (suramin sodium)

medications *(cont.)*
Naropin (ropivacaine)
Nashville Rabbit Antithymocyte Serum (lymphocyte immune globulin, antithymocyte [rabbit])
nateglinide
Natural Vegetable (psyllium hydrophilic mucilloid)
Nature's Remedy (cascara sagrada)
Nausea Relief (phosphorated carbohydrate solution)
Nausetrol (phosphorated carbohydrate solution)
NC-503 (Fibrillex)
Neo-Cultol (mineral oil)
Neo-Diaral (loperamide)
Neocate One +
Neoloid
Neomark (broxuridine)
neomycin sulfate
Neoral (cyclosporine; alcohol)
Neotrace-4 (multiple trace elements)
Neovastat
NE-0080
Nephrox (aluminum hydroxide; mineral oil)
Neuprex
neutral insulin
neutral protamine Hagedorn (NPH) insulin
Nexium (esomeprazole magnesium)
niacin
Niaspan (niacin)
nicotinamide
Nilstat
9-nitro-20-(S)-camptothecin (9-NC)
nitrofural
nitrofurazone
nitroglycerin
nitroglycerin ointment
Nitrolan
nitrous oxide
nizatidine
Nizoral

medications *(cont.)*
No Pain-HP (capsaicin)
nolinium bromide
Nolvadex (tamoxifen citrate)
Norco (hydrocodone bitartrate; acetaminophen)
Normal Stool Formula
Normal Stool Formula-IB (NSF-IB)
Normosol-M and 5% Dextrose
Normosol-R and 5% Dextrose
Normosol-R pH 7.4 (combined electrolyte solution)
Novamine 15% (amino acids)
Novo-Domperidone (domperidone maleate)
Novocain (procaine HCl)
Novolin L (insulin)
Novolin N PenFill
Novolin N Prefilled (insulin)
Novolin R PenFill
Novolin R Prefilled (insulin)
Novolin 70/30 PenFill
Novolin 70/30 Prefilled
Novolin 85/15 PenFill (insulin)
NovoLog (insulin aspart)
Novopaque (barium sulfate)
NovoRapid (insulin)
NPH (neutral protamine Hagedorn) insulin
NPH Iletin II insulin
NPH-N insulin
NSF-IB (Normal Stool Formula-IB)
NuLytely (polyethylene glycol-electrolyte solution)
Numorphan (oxymorphone HCl)
Nupercainal
Nutraloric
Nutren 1.0, 1.5, 2.0
Nutrilan
Nutrilyte II (combined electrolyte solution)
Nutropin (somatropin)
Nutropin Depot (somatropin)
nystatin suspension

medications *(cont.)*
Nystex
OCL (polyethylene glycol electrolyte solution)
Octamide PFS (metoclopramide)
Octastatin (vapreotide)
octatropine methylbromide
Octocaine HCl (lidocaine HCl; epinephrine)
OctreoScan imaging agent
octreotide, octreotide acetate
oestradiol (estradiol)
oestrone (estrone)
ofloxacin, Floxin
OGT-918
OKT3
olsalazine sodium
omega-3 fatty acid
omeprazole sodium
omeprazole plus amoxicillin
Omnicef (cefdinir)
Omnipaque iohexol)
Omniscan (gadodiamide)
Onco TCS
Onconase (p30 protein)
Oncophage vaccine
OncoScint CR/OV (^{111}In satumomab pendetide)
OncoScint CR103 (colorectal) imaging agent
OncoVax-P
Oncovin (vincristine sulfate)
ondansetron HCl
Operand (povidone; iodine)
opium tincture
OptiMARK (gadoversetamide injection)
Optison contrast medium
Oralgen
Orgaran (danaparoid sodium)
orlistat
Orzel (UFT/leucovorin calcium)
Ostavir vaccine
OvaRex

medications *(cont.)*
ox bile extract
oxaliplatin
oxamniquine
Oxandrin (oxandrolone)
oxidized bile acids
Oxiplex
oxybuprocaine
oxycodone and acetaminophen
oxycodone HCl
oxycodone terephthalate/aspirin
OxyContin (oxycodone HCl)
oxymorphone HCl
oxyphencyclimine HCl
oxyphenisatin, oxyphenisatin acetate
oxyphenonium
p10 protein
p30 protein
paclitaxel
Pafase
palmoxirate sodium
palmoxiric acid
palonosetron HCl
PALS tablets (chlorophyllin copper complex)
pamidronate disodium
Pamine (methscopolamine bromide)
Pamisyl (aminosalicylic acid)
Pan-HER
Panafil enzymatic debriding agent
Panafil White ointment
pancopride
Pancrease, Pancrease MT 4, Pancrease MT 10, Pancrease MT 16, Pancrease MT 20 (lipase; protease; amylase)
pancreatic enzyme therapy
Pancreatin 8X (pancreatin; lipase; protease; amylase)
Pancrecarb MS-8 (lipase; protease; amylase; pancrelipase)
pancrelipase
Pancrex

medications *(cont.)*
Pancrezyme 4X (pancreatin; lipase; protease; amylase)
pancuronium bromide
Panretin (alitretinoin)
Pantoloc (pantoprazole)
pantoprazole
Pantozol (pantoprazole)
papain
Papaya Enzyme (papain; amylase)
paregoric (PG)
Parepectolin (attapulgite)
paricalcitol
paromomycin sulfate
Pathibamate-200
Pathilon (tridihexethyl chloride)
Pavulon (pancuronium bromide)
Paxene (paclitaxel)
Pazo Hemorrhoid (ephedrine sulfate; zinc oxide)
PCA (prezatide copper acetate)
pectin
Pedialyte (sodium, potassium, and chloride electrolytes)
PedTE-Pak-4 (multiple trace elements)
Pedtrace-4 (multiple trace elements)
PEG (polyethylene glycol)
PEG-interferon alfa-2a
PEG-interferon alfa-2b
PEG-Intron (PEG-interferon alfa-2b)
PEG-Intron A (interferon alfa 2b in a polyethylene glycol carrier)
Pegasys (PEG-interferon alfa-2a)
pegvisomant
pegylated interferon
Pentacea
pentagastrin
Pentasa (mesalamine)
Pepcid AC
Pepcid Complete
Pepcid RPD (famotidine)
Peptavlon (pentagastrin)

medications *(cont.)*
Pepto-Bismol (bismuth subsalicylate)
Pepto Diarrhea Control (loperamide)
Perdiem (psyllium husks; senna extract)
perflenapent
perflutren
Peri-Colace (casanthranol; docusate sodium)
Peri-Dos (casanthranol; docusate sodium)
Peruvian balsam
pexiganan acetate
PG (paregoric)
PG-TXL (polyglutamic acid paclitaxel)
PGG glucan
Phazyme (simethicone)
Phazyme-125
Phazyme-PB
Phenergan Fortis (promethazine HCl)
phenobarbital
Phenolax (phenolphthalein)
phenolphthalein
phentermine
Phillips' Milk of Magnesia (M-O) (magnesium hydroxide)
Phosphaljel
Photofrin (porfimer)
pimagedine HCl
Pink Bismuth (bismuth subsalicylate)
Pin-Rid (pyrantel pamoate)
Pin-X (pyrantel pamoate)
pioglitazone HCl
piperamide, piperamide maleate
piperazine, piperazine calcium edetate, piperazine edetate calcium
pirenzepine HCl
piritrexim
piroglitride, piroglitride tartrate
Pitressin
Pitressin Synthetic (vasopressin)

medications *(cont.)*
- Pivanex
- podophyllum
- polidocanol
- Polocaine (mepivacaine)
- poloxamer 188
- polyethylene glycol (PEG)
- polyethylene glycol-electrolyte solution
- polyethylene glycol 3350
- polyglutamic acid paclitaxel
- Pondimin (fenfluramine)
- porcine islet preparation, encapsulated
- porfimer sodium
- Portagen
- potassium iodide
- PPMA (polymethylmethacrylate-copolymer) beads
- pramlintide acetate
- Pramoxine HC (hydrocortisone acetate; pramoxine)
- Prandase (acarbose)
- Prandin (repaglinide)
- praziquantel
- Precedex (dexmedetomidine)
- Precose (acarbose)
- prednisolone
- prednisone
- Premarin (conjugated estrogens)
- Preparation H anorectal cream
- Preparation H cleansing tissues
- Preparation H Cooling Gel
- Preparation H rectal suppositories
- Prepodyne solution
- Prevacid (lansoprazole)
- Prevacid triple therapy
- Prevalite (cholestyramine resin)
- Prevatac (exisulind)
- Prevenzyme
- Prevpac (lansoprazole; clarithromycin; amoxicillin)
- priliximab
- Prilosec (omeprazole)

medications *(cont.)*
- Pro-Banthine (propantheline bromide)
- Pro-Cal-Sof (docusate sodium)
- prochlorperazine
- Proctocort (hydrocortisone)
- ProctoCream HC (hydrocortisone acetate)
- Procto-Esthesia
- ProctoFoam NS (pramoxine HCl)
- Proderm Topical (castor oil; Peruvian balsam)
- profiromycin
- Prograf (tacrolimus)
- Proleukin (aldesleukin)
- promethazine HCl
- Promycin (porfiromycin)
- propantheline bromide
- Prophyllin (sodium propionate; chlorophyll derivatives)
- Propimex-2
- propiram
- propofol
- ProSol 20% (amino acids)
- prostaglandin E1
- ProstaScint (CYT-356 radiolabeled with ^{111}In indium chloride) imaging agent
- Prostigmin
- protamine zinc insulin
- protease digestive enzyme
- ProTec (isofylline)
- protein pump inhibitor
- Protenate (plasma protein fraction)
- Prothecan
- protirelin
- Protonix (pantoprazole)
- Protostat
- Provir
- Prulet (white phenolphthalein)
- psyllium hydrophilic mucilloid
- psyllium seed husks
- Purge (castor oil)
- Pylorid (ranitidine bismuth citrate)

medications *(cont.)*
pyrantel pamoate
Pyridium
PZI (protamine zinc insulin)
Quarzan (clidinium bromide)
quassia (amargo; amara)
Questran (cholestyramine)
quiflapon sodium
Quilimmune-M
quinacrine HCl
quinupristin/dalfopristin
rabeprazole sodium
raltitrexed
ramoplanin
ranitidine
ranitidine bismuth citrate
rapacuronium bromide
Rapamune (sirolimus)
rapamycin
Rebetol (ribavirin)
Rebetron (interferon alfa-2b injection)
Rebetron (ribavirin and interferon alfa-2b)
Reclomide (metoclopramide HCl)
Recombivax HB
Rectacort (hydrocortisone acetate)
Rectagene (live yeast cell derivative; shark liver oil)
Rectolax (bisacodyl)
Reducin (somatostatin)
Redux (dexfenfluramine)
Reese's Pinworm (pyrantel pamoate)
ReFacto (factor VIII SQ, recombinant)
Reglan (metoclopramide HCl)
Regranex (becaplermin)
Regranex gel (becaplermin)
Regulace (docusate sodium)
Regular Iletin II (insulin)
Regular Iletin II U-500 (concentrated insulin)
Regular Purified Pork Insulin
Regulax SS (docusate sodium)

medications *(cont.)*
Reguloid (psyllium hydrophilic mucilloid)
Regutol
Rehydralyte (electrolyte solution)
Remegel
Remicade (infliximab)
remifentanil
Renacidin
repaglinide
Resol
retinoid
Rezipas (aminosalicylic acid)
Rezulin (troglitazone)
Rezyme
Rheaban (activated attapulgite)
Rheomacrodex (dextran 40)
rhesus rotavirus-tetravalent vaccine (RRV-TV)
ribavirin
ribavirin and interferon alfa-2b
rifaximin
Riopan (magaldrate)
Riopan Plus 2
Ro-Bile
Robinul Forte (glycopyrrolate)
Rocaltrol (calcitriol)
rofecoxib
Rolaids, Calcium Rich
ropivacaine
rosiglitazone maleate
rosuvastatin
RotaShield vaccine
Rowasa (mesalamine)
roxatidine, roxatidine acetate HCl
Roxicodone (oxycodone)
Roxin (roxatidine acetate HCl)
RRV-TV (rhesus rotavirus-tetravalent) vaccine
rubitecan
RuLox (aluminum hydroxide; magnesium hydroxide)
sacrosidase
salazosulfapyridine

medications *(cont.)*
- Salofalk (mesalamine)
- Sal-Tropine (atropine sulfate)
- Sandimmune (cyclosporine)
- Sandostatin
- Sandostatin LAR Depot (octreotide acetate)
- SangCya (cyclosporine; alcohol)
- Sani-Supp (glycerin)
- Saratoga (zinc oxide; boric acid; eucalyptol)
- sargramostim
- Satietrol Complete
- Satric-500
- satumomab pendetide
- SCCS (simethicone-coated cellulose suspension)
- Scleromate
- sclerosant
- Sclerosol
- scopolamine
- seabuckthorn seed oil
- secretin
- Secretin Ferring (secretin)
- SelCID (selective cytokine inhibitory drug)
- selenium-75 (^{75}Se) radioisotope
- Senexon (senna concentrate)
- senna concentrate
- Senna-Gen (senosides)
- Senokot (senna concentrate)
- Senokot-S
- Senokot X-prep
- Senokotxtra (senna concentrate)
- senosides
- Sensorcaine MPF (bupivacaine)
- Sepracoat coating solution
- Sepragel bioresorbable gel
- Septopal beads
- Septra
- sermorelin acetate
- Serutan
- shark cartilage
- shark liver oil

medications *(cont.)*
- short chain fatty acids
- sibutramine HCl
- Silace-C (docusate sodium)
- Silvadene (silver sulfadiazine)
- silver sulfadiazine (SSD, SSD AF)
- Simaal Gel 2 (aluminum hydroxide; magnesium hydroxide; simethicone)
- simaldrate
- Simeco
- simethicone
- simethicone-coated cellulose suspension (SCCS)
- Simulect (baxiliximab)
- sincalide
- sirolimus
- 6-mercaptopurine (6-MP)
- SMX-TMP (sulfamethoxazole and trimethoprim)
- sodium bicarbonate
- sodium citrate
- sodium morrhuate
- sodium oxybate
- sodium perborate
- sodium phosphate
  - dibasic
  - monobasic
- sodium stibogluconate
- sodium tetradecyl (STD) sulfate
- sodium tetradecyl sulfate (sclerosant)
- sodium tyropanoate
- SomatoKine (IGF-BP3 complex)
- somatostatin
- somatropin
- somatropin & glutamine
- somatropin lyophilized powder
- Somavert (pegvisomant)
- SonoRx (simethicone-coated cellulose suspension)
- Sotradecol (sodium tetradecyl sulfate)
- Sparkles (sodium bicarbonate; citric acid; simethicone)

medications *(cont.)*
Spasmolin (atropine sulfate; scopolamine hydrobromide; hyoscyamine hydrobromide; phenobarbital)
Spasmophen
Spastosed (calcium carbonate; magnesium carbonate)
Spexil (trospectomycin)
spironolactone
Sporanox (itraconazole)
Sporidin-G (bovine immunoglobulin concentrate)
Sporidin-G (*Cryptosporidium parvum* bovine colostrum IgG concentrate)
S-P-T (thyroid, desiccated porcine)
squalamine (shark cartilage powder)
SS (somatostatin)
SSD, SSD AF (silver suladiazine)
St. John's wort (amber; amber touch-and-heal)
St. Joseph Anti-Diarrheal for Children (attapulgite)
stannous sulfur colloid
Starlix (nateglinide)
steroid
stillingia
stool softener
streptozocin
Stresstein (multiple branched-chain amino acids)
Stromagen
Stromectol (ivermectin)
Strong Iodine (iodine; potassium iodide)
SU-5416
sucralfate
Sulfalax Calcium (docusate sodium)
Sulfamylon (mafenide acetate)
sulfasalazine
sulfonylurea
SuperChar
suppository

medications *(cont.)*
suramin sodium
SureLac (lactose enzyme)
Surfak (docusate calcium)
Surgi–Prep (Betadine, povidone-iodine)
sutilains
Syllact
Symlin (pramlintide acetate)
Synercid (quinupristin/dalfopristin)
Synsorb Cd
Synsorb-PK
synthetic ^{13}C urea lyophilized powder
Synthroid (levothyroxine sodium)
syrup of ipecac
tacrolimus
Tagamet, Tagamet HB (cimetidine)
tamoxifen citrate
taurolidine
Taxol (paclitaxel)
Taxotere (docetaxel)
Tazocin
tazofelone
TBZ (thiabendazole)
Tebamide (trimethobenzamide HCl)
technetium macroaggregated albumin (^{99m}Tc MAA)
technetium ^{99m}Tc pertechnetate
technetium sulfur colloid (^{99m}Tc-SC)
tegaserod
Telepaque (topanoic acid)
telithromycin
Tempo (aluminum hydroxide; magnesium hydroxide; calcium carbonate; simethicone)
Ten-K
Tensilon
Tenuate
Tepanil
terlipressin
Tesamone (testosterone)
Teslac (testolactone)
testosterone

medications *(cont.)*
Testred (methyltestosterone)
tetracaine, tetracaine HCl
tetradecyl sulfate
tetrahydrocannabinol (THC)
T-Gen (trimethobenzamide)
thalidomide
Thalomid (thalidomide)
theraccine
Theragyn
Theralax
Theratope-STn
Theratope vaccine
Therevac-Plus (docusate sodium; benzocaine)
Thermazene (silver sulfadiazine)
thiabendazole (TBZ)
thiazolidinedione
thiethylperazine
Thioplex (thiotepa)
thiosalan
thiotepa
Thrombin-JMI (thrombin)
thrombin-Keflin-sotredechol
Thrombogen (thrombin)
Thrombostat (thrombin)
thymalfasin
Thymitaq (nolatrexed dihydrochloride)
thymosin alpha 1
Thypinone (protirelin)
Thyrar (thyroid, desiccated bovine)
Thyrel-TRH (protirelin)
Thyro-Block (potassium iodide)
Thyrogen (thyrotropin alfa)
thyroglobulin
thyroid
thyroid-stimulating hormone
Thyrolar (liotrix)
thyromedan HCl
thyrotrophic hormone
thyrotropin alfa
thyrotropin-releasing hormone (TRH)

medications *(cont.)*
thyroxine
Thytropar (thyrotropin)
tiabendazole
Ticlid (ticlopidine)
ticlopidine
Ticon (trimethobenzamide HCl)
Tigan (trimethobenzamide HCl)
tincture of benzoin
tincture of opium
tinzaparin sodium
tirolimus
Titralac
tolazamide
tolbutamide sodium
Tolinase (tolazamide)
tolrestat
Tomudex (raltitrexed)
Tonalin (conjugated linoleic acid)
topical bovine thrombin
Torecan
toremifene citrate
tositumomab
Transderm Scop (scopolamine hydrobromide)
transmucosal fentanyl citrate oral
Transplatin (oxaliplatin)
trastuzumab
Travasol in Dextrose
Travasol with electrolytes
Triacana (tiratricol; levothyroxine sodium)
Triban (trimethobenzamide HCl; benzocaine)
tridihexethyl chloride
Trimazide (trimethobenzamide HCl)
trimethobenzamide
trimethoprim-sulfamethoxazole
Triptone (dimenhydrinate)
Tritec (ranitidine bismuth citrate)
Trizivir
Trizyme (amylase; protease; cellulase)
troglitazone

medications *(cont.)*
Tronolane (pramoxine HCl)
tropisetron
trospectomycin
trovafloxacin
Trovan (trovafloxacin)
Trovax
troxacitabine
Tru-Scint AD imaging agent
trypsin
Tucks ointment
Tums
Twinrix vaccine
Tylenol No. 3
UDCA (ursodeoxycholic acid)
UFT (uracil plus tegafur)
Unilax (phenolphthalein; docusate sodium)
Unithroid (levothyroxine sodium)
uracil plus tegafur (UFT)
Urso (ursodiol)
ursodeoxycholic acid (UDCA)
ursodiol
V-Lax (psyllium hydrophilic mucilloid)
Valium (diazepam)
Valpin 50
Vansil (oxamniquine)
vapreotide
Vaqta (hepatitis A vaccine, inactivated) vaccine
vasoactive intestinal polypeptide (VIP)
vasopressin
vasopressin with nitroglycerin
Velban (vinblastine sulfate)
Velosulin Human BR (insulin)
Verluma (nofetumobab)
Vermox (mebendazole)
Versabran
Versed (midazolam HCl)
Vianain (ananain; comosain; bromelains)
Vicodin

medications *(cont.)*
VIMRxyn (synthetic hypericin)
vinblastine sulfate
Viokase
Vioxx (rofecoxib)
Virilon (methyltestosterone)
Virulizin
viscous lidocaine
viscous Xylocaine gargle
Visicol bowel prep
Vistaril
Vita-PMS, Vita-PMS Plus
vitamin K
VX-497
warfarin potassium
warfarin sodium
Welchol (formerly Cholestagel)
Wellferon (interferon alfa-n1)
wetting agents
white phenolphthalein
WinGel
Wyanoids Relief Factor (cocoa butter; shark liver oil)
Xcytrin (motexafin gadolinium)
Xeloda (capecitabine)
Xenical (orlistat) capsules
X-Prep
Xylocaine (lidocaine)
Xylocaine topical anesthetic
Xylo-Pfan (xylose)
xylose
yellow phenolphthalein
Zacutex (lexipafant)
zamifenacin
Zanosar (streptozocin)
Zantac, Zantac 75 (ranitidine)
Zantac EFFERdose
Zantac GELdose
Zeffix (lamivudine)
Zelmac (tegaserod)
Zemplar (paricalcitol)
Zenapax (daclizumab)
zinc acetate
Zixoryn (flumecinol)

medications *(cont.)*
Zofran (ondansetron HCl)
Zofran ODT (ondansetron)
Zoladex (goserelin acetate)
zoledronic acid
Zometa (zoledronic acid)
zopolrestat
Zosyn (piperacillin sodium; tazobactam sodium)
Zydone (hydrocodone bitartrate/ acetaminophen)
Zypan
Zyvox (linezolid)
MedCam Pro Plus video camera
Medco Adson tissue forceps
Medco Allis tissue forceps
Medco Babcock forceps
Medco Bozeman uterine forceps
Medco Brown Adson forceps
Medco Carmalt splinter forceps
Medco Crile forceps
Medco eye dressing forceps
Medco Foerster sponge forceps
Medco forceps
Medco Halstead mosquito forceps
Medco Lister bandage scissors
Medco Schroder tenaculum forceps
Medco splinter forceps
Medco thumb dressing forceps
Medco tissue thumb forceps
Medebar Plus (barium sulfate)
Med-E-Jet inoculator injector
MED endoscope
Medescan (barium sulfate)
Medex Protégé 3010 syringe infusion pump
Medfusion 2001 syringe infusion pump
media (pl. of medium), contrast
medial cystic necrosis
medial genicular position
medial incision
medial parapatellar incision
medial pectoral nerve
medial thoracic nerve
medial to pectoral minor muscle
medial umbilical fold
median arcuate ligament
median incision
median length of survival
median lobe of prostate
median lymph node dissection
median parapatellar incision
mediastinal crunch
mediastinal cyst
mediastinal emphysema
mediastinal lymphadenectomy
mediastinal lymphatic and fibrofatty tissue
mediastinal lymphatics
mediastinal thickening
mediastinitis
mediastinodiaphragmatic pleural reflection
mediastinoscope
mediastinoscopy aspirating needle
mediastinum
mediated by gastrin
medical adhesive
medical blockade
medical therapy
medical vagotomy
medicated urethral system for erection (MUSE)
Medicina percutaneous button
Medicone (benzocaine)
Medicon-Jackson rectal forceps
Medicut catheter
Medicut shears
Medifil dressing
Mediflex-Gazayerli retractor
Mediflex video camera system
Medi-Ject needle-free insulin injection system
Medi-Jector Choice needle-free insulin injection system
Medilas laparoscope
Medina ileostomy catheter
mediolateral oblique view

medionodular cirrhosis
Medi plaster scissors
Medipore Dress-it surgical dressing
Mediskin hemostatic sponge
Medi-Tech bipolar probe
Medi-Tech catheter
Mediterranean fever
Mediterranean lymphoma
Medi-therm II Freon free unit
medium chain acyl-CoA dehydrogenase (MCAD) deficiency
medium chain fatty acids (MCFA)
medium chain triglycerides (MCT)
medium pressure catheter
medium pressure shunt
medius, scalenus
Medi-Vac bulk tubing
Medi-Vac CRD suction liner
Medi-Vac critical measurement unit
Medi-Vac Flex Advantage suction liner
Medi-Vac Flexi-Clear suction handle
Medi-Vac Yankauer suction handle
Medi-Vu endoscope
Medix anoscope
Medoc-Celestin endoprosthesis
Medoc-Celestin pulsion tube
Medoff sliding plate
MedPulser device
Medrad Mrinnervu (also MRinnervu) endorectal colon probe
Medstone STS lithotriptor
Medstone STS-T transportable lithotripsy system
MedSystem III infusion pump
Med-Tech Teflon dilator
Medtronic Previa
Meduck anesthesia monitor
medulla (pl. medullas, medullae)
  adrenal
  dusky
  lymphatic
  ovarian
  renal
  spinal
medulla oblongata
medulla of bone
medulla of kidney
medulla of lymph node
medulla of thymus
medullary artery
medullary bone
medullary bone graft
medullary canal
medullary canal reamer
medullary carcinoma
medullary carcinoma of the thyroid (MTC)
medullary cavity
medullary cord
medullary nail
medullary ray
medullary sarcoma
medullary sinus
medullary sponge kidney
medullary substance
medullary thyroid cancer (MTC)
medullary thyroid carcinoma
medullary zone
medullated corneal nerve fibers
medulloadrenal hyperfunction
medulloblastoma
medusae, caput
Meeker forceps
Meeker gallbladder clamp
Meeker intestinal forceps
Mefoxin
Megace (megestrol acetate)
megacolon
  acquired
  congenital
  idiopathic
  toxic
megacystis-microcolon-intestinal hypoperistalsis syndrome
megaduodenum
MegaDyne all-in-one hand control
megaesophagus
megakaryocyte

Megalink biliary stent
"mega-pocket" augmentation mammoplasty
megarectum
megestrol acetate
meglumine diatrizoate contrast medium
meglumine iocarmate
meglumine iothalamate
meglumine iotroxate contrast medium
meglumine ioxaglate
Meigs syndrome
melanocytes
melanoma
- acral-lentiginous
- amelanotic
- anorectal
- benign juvenile
- benign uveal
- desmoplastic malignant
- halo
- intraocular
- juvenile
- lentigo maligna
- malignant
- malignant lentigo
- minimal deviation
- mucosal
- nodular
- ocular
- staging of malignant
- subungual
- superficial spreading
- uveal

melanomatosis
melanophage
melanoplakia-intestinal polyposis
melanosis
melanosis coli
melanotic cancer
melanotic carcinoma
melanotic pigmentation
MELAS (mitochondrial encephalomyopathy, lactic acidosis, and stroke-like episodes)
melena
melenic stool (*not* melanotic)
- basement
- peritoneal
- phrenoesophageal
- pleuroperitoneal
- TefGen guided tissue

membrane lipid composition
membrane phospholipid
membrane-puncturing forceps
membranous colitis
Memotherm colorectal stent
Memotherm endoscopic biliary stent
Memotherm Flexx biliary stent
Memotherm nitinol self-expanding stent
MEN (multiple endocrine neoplasia) syndrome
MEN 1 (multiple endocrine neoplasia, type 1) syndrome
MEN 2 (multiple endocrine neoplasia, type 2b or IIB, syndrome
menarche, early
Mendelsohn maneuver
Menest (esterified estrogens)
Menetrier disease
Menghini "one second" technique
Menghini liver biopsy needle
Menghini percutaneous liver biopsy technique
menginococcal septicemia
Meni-D (meclizine HCl)
meningeal adhesion
meningeal carcinoma
meningioma of the cribriform plate
meningitis
meningococcus
MENIN tumor
meniscal trimmer blade
meniscectomy blade
meniscectomy scissors
meniscotomy chisel
meniscotomy knife
meniscus clamp
meniscus forceps

meniscus hook
meniscus knife
meniscus retractor
meniscus scissors
meniscus sign
meniscutome
Menkes disease (kinky hair syndrome)
menopausal syndrome
menopause, early or late
mental status changes
Mentor breast implant
mentor tubing
Mentor wet-field electrocautery
mepenzolate bromide
meperidine
Mepiform
Mepilex self-adherent foam dressing
Mepitel contact-layer wound dressing
mepivacaine HCl
Mepore absorptive dressing
mercaptans
Mercator atrial high-density array
 catheter
Mercedes Benz sign, reversed
Mercedes cannula
Mercedes microtip
Mercedes One Piece cannula
Mercedes tip cannula
Mercedes Toomey syringe cannula
Merchant view
mercury-containing balloon
mercury-filled bougie
mercury-filled dilator
mercury-weighted dilator
mercury-weighted tube
Meriam dissecting forceps
Meridia (sibutramine HCl)
Merindino operation
Meritene liquid feeding
Merkel cell carcinoma
Merogel nasal dressing and stent
meropenem
Merrem (meropenem)
Mersilene braided nonabsorbable suture
Mersilene polyester fiber mesh
Mersilene polyester fiber suture
Mersilene suture
Mersilene tape
Mersilk braided silk suture
merycism
mesalamine delayed-release tablets
mesalamine enema
mesalazine
Mesalt ribbon dressing
mesenchymal tumor
mesenchyme
mesenteric abscess
mesenteric adenitis
mesenteric angina
mesenteric apoplexy
mesenteric artery syndrome
mesenteric attachment of colon
mesenteric cyst
mesenteric embolism
mesenteric fat creeping onto the
 antimesenteric border
mesenteric fat stranding (on CT scan)
mesenteric fistula
mesenteric gland
mesenteric infarction
mesenteric infiltration
mesenteric ischemia
mesenteric lymph node
mesenteric lymphadenitis
mesentericoparietal fossa
mesenteric rupture
mesenteric stranding
mesenteric tear
mesenteric thrombosis
mesenteric triangle
mesenteric vascular insufficiency
mesenteric vascular lesion
mesenteric vessel rupture
mesenteritis, retractile
mesenteropexy
mesentery
 appendiceal
 ileal

mesentery *(cont.)*
- jejunal
- plication of
- small bowel
- small intestine (SIM)

mesentery is divided
mesentery of appendix
mesentery of ileum
mesentery of jejunum
mesentery of small bowel
mesh
- Altex polypropylene
- Bard Composix
- Bard Sperma-Tex preshaped
- Bard Visilex
- bilayer polypropylene
- BioMesh
- Brennen biosynthetic surgical
- Composix
- Dacron
- Dexon polyglycolic acid
- freeform prosthetic
- Gore-Tex DualMesh Plus
- Gore-Tex MycroMesh Plus
- Guidor
- Hermesh-3
- Herniamesh surgical
- Hertra-2
- Marlex
- Marlex propylene
- Mersilene
- Mersilene polyester fiber
- monofilament microporous
- Omniderm
- Parietex composite
- Paritene
- PerFix Plus Plug
- polyglactin
- polyglycolic acid
- polypropylene
- preformed prosthetic
- Prolene polypropylene hernia
- prosthetic
- Resolut

mesh *(cont.)*
- Sepramesh Biosurgical Composite
- Sepramesh prosthetic surgical
- Sperma-Tex preshaped
- Surgipro
- SurgiSis sling
- synthetic
- Tramex
- Trelex
- Trelex mesh
- Vicryl knitted
- Vicryl woven polyglactin
- Visilex polypropylene

mesh plug hernioplasty
mesoappendicitis
mesoappendix
mesoatrial shunt
mesocaval anastomosis
mesocaval H-graft shunt
mesocaval interposition shunt
mesocaval shunt
mesocolic band
mesocolic gland
mesocolic shelf
mesocolic window
mesocolonic vessel
mesocolon, transverse
mesodermal cell
mesodermal cortex
mesoenteric vein
mesogastric fossa
mesophilic bacteria
mesorectum
mesosigmoid colon
mesosigmoiditis
mesothelioma, peritoneal
messenger RNA (mRNA)
MET-Rx
metabolic acidosis, intractable
metabolic alkalosis
metabolic calculus
metabolic cirrhosis
metabolic decompensation
metabolic deficiency

metabolic derangement
metabolic derangement from vomiting
metabolic encephalopathy
metabolic energy production
metabolic pathway
metabolic process
metabolic stone
metabolic waste
metabolism
  acid-base
  bacterial (in intestines)
  bilirubin
  calcium
  defect of
  drug
  estrogen
  fat
  fatty-acid
  glucose
  impaired fat
  liver
  nitrogen
  pyrrole
metabolite
metabolite level
metabolize
metacarpal retractor
metacarpal saw
metal clamp
Metalite + A4270
metallic clamp
metallic clip
metallic pin
metallic staple
metallic stent placement
metal needle
metal olive
metal prosthetic graft
metal-weighted Silastic feeding tube
metamass
Metamucil (psyllium hydrophilic mucilloid; sodium bicarbonate; potassium bicarbonate)
metanephrine
metaphyseal abscess
metaplasia
  apocrine
  columnar
  intestinal
  myeloid
  specialized intestinal
  squamous
metaplastic polyp
metastasis (pl. metastases)
  advanced
  bone
  brain
  breast skin satellite
  distal lymph node
  distant
  extrahepatic (EHM)
  far-away
  focus of
  liver
  lung
  lymph node
  nodal
  nonskeletal
  peritoneal
  pleural
  port-site
  positive nodal
  satellite
  shunt-related
  skeletal
metastasis to liver
metastatic abscess
metastatic carcinoid syndrome
metastatic carcinoma
metastatic cascade
metastatic colorectal cancer
metastatic disease
metastatic gastric cancer
metastatic malignancy
metastatic polyp
metastatic septicopyemia
metastatic trophoblastic disease (MTD)
metastatic tumor

metatarsal head extractor
metatypical carcinoma
METAVIR classification of chronic hepatitis C (0–4)
meteorism
meter (see *blood glucose monitor*)
metformin HCl
methanethiol
methantheline
methantheline bromide
methicillin-resistant *Staphylococcus aureus* (MRSA, pronounced "mer-sah")
methimazole
method
  Benedict-Talbot body surface area
  Brown dietary (for colon preparation)
  Cherry-Crandall (for testing serum lipase)
  dye scattering
  EMR (endoscopic mucosal resection) suction cap
  Gallego
  leading cord (of colonofibroscopy)
  modified Papanicolaou
  Morison
  Papanicolaou
  Parker-Kerr closed (of end-to-end enteroenterostomy)
  Siffert
  staging
  strip biopsy
  suction cap
methohexital sodium
methotrexate
methoxamine
methoxyflurane
methscopolamine bromide
methylcellulose
methylene blue dye
methylene blue enema
methylene blue instillation
methylene blue stain
methylmethacrylate adhesive
methylprednisolone acetate
methylprednisolone sodium succinate
methyl red test
methyl tertiary butyl ether (MTBE)
methyltestosterone
methyltestosterone-induced cholestasis
meticulous apposition
meticulous hemostasis
metoclopramide nasal spray
metocurine iodide
metopic cranial suture
MetraGrasp ligament grasper
MetraPass suture passer
MetraTie knot pusher
metrizamide
metrizoate sodium
Metro I.V. (metronidazole)
metronidazole
Metryl 500
mets (metastases)
Metubine Iodide (metocurine iodide)
MetXia
"Metz" or "Mets" (slang for Metzenbaum scissors)
Metzenbaum chisel
Metzenbaum dissecting scissors
Metzenbaum gouge
Metzenbaum scissors, curved, double-action
Metzenbaum-TC scissors
Meurig Williams plate
Mewi-5 sidehole infusion catheter
Meyerding chisel
Meyerding curved gouge
Meyerding finger retractor
Meyerding laminectomy blade
Meyerding laminectomy retractor
Meyerding mallet
Meyerding-Scoville blade
Meyerding self-retaining retractor
Meyer vein stripper
MFG (manofluorography)
Mg (magnesium)

MGB (mini-gastric banding)
$MgSO_4$ (magnesium sulfate)
M.G.H. needle holder
M.H.G. elevator
MH needle
MHV (middle hepatic vein)
MIBB breast biopsy system
MIC gastroenteric tube
MIC jejunostomy tube
MIC-Key G gastrostomy tube
MIC-Key J gastrostomy tube
MIC Thermal Option disposable biopsy forceps
MIC-TJ transgastric jejunal tube
micelle formation
Michel aortic clamp
Michel applying and removing forceps
Michel clip
Michel clip-removing forceps
Michele vertebral biopsy
Michel wound clip
Micral chemstrip urine test
Micral urine dipstick test
Micrins microsurgical suture
microabscess
microadhesiolysis
MicroAire blade
MicroAire drill
MicroAire oscillating saw
MicroAire power-assisted lipoplasty device
MicroAire reamer
micro artery forceps (see *forceps*)
micro balloon probe
Microban drape
micro bipolar forceps (see *forceps*)
Microblater ArthroWand
microbubble contrast agent
microcalcifications, clustered
microchromoendoscopy
microclip or micro clip (see *clip*)
micro cross-action bulldog clamp
microcyst formation
microcyst, lymphatic
microcytic anemia
Microdermabrader
Micro Diamond-Point microsurgery instruments
Micro dissecting forceps, fenestrated, double-action
microdissection of the cervical lymph node compartments
micro dissector or microdissector
Microdot technique for precision suture placement
micro dural hook
Microelectrode MI-506 small-caliber pH electrode
microerosion
microfibrillar collagen hemostat
microfixation plate
MicroFlow needle
MicroFlow phacoemulsification needle
Microfoam dressing
Microfoam surgical tape
micro forceps or microforceps (see *forceps*)
Microgyn resectoscope sheath
micro Halsted mosquito forceps
micro hook or microhook (see *hook*)
micro instruments, surgical
microinvasive carcinoma
micro irrigating cannula (see *cannula*)
Micro Jaw rotatable dissecting forceps
micro jaw rotatable Kelly (Metzenbaum, grasping, etc.) dissecting forceps
Micro-Kerrison rongeur
MicroKlenz wound cleanser
Microknit vascular graft
micro laminectomy rongeur (see *rongeur*)
MicroLap and Microlap Gold micro-laparoscopy system
micro laryngeal instruments
Microlase transpupillary diode laser
Microlet Vaculance
Microlight 830 laser
microlithiasis

microlobular cirrhosis
MicroMark clip
MicroMark tissue marker
micromelena
micrometastatic disease
MicroMewi multi-sidehole infusion catheter
MicroMite suture anchor
Micronase (glyburide)
Micron needle holder
micro needle or microneedle (see *needle*)
micro nerve hook (see *hook*)
micro neurosurgical scissors (see *scissors*)
Micronized Glyburide (glyburide)
micronodular cirrhosis of liver
micronodular fibrotic pattern
Micro-One dissecting forceps
Micro-One hook
Micro-One needle holder
Micro-One scissors
Micro-optical forceps
micro oscillating saw
micropapillary carcinoma
microperforation
micro pin or micropin (see *pin*)
micro plate or microplate
  C-shaped
  H-shaped
  half-circle
  Howmedica
  Leibinger
  L-shaped
  Luhr
  Microfixation cranial
  Storz Microsystem
  Synthes Microsystems
  T-shaped
  X-shaped
  Y-shaped
micropoint-reverse cutting
micropoint spatula
microport or micro port
Microprobe laser
Micro-Probe microdissection tip
micro probe or microprobe (see *probe*)
Micro QuickAnchor
Micropuncture Peel-Away introducer
microradiograph
micro rasp or microrasp (see *rasp*)
Micro-Retractor
microreamer or micro reamer
micro sagittal saw
microsatellite instability (MSI)
microsaw or micro saw (see *saw*)
micro scissors or microscissors (see *scissors*)
microscope
  darkfield
  double binocular operating
  electron
  Grenoble-Paris-Rennes (GPR) robot
  Leica Aristoplan laser-scanning
  light
  monocular
  Olympus OME-8000 dual stereo surgical
  operating
  phase-contrast
  robot neurosurgical
  stereotactic (or stereotaxic) operating
  Zeiss operating
  Zeiss OPMI surgical
microscopic blood in stool
microscopic colitis
microscopic diagnosis
microscopic dissecting needle
microscopic extension of tumor cells
microscopic hemorrhage of ligament
microscopic multicentric lesion
microscopic multifocal medullary carcinoma
microscopic scissors (see *scissors*)
microscopy
  darkfield
  electron

microscopy *(cont.)*
 electronic
 endoscopic confocal
 immune electron
 immunofluoresence
 light
 polarized light
 scanning electron
microscopy of gastric biopsy
microscrew (see *screw*)
Microscribe 3DX digitizer
Micro Series wire driver
microsphere
Microspike approximator clamp
microstaple or micro staple (see *staple*)
microsurgery
 computer-assisted
 guided
 stereotactic laser
 transanal endoscopic (TEM)
 video-endoscope-assisted
microsurgery drill (see *drill*)
microsurgery forceps (see *forceps*)
microsurgery or microsurgical scissors
microsurgical decompression
microsurgical dissection
microsurgical DREZ-otomy
microsurgical epididymovasostomy (MSEV)
microsurgical free flap
microsurgical free tissue transfer
microsurgical technique
microsuture or micro suture (see *suture*)
Microtainer lancet
micro tear
Microtek Medical
microtelangiectasia
MicroTeq portable belt
Micro-Three microsurgery instruments
microthrombus
microtome object disc
microtrabecular hepatocellular carcinoma
Micro-Two forceps
Micro-Two needle holder
Micro-Two scissors
microvascular anastomosis
microvascular clamp
microvascular decompression
microvascular disease
microvascular flap transfer
microvascular forceps
microvascular hemodynamics
microvascular knife
microvascular scissors
microvascular transfer
microvasculature
microvasculopathy
microvasive endoscopic balloon
Microvasive Glidewire
Microvasive Mini Button low-profile balloon
Microvasive Rigiflex TTS balloon
Microvasive sclerotherapy needle
Microvasive stiff piano wire guidewire
MicroVent Resuscitator
microvesicular fat
microvilli of intestine
microvillus (pl. microvilli)
midabdominal transverse incision
midabdominal wall
Midas Rex craniotomy saw
Midas Rex knife
Midas Rex rongeur
midaxillary line
midaxillary line incision
midazolam HCl
midcolon
Middeldorpf retractor
middle colic artery
middle extrahepatic bile duct
middle hemorrhoidal artery
middle thyroid vein
midepigastric area
midepigastrium
midesophagus
midgut volvulus
midgut volvulus with malrotation

midinfrared laser
midline abdominal crease
midline abdominal incision
midline adducted position
midline incision
midline mass
midline mass below hyoid bone
midline small of back pain
midpalmar abscess
midrectal area
midsection
midsigmoid colon
midzonal necrosis
Mielke BT (bleeding time)
miglitol
migraine headache
migrating motor complex (MMC)
migration of pain
migration of shunt
migration of the spleen
Mik (Mikulicz)
Mikhail design
Mik pad (Mikulicz pad)
Mikulicz abdominal retractor
Mikulicz clamp
Mikulicz drain
Mikulicz exteriorization and resection of bowel
Mikulicz fiberoptic retractor
Mikulicz gastrostomy tube
Mikulicz pad (Mik pad)
Mikulicz peritoneal forceps
Mikulicz pyloroplasty
Mikulicz retractor
Milan curette
Milch plate
mild fever
mild hematuria
Miles abdominoperineal resection
Miles bone chisel
miliary pattern
milk
  acidophilus
  breast

milk *(cont.)*
  cow's
  goat
  intolerance of
  soy
  unpasteurized
milk-alkali syndrome
milk diet
milk-filled cyst
milking of intestine
Milkinol (mineral oil)
milk intolerance
milk line
milk of magnesia (MOM)
Milk of Magnesia–Cascara, Concentrated
milk protein antibody
milky ascites
milky fluid
milky nipple discharge
Millar MPC-500 catheter
Millenia balloon catheter
Millennium MLC-120 multileaf collimator
Millennium ultrasonic aspirator
Miller-Abbott intestinal tube
Miller-Abbott long gastrointestinal tube
Miller laryngoscope
Miller laryngoscope blade
miller's lung
Miller rasp
Miller rectal forceps
Miller rectal scissors
Miller-Senn retractor
Milligan-Morgan hemorrhoidectomy
Milligan-Morgan technique for treating hemorrhoids
Millin bladder neck spreader
milliner's needle
Millin forceps
Millin ligature-holding forceps
Millin retropubic retractor
Mills arteriotomy scissors
Mills dressing

Mills vascular scissors
Miltex diagnostic instruments
Miltex ear loop
Miltex edge scissors sharpener
Miltex forceps
Miltex instrument guard
Miltex-Kerrison cervical rongeur
Miltex mallet
Miltex needle holder
Miltex punch
Miltex scissors
Miltex speculum
Miltex tendon-pulling forceps
Miltex tissue twist hook
minalrestat
mineral oil
mineralocorticoid
miner's lung
Ming classification of gastric carcinoma
mini applier
miniature stomach
Mini-CABG instrument set
Mini Crown stent
mini fragment plate
mini gastric bypass (MGB)
Mini GLS anchor
mini Hohmann podiatric retractor
minilap (minilaparotomy)
mini laparoscope, Storz
minilaparotomy incision
mini-Lexer gouge
minimal deviation melanoma
minimally invasive esophagectomy
minimally invasive surgery (MIS)
minimal urine output
MiniMed insulin pump
Minimedicut
mini meniscus blade
mini Metzenbaum scissors
mini papillotome or minipapillotome
Mini QuickAnchor anchor
Mini-Revo Screw suture anchor
mini Roux retractor
mini Ruskin rongeur
MiniSite laparoscope
MINI 6600 C-arm
Mini Virobac filter
Minnesota tube, modified
minor crossmatch
minor duodenal papilla
Mintezol (thiabendazole)
Mintox, Mintox Plus
minute bleeding mucosal ulcer
minute papule
minute ventilation
Mira cautery
Mirage ostomy appliance
MiraLax (polyethylene glycol 3350)
Miralene suture
Miraluma (technetium ^{99m}Tc sestamibi kit)
Miraluma nuclear breast imaging
Mira Mark III cranial drill
Mira reamer
Mirizzi syndrome
mirror
  Bramber head
  laryngeal
  Ziegler head
mirror image breast biopsy
MIS (minimally invasive surgery)
MIS Source colonoscope
MIS Source duodenoscope
MIS Source flexible endoscope
MIS Source gastroscope
MIS Source sigmoidoscope
Miskimon cerebellar retractor
misoprostol
missed accessory spleen
missile track abscess
MIST insufflator
MIST video camera system
Mitek bone anchor
Mitek GII suture anchor
Mitek knotless suture anchor
Mitek Mini GII suture
Mitek staple
Mitek Superanchor suture anchor

Mitek suture
Mitek suture anchor
Mitek Vapor probe
Mitek VAPR system
Mitek VAPRTM T thermal electrode
mitochondrial antibody
mitochondrial oxidative
  phosphorylation
MitoExtra
mitogen-activated protein kinase
  (MAPK) cascade
mitomycin
Mitraflex dressing
Mitraflex Plus dressing
Mitraflex SC dressing
Mitraflex SC sacral dressing
mitral orifice
mitral stenosis
mitral valve homograft
Mitrofanoff appendicovesicotomy
Mitrofanoff neourethra procedure
Mitrolan (calcium polycarbophil)
Mitscherlich test
Mittelman nasal cartilage graft kit
mittelschmerz
Mitutoyo digital calipers
Mivacron (mivacurium chloride)
mivacurium chloride
mixed cell Hodgkin disease
mixed cell sarcoma
mixed cell thymoma
mixed cell tumor
mixed-cholesterol gallstone
mixed elemental-fat diet
mixed growth on culture
mixed hemorrhoids
mixed hepatocholangiocellular
  carcinoma
mixed hiatal hernia
mixed infection
mixed lesion
mixed neuropathic picture
mixed protein-fat diet
mixed venous blood
Mixter artery forceps
Mixter clamp
Mixter dilating probe
Mixter dissecting forceps, 90° angle,
  double-action
Mixter-O'Shaughnessy artery forceps
Mixter right-angle clamp
Mixter thoracic forceps
Mixter ventricular needle
Mladick concave cannula
Mladick convex cannula
Mladick liposuction cannula
MLT microlaryngeal tracheal tube
MMC (migrating motor complex)
MMF (mycophenolate mofetil)
MMMP (mucosal neuroma, medullary
  thyroid carcinoma, marfanoid body
  habitus, pheochromocytoma)
mmol/L (millimole per liter)
MM virus
MoAb monoclonal antibody
Mobetron electron accelerator
mobile axillary node
mobile gallbladder
mobile suction cart
mobilization of breast
mobilization of cecum
mobilization of gastric fundus
mobilization of small intestine through
  the mesocolon
mobilization of upper pole of thyroid
mobilize the duodenum and pancreas
mobilizer, Derlacki
MOC (metronidazole, omeprazole,
  clarithromycin)
Moctanin (monoctanoin)
Modane Bulk
Modane Plus
Modane Soft
Modane Versabran
model
  Claus breast cancer
  Gail breast cancer
  Markov simulation

moderate ductal hyperplasia
moderately differentiated adenoma
moderately well-differentiated carcinoma
moderate-size polymorphic inflammatory cell infiltrate
modified Allis grasping forceps, double-action
modified barium swallow
modified Bassini inguinal hernia repair
modified Delphi technique
modified dorsal lithotomy position
modified double Allis grasping forceps, double-action
modified Dukes staging (A-D)
modified Kessler suture
modified lithotomy position
modified Minnesota tube
modified neck dissection
modified Papanicolaou method
modified radical mastectomy
modified Robert Jones dressing
modified Shouldice hernioplasty
modified TAPP hernioplasty
modified tumescent technique
modified Whitehead hemorrhoidectomy
MODM (maturity-onset diabetes mellitus)
Modny pin
MODS (multiorgan [multiple organ] dysfunction syndrome)
Modudose A4398 unit dose saline vial
Modulap probe
Modulith SL 20 lithotriptor
MODY (maturity-onset diabetes of the young)
Moe distraction rod
Moe gouge
Moe intertrochanteric plate
Moe-modified Harrington rod
Moe spinal hook
Moe square-ended hook
MOF (multiple organ failure)
Mogen circumcision clamp
Mohr test
Mohs fresh tissue chemosurgery
moist sponge on ring forceps
molar mass
molar pregnancy (hydatidiform mole)
molecular death
molecular lesion
molecular marker
molecular mass
molecule
  antibody
  filtered
  middle
  PEG (polyethylene glycol)
  RNA
  secreted
moleskin dressing
moleskin scissors
moleskin strips dressing
Mollelast bandage
Mollison retractor
molluscum contagiosum
molluscum contagiosum virus
MOLLY bipolar forceps
Molt mouth gag
Molt periosteal elevator
Molypen (ammonium molybdate tetrahydrate)
MOM (milk of magnesia)
Mon-a-therm esophageal stethoscope temperature sensor
Mon-a-therm Foley catheter
Mon-a-therm skin temperature sensor
Mondor disease
mongolian spot-like lesion
monilial infection
monitor, monitoring (see also *blood glucose monitor)*
  Biotrack coagulation
  Cardiocap 5
  chronicle implantable hemodynamic
  Diasensor 1000 glucose
  Digital Response (DRx)
  DRx (Digital Response)

monitor *(cont.)*
- Duet glucose control
- esophageal pH
- FastTake blood glucose
- gastric pH
- Glycosal diabetes
- Health Buddy
- HealthCheck
- hemodynamic
- HemoMatic
- HERMES surgery
- Hewlett Packard temperature
- high-resolution video
- HomMed Sentry/Observer
- incuTemp
- IVAC
- Laserflo blood perfusion (BPM)
- Licox
- LifeShirt
- Lifestream Personal Cholesterol Monitor
- Meduck anesthesia
- Optical Sensors blood gas
- Prestige Smart System (PSS) glucose
- PSA 4000 anesthesia
- SureStep glucose
- TD Glucose
- 24-hour ambulatory esophageal pH

monitored anesthesia care (MAC)
monitoring lumen
monocautery cable
monoclonal antibody (see *medication*)
- altumomab (^{111}In altumobab pentetate)
- altumomab pentetate (^{111}In altumobab pentetate)
- anti-HER2
- anti-HER2 humanized
- basiliximab
- B43.13 (BrevaRex) vaccine for solid tumors
- BTI-322
- cA2

monoclonal *(cont.)*
- Campath
- CB-45RB
- CEA-Cide
- cedelizumab
- Cotara
- CTLA4-Ig
- dacliximab (daclizumab)
- Ha1A
- Herceptin (trastuzumab) anti-HER2
- IgG 2A
- Immurait (IgG 2A)
- ^{111}In altumomab pentetate
- infliximab
- MAb
- MAb-170
- MoAb
- murine
- muromonab-CD3
- Orthoclone OKT3
- Ostavir (tuvirumab)
- satumomab pendetide
- Simulect (baxiliximab)
- technetium ^{99m}Tc solesomab
- Therex (huHMFG1)
- trastuzumab

monoclonal antibody to CEA, humanized
monoclonal antibody to hepatitis B virus, human
monoclonal B cell proliferation
- Muromonab-CD3

Monocryl (poliglecaprone 25) suture
monoctanoin
monocular microscope
monocytes
monofilament absorbable suture
monofilament microporous mesh
monofilament nylon drain
monofilament nylon suture
monofilament polypropylene suture
monofilament stainless steel suture
Monojector fingerstick device
monojet Toomey syringe

monolobular cirrhosis
mononeuropathy, diabetic
mononuclear infiltrate
mononucleosis
  acute
  chronic
  cytomegalovirus
  infectious (IM)
  post-transfusion
monooctanoin
mono-oxygenase, flavin-containing
monopolar cable
monopolar coagulation
monopolar dissector
monopolar electrocoagulation
monopolar and bipolar cords and electrodes
monoscopic endoscope
Monoscopy locking trocar with Woodford spike
Monosof monofilament nylon suture
monotherapy, interferon
Monsel hemostatic solution
monster rongeur
Monte Carlo analysis
Montenovesi rongeur
Montevideo unit
Montezuma's revenge
Montgomery abdominal strap
Montgomery gland
Montgomery tape
Moolgaoker forceps
moon face or facies
Moon rectal retractor
Moore bone elevator
Moore bone reamer
Moore gallstone scoop
Moore hand drill
Moore nail
Moore pin
Moore prosthesis extractor
Moore sliding nail plate
Moorfield stitch-removing forceps
Morais retractor
morantel
morantel tartrate
morbidity
morbidity and mortality
morbidity following biopsy
morbid obesity
morcelized bone graft
morcellation of tissue
morcellation, tissue
morcellator
Moreira plate
morgagnian cyst
Morgagni appendix
Morgagni, column of
Morgagni crypt
Morgagni gland
Morgagni hernia
Morgagni hydatid
Morgagni nodule
Morgagni ventricle
Morganella morganii
Mori knife
Morinaga hemorrhoidectomy
Morison method
Morison pouch
Morphelan (oral morphine)
MorphiDex
morphine
morphine sulfate
morphology
morrhuate sclerosant
Morris aorta clamp
Morris retractor
Morrison tissue forceps
Morscher cervical plate
morselized (morcellized) bone graft
mortality
mortar kidney
mortise view
mortising chisel
mosaic pattern of duodenal mucosa
Mosher life-saving tube
mosquito-borne virus
mosquito clamp

mosquito forceps
mosquito hemostat
Moss decompression feeding catheter
Mosse syndrome
Moss gastrostomy tube (G-tube)
Moss G-tube PEG kit
Moss hook
Moss nasal tube, Mark IV
Moss rod
Moss Suction Buster tube
Moss T-anchor needle introducer gun
moth-eaten appearance (on imaging)
mother cyst
mother/daughter endoscope
Mother Jones (modified Robert Jones) dressing
motility
- colonic
- cornflake esophageal
- esophageal
- gastrin-stimulated intestinal
- GI
- intestinal
- primary esophageal

motility disorder
- esophageal
- gastric
- intestinal
- nonspecific esophageal motility (NEMD)
- smooth-muscle
- primary esophageal

Motilium (domperidone maleate)
motion pain
motion sickness
Motofen (difenoxin HCl; atropine sulfate)
motorized gouge
motor meal barium GI series
motor oil peritoneal fluid
motor test meal
mottled appearance
moulage for breast implant
moulage for custom breast implant
moulage sign
Mount laminectomy rongeur
Mouradian rod
mouse, peritoneal
Mousseaux-Barbin intraluminal tube
Mousseaux-Barbin prosthetic tube
mouth gag
- Ackland
- Crowe-Davis
- Davis
- Denhardt
- Dingman
- Doyen-Jensen
- Jennings
- McIvor
- Molt

mouth guard
mouth to anus
movable kidney
movement, bowel (BM)
moxifloxacin
Moynihan artery forceps
Moynihan bile duct probe
Moynihan forceps
Moynihan gall duct forceps
Moynihan gallstone probe
Moynihan gallstone scoop
Moynihan test
Moynihan towel clamp
MPC scissors
MPD (main pancreatic duct) stent
MPEC (multipolar electrocoagulation)
MPH (medullary thyroid carcinoma, pheochromocytoma, hyperparathyroidism)
MPI 5020
MPM hydrogel dressing
MPT (multiple parameter telemetry)
MRC (magnetic resonance cholangiography)
MRCP (magnetic resonance cholangiopancreatography)
MRCP using HASTE with a phased array coil

MRI (magnetic resonance imaging)
MRM (magnetic resonance mammography)
MRN (magnetic resonance neurography)
MRP (magnetic resonance pancreatography)
MR peritoneography
MRSA (pronounced "mer-sah") (methicillin-resistant *Staphylococcus aureus*)
MS Classique balloon dilatation catheter
MSA (microsomal antibody)
MSEV (microsurgical epididymovasostomy)
MSI (microsatellite instability)
MSOF (multisystem organ failure)
MS-1 hepatitis
MS-2 hepatitis
MS-325 imaging agent
MTBE (methyl tertiary butyl ether)
mtDNA (mitochondrial DNA)
M2A Swallowable Imaging Capsule
M-25 virus
mucin clot formation
mucin clot test
mucin, gastric
mucinoid degeneration
mucinosis
  follicular
  papular
mucinous adenocarcinoma
mucinous adenoma
mucinous carcinoma
mucinous cystadenocarcinoma
mucinous degeneration
mucinous nest
mucocele, appendiceal
mucocele of gallbladder
mucocutaneous hemorrhoids
mucocutaneous junction
mucocutaneous line
mucocutaneous pigmentation of Peutz-Jeghers syndrome
mucoepidermal carcinoma
mucoepidermoid carcinoma
mucoid material
mucoid secretion
mucoid stool
Mucomyst
Mucopolysaccharidoses
mucopurulent drainage
mucormycosis
mucosa
  alimentary
  alveolar
  anorectal
  antral
  auditory
  Barrett
  blanching of
  bronchial
  buccal
  bulging of
  burned out (on x-ray)
  cardiac (of stomach)
  cobblestone
  cobblestoning of
  colorectal
  denuded
  discolored
  ectopic gastric
  edematous
  endocervical
  esophageal
  foveolar gastric
  foveolosulciolar gastric
  friable
  fundic
  gallbladder
  gastric antral
  gastrointestinal
  gingival
  hemorrhagic
  honeycomb

mucosa *(cont.)*
 hyperemic
 hyperplastic
 hypertrophied
 intestinal
 irregular
 Neisseria
 normal-appearing
 outpouching of
 oxyntic
 polyp of hypertrophied
 protrusion of the
 pyloric
 rectal
 sloughing of
 small bowel
 spiraling of rectal
 sulciolar gastric
 thumbprinting of
 tracheobronchial
 urinary
 vaginal
mucosal abnormality
mucosal advancement
mucosal atrophy
mucosal bridge
mucosal disease virus
mucosal folds
mucosal guideline pattern
mucosal hyperemia
mucosal hyperplasia
mucosal ileal diaphragms
mucosal immune system
mucosal injection
mucosal involvement
mucosal island (on x-ray)
mucosal junction, squamocolumnar
mucosal melanoma
mucosal necrosis
mucosal neuroma syndrome (MEA type III)
mucosal neuromas
mucosal patch
mucosal pattern
mucosal proctectomy
mucosal ring, esophageal
mucosal sleeve resection
mucosal surface
mucosal suspensory ligament
mucosal ulcer
mucosal ulceration
mucosal view
mucosal zone
mucosanguineous discharge
mucosectomy, rectal
mucoserous cell
mucositis
 candida
 cytolomegalovirus
 herpes
mucous (adj.)
mucous carcinoma
mucous cell
mucous colic
mucous colitis
mucous cyst
mucous degeneration
mucous diarrhea
mucous fistula
mucous gland of duodenum
mucous lake of stomach
mucous membrane
mucous neck cell
mucous plug
mucous polyp
mucous salivary gland
mucous shred
mucous stool
mucous strand
mucous surface
mucoviscidosis
mucus (noun); mucous (adj.)
mucus per rectum
mucus plug
mucus plugging
mucus-secreting cell
mucus-secreting gland
mud, biliary

Mueller (Müller)
Mueller compression blade plate
Mueller maneuver
Mueller rongeur
Mueller saw
Mueller 0° 5 mm rigid laparoscope
"muffs" bandage
Muir hemorrhoid forceps
mulberry calculus
mulberry gallstone
mule-spinner's cancer
Mulholland sphincterotomy
Muller pediatric clamp
Müller (see *Mueller*)
Mullins catheter introducer
MultAport cannula
MultApplier device
MultApump device
MultAvalue laparoscopic device
MulTE-Pak-4: MulTE-Pak-5 (multiple trace elements [metals])
multi-agent therapy
Multibite biopsy forceps
multicellular organism
multicentric lesion
multicentric thyroid
multicentricity
Multiclip ligating clip device
Multidex hydrophilic powder dressing
Multidex wound-filling material
multidisciplinary transplant team
multidrug resistant (MDR)
multidrug systemic chemotherapy
multifactorial etiopathogenesis
multifilament suture
Multifire Endo GIA stapler
Multifire Endo Hernia clip applicator
Multifire Endo Hernia stapler
Multifire GIA surgical stapler
Multifire TA surgical stapler
Multifire VersaTack stapler
multiflanged Portnoy (for hydrocephalus shunt) catheter
Multi-Flex stent
multifocal lesion
multifocal tumor
multifunction port
Multikine
Multikuf sphygmomanometer
Multi-Link Tetra coronary stent system
multilobular cirrhosis
multilocular mass
multiloculated tumor
multilumen probe
Multilyte-40 (combined electrolyte solution)
multimodal therapy
multinodular gland
multinodular goiter
multinodular mass
Multi-Operatory Dentalaser (MOD) laser
multiorgan dysfunction syndrome (MODS)
multiorgan failure
multiplanar fluoroscopic stress view
multiple abscess formation
multiple colloid adenomatous goiter (MCAG)
multiple cysts
multiple dysplastic nevi
multiple endocrine adenomatosis (MEA) syndrome, type 2
multiple endocrine deficiency syndrome, type 2
multiple endocrine neoplasia, type 2B
multiple familial polyposis
multiple hamartoma syndrome
multiple hamartomatous polyps
multiple idiopathic hemorrhagic sarcoma
multiple inert gas elimination techniques (MIGET)
multiple infarcts
multiple inflammatory fibrous thickenings
multiple intestinal polyposis
multiple myeloma

multiple myositis
multiple neuritis
multiple nodules
multiple organ dysfunction
multiple organ dysfunction syndrome (MODS)
multiple organ failure (MOF)
multiple organ failure syndrome (MOFS)
multiple organ involvement
multiple pain afferents
multiple parameter telemetry (MPT)
multiple polyp
multiple previous surgical procedures
multiple proinflammatory cytokines
multiple sclerosis
multiple-strand suture
multiple thyroid nodules
multiple transfusions
multipolar coagulation
multipolar electrocautery
multipolar electrocoagulation (MPEC) therapy (MECT)
Multipurpose-SM catheter
multiseptate gallbladder
multisized reamer
multistep carcinogenesis
multistrand
multisystem disease
multisystem organ failure (MOM)
Multitak SS suture anchor
multivariate analysis
multiverrucous friable lesion
multivisceral transplantation
mumps hepatitis
mumps pancreatitis
mumps virus
Munchausen syndrome
Munro point
mural kidney
mural thickening
MUR (multiuse reposable) clip applier
murine leukemia virus
murine monoclonal antibody
Murless fetal head extractor
muromonab-CD3 monoclonal antibody
Murphy common duct dilator
Murphy eye
Murphy gallbladder retractor
Murphy gouge
Murphy-Lane bone skid
Murphy retractor
Murphy sign
Murphy tip
Murray Valley encephalitis virus
muscle biopsy
muscle biopsy clamp
muscle carnitine deficiency
muscle fasciculation
muscle guarding
muscle hook
muscle necrosis
muscle pedicle
muscle-splitting incision
muscle-to-bone suture
muscle wasting
muscular propria
muscular ring, esophageal
muscularis
musculature, intra-abdominal wall
musculoaponeurotic band
musculoaponeurotic sheath tumor
MUSE (medicated urethral system for erection)
mushroom catheter
mushroom gastrostomy tube
mushroom-shaped mass
mushy stools
musical bowel sounds
Mustang steerable guidewire
Mutamycin (mitomycin)
mutation
  BRCA
  gene
  P53
MVR blade
Mya hook
myalgia

myasthenia gravis
mycobacterial antibody
mycobacterial spheroplast
Mycobacterium avium-intracellulare (MAI) complex
Mycobacterium gordonae
Mycobacterium tuberculosis
mycophenolate mofetil (MMF)
Mycoplasma pneumoniae
mycosis, gastric
Mycostatin
mycotoxin aflatoxin
MycroMesh biomaterial graft
myelin kidney
myelogenic sarcoma
myelogenous leukemia
myeloid metaplasia
myeloid sarcoma
myeloma kidney
myelophthisic splenomegaly
myeloproliferative disorder
myelosuppression
myelotomy knife
myenteric plexus
Myers-Fine test
Myers knee retractor
Mylagen, Mylagen II (aluminum hydroxide; magnesium hydroxide; simethicone)
Mylanta (calcium carbonate; magnesium hydroxide; simethicone)
Mylanta Natural Fiber Supplement (psyllium hydrophilic mucilloid)
Mylanta-II
Mylar patch
Mylicon (simethicone)
Mylius test
myoblastoma, granular cell
myocardial necrosis
Myocet (liposome encapsulated doxorubicin citrate complex)
myocutaneous flap
myocutaneous graft
myodesis suture
myoelectric dysrhythmia
myofibroblast
myofibroma
myolysis
myoma
myomatous polyp
myomectomy, anorectal
myoneural junction
myoneural necrosis
myopathic carnitine deficiency
myopathic electromyography
myopathy
  infantile mitochondrial
  inflammatory
  ipecac-induced
  myxedema
  steroid
  thyrotoxic
  toxic
myopectineal opening of Fruchaud
myopectineal orifice (MPO)
myotomy
  circular
  cricoid
  cricopharyngeal
  esophageal
  extramucosal
  Heller
  laparoscopic
  longitudinal
myotonic dystrophy
myxedema ascites
myxedema coma
myxedema madness
myxedema myopathy
myxedema, pretibial
myxofibroma
myxoid material
myxomatous tumor
myxorrhea gastrica
myxovirus

N, n

N (nitrogen)
NA (Narcotics Anonymous)
Na (sodium)
Nabi-Altastaph vaccine
Nabi-HB (hepatitis B immune globulin [human])
Nabi NicVAX vaccine
Nabi-StaphVAX vaccine
nabothian gland
NABS (normoactive bowel sounds)
N-acetylcysteine (NAC)
NaCl (sodium chloride)
Nadler coaptation bipolar forceps
Naganol (suramin sodium)
nagging pain
nail
  adjustable
  Ainsworth modification of Massie
  antegrade femoral
  AO slotted medullary
  AP
  Augustine boat
  Bailey-Dubow
  Barr
  Bickel intramedullary
  Bionx SmartNail
  blind medullary
  boat

nail *(cont.)*
  Brooker femoral
  Brooker-Wills
  cannulated
  Chick
  Christensen interlocking
  closed
  closed Küntscher (Kuentscher)
  closed unlocked
  cloverleaf intramedullary
  cloverleaf Küntscher (Kuentscher)
  condylocephalic
  crutch-and-belt femoral closed
  Curry hip
  Derby
  Deyerle pin
  diamond-shaped medullary
  Dooley
  double-ended
  double-hollow
  dynamic locking
  elastic stable intramedullary (ESIN)
  Ender
  Ender flexible medullary
  Engel-May
  extension
  femoral neck
  fixator-augmented

nail *(cont.)*
- fluted titanium
- four-flanged
- gamma locking
- Grosse-Kempf interlocking medullary
- Hagie pin
- Hahn bone
- half-and-half
- hallux
- Hansen-Street
- Harris condylocephalic
- Harris hip
- Harris medullary
- Holt
- hooked intramedullary
- hooked medullary
- Huckstep
- ingrown (onychocryptosis)
- INRO surgical
- interlocking
- interlocking intramedullary
- intramedullary (IM)
- Inyo
- Jewett
- Johannson hip
- Kaessmann
- Ken
- Ken sliding
- Knowles
- Küntscher (Kuentscher) medullary
- left-sided
- Lewis
- locked intramedullary
- locking
- Lottes triflanged medullary
- Massie II
- Massie sliding
- McKee tri-fin
- McLaughlin
- medullary
- Moore
- nailing
- nested

nail *(cont.)*
- Neufeld
- noncannulated
- Nylok self-locking
- open
- OrthoSorb pin
- Palmer bone
- PGP
- Pidcock
- pre-bent
- Pugh sliding
- reconstruction
- retrograde femoral
- Richards reconstruction
- right-sided
- Rush flexible medullary
- Rush pin
- Russell-Taylor (R-T) interlocking medullary
- Rydell
- Sage triangular
- Sampson medullary
- Sarmiento
- Schneider medullary
- Seidel humeral locking
- self-broaching
- self-locking
- Slocum
- SmartNail
- Smillie
- Smith-Petersen femoral neck
- Smith-Petersen transarticular
- spring-loaded
- static locking
- Steinmann extension
- Street
- Sven-Johansson femoral neck
- telescoping
- Temple University
- Terry
- Thatcher
- Thornton
- Tiemann
- titanium

nail *(cont.)*
triangular medullary
triflange
triflanged Lottes
Uniflex intramedullary
Venable-Stuck
Vesely-Street split
Vitallium Küntscher (Kuentscher)
V-medullary
Watson-Jones
Webb
Z fixation
Zickel intramedullary
Zickel subtrochanteric
Zickel supracondylar medullary
nail assembly, Massie
nail atrophy
nail bed
nail driver
nail-extracting hook
nail nipper
nail plate
nail-pulling forceps
nail rotational guide
nail scissors
nail splitter
nail-splitting scissors
Nakao snare I and II
Nakayama test
Namalwa cell
NANB (non-A, non-B) hepatitis (now hepatitis C)
nandrolone phenpropionate
N&V (nausea and vomiting)
NAP hepatitis B virus (HBV) quantitative panel
Naphuride (suramin sodium)
napkin-ring annular lesion
Narco esophageal motility machine
narcotic addiction
Narcotics Anonymous (NA)
Nardi test (morphine-prostigmine)
Naropin (ropivacaine)
narrow blade retractor
narrow neck mini Hohmann retractor
narrowing of thoracic aorta
nasal dressing sponge
nasal elevator
nasal instrumentation
nasal intubation
nasal olives glass
nasal polyp
Nasal RAE uncuffed tube
nasal septal hematoma
nasal smear
nasal sponge
nasal suction/irrigator with sheath
NASH (nonalcoholic steatohepatitis)
Nashold biopsy needle
Nashville Rabbit Antithymocyte Serum (lymphocyte immune globulin, antithymocyte [rabbit])
nasobiliary catheter
nasobiliary drain
nasobiliary drainage
nasobiliary drainage catheter
nasobiliary drainage tube
nasoduodenal feeding tube
nasoendoscopy
nasogastric (NG)
nasogastric feeding tube
nasogastric suction
nasogastric aspirate
nasogastric drainage
nasogastric intubation
nasogastric tube
nasogastric tube suction
nasojejunal (NJ) feeding tube
nasolabial fistula
nasolaryngopharyngoscope
nasopancreatic drainage
nasopancreatic drainage tube
nasopancreatic tube
nasopharyngeal carcinoma
nasopharyngeal hemorrhage
nasopharyngeal reflux
nasopharynx
nasotracheal intubation

nasotracheal tube
nateglinide
National Cancer Institute (NCI)
National Diabetes Data Group (NDDG)
National Digestive Diseases Information Clearinghouse (NDDIC)
National Donor Family Council (NDFC)
National Hospital percussor
National Institute of Diabetes and Digestive and Kidney Diseases (NIDDK)
National Kidney Foundation
National Organization for Rare Disorders, Inc.
native vasculature
Native American heritage
native tissue Harmonic imaging (NTHI)
natural body fluid
natural death
natural killer (NK) antigen
natural killer cell
natural resin, propolis
Natural Vegetable (psyllium hydrophilic mucilloid)
Nature's Remedy (cascara sagrada)
Naunton Morgan proctoscope
Naunton Morgan rectal speculum
nausea and vomiting (N/V, N&V)
nausea, postprandial
Nausea Relief (phosphorated carbohydrate solution)
nauseous
Nausetrol (phosphorated carbohydrate solution)
NAVEL (nerve, artery, vein, extralymphatic material, lymphatics)
navicular shoe cookie (pad)
navicular view
Navigator flexible endoscope
Navigator system for lymph node detection
Naviguide introducer
Navion BioNavigation system
Naviport catheter
Naviport deflectable tip-guiding catheter
Navi-Star catheter
Navitrack system
Navratil retractor
NBT (nitroblue tetrazolium)
NBT-PABA test
NCCH (National Cancer Center Hospital)
NCI (National Cancer Institute)
NCPF (noncirrhotic portal fibrosis)
NDDG (National Diabetes Data Group)
NDDIC (National Digestive Diseases Information Clearinghouse)
NDFC (National Donor Family Council)
Nd:YAG (neodymium:yttrium-aluminum-garnet) laser
Neal fallopian cannula
near-anatomic position
near-far suture
near-infrared spectroscopy (NIRS)
Nearly Me breast prosthesis
near-syncopal episode
near-syncope
near-total esophagectomy
near-total pancreatectomy
near-total removal
near-total thyroidectomy
nebulizer
  handheld
  large-volume
  ultrasonic
NEC (necrotizing enterocolitis)
Necator americanus
neck crepitus
neck exploration
neck hematoma
neck irradiation
neck masses
neck of gallbladder
neck of pancreas
necrosectomy

necrosis
- acute sclerosing hyaline (ASHN)
- acute tubular
- aseptic
- avascular (AVN)
- bacillary
- Balser fatty
- bilateral cortical
- biliary piecemeal
- blood vessel
- bloodless zone of
- bone
- bony
- bowel
- bridging
- caseous
- central
- centrilobular
- cerebral radiation (CRN)
- cheesy
- coagulation
- colliquative
- colonic
- contraction band
- cortical
- cystic medial
- diffuse
- dry
- embolic
- epiphyseal ischemic
- Erdheim cystic medial
- exanthematous
- extensive pancreatic
- fat
- fatty
- femoral head
- fibrinoid
- fibrosing piecemeal
- focal
- focal hepatic
- frank
- gallbladder
- gangrenous
- gangrenous pulp

necrosis *(cont.)*
- hemorrhagic
- hemorrhoidal
- hepatic
- hepatocellular
- hyaline
- indurative
- infected
- infectious pancreatic
- intestinal
- liquefaction
- liver
- localized
- malarial
- Marcus grading scale for avascular
- massive hepatic
- massive ischemic
- medial cystic
- midzonal
- mucosal
- muscle
- myocardial
- myoneural
- neuronal
- Paget quiet
- pancreatic
- papillary
- peripheral
- peripheral hepatic
- phosphorus
- piecemeal
- postpartum pituitary
- postreduction ischemic
- pressure
- progressive emphysematous
- radiation
- renal tubular
- segmental
- septic
- skin
- small bowel
- soft tissue
- sterile pancreatic
- stomal

necrosis *(cont.)*
- strangulation
- stromal
- subacute
- subacute hepatic
- subcutaneous fat
- submassive
- submassive hepatic
- superficial
- syphilitic
- thermal
- tissue
- total
- tracheobronchial mucosal
- tumor
- Zenker
- zonal

necrosis and perforation
necrosis of bladder epithelium
necrosis of bladder mucosa
necrosis of ductal epithelium
necrosis of gallbladder wall
necrosis of hepatocyte
necrosis of muscle
necrosis of muscle cells
necrosis of small bowel mucosa
necrosis of tissue
necrotic abscess
necrotic "anchovy paste" material
necrotic bone
necrotic bowel
necrotic debris
necrotic fibroid
necrotic hemorrhoids
necrotic inflammation
necrotic lesion
necrotic segment
necrotic tissue
necrotic tumor
necrotic ulceration
necrotizing arteriolitis in kidney
necrotizing arteritis
necrotizing arteritis associated with hepatitis B infection
necrotizing enterocolitis (NE, NEC)
necrotizing fasciitis
necrotizing gastritis
necrotizing gingivitis
necrotizing glomerulonephritis
necrotizing granulomatous lymphadenitis
necrotizing migratory erythema
necrotizing nephrosis
necrotizing pancreatitis
necrotizing papillitis
necrotizing pneumonia
necrotizing vasculitis of bowel
NED (no evidence of disease)
needle
- Abrams
- Abrams biopsy
- Accucore II core biopsy
- Adson aneurysm
- Adson scalp
- Ailee
- Aldrete
- AMC
- aneurysm
- aortic root perfusion
- Arruga
- Arthrotek RC
- aspirating
- aspiration
- aspiration injection
- Atraloc surgical
- Backlund biopsy
- band circling
- Barraquer
- B-D spinal
- B-D Weiss epidural with fixed wings
- Becton Dickinson Teflon-sheathed
- Bengash-type
- beveled thin-walled
- Beyer paracentesis
- Bier lumbar puncture
- Bierman
- BiLAP bipolar needle electrode

needle *(cont.)*
biopsy
Biopty cut
bone biopsy
bone round
Bonney
bore
Bouge
Boynton
BRK series transseptal
Brockenbrough transseptal
Bunnell tendon
butterfly
BV-2
BV130-5
cardioplegic
Cardiopoint
Castroviejo
Castroviejo-Mayo
cataract
Charles flute
Chiba
Chiba aspiration biopsy
Chiba cholangiography
Cibis ski
CIF-4
coaxial sheath cut-biopsy
Cobb-Ragde
Colapinto curved
Colapinto transjugular liver biopsy
Colorado microdissection
cone biopsy
cone ventricular
Control-Release pop-off
conventional cutting-sternum
Cook aspiration biopsy
Cook endoscopic curved
Cope biopsy
core biopsy
Core aspiration/injection
Core CO_2 insufflation
Core laparoscopic aspiration/ injection
Cournand arteriogram

needle *(cont.)*
Cournand-Grino arteriogram
Craig biopsy
Crawford
Crile-Wood
C-type acupuncture
culposuspension
Cushing ventricular
cut-biopsy
cutting
cutting biopsy
cyst aspiration
Dandy ventricular
DeBakey
Derf
Derf-TC
D'Errico ventricular
Deschamps
Deschamps ligature
Dieckmann intraosseous
discission
DLP cardioplegic
docking
Dos Santos
double-pointed
D-TACH removable
dural
Echo-Coat ultrasound biopsy
electrode
EMG (electromyogram)
Endoknot suture
Endopath Ultra Veress
Estridge biopsy
Ethalloy TruTaper cardiovascular
Ethibond
ExtreSafe
eye
Feild-Lee brain biopsy
fine
Finochietto
fistula
Framer tendon-passing
Franklin-Silverman liver biopsy
Franseen stereotactic

needle *(cont.)*
- Frazier ventricular
- French-eye
- Gabriel hemorrhoidal
- Gallie
- gastrointestinal
- Gillies
- GraNee
- Greene biopsy
- Gripper
- Gynex extended-reach
- Hagedorn
- Halsy
- Hariri-Heifetz
- Hawkeye suture
- Hawkins
- Hegar-Baumgartner
- Hemo-Drain
- Hoen ventricular
- hollow
- House
- House-Barbara shattering
- House-Rosen
- Howell biopsy aspiration
- hubbed
- Huber
- hypodermic
- insufflation
- Intracath
- J
- Jamshidi liver biopsy
- Jelco
- Jordan
- Kalt
- Keith
- Keith abdominal
- Klatskin liver biopsy
- Klima-Schleicher biopsy
- Knight needle
- Kobak pudendal block
- Koch nucleus hydrolysis
- Kopans breast lesion localization
- Kronecker aneurysm
- laparoscopy

needle *(cont.)*
- large bore
- large-bore slotted aspirating
- Lee cutting biopsy
- Lewis Pair-Pak
- Lewy-Holinger Teflon injection
- Lewy-Rubin Teflon glycerine mixture injection
- Lichtenberg
- ligature
- liver and peritoneum biopsy
- liver biopsy
- lumbar puncture
- Maciol laparoscopic suture
- Madayag biopsy
- MAGneedle controller
- Maho-Hegar
- Martin
- Martin cutting
- Mathieu
- Mayo Hegar
- Mayo noncutting
- Mayo trocar-point
- mediastinoscopy aspirating needle
- Menghini liver biopsy
- metal
- MH
- micro
- MicroFlow
- microscopic dissecting
- Microvasive sclerotherapy
- milliner's
- Mixter ventricular
- Nashold biopsy
- Neivert
- nonferromagnetic
- Nordenstrom biopsy
- Nottingham
- olive-tipped
- Olsen-Hegar
- OmniTip laser
- Optivis
- Pace ventricular
- Paparella straight

needle *(cont.)*
Parhad-Poppen arteriogram
Parham band-circling
PC-7
P.D. Access
Pencan spinal
Penfine
PercuCut cut-biopsy
percutaneous cutting
Pereyra
pericardiocentesis
peritoneal biopsy
P-4
phacoemulsification
Pitkin spinal
pleural biopsy
Plum-Blossom
PMT biopsy
Pneu-Stick abdominal
pneumoinsufflation
pneumoperitoneum
Poppen ventricular
port closure
postmortem
  double-curve cutting-edge
  half-curved cutting-edge
Potts-Cournand
pressure (teishein)
Protect Point
Punctur-Guard
Quincke lumbar puncture
Quincke spinal
Redon wound drainage
Reichert-Mundinger biopsy
Retter aneurysm
Reverdin suture
Rhoton
Riza-Ribe grasper
root
Rosch-Uchida transjugular liver
  access needle-catheter
Rosen
Rosenthal
Rotex cutting biopsy

needle *(cont.)*
Rotex II biopsy
Ruskin antrum trocar
Ryder
Sabreloc spatula
SafeTap tapered spinal
Safetrak epidural
Safety AV fistula
Sahli biopsy and aspiration needle
SampleMaster biopsy needle
Sarot
scalp
sclerotherapy
SC-1
Scoville ventricular
Seldinger
Seldinger gastrostomy
self-aspirating cut-biopsy
Sensi-Touch anesthesia
Shambaugh palpating
Shaw aneurysm
Sheldon-Spatz vertebral arteriogram
side-aspirating biopsy
side-cutting spatulated
Sieman irrigation injection
Silverman
Silverman-Boeker
Simcoe
skinny
skinny Chiba
slotted
SmallPort
SmartNeedle
Smiley-Williams arteriogram
Solitaire
spatulated half-circle
spinal
Spinell biopsy
spinocan spinal
Sprotte
Stamey
steel-winged butterfly
Steis
stereotactic biopsy

needle *(cont.)*
- Stifcore aspiration
- straight cutting
- Stratte
- Sureshot metal sheathed injection
- Surgalloy
- Surgineedle pneumoperitoneum
- suture
- SutureLoop
- suture-release
- swaged
- swaged-on
- Swedish
- Syme aneurysm
- Szabo-Berci needle driver
- tapered
- taper point
- teasing
- Teflon-coated hollow-bore
- teishein
- tendon-passing
- Terry-Mayo
- THI
- Thomas
- thoracentesis
- transjugular access
- transseptal
- Troutman
- Tru-Cut biopsy
- Tru-Cut cutting biopsy
- Tru-Cut liver biopsy
- Tru-Cut/Vim Silverman
- Tuohy epidural
- Tuohy lumbar puncture
- Tuohy point
- Tuohy thin-wall
- Turner biopsy
- ultrasound biopsy
- UMI
- Unimar J-Needle
- venting aortic Bengash-type
- ventricular
- ventriculostomy
- Verbrugge

needle *(cont.)*
- Veress (not Verres)
- Vim-Silverman
- Visi-Black surgical
- Voorhees (do not confuse with Veress)
- Wangensteen
- Waterfield
- Webster
- Westcott cutting biopsy
- Westerman-Jensen
- Whitacre spinal
- wire circling
- Wright
- Yankauer

NeedleAid device

needle and spud

needle aspiration, fine-

needle aspiration for culture

needle biopsy (see *biopsy*)
- confirmatory
- core
- CT-directed
- CT-scan directed
- fine-
- guided
- random
- stereotactic core needle (SCNB)
- transthoresis (TNB)
- ultrasound-guided
- Vim/Silverman

needle case

needle catheter jejunostomy

needle core biopsy

needle drainage

needle driver, Zsabo-Berei

needle electro probe

needle EMG

needle guide
- Iowa trumpet
- Site~Rite

needle holder
- Adson dural
- Ayers

needle holder *(cont.)*
- Barraquer
- Baumgartner-TC
- Berry sternal
- boomerang
- Boynton
- Bozeman Thomas Walker
- Brown
- Castroviejo
- Castroviejo-Mayo
- Castroviejo-TC
- Castroviejo-TC spring
- Collier
- Converse-TC
- Crile-Wood
- DeBakey-TC
- Derf, Derf-TC
- Diethrich-TC
- Donaghy angled suture
- Dubecq-Princeteau angulating
- Foster-TC
- Fukushima-Giannotta
- Gillies
- Gillies-Finochietto
- Halsey-TC
- Heaney
- Jacobson microvascular
- Jacobson-TC
- Kalman
- Kilner-TC
- Lichtenberg-Ryder
- Masson
- Mathieu-TC
- Mayo-Hegar
- M.G.H.
- Micro-One
- Micron
- Miltex
- Neivert-TC
- New Orleans
- Olsen-Hegar-TC
- Olsen-Mathieu-TC
- Parell-TC
- Parks-TC

needle holder *(cont.)*
- ratchet-on-demand
- Ryder-TC
- Ryder micro
- Sarot-TC
- Stevens
- Stratte-TC
- TC (tungsten carbide)
- Thomson
- Thomson Walker-TC
- titanium microsurgical
- Twisk
- Vantage
- Vickers
- Vital Cooley microvascular
- Vital Ryder microvascular
- Wangensteen
- Ward
- Webster
- Webster-TC
- Wright
- Young-Millin boomerang holder

needle holder+A4654 with tungsten carbide (TC) inlays
needle hub
needle inserted under fluoroscopic control
needle introducer
needle knife
needle-knife sphincterotome
needle lavage
needle localization, mammographically guided
needle localization of breast lesion
needle manometer technique
needle-nose dissecting forceps, double-action
needle-nose pliers
needlepoint electrocautery
needle-pulling forceps
needle puncture
needle puncture wound
needle raiser
needlescope
needlescopic TAPP hernia repair

needle sprotte
needlestick exposure
needle thoracostomy
needle-tip electrocautery
needle with Hustead wing
needle with tungsten carbide (TC)
  inserts, double-action
Neer lateral view
Neer transscapular view
Neff meniscus knife
negative antibody screen
negative appendectomy
negative breast biopsy
negative feedback
negative inotropic effect
negative inspiratory pressure
negative margin
negative pleural space pressure
negligible blood loss
Negus rigid esophagoscope
Neisseria
Neivert needle
Neivert polyp hook
Neivert-TC needle holder
Nélaton fold
Nélaton rubber tube drain
Nélaton sphincter
Nelson cannula
Nelson forceps
Nelson rib retractor
Nelson scissors
Nelson syndrome
Nelson thoracic trocar
Nelson tissue forceps
Nelson trocar
NEMD (nonspecific esophageal
  motility disorder)
neobladder construction following total
  cystectomy
Neocate One +
neocholangiole
Neo-Cultol (mineral oil)
NeoCure Cryoablation System
NeoDerm
Neo-Diaral (loperamide)
neodymium-YAG laser
neodymium:yttrium-aluminum-garnet
  (Nd:YAG) laser
Neoflex bendable knife
Neoflex bendable-knife electrocautery
Neoloid
Neomark (broxuridine)
Neomark-BU (broxuridine) test
Neo-Med cautery unit
Ne-Osteo bone morphogenic protein
  (BMP)
Neo-Sert umbilical vessel catheter
neotherm probe
Neo tracheal tube
neomycin sulfate
neonatal diabetes mellitus
neonatal diagnosis
neonatal diaphragmatic hernia
neonatal hepatitis
neonatal hyperbilirubinemia
neonatal hypoglycemia
neonatal hypoparathyroidism
neonatal intestinal obstruction
neonatal jaundice
neonatal lupus
neonatal lymphedema
neonatal thyrotoxicosis
neoplasia, anal epithelial
neoplasm (see also *tumor*)
  benign
  breast
  encapsulated
  firm
  functioning
  gonadal
  grading
  hormone-dependent
  Hürthle cell
  invasive
  islet cell
  lethal
  malignant
  ovarian

neoplasm *(cont.)*
  periampullary
  premalignant
  spherical
  staging
  thyroid
  well-circumscribed
neoplastic disease
neoplastic disorder
neoplastic extension
neoplastic polyp
Neoprobe 100 gamma-detection probe
Neoral (cyclosporine; alcohol)
neorectum
neostigmine
NeoTect disease-specific imaging agent
NeoTect kit
Neotrace-4 (multiple trace elements)
neovagina, rectal
Neovastat
nephritic calculus
nephritic colic
nephritis, interstitial
nephrogenic ascites
nephrogenic diabetes insipidus
nephroscope, Pentax ECN-1530 choledochonephroscope
nephrostomy-type catheter
nephrotic syndrome
nephrotoxic agent
Nephrox (aluminum hyroxide; mineral oil)
NERD (nonerosive reflux disease)
nerve biopsy
nerve block anesthesia
Nerve Block Infusion Kit
nerve block, percutaneous celiac
nerve graft
nerve hook
nerve hook plain
nerve of Latarjet
nerve root retractor
nerve suture
nervous gut
nervous vomiting
Nesacaine MPF (chloroprocaine)
nesidioblastosis
nested nail
Neufeld nail
Neufeld plate
Neukomm test
Neupogen (filgrastim) recombinant G-CSF
Neuprex
neural cell adhesion molecule (NCAM) expression
neural tube
neuralgia
neurinoma
neuroblockage
NeuroCol sponge
NeuroDrape surgical drape
neuroectoderm
neuroectodermal dysplasia
neuroendocrine C cells of the thyroid
neuroendocrine carcinoma of skin
neuroendocrine malignancy
neurofibroma, gastrointestinal
neurofibromatosis
neurogastroenterology
neurogenic arthropathy
neurogenic dysphagia
neurogenic intestinal obstruction
neurogenic sarcoma
neurohypophysis
neuroimmune dysfunction
neurolimmoma, malignant
neurologic gut dysfunction
neurological hammer
neurological insulin
neurological or neurosurgical scissors
neurolytic drug
neuroma, mucosal
Neuromeet nerve approximator
neuromuscular actions of catecholamines
neuromuscular irritability
neuromuscular transmission

neuronal necrosis
neuronoma, VIP-secreting
neuropathy
  alcoholic
  angiopathic
  ascending
  Dejerine-Sottas
  Denny Browne (Denis Browne)
  descending
  diabetic
  entrapment
  familial visceral
  peripheral
  peripheral autonomic
  postherniorrhaphy
  postoperative
  somatic
  visceral
Neuro-Patties sponge
neuroplasty fat graft
neuroplexus block
neurosurgical chisel
neurosurgical needle holder with tungsten carbide (TC) inlay
Neurotone multipurpose instrument
neurotransmitter
Neurotrend probe
neurovascular bundle
neurovascular island graft
neurovascular stent
NeuroVasx (Sub-Microinfusion) catheter
neutral and load drill guide
neutral calcaneal stance position
neutral drill guide
neutral hip position
neutral protamine Hagedorn (NPH) insulin
neutral spine position
neutralization plate
neutropenia
neutrophil activation
neutrophilic infiltration
Neville-Barnes forceps
nevus (pl. nevi), spider
Nevyas drape retractor
newborn hepatitis
newborn jaundice
newborn pneumonitis virus
Newcastle disease virus
New Eder Corporation trocar
Newman anoscope
Newman plate
Newman proctoscope
new-onset constipation
New Orleans needle holder
NEW Speaking Tube
New York Glass suction tube
new variable stiffness (VS) colonoscope
Nexium (esomeprazole magnesium)
NexStent carotid stent
Nexus 2 linear ablation catheter
Nezhat-Dorsey Trumpet Valve
NFkB-dependent gene activation
NG (nasogastric)
NG aspirate
NG feeding tube
NG suction as needed
NG tube decompression
NGT (nasogastric tube)
NGT aspiration
NGT suction
N High Sensitivity CRP (C-reactive protein) assay
niacin
Niaspan (niacin)
Nibbler device for dissection, morcellation, suction, and irrigation
Nibblit laparoscopic device
Nibs mapping pen
NIC (Nursing Interventions Classification)
nick, nicking (of fascia)
Nicola forceps
Nicola pituitary rongeur
Nicola rasp
Nicola scissors
Nicoll cancellous bone graft

Nicoll extractor
Nicoll graft
Nicoll plate
Nicoll rasp
nicotinamide
NIDDK (National Institute of Diabetes and Digestive and Kidney Diseases)
NIDDM (non-insulin-dependent diabetes mellitus)
Nidek EC-5000 excimer laser
nidus of inflamed tissue
nidus of necrotic tissue
nidus of stone formation
Niedner anastomosis clamp
Niemann-Pick disease
Niemeier classification of gallbladder perforation
Niemeier gallbladder perforation
night sweats, chills, and fever
Nigro protocol
NIH mitral valve forceps
Nilstat
Niopam contrast medium
nipple (pl. nipples)
  accessory
  cracked
  everted
  inverted
  level of
  slough of
  supernumerary breast
  ulcer of
nipple-areola complex
nipple change
nipple discharge
  bloody
  guaiac-positive
  milky
  persistent
  spontaneous
nippled stoma
nipple eversion
nipple exploration with excision
nipple-flap duct resection
nipple inversion
nipple lesion
nipple level
nipple rash
nipple reconstruction
nipple retraction
nipple valve
Niro bone-cutting forceps
NIR ON Ranger premounted stent system
NIR Primo Monorail stent system
Niro wire-twisting forceps
Niroyal Elite Monorail stent
NIRS (near-infrared spectroscopy)
Nissen antireflux operation
Nissen fundoplasty
Nissen fundoplication wrap
Nissen gall duct forceps
Nissen laparoscopic fundoplication
Nissen technique and partial posterior hemifundoplication (Toupet and Lind techniques)
Nissen 360° wrap fundoplication
Nissen wrap
nitinol mesh-covered frame
nitinol stent
nitrazoxanide
nitric oxide (NO)
nitrofural
nitrofurazone
nitrogen (N)
nitrogen balance
  negative
  positive
nitrogen partition test
nitroglycerin (NTG)
nitroglycerin I.V. (IV) drip
nitroglycerin ointment
Nitrolan
nitroprusside
nitrosamine
nitrous oxide
nitrous oxide insufflator
nizatidine

Nizoral
NJ (nasojejunal) feeding tube
NK (natural killer) cell
NKHHC (nonketotic hyperglycemic-hyperosmolar coma)
NL fasting
NLH (nodular lymphoid hyperplasia)
NO (nitric oxide)
no-angulation view
Noble bowel plication
Noble surgical plication of bowel
Nocardia
nocturia x 3 (times 3)
nocturnal gastric reflux
nocturnal pain
nocturnal regurgitation
nodal involvement
nodal metastasis
nodal status
nodal tissue
nodal tumor
node (see also *lymph node*)
  axillary lymph
  Calot
  celiac lymph
  Cloquet
  common iliac
  enlarged lymph
  fixed axillary
  gastroduodenal
  iliac lymph
  infraclavicular
  inguinal
  interjugular
  internal mammary lymph
  interpectoral lymph
  ipsilateral internal mammary lymph
  ipsilateral supraclavicular
  Irish
  local
  lymph
  matted
  mesenteric lymph
  para-aortic

node *(cont.)*
  paratracheal
  pelvic lymph
  periaortic lymph
  pericholedochal lymph
  perirectal lymph
  periumbilical lymph
  retrorectal lymph
  Rotter
  sentinel
  shotty lymph
  Sister Mary Joseph lymph
  splenic hilar lymph
  subcarinal
  superficial inguinal lymph
  supraclavicular lymph
  tracheoesophageal groove
  Troisier
  Virchow
  Virchow sentinel
  Virchow-Troisier
node dissection
node-negative patient
node-positive patient
node sampling
nodular cirrhosis
nodular fullness
nodular goiter
nodular HCC
nodular lesion
nodular liver
nodular lymphoid hyperplasia (NLH)
nodular lymphoma
nodular mass
nodular melanoma
nodular nonsuppurative panniculitis
nodular regenerative hyperplasia (NRH)
nodular sclerosing Hodgkin disease
nodular thyroid disease
nodular thyroid enlargement
nodularity, surface
nodule
  autonomously hyperfunctioning
  benign thyroid

nodule *(cont.)*
cold
ectopic thyroid
encapsulated
fibroadenomatous
freely movable
HCC
hot
infiltration of
lymphoid tissue
malignant thyroid
Morgagni
multiple thyroid
nondiscrete
palpable
regenerative cirrhotic
rubbery
satellite
solitary thyroid
subcutaneous
thyroid
nodule uptake of intravenous ^{131}I or ^{99m}Tc
no evidence of disease (NED)
nolinium bromide
Nolvadex (tamoxifen citrate)
NOMSI (nonoperative management of splenic injury)
nonabsorbable blue monofilament suture
nonabsorbable dark blue braided stainless steel suture
nonabsorbable green and white braided suture
nonabsorbable green braided Ethibond suture
nonabsorbable steroid
nonabsorbable surgical suture
nonabsorbable white braided suture
nonadherent gauze dressing
nonadhesive bandage
nonadhesive dressing
nonadrenal tumor
nonalcoholic cirrhosis
nonalcoholic patient
nonalcoholic steatohepatitis
non-alpha, non-beta pancreatic islet cell
nonan malaria
non-A, non-B hepatitis (now hepatitis C)
nonbacterial gastroenteritis
nonbilious vomiting
nonbeta islet cell tumor of the pancreas
nonbloody stools
noncalcified stone
noncannulated nail
noncaseating tubercle-like granuloma
noncellular material
noncholecystokinin substance
noncirrhotic hepatitis C
noncirrhotic liver
noncirrhotic portal fibrosis (NCPF)
noncirrhotic portal hypertension
nonclinical diabetes
noncompliant patient
noncompliant ventricle
nonconductive tubing
noncontrast-enhanced CT scan
noncrushing bowel clamp
noncrushing vascular clamp
noncutaneous region
noncyclic pain
nondiabetic gastroparesis
nondiabetic insulin coma
nondiscrete nodule
nondistended abdomen
nondistensible
nondysenteric colitis
nonepithelial wall
nonerosive nonspecific gastritis
nonerosive reflux disease (NERD)
noneverting suture
nonfamilial intestinal pseudo-obstruction
nonferromagnetic needle
nonfibrous material
nonfilling gallbladder

nonfunctioning adrenal mass
nonfusion of cranial suture
nonhealing ulcer
non-heart-beating donor
nonhemolytic jaundice
nonhemolytic strep (streptococcus)
non-Hodgkin lymphoma
noniatrogenic cause
nonicteric sclerae
nonicteric skin
noninfectious colitis
noninfectious hepatitis
noninfective endocardial lesion
noninfiltrating lobular carcinoma
non-insulin-dependent diabetes mellitus (NIDDM)
non-Lynch syndrome
nonmedullary thyroid cancer
noninvasive carcinoma
noninvasive exploration of biliary tract
noninvasive imaging study
noninvasive localization study
nonionic contrast media
nonislet cell tumor
nonketotic coma
nonketotic hyperglycemic-hyperosmolar coma (NKHHC)
nonketotic hypoglycemia and carnitine deficiency due to MCAD deficiency
nonmalodorous fluid
nonmucosal hemorrhoidectomy
nonmutagenic surgical suture
nonobstructive hepatic parenchymal disease
nonobstructive ileus
nonocclusive intestinal infarction
nonocclusive mesenteric thrombosis
nonopaque stone
nonoperative management of splenic injury (NOMSI)
nonoperative therapy
nonoptical rigid bronchoscope
nonorganic dyspepsia
nonoxygenated blood
nonpalpable mass on mammogram
nonpalpable parathyroid
nonpathogenic organism
nonpenetrating wound
nonperforated appendicitis
nonperforated appendix
nonpliable
nonpuerperal breast abscess
nonrebreathing anesthesia
nonreducible mass
nonreflux esophagitis
nonrigid technique reduction mammoplasty
nonskeletal metastases
non-small cell lung cancer
nonspecific colitis
nonspecific enteritis
nonspecific esophageal motility disorder (NEMD)
nonspecific gas pattern
nonspecific ulcerative proctitis
nonstanding lateral oblique view
Nonsterile Guedel Airways
nonsteroidal anti-inflammatory drug (NSAID)
Non-Stix sponge
nonsuppurative cholangitis
nonsuppurative thyroiditis
nontender gallbladder
nonthyroidal neck mass
nontoxic diffuse goiter
nontoxic nodular goiter
nontraumatic hernia
nontropical sprue
nontubed closed distant flap graft
nontubed open distant flap graft
nonulcer dyspepsia (NUD)
nonventilated patient
nonviable bowel
nonviable tissue
nonvisualization of gallbladder
nonweightbearing view
Noon AV fistula clamp
No Pain-HP (capsaicin)

no peritoneal signs
NoProfile balloon catheter
Norco (hydrocodone bitartrate; acetaminophen)
Nordenstrom (Rotex II) biopsy needle
Nordt knot tightener
norepinephrine (NE)
norepinephrine analog
norepinephrine level
Norfolk-Norwich retractor
normal active bowel sounds
normal adrenal physiology
normal anatomic position
normal appendix
normal bile duct
normal calcitonin concentration
normal caliber duct
normal carrier hepatitis
normal colonic epithelium
normal flora
normal gas exchange in lung
normal gastric slow wave
normal hepatocyte
normal intestinal microflora
normal negative feedback loop
normal rectal exam
normal saline
normal saline drip
normal saline solution
Normal Stool Formula-IB (NSF-IB)
normal-appearing mucosa
normally apposed parietal and visceral pleura
normetanephrine
Normigel hydrogel dressing
normoactive bowel sounds
normochloremic metabolic acidosis
normochlorhydria
normocytic
normoglycemia, absolute
Normosol-M and 5% Dextrose
Normosol-R and 5% Dextrose
Normosol R pH 7.4 (combined electrolyte solution)
Northbent stitch scissors
North-South retractor
Norton ball reamer
Norwalk agent
Norwalk gastroenteritis
Norwalk virus
Norwood rectal snare
nosocomial infection
No Sting Barrier Film
not amenable to percutaneous drainage
notchplasty blade
notch, suprasternal
notch view
"no-trocar" zone (in path of epigastric arteries or immediately under costal margins)
Nottingham colposuspension needle
Nottingham introducer, semirigid
Nottingham Key-Med introducing device
NovaCath multi-lumen infusion catheter
Novafil suture
NovaGold breast implant
Novak suction curette
NovaLine Litho-S DUV excimer laser
Novamine 15% (amino acids)
NovaPulse CO_2 laser
NovaSaline inflatable saline breast implant
NovaSaline pre-filled breast implant
Novocain (procaine HCl)
Novo-Domperidone (domperidone maleate)
Novofil suture
Novolin L (insulin)
Novolin N PenFill
Novolin N Prefilled (insulin)
NovolinPen insulin device
Novolin R PenFill
Novolin R Prefilled (insulin)
Novolin 70/30 PenFill
Novolin 70/30 Prefilled (insulin)
Novolin 85/15 PenFill (insulin)
NovoLog (insulin aspart)

Novopaque (barium sulfate)
NovoRapid (insulin)
Noyes alligator forceps
Noyes iris scissors
Noyes microscopic scissors
NP-59 (cholesterol analog) scanning
NPH (neutral protamine Hagedorn) insulin
NPH Iletin II insulin
NPH-N insulin
n.p.o. or NPO (nothing by mouth)
NRH (nodular regenerative hyperplasia)
NSAID (nonsteroidal anti-inflammatory drug)
NSAID enteropathy
NSAID-induced gastropathy
NSF-IB (Normal Stool Formula-IB)
N-shaped sigmoid loop
NTC (normal transit constipation)
NTHI (native tissue Harmonic imaging)
Nu-Brede packing and debridement sponge dressing
Nuck, canal of
nuclear bleeding scan
nuclear enema
nuclear factor NF-kB
nuclear hepatobiliary imaging
nuclear medicine
nuclear medicine procedure
nuclear medicine scan
nuclear-tagged cell
nuclear-tagged red blood cell bleeding study
nuclear technetium ^{99m}Tc study
nuclear transfer
nucleoside analog
Nucleotome aspiration probe
Nucleotome Flex II cutting probe
Nu-Comfort ostomy appliance
NuDerm hydrocolloid dressing material
Nu-Derm foam island dressing
Nu Gauze dressing
Nu Gauze gauze
Nu Gauze occlusive hydrogel dressing
Nu Gauze sponge dressing
Nu Gauze sterile gauze bandage
Nu-Gel clear hydrogel wound dressing
Nu-Gel dressing
Nu-Hope Convex Insert
Nu-Hope ileostomy pouch
Nu-Hope Nu-Self drainable pouch
Nu-Hope Protective Skin Barrier (for ostomy skin)
nulliparity
Nullo deodorant tablets
NuLytely (polyethylene glycol-electrolyte solution) bowel prep
NuMA test kit
numbness and tingling, circumoral
Numorphan (oxymorphone HCl)
Nupercainal
Nuport PEG tube
Nurolon braided nylon suture
nurses scissors
Nursing Interventions Classification (NIC)
Nursoy formula
Nussbaum forceps
Nussbaum intestinal clamp
nutcracker esophagus
Nu-Tip disposable scissor tip
nutmeg appearance of cut surface of liver
nutmeg liver
nutmeg pattern
Nutraloric enteral nutritional therapy
Nutramigen formula
Nutren
Nutricath catheter
Nutrilan enteral nutritional therapy
Nutrilyte II (combined electrolyte solution)
nutrition
- altered
- enteral (EN)
- home parenteral (HPN)
- parenteral
- support parenteral (SPN)
- total parenteral (TPN)

nutritional autonomy
nutritional cirrhosis
nutritional deficiency
nutritional deficit
nutritional/electrolyte therapy
  5% Dextrose and Electrolyte #48
  5% Dextrose and Electrolyte #75
  10% Dextrose and Electrolyte #48
  50% Dextrose with Electrolyte
    Pattern A (or N)
nutritional index
nutritional rehabilitation
nutritional status
nutritional supplement
nutritional support
nutritional therapy (see *medication*)
Nutropin (somatropin)
Nutropin Depot (somatropin)
NUVO barrier film
Nuvolase 660 laser
Nyhus classification of groin hernias
  (types 1, 2, 3a, 3b, 3c, and 4)
Nyhus-Nelson gastric decompression
  and jejunal feeding tube
Nylok self-locking nail
nylon insulated coating
nylon mesh graft
nylon suture
nylon threads as drain
Nystagmus testing spectacles
nystatin suspension
Nystex (nystatin)

O, o

O_2 (oxygen)
O&P (ova and parasites) test
Oasis One Action stent introducer
Oasis wound dressing
oat cell carcinoma of lung
oat cell tumor of lung
O'Beirne sphincter
O'Brien rib hook
O'Brien staple
Oberhill laminectomy retractor
obesity
  adult-onset
  alimentary
  endogenous
  exogenous
  hyperinsulinar
  hyperinterrenal
  hyperplasmic
  hyperplastic
  hyperplastic-hypertrophic
  hypertrophic
  hypogonad
  hypoplasmic
  hypothyroid
  lifelong
  morbid
  simple
  truncal
obesity-associated diabetes
obesity hypoventilation syndrome (OHS)
obesity index
oblique course
oblique film
oblique hernia
oblique incision
oblique view
obliterated umbilical vein
obliteration of diverticulum
obliteration, percutaneous transhepatic
oblong-shaped onlay component
OBL RC5 soft tissue anchor
O_2 (oxygen) Boot
O'Brien scissors
Obrinsky syndrome
observation
obstipation
obstructed shunt tube
obstruction
  adynamic intestinal
  airway
  appendiceal lumen
  arterial
  bilateral ureteral (BUO)
  bile duct
  biliary

obstruction *(cont.)*
- bowel
- cardiac
- closed-loop bowel
- closed-loop intestinal
- colonic
- common bile duct
- common duct
- common hepatic duct
- complete (of cystic duct)
- complete (of lumen)
- complete bowel
- cystic duct
- distal bile duct
- esophageal
- extrahepatic
- extrinsic
- false colonic
- fecal
- focal small bowel
- food bolus
- functional bowel
- functional cystic duct
- functional intestinal (in infancy)
- gallstone (of main pancreatic duct)
- gastric
- gastric outflow
- gastric outlet (GOO)
- gastrojejunal loop
- hepatic
- hepatic venous outflow (HVOO)
- high-grade
- high small bowel
- hilar
- idiopathic
- inferior vena cava
- intestinal
- large-bowel
- lower tract
- low small bowel
- lymphatic
- malignant biliary
- mammary duct
- mechanical

obstruction *(cont.)*
- mechanical biliary
- mechanical bowel
- mechanical duct
- mechanical extrahepatic
- mechanical intestinal
- mechanical small bowel
- neonatal intestinal
- neurogenic intestinal
- Ogilvie
- otic
- pancreatic duct
- paralytic colonic
- paralytic intestinal
- partial bowel
- pyloric channel
- pyloric outlet
- pyloroduodenal
- renal
- respiratory
- simple mechanical
- small bowel (SBO)
- strangulated bowel
- strangulation
- subacute
- tumbling
- urinary
- venous

obstruction of appendiceal lumen
obstruction of bile flow to duodenum
obstruction of hollow viscus
obstruction of pancreatic duct
obstructive appendicitis
obstructive biliary cirrhosis
obstructive dysfunctional ileitis
obstructive jaundice
obstructive pneumonia
obstructive symptoms
obstructive uropathy
obtundation
obtunded
obturator
- Auto Suture Soft Thoracoport
- Endopath Optiview optical surgical

obturator *(cont.)*
Frazier suction tube
LaparoSAC single-use
Soft Thoracoport
Versaport
obturator canal
obturator fossa
obturator hernia
obturator node
obturator sign
obturator test
occipital suture
occipital view
occipitoanterior position
occipitocervical plate
occipitomastoid suture
occipitoparietal suture
occipitoposterior position
occipitosphenoid suture
occipitotransverse position
occluding clamp
occlusion
balloon
blood outflow line
hepatic vein
rectal
splenic vein
occlusion clamp
occlusive dressing
occlusive ileus
occlusive lesion
occult blood
occult blood in stool
occult blood in urine
occult blood, positive test for
occult cancer
occult hepatitis
occult lesion
OCG (oral cholecystogram)
Ochsner artery forceps
Ochsner flexible spiral gallstone probe
Ochsner gall duct probe
Ochsner gallbladder probe
Ochsner gallbladder trocar
Ochsner hemostat
Ochsner ribbon retractor
Ochsner ring
OCL (polyethylene glycol electrolyte solution) bowel prep
o'clock (position, i.e., 9 o'clock position)
OCP (oral contraceptive pills)
ocrylate tissue adhesive (also ocrilate)
Ocrilon
OCT (optical coherence tomography) surgical imaging probe
Octamide PFS (metoclopramide)
Octastatin (vapreotide)
octatropine methylbromide
Octocaine HCl (lidocaine HCl; epinephrine)
Octopus tissue stabilizer
OctreoScan 111 (^{111}In pentetreotide)
octreotide
octreotide acetate
octreotide scan
ocular infection
ocular melanoma
ocular myasthenia
OcuLight SL diode laser
oculopharyngeal muscular dystrophy
OD (overdose)
Oddi sphincter
Oder-Weber-Rendu telangiectasia
O'Donoghue dressing
odontoid view
odynophagia
Oehler tissue and needle-pulling forceps
oestradiol (estradiol)
oestrone (estrone)
Oettingen abdominal retractor
Officer sigmoidoscope biopsy forceps
Officer tissue forceps
ofloxacin
OFS (organ failure score)
O'GAWA two-way cataract aspirating cannulas
Ogden anchor

Ogden plate
Ogilvie obstruction
Ogilvie pseudo-obstruction
Ogilvie syndrome (pseudo-obstruction of colon)
OGT (oral gastric tube)
OGT-918
Ogura tissue and cartilage forceps
O'Hanlon intestinal clamp
Ohio air
OHS (obesity hypoventilation syndrome)
oil
  castor
  evening primrose
  MCT (medium chain triglyceride)
  mineral
  oil-red-O
  peppermint
  rice bran
  seabuckthorn seed
  shark liver
oil enema
oil-red-O stain
oil retention enema
oily stools
OKT3 antibody
Okuda staging classification
Okuda transhepatic obliteration of varices
Oldberg brain retractor
Oldberg intervertebral disk rongeur
Oldberg pituitary forceps
Oldberg pituitary rongeur
Oldfield syndrome
Olds pin
O'Leary gastroplasty
O'Leary lesser curvature gastroplasty
Olerud PSF rod
oligomerization
Oligon catheter
olive (instrument)
  Eder-Puestow
  expandable
olive *(cont.)*
  metal
  palpable pyloric
Olivecrona clip-applying and removing forceps
Olivecrona dissector
Olivecrona dural scissors
Olivecrona-Gigli saw
Olivecrona rasp
Olivecrona rongeur
Olivecrona-Toennis clip-applying forceps
Olivecrona trigeminal knife
Olivecrona trigeminal scissors
olive over guidewire
olive-tipped needle
Olivier retractor
Ollier incision
Ollier rake retractor
Ollier thick split free graft
Ollier-Thiersch skin graft
OLM (ophthalmic laser micro-endoscope)
olsalazine sodium
Olsen cholangiogram clamp
Olsen-Hegar needle
Olsen-Hegar needle holder with tungsten carbide (TC) inlays
Olsen-Mathieu-TC needle holder
OLT (orthotopic liver transplant or transplantation)
Olympus (see *endoscope*)
Olympus clip applier
Olympus heat probe
Olympus hot biopsy forceps
Olympus hysteroscope
Olympus laparoscope
Olympus ligator
Olympus lithotriptor
Olympus monopolar cannula
Olympus needle-knife papillotome
Olympus OME-8000 dual stereo surgical microscope
Olympus One-Step Button gastrostomy tube

Olympus reusable hot biopsy forceps
Olympus rotatable clip applicator
Olympus rectal probe
Olympus SonoSurg ultrasonic cutting and coagulation
Olympus sphincterotome
Ombredanne forceps
Ombredanne mallet
Omed bulldog vascular clamp
omega-shaped incision
omega sign
omega-3 fatty acid
omental abscess
omental adhesion
omental band
omental bursa
omental cyst
omental flap
omental pack
omental patch (Graham closure)
omental pedicle
omental studding
omental wrapping
omentectomy
omentopexy
omentum
  colic
  gastric
  gastrocolic
  gastrohepatic
  gastrosplenic
  greater (omentum majus)
  incarcerated
  lesser (omentum minus)
  pancreaticosplenic
  splenogastric
  viable
omeprazole, omeprazole sodium
omeprazole plus amoxicillin
Omiderm dressing
Omiderm plain and mesh occlusive dressing
Omiderm transparent adhesive film dressing
Ommaya ventriculoperitoneal shunt
Omnican Piston syringe
OmniCath atherectomy catheter
Omnicef (cefdinir)
OmniFilter
Omni-Lift retractor
Omnipaque (iohexol)
OmniPulse holmium pulsed laser
OmniPulse-MAX holmium laser
Omni retractor
Omniscan (gadodiamide)
OmniStent
OmniTip laser needle
Omni-Tract adjustable wishbone retractor
omphalectomy
omphalocele
omphalomesenteric duct
Omsk hemorrhagic fever virus
Onchocerca volvulus
OncoChek immunoassay
oncogene
  Bc1-2
  c-erb B-2
  c-fos
  HER2/neu
oncogenesis
oncogenic virus
On-Command (male and female) catheter
Onconase (p30 protein)
Oncophage vaccine
OncoScint CR/OV (^{111}In satumomab pendetide)
OncoScint CR103 (colorectal) imaging agent
OncoScint OV103 imaging agent
oncosuppressor gene
Onco TCS
OncoVax-P
Oncovin (vincristine sulfate)
oncovirus
OnCyte assay
ondansetron HCl

one-chip camera
one-hour glucose tolerance test
O'Neill clamp
one-piece ostomy pouch
One Piece cannula
one-piece shunt
one-quadrant hemorrhoidectomy
One Touch Basic blood glucose monitor
One Touch FastTake blood glucose monitor
One Touch Profile blood glucose monitor
One Touch II blood glucose monitor
One Touch Ultra blood glucose monitor
On-Q anesthesia delivery system
On-Q postoperative pain management system
One-Shot anastomotic instrument
One Shot vascular clip applier
one-stage enterolithotomy and cholecystectomy
one-stage operation
One Touch Basic blood glucose monitor
One Touch blood glucose monitor
One Touch FastTake blood glucose monitor
One Touch Profile glucose monitor
One Touch reagent strips
One Touch II blood glucose monitor
One Touch II glucose monitor
one-tube cuff
onion bulb changes (on biopsy)
onion peel appearance
onion scale lesion
onion-shaped dilatation (of the duodenum)
onionskin appearance
onionskin lesion
onlay cancellous iliac graft
onlay mesh graft
onset of pain
OnSite stainless steel instrument repair
oophoropexy
ooze
oozing (of blood or fluid)
oozing, venous
opacification
  complete
  incomplete
  poor
Opal R.F. tissue ablation device
opaque calculi
opaque meal
Opdima digital mammography system`
open anesthesia
open biopsy
open brain biopsy
open diathermy-excision hemorrhoidectomy
open drainage
open drop anesthesia
opened in direction of its fibers
open-end ostomy pouch
open esophagectomy
open gastric banding procedure
opening of ampulla of Vater
open investing peritoneum over the internal inguinal ring
open laparoscopy cannula adapter
open laparotomy
open liver biopsy
open loop reflex
open mesh-plug hernioplasty
open-mouth odontoid view
open nail
open periprosthetic capsulotomy, breast
open pin
open pneumothorax
open posterior approach
open procedure
Open Sky MRI
open weave mesh graft
open wedge biopsy of the liver
open wound
Operand (povidone; iodine)
operating laparoscope
operating microscope

operating scissors (see *scissors*)
operating thorascope
operation or procedure (quick-reference list of diagnostic procedures and studies, and surgical procedures, approaches, maneuvers, methods, techniques, and therapies)
  Abbe
  Abbott esophagogastrostomy
  abdominal colectomy
  abdominal exploration
  abdominal pull-through
  abdominal-sacral colpoperineopexy
  abdominoperineal or abdominal-perineal resection (APR)
  Acucise retrograde procedure for incision of ureteral stricture and ureteropelvic junction obstruction
  afferent jejunostomy
  Albert-Lembert gastroplasty
  Alden loop gastric bypass
  Allison gastroesophageal reflux
  Alliston GE reflux correction
  Altemeier repair of rectal prolapse
  ampullectomy
  Amussat
  anal anastomosis
  anal stretch
  antireflux
  argon plasma coagulation
  anoplasty
    Martin
    posterior sagittal and 3-flap
  anorectoplasty, Laird-McMahon
  anorectovaginoplasty
  antecolic anastomosis
  anterior colon resection
  antiperistaltic
  antireflux
  antrectomy
  antrostomy
  antrotomy
  appendectomy
  appendicovesicotomy

operation *(cont.)*
  APR (abdominoperineal resection)
  Aries-Pitanguy correction of mammary ptosis
  Auchincloss modified radical mastectomy
  augmentation mammoplasty
  autologous bone marrow transplantation
  autotransplantation of parathyroid to forearm
  axillary approach in augmentation mammoplasty
  axillary dissection
  axillary endoscopic reduction
  Aylett
  Baldy-Webster operation
  Ball operation for treatment of pruritus ani
  balloon tamponade
  BAMBI (breast augmentation mammoplasty by injection)
  banding (hemorrhoidal)
  band ligation of esophageal varices
  band sigmoidopexy
  band-snare technique
  bariatric
  Barron hemorrhoidal banding technique
  Bassini hernia repair
  Bassini herniorrhaphy
  Battle
  "belly button" augmentation mammoplasty
  Belsey antireflux Mark IV
  Belsey IV fundoplasty
  Belsey Mark IV 240° fundoplication
  Belsey two-thirds wrap fundoplication
  Benelli mastopexy
  bilateral inguinofemoral lymphadenectomy
  bilayer patch hernia repair
  biliary enteric anastomosis

operation *(cont.)*
- biliary sphincterotomy and stent placement
- biliointestinal bypass (BIB)
- biliopancreatic bypass (BPB)
- Billroth gastroenterostomy
- Billroth I (truncal vagotomy, antrectomy, gastroduodenostomy)
- Billroth II (truncal vagotomy, antrectomy, gastrojejunostomy)
- Billroth II-type gastrectomy
- Bishop-Koop ileostomy
- blind esophageal brushing (BEB)
- Bloch-Paul-Mikulicz
- Blumgart technique for hepaticojejunostomy
- blunt dissection
- Boerema anterior gastropexy
- Boerema hernia repair
- Brackin ureterointestinal anastomosis
- Braun anastomosis
- Braun-Jaboulay gastroenterostomy
- breast augmentation mammoplasty by injection (BAMBI)
- breast reconstruction during mastectomy
- breast reconstruction with latissimus dorsi flap
- breast reduction
- Bricker ureteroileostomy
- Brooke ileostomy
- Brunschwig
- Burch colposuspension
- Burch iliopectineal ligament urethrovesical suspension
- Burch laparoscopic procedure
- Burhenne biliary duct stone extraction
- buttonhole puncture technique for hemodialysis needle insertion
- buttonpexy fixation for stomal prolapse
- CAGEIN (catheter-guided endoscopic intubation)

operation *(cont.)*
- Camey ileocystoplasty
- capsulectomy of breast
- cardiomyotomy (stomach)
- CASH (classic abdominal Semm hysterectomy)
- catheter balloon valvuloplasty
- catheter-directed thrombolysis and endovascular stent placement
- cecopexy
- cecorrhaphy
- cecostomy
- central cone technique reduction mammoplasty
- cervical esophagotomy
- Child pancreaticoduodenostomy
- Childs-Phillips bowel plication
- cholecystectomy, three-trocar technique
- cholecystoduodenostomy
- cholecystoenterostomy
- cholecystojejunostomy
- choledochoduodenostomy
- choledochoenterostomy
- choledochojejunostomy
- choledochostomy
- choledochotomy
- cholelithotripsy
- Clagett-Barrett esophagogastrostomy
- “cleavoplasty” augmentation mammoplasty
- Coblation-Channeling
- Coffey ureterointestinal anastomosis
- colectomy, total abdominal (TAC)
- Collis antireflux
- Collis gastroplasty
- Collis-Nissen fundoplication
- Collis-Nissen gastroplasty
- coloanal anastomosis
- colocolostomy
- colopexy
- coloplasty procedure
- coloproctostomy

operation *(cont.)*
- colorrhaphy
- colosigmoid resection
- colostomy
- combined Collis gastroplasty-fundoplication for scleroderma reflux esophagitis
- combined liver and intestinal transplantation
- Commando glossectomy
- common bile duct exploration
- complete wrap Nissen
- composite
- conductive keratoplasty (CK)
- continent ileostomy
- contralateral subtotal thyroid lobectomy
- Cooper ligament repair
- Cordonnier ureteroileal loop
- corner mouth lift
- Courvoisier gastroenterostomy
- cricopharyngeal myotomy
- "cross-the-heart" augmentation mammoplasty
- cryptectomy
- CT cholangiography
- CT PEG (CT-guided percutaneous endoscopic gastrostomy)
- culdolaparoscopy
- curative
- cut-back
- cystogastrostomy
- cystojejunostomy
- cystopericystectomy
- decompression
- defatting of panniculus
- Delorme rectal prolapse
- Dennis-Brooke ileostomy
- Dennis-Varco pancreaticoduodenostomy
- Depage-Janeway gastrostomy
- Devine
- DGHAL (Doppler-guided hemorrhoidal artery ligation)

operation *(cont.)*
- diagnostic laparoscopy
- dilatation of stenotic hepaticojejunostomy
- distal gastrectomy with excision of ulcer
- distal near-total pancreatectomy
- distal pancreatectomy
- distal Roux-en-Y gastric
- distal subtotal pancreatectomy
- diverticulectomy
- donut mastopexy
- Doppler-guided HAL (hemorrhoid artery ligation) (DGHAL)
- Doubilet sphincterotomy
- double seton modified surgical approach to transsphincteric anal fistula repair
- double-wrap graciloplasty
- Douglas procedure
- Douglas suture of tongue for micrognathia
- drainage
- duct-to-duct anastomosis
- Duecollement hemicolectomy
- Duhamel laparoscopic pull-through
- duodenal diversion
- duodenal seromyectomy
- duodenoenterostomy
- duodenoileal bypass (DIB)
- duodenojejunostomy
- duodenotomy
- Duval distal (caudal) pancreaticojejunostomy
- Duval pancreaticojejunostomy
- dynamic graciloplasty
- Eckhout gastroplasty
- Eckhout vertical gastroplasty
- elective shunt procedure
- elective sigmoid resection
- electrohydraulic lithotripsy for bile duct stone
- emergency
- emergency laparotomy

operation *(cont.)*
emergency tracheostomy
en bloc augmentation mammoplasty
en bloc distal pancreatectomy
en bloc resection
en bloc vein resection
Endo Lumenal gastroplication procedure (ELGP)
endorectal ileal pull-through
endoscopic antireflux procedure
endoscopic-assisted transumbilical augmentation mammoplasty
endoscopic cryoablation
endoscopic cryotherapy
endoscopic cystogastrostomy
endoscopic gastroplasty
endoscopic injection
endoscopic laser cholecystectomy
endoscopic mucosal ablation
endoscopic mucosal resection (EMR)
endoscopic mucosectomy
endoscopic papillectomy (EP)
endoscopic papillotomy
endoscopic resection
endoscopic retrograde balloon dilation
endoscopic retrograde cholangiography (ERC)
endoscopic retrograde cholangiopancreatogram (ERCP)
endoscopic sphincterotomy (ES)
endoscopic stent placement
endoscopic transpapillary catheterization of the gallbladder (ETCG)
endoscopic Zenker diverticulectomy
endoscopy with tumor ablation
enteroenterostomy
enterolithotomy
enterotomy
end-to-back bowel anastomosis
end-to-end anastomosis
end-to-end jejunoileal bypass
end-to-side anastomosis

operation *(cont.)*
end-to-side choledochojejunostomy
end-to-side jejunoileal bypass
epiploectomy
esophageal-jejunal anastomosis
esophageal sling procedure
esophageal transection with para-esophagogastric devascularization
esophagectomy
esophagoduodenostomy
esophagoenterostomy
esophagogastrectomy
esophagogastric anastomosis
esophagogastric fundoplasty with fundic patch (Thal-Nissen procedure)
esophagogastric tamponade
esophagogastrostomy
esophagojejunostomy
esophagomyotomy (Heller type)
esophagostomy
EUS-guided fine-needle aspiration
exclusion bypass
explantation of breast implant
exploratory celiotomy
exploratory laparotomy
extended right hepatectomy
extended right hepatic lobectomy
external fistulization of intestine
extracorporeal shock-wave lithotripsy
extramucosal myotomy
failed shunt surgery
femoral hernia repair
Finney pyloroplasty
fissurectomy
fistulectomy
fistulotomy
floppy Nissen fundoplication
Fobi pouch
formal laparotomy
Fredet-Ramstedt pyloromyotomy
free nipple transposition technique reduction mammoplasty

operation *(cont.)*
frenoplasty
fundic mobilization in Nissen fundoplication
fundoplasty
fundoplication
gasless laparoscopic-assisted colostomy
gastrectomy
gastric bypass (GBP)
gastric loop-type bypass
gastric neobladder procedure
gastric partitioning
gastric resection
gastric restrictive procedure
gastric stapling
gastroduodenopancreatectomy
gastroduodenostomy
gastroenterostomy
gastrogastrostomy
gastrojejunal anastomosis
gastrojejunostomy
gastropexy
gastroplasty
gastrorrhaphy
gastrostomy
Gauderer-Ponsky PEG
Gauderer-Ponsky-Izant PEG
gift-wrap suture technique
glossectomy
Goligher ileostomy
Gomez fundoplasty
Gomez gastroplasty
Gore-Tex banding of sigmoid colon to abdominal wall
Goulian mammoplasty
gracilis muscle transposition
graciloplasty
Greenville gastric bypass
Griffen Roux-en-Y bypass
groin dissection
Grondahl-Finney esophagogastroplasty
Gross

operation *(cont.)*
HAL (hemorrhoid arterial ligation), Doppler-guided
HALS (hand-assisted laparoscopic surgery)
Halsted-Bassini herniorrhaphy
Halsted inguinal herniorrhaphy
hand-assisted laparoscopic colectomy
hand-assisted laparoscopic gastrectomy
hand-assisted laparoscopy
hand-assisted sigmoidectomy
Harrington esophageal diverticulectomy
Hartmann pouch
Hartmann resection of bowel
Hasson technique
Heineke-Mikulicz gastroenterostomy
Heineke-Mikulicz pyloroplasty
Heller-Belsey operation for achalasia of esophagus
Heller cardiomyotomy
Heller-Dor operation for achalasia of esophagus
Heller esophagomyotomy
Heller myotomy
hemicolectomy
hemigastrectomy
hemorrhoid arterial ligation (HAL)
hemorrhoidal banding
hemorrhoid cryotherapy
hemorrhoid infrared photocoagulation
hemorrhoid laser excision
hemorrhoid sclerotherapy
hemorrhoid vaporization
hemorrhoidectomy
hepatectomy
hepatic lobectomy
hepatic resection
hepatic segmentectomy
hepaticojejunostomy with cutaneous stoma

operation *(cont.)*
- hepatopancreatoduodenectomy
- hepatoportoenterostomy
- hepatorrhaphy
- hepatotomy
- herniorrhaphy
- Higgins technique for uretero-intestinal anastomosis
- highly selective vagotomy
- Hill antireflux
- Hill cluster harvest technique
- Hill fundoplasty
- Hill gastropexy
- Hill hiatus hernia
- Hill median arcuate repair
- Hill repair for esophageal reflux
- Hofmeister anastomosis
- Hofmeister gastroenterostomy
- Horsley anastomosis
- Horsley gastrectomy
- Hunt-Lawrence pouch
- hydrocelectomy
- hypophysectomy
- ileal pouch-anal anastomosis
- ileal pull-through
- ileal resection
- ileectomy
- ileoanal anastomosis
- ileoanal endorectal pull-through
- ileocolectomy
- ileocolic resection
- ileocolostomy
- ileocystoplasty
- ileogastrostomy
- ileo-ileal anastomosis
- ileoproctostomy
- ileorectal anastomosis (IRA)
- ileorectostomy
- ileostomy
- Indiana pouch
- inferior central pedicle reduction mammoplasty
- inferior pedicle technique reduction mammoplasty

operation *(cont.)*
- infrahepatic caval anastomosis
- inframammary approach in augmentation mammoplasty
- inguinal exploration
- inguinal lymphadenectomy
- intestinal anastomosis
- intestinal bypass
- intestinal transplantation
- intracorporeal shock-wave lithotripsy (ISWL)
- intrahepatic cholangioenterostomy
- intrahepatic transjugular portosystemic shunt
- intraoperative cholangiography (IOC)
- intraperitoneal onlay mesh (IPOM) hernia repair
- inversion-ligation appendectomy
- inverted U-pouch ileal reservoir
- IPAA (ileal pouch-anal anastomosis)
- ipsilateral thyroid lobectomy
- isoperistaltic anastomosis
- isthmusectomy
- Ivalon rectopexy
- Ivalon sponge-wrap
- Ivor Lewis esophagectomy
- Ivor Lewis esophagogastrectomy
- Jaboulay gastroduodenostomy
- Jaboulay pyloroplasty
- Janeway procedure
- jejunoileal bypass
- jejunoileostomy
- jejunojejunostomy
- jejunostomy
- Jenckel cholecystoduodenostomy
- Johnson esophagogastrostomy
- Judd ventral hernia repair
- Kader gastrostomy
- Karydakis pilonidal cyst excision
- Kasai portoenterostomy
- Kiricuta breast reconstruction
- Kocher anastomosis
- Kocher pylorectomy

operation *(cont.)*
Kocher pyloromyotomy
Kock ("coke") ileostomy
Kock pouch modified procedure
Kugel hernia repair
Kugel patch
Kuzmak gastric banding
Kuzmak gastroplasty
Ladd correction of malrotation of the bowel
Lane
laparoscopic adrenalectomy
laparoscopically assisted colorectal resection
laparoscopically assisted sigmoid resection
laparoscopic anterior fundoplication
laparoscopic antireflux surgery
laparoscopic appendectomy ("lap appy")
laparoscopic approach
laparoscopic-assisted procedure
laparoscopic-assisted vaginal hysterectomy
laparoscopic bile duct exploration
laparoscopic biopsy of liver
laparoscopic bladder neck suture suspension procedure
laparoscopic bowel resection
laparoscopic Burch procedure
laparoscopic cholecystectomy ("lap chole")
laparoscopic colectomy
laparoscopic common bile duct exploration
laparoscopic dissection
laparoscopic distal pancreatectomy
laparoscopic duct exploration
laparoscopic esophagogastroplasty with Nissen fundoplication
laparoscopic exploration of common bile duct
laparoscopic fundoplication
laparoscopic Heller myotomy

operation *(cont.)*
laparoscopic hernia repair
laparoscopic herniorrhaphy
laparoscopic Kittner
laparoscopic laser cholecystectomy (LLC)
laparoscopic liver biopsy
laparoscopic lysis of adhesions
laparoscopic micro scissors
laparoscopic monopolar scissors
laparoscopic Nissen and Toupet fundoplication
laparoscopic Nissen fundoplication
laparoscopic Nissen fundoplication with esophageal lengthening
laparoscopic paraesophageal hernia repair (LPHR)
laparoscopic placement of peritoneal dialysis catheter
laparoscopic pneumodissection
laparoscopic posterior hemi-fundoplication
laparoscopic radical prostatectomy
laparoscopic repair of para-esophageal hernia (LRPH)
laparoscopic retroperitoneal lymphadenectomy
laparoscopic Roux-en-Y gastric bypass procedure (LRYGBP)
laparoscopic supracervical hysterectomy (LASH)
laparoscopic surgery for peptic ulcer disease
laparoscopic Toupet fundoplication
laparoscopic transcystic duct exploration
laparoscopic transcystic papillotomy
laparoscopic tubal ligation
laparoscopic urinary diversion
laparotomy
laparotomy with splenectomy
laparotomy with splenorrhaphy
Lap-Band adjustable gastric banding (LAGB)

operation *(cont.)*
"lap chole" (laparoscopic cholecystectomy)
lap Nissen (laparoscopic Nissen fundoplication)
LAP-TAPP (laparoscopic transabdominal preperitoneal) hernioplasty
LAR/CAA (low anterior resection in combination with coloanal anastomosis)
large-volume paracentesis
LARS (laparoscopic antireflux surgery)
laryngopharyngectomy
laser ablation
laser-assisted spinal endoscopy (LASE)
laser-assisted tissue welding technique
laser-assisted uvulopalatoplasty (LAUP)
laser biomicroscopy
"Laser Bra" (see *L.I.F.T.*)
laser correlational spectroscopy (LCS)
laser Doppler flowmetry (LDF)
laser hemorrhoidectomy
laser image custom arthroplasty (LICA)
laser-induced thermotherapy (LITT)
laser lithotripsy
laser myringotomy
laser nucleotomy
laser photoablation
laser reduction mammoplasty
laser thermal keratoplasty (LTK)
laser trabeculodissection (LTD)
laser uterosacral nerve ablation (LUNA)
LASH (laparoscopic supracervical hysterectomy)
lateral cervical lymphadenectomy
lateral cervical node dissection

operation *(cont.)*
lateral crural steal (LCS)
Latzko vesicovaginal fistula repair
LAUP (laser-assisted uvulopalatoplasty)
LAVH (laparoscopically assisted vaginal hysterectomy)
Laws gastroplasty
Lazaro da Silva continent perineal colostomy creation technique
Lazarus-Nelson pneumoperitoneum technique
Leadbetter-Politano ureterovesicoplasty
LeDuc anastomosis
LeDuc-Camey ileocolostomy
LeDuc-Camey ileocystoplasty
LEEP (loop electrosurgical excision procedure)
LeFort urethral sound
left hepatic lobectomy
left-to-right subtotal pancreatectomy
LeJour technique of reduction mammoplasty
LeJour-type breast reduction
LESA (lower esophageal sphincter augmentation)
Lester Martin modification of Duhamel procedure
levator muscle imbrication
Lewis-Tanner subtotal esophagectomy and reconstruction
Lich-Gregoire kidney transplant surgery
Lichtenstein herniorrhaphy
Lich ureteral implantation in transplantation surgery
L.I.F.T. (laser-assisted internal fabrication) of breast
ligamentum teres cardiopexy
lip lift
Lipostructure technique
LLETZ (large loop excision of the transformation zone)

operation *(cont.)*
lobectomy
long limb gastric bypass
Longmire-Gutgemann gastric reconstruction
Longo hemorrhoidectomy
loop choledochojejunostomy
loop-end ileostomy
Lord hemorrhoidectomy
Lortat-Jacob hepatic resection
low anterior resection
low-intensity laser therapy (LILT)
LRYGBP (laparoscopic Roux-en-Y gastric bypass procedure)
LULA (laparoscopy under local anesthesia)
lumpectomy of breast
LUNA (laparoscopic uterine nerve ablation)
lung tumor resection
lung volume reduction surgery (LVRS)
lymph node dissection
Macewen herniorrhaphy
Madden herniorrhaphy
Madden repair of incisional hernia
Madigan prostatectomy
Magerl screw placement in lower cervical spine
magnetic resonance cholangiography (MRC)
magnetic resonance cholangiography with HASTE
magnetic resonance cholangiopancreatography (MRCP)
magnetic resonance mammography (MRM)
MAGPI (meatal advancement, glanuloplasty, penoscrotal junction meatotomy)
Maki pylorus-preserving gastrectomy
Mallory-Weiss procedure
Marlex mesh rectopexy

operation *(cont.)*
Martin anoplasty
Mason abdominotranssphincteric resection
Mason vertical-banded gastroplasty
mastotomy
Maunsell-Weir
Mayo
McBurney
McVay herniorrhaphy
mechanical lithotripsy for bile duct stone
Meckel diverticulectomy
mediastinal lymphadenectomy
"mega-pocket" augmentation mammoplasty
Menthini "one second" technique
Merindino
mesenteropexy
mesh plug hernioplasty
mesocaval anastomosis
Miles abdominoperineal resection
minilaparotomy
minimally invasive esophagectomy
mirror-image breast biopsy
Mitrofanoff appendicovesicotomy
Mitrofanoff neourethra procedure
modified Bassini inguinal hernia repair
modified radical mastectomy
Mohs fresh tissue chemosurgery
Morinaga hemorrhoidectomy
MR peritoneography
mucosal sleeve resection
mucosectomy
Mulholland sphincterotomy
multipolar electrocoagulation therapy (MECT)
multivisceral transplantation
necrosectomy
needle biopsy
needle catheter jejunostomy
needlescopic TAPP hernia repair
Newman procedure

operation *(cont.)*
nipple-flap duct resection
Nissen antireflux
Nissen fundoplasty
Nissen fundoplication
Nissen laparoscopic fundoplication
Noble bowel plication
noninvasive exploration of the biliary tract
nonrigid technique reduction mammoplasty
O'Leary gastroplasty
omentectomy
omentopexy
omphalectomy
open diverticulectomy
open esophagectomy
open gastric banding procedure
open mesh-plug hernioplasty
open wedge biopsy of the liver
one-stage
optical coherence tomography
Oriental V-Y flap technique
Orr-Loygue transabdominal proctopexy
Orr rectal prolapse repair
Owl incision technique reduction mammoplasty
palliative resection
palliative surgical
pancreas after kidney (PAK) transplantation
pancreas-preserving total gastrectomy
pancreas transplantation
pancreatectomy
pancreatic islet cell transplantation
pancreaticobiliary
pancreaticocystostomy
pancreaticoduodenectomy
pancreaticoduodenostomy
pancreaticogastrostomy
pancreaticojejunal anastomosis
pancreaticojejunostomy
pancreatoduodenectomy

operation *(cont.)*
pancreatoscopy
percutaneous endoscopic gastrojejunostomy
percutaneous transhepatic cholangiography (PTC)
plication of mesentery (mesenteropexy)
proctocolectomy
pancreas-preserving total gastrectomy
pancreatorrhaphy
pancreatotomy
panproctocolectomy
pants-over-vest hernia repair
papillectomy
papillotomy transection of the sphincter of Oddi
paracentesis
paraesophageal hernia, type 2
parietal cell vagotomy
Parker-Kerr enteroenterostomy
Parks fistulotomy
Parks ileoanal anastomosis
Parks posterior anal repair
Parks sphincterotomy
Parks transanal anastomosis
partial distal gastrectomy
partial ileal bypass
partial pancreatectomy
Partipilo gastrostomy
Paul-Mikulicz resection
Payne-DeWind jejunoileal bypass
PCTCL (percutaneous transhepatic cholecystolithotomy)
pedicle technique reduction mammoplasty
PEG (percutaneous endoscopic gastrostomy)
PEJ (percutaneous endoscopic jejunostomy)
per anum intersphincteric rectal dissection and coloanal anastomosis

operation *(cont.)*
percutaneous catheter cecostomy
percutaneous cholecystostomy
percutaneous choledochoscopy
percutaneous deflation of sigmoid loop
percutaneous endoscopic gastrojejunostomy
percutaneous endoscopic gastrostomy (PEG)
percutaneous endoscopic jejunostomy (PEJ)
percutaneous gastroenterostomy (PGE)
percutaneous gastrostomy (PG)
percutaneous nephrostolithotomy (PCNL)
percutaneous stone dissolution
percutaneous transfemoral dilatation
percutaneous transhepatic cholangiogram (PTC)
percutaneous transhepatic cholangiography (PTC)
percutaneous transhepatic cholangioscopy (PTCS) tube stenting
percutaneous transhepatic cholangioscopy and lithotripsy for complicated hepatolithiasis
percutaneous transhepatic cholangioscopy tube stenting through a mature T-tube tract
percutaneous transhepatic choledochoscopic electrohydraulic lithotripsy (PTCS-EHL)
periareolar augmentation mammoplasty
periprosthetic capsulectomy of breast
peritoneocentesis
pharyngoesophageal repair
pharyngogastrostomy
pharyngostomy (fistulization of pharynx)
plication of bowel

operation *(cont.)*
plug-and-patch hernia repair
Polya gastrectomy
polypectomy
polyvalent pneumococcal vaccine postsplenectomy
Ponka herniorrhaphy
portacaval anastomosis
portal systemic anastomosis
portoenterostomy
portoportal anastomosis
portosystemic anastomosis
posterior diaphragmatic gastropexy
posterior repair of the diaphragmatic hiatus
posterior sagittal and 3-flap anoplasty
PPPD (pylorus-preserving pancreatoduodenectomy)
precut sphincterotomy
preperitoneal approach
preperitoneal hernioplasty
preperitoneal prosthetic mesh repair of hernia via laparoscopy
Pringle maneuver for clamping the hepatic pedicle
proctectomy, mucosal
proctocolectomy
proctopexy
Prolene Hernia System (PHS) bilayer patch repair
prophylactic cholecystectomy
prophylactic gastrojejunostomy
proximal duct excision
proximal gastric vagotomy
proximal subtotal pancreatectomy
Puestow pancreaticojejunostomy
Puestow-Gillesby
pull-through
push enteroscopy
pyeloileocutaneous anastomosis
pylorectomy
pyloromyotomy
pyloroplasty

operation *(cont.)*
pylorotomy
pylorus-preserving modification
pylorus-preserving pancreato-duodenectomy (PPPD)
pylorus-preserving resection
pylorus-preserving Whipple
pylorus-sparing Whipple procedure
radical mastectomy
radioguided parathyroidectomy
radioiodide ablation
Ramstedt-Fredet pyloromyotomy
Ramstedt pyloroplasty
rapid pull-through (RPT)
reconstructive mammoplasty
rectal mucosectomy
rectal prolapse repair
rectal sleeve advancement
rectopexy
rectosigmoidectomy
rectovaginopexy
reduction mammoplasty
Rehne-Delorme plication
resection and primary anastomosis of bowel
resection with Roux-en-Y hepatico-jejunostomy
retrocolic choledochojejunostomy
retropharyngeal approach
retropubic prostatectomy
right colectomy with ileostomy
right hepatic lobectomy
Ripstein rectal prolapse repair
Ripstein rectopexy
robot-assisted
Rodney Smith biliary stricture
Roux-en-Y anastomosis
Roux-en-Y chimney surgical technique
Roux-en-Y choledochojejunostomy
Roux-en-Y cystojejunostomy
Roux-en-Y esophagojejunostomy reconstruction
Roux-en-Y gastric bypass
Roux-en-Y gastrojejunostomy

operation *(cont.)*
Roux-en-Y hepaticojejunostomy
Roux-en-Y jejunoileostomy
Roux-en-Y pancreaticojejunostomy
Roux-en-Y reconstruction
Roux-Y (see *Roux-en-Y*)
rubber band hemorrhoid ligation
Russell percutaneous endoscopic gastrostomy
Rutkow sutureless plug and patch repair for inguinal hernia
sacroabdominoperineal pull-through
sacrofixation
sacrospinous
SBE (small bowel enteroscopy)
Schoemaker anastomosis
Schwartz-Pregenzer urethropexy
Scopinaro pancreaticobiliary bypass
Scott jejunoileal bypass
second-look laparotomy
segmental bowel transplantation
segmental colon resection
segmental mastectomy
segmental reduction and split-graft techniques
segmental resection of bowel
segmentectomy
SEPS (subfascial endoscopic perforator surgery)
serosal patch repair
shoelace technique for delayed primary closure of fasciotomy
short-scar procedure in breast reduction
short-scar tumescent reduction mammoplasty
Shouldice hernia repair
Shouldice herniorrhaphy
sialodochoplasty
sialolithotomy
side-to-side anastomosis
sigmoid colectomy
sigmoid colostomy
sigmoidoscopic decompression of volvulus

operation *(cont.)*
- sigmoidoscopic reduction of volvulus
- Simonsen technique for large rectovaginal fistula repair
- simple mastectomy
- Sistrunk procedure
- small bowel resection
- snare resection (band and snare)
- Soave abdominal pull-through
- Soave endorectal pull-through
- solid organ transplantation
- sphincterotomy of papilla
- sphincterotomy with stone extraction
- sphincter-saving procedure
- Stretta
- splenectomy
- splenorrhaphy
- Ssabanejew-Frank gastrostomy
- staging
- staging laparotomy
- Stamm gastrostomy
- standard Whipple pancreatico-duodenectomy
- stapler-facilitated rectal eversion
- stapling esophago-diverticulostomy by endoscopy
- stapling off of small gastric pouch
- State end-to-end anastomosis
- station pull-through
- stereotactic transsphenoidal hypophysectomy
- stereotaxic core needle biopsy
- Stoppa posterior approach
- Stoppa-Rives giant prosthetic repair of the visceral sac
- stricturoplasty
- subcutaneous mastectomy
- subfascial endoscopic perforator surgery (SEPS)
- subglandular augmentation mammo-plasty
- submucosal tunnel technique
- subserosal needle catheter jejunostomy

operation *(cont.)*
- subtotal colectomy
- subtotal pancreatectomy
- subtotal thyroidectomy
- suction-assisted lipectomy (SAL)
- Sugiura esophageal varices procedure
- superior pedicle technique reduction mammoplasty
- superwet reduction mammoplasty
- suprahyoid neck
- sutureless plug and patch repair for inguinal hernia
- Swenson abdominal pull-through
- Tanner
- TAPP (transabdominal preperi-toneal) hernia repair
- TAPP (transabdominal preperi-toneal) laparoscopic hernioplasty
- Teflon sling repair
- temporary colostomy
- temporary ostomy
- tension-eliminating repair
- tension-free anastomosis
- tension-free hernia repair
- tension-free prosthetic repair
- TEP (totally extraperitoneal) laparo-scopic hernioplasty
- T-fastener gastropexy
- Thal esophageal stricture repair
- Thal esophagogastrostomy
- Thal stricturoplasty
- Thal-Nissen fundoplasty
- Thiersch anal incontinence proce-dure
- thoracoabdominal esophagectomy
- thoracophrenolaparotomy
- thoracoscopic esophagomyotomy
- thorascopic esophagomyotomy
- three-trocar technique of cholecys-tectomy
- thymectomy
- TIPS (transjugular intrahepatic portal shunt procedure)

operation *(cont.)*
total abdominal colectomy (TAC)
total abdominal evisceration (TAE)
total colectomy
total esophagectomy
total fundic wrap (Nissen-Rossetti)
total gastrectomy
total hepatectomy
total lobectomy
totally (or total) extraperitoneal laparoscopic hernioplasty
total mastectomy
total mesorectal excision (TME)
total pancreatectomy
total parathyroidectomy
total protocolectomy and ileostomy
total sac excision
total thoracic esophagectomy
total thyroidectomy
Toupet (partial posterior) fundoplication
Toupet fundoplasty
Toupet fundoplication
transabdominal preperitoneal laparoscopic hernioplasty
transabdominal repair
transabdominal retroperitoneal lymph node dissection
transanal deflation of sigmoid volvulus
transanal endoscopic microsurgery (TEM)
transanal pouch advancement
transaxillary subpectoral mammoplasty
transcystic common bile duct exploration
transcystic duct/common bile duct exploration (TCD/CBDE)
transduodenal sphincterotomy
transected vertical gastric bypass with Silastic ring band and gastrostomy
transection of esophagus
transectomy of vagus nerves

operation *(cont.)*
transhiatal esophagectomy
transhiatal pyloroplasty
transjugular intrahepatic portosystemic shunt procedure (TIPS)
transomental posterior gastroenterostomy
transpapillary endoscopic cholecystotomy
transthoracic Nissen fundoplication
transumbilical augmentation mammoplasty
transumbilical breast augmentation (TUBA)
transurethral balloon Laserthermia prostatectomy
transurethral laser-induced prostatectomy (TULIP)
transverse colectomy
transverse wedge
transversostomy
Traverso-Longmire technique
T-tack gastropexy
TUBA (transumbilical breast augmentation)
tube duodenostomy with feeding jejunostomy
tumescent liposuction technique
Turbinger gastric reconstruction
Turnbull multiple ostomy
typhlorrhaphy
umbilectomy
unilateral adrenalectomy
unilateral groin dissection
UPPP (uvulopalatopharyngoplasty)
Urban
ureteral reimplantation
ureteroileocutaneous anastomosis
ureteroileostomy
uvulopalatopharyngoplasty (UPPP)
vaginal lengthening
vagotomy
venovenous bypass
vermilionectomy
vertical-banded gastroplasty (VBG)

operation *(cont.)*
vertical bipedicle flap technique reduction mammoplasty
vertical reduction mammoplasty
vest-over-pants hernia repair
V-excision
video-assisted thoracic surgery (VATS)
videoendoscopic augmentation mammoplasty
videoscopic fundoplication
Von Haberer-Finney anastomosis
Von Haberer gastroenterostomy
WAMBA (Wise areola mastopexy breast augmentation)
Waugh Clagett pancreatico-duodenostomy
wedge resection
weight reduction
Weinberg pyloroplasty
Wells rectopexy
wet-technique breast reduction with liposuction
Wheeless surgical construction of J rectal pouch
Whipple pancreaticoduodenectomy
Whitehead hemorrhoidectomy
Wise pattern for reduction mammoplasty
Witzel duodenostomy
Witzel gastrostomy
Witzel jejunostomy
Womack procedure
xanthogranulomatous cholecystitis
Y-V anoplasty
Y-V plasty
zipper sphincterotomy
operative biliary bypass
operative cholangiogram
operative cholangiogram catheter
operative debridement and placement of drain
operative diagnosis
operative drainage
operative field
operative laparoscope
operative stone removal
operculectomy
OpEX instrument service
ophthalmic retractor
opiates
Opisthorchis sinensis
opisthotonic position
Opmi microscope drape
Opmilas 144 Plus laser
Opmilas CO_2 multipurpose laser
OP-1 implant graft
opportunistic infection
Opraflex incise drape
OpSite dressing
OpSite Flexigrid transparent adhesive film dressing
OpSite occlusive dressing
opsonin production
Opteform 100HT bone graft
Op-Temp cautery
optical biopsy
optical biopsy forceps
optical biopsy instruments
Optical Biopsy system
optical bronchoscopes
optical coherence tomography (OCT)
optical forceps
optical retractor
Optical Sensors blood gas monitor
Optical Tracking System (OTS)
Optik rigid laparoscope
Optima fabric
optimal tracheal seal
OptiMARK (gadoversetamide injection)
optimized serum pancreolauryl test
option, therapeutic
OptiPen insulin delivery pen
OptiPen Pro insulin delivery pen
Optipore sponge dressing
Optipore wound-cleaning sponge
Opti-Port right-angle, double-swivel connector

OptiQue sensing catheter
Optiray 350 (ioversal)
OptiSet insulin delivery pen
Optison contrast agent
Opti-Sorb reinforcement
Optistar MR contrast delivery system
Optistat power injector
Optiva I.V. catheter
Optivis needle
Oracle Focus catheter
Oracle Megasonics catheter
Oracle Micro catheter
Oracle Micro Plus catheter
Oragrafin contrast medium
Oragrafin Sodium (ipodate sodium)
oral airway
oral calcium
oral cholecystogram (OCG)
oral contraceptive
oral gastric calibration tube
oral gastric tube (OGT)
oral hypoglycemic agent
  biguanide
  sulfonylurea
oral intubation
oral papilloma
oral propanolol
oral purge
oral sepsis
oral smear
oral transmission
oral ulcer
Oral RAE uncuffed tube
Oralgen oral aerosol insulin
orange peel appearance (peau d'orange)
Oratec electrocautery probe
orbital plate
orbital reducer seal
orbital retractor
orbital rim dissector
Oreopoulos-Zellerman catheter
Oretorp arthroscopy knife
organ
  ancestral
  cadaveric
organ *(cont.)*
  distant
  donor
  extraperitoneal
  failure of
  glandular
  harvesting of
  inadequate perfusion of
  recipient of
  reticuloendothelial
  retroperitoneal
  target
  Zuckerkandl
organ donation
organ donor registry
organ harvesting
organic acids
organic lesion
organism
  acid-fast
  blood-borne
  gram-negative
  intracellular
  multicellular
  nonpathogenic
  pathogenic
    bacterium
    fungus
    parasite
    rickettsia
    virus
  pleuropneumonia-like (PPLO)
  pyogenic
  unicellular
  urease-producing
  virulent
Organización Nacional de Transplantes (Spain)
organized clot
organized thrombus
organoaxial gastric volvulus
organomegaly
organ procurement agency
organ recipient
organ recovery

organ-sparing surgery
Orgaran (danaparoid sodium)
ORI electronic endoscopy system
Oriental cholangiohepatitis
Oriental V-Y flap technique
orienting reflex
orienting suture
orifice
  anal
  aortic
  appendiceal
  atrioventricular
  cardiac
  esophagogastric
  external urethral
  gastroduodenal
  golf-hole ureteral
  hernial
  ileocecal
  internal urethral
  mitral
  myopectineal (MPO)
  pharyngeal
  pulmonary
  pyloric
  tricuspid
  ureteral or ureteric
  urethral
  vaginal
orifice of appendix
Origin balloon
Origin distention balloon system
Origin Medsystems trocar
Origin Tacker laparoscopic tacking device
Origin trocar
Oris pin
orlistat
Ormond disease
Ormon rectal scissors
oroendotracheal tube
orofacial fistula
orofacial herpes
orogastric tube
OR1 electronic endoscopy system
oropharyngeal anesthesia
oropharyngeal cancer
oropharyngeal dysphagia
  from esophageal dysphagia
oropharyngeal hemorrhage
oropharyngeal tumor
orotracheal intubation
Orozco cervical plate
orphan virus
Orr gall duct forceps
Orr-Loygue transabdominal proctopexy
Orr rectal prolapse repair
Orthair oscillating saw
Orthoairtome wire driver
Orthoclone OKT3 monoclonal antibody
orthogonal view
Ortholav stand
orthopedic mallet
orthosis, Gillette joint
OrthoSorb absorbable fixation pin
OrthoSorb pin nail
orthostasis
orthostatic blood pressure
orthostatic change
orthostatic hypotension
Orthotec handpiece and tubing
Orthotec pulsed irrigation
orthotic plate
orthotopic liver transplant (transplantation) (OLT)
Ortho-Trac adhesive bandage
Ortho-Vent nonadhesive bandage
Orzel (UFT/leucovorin calcium)
O_2 (oxygen) saturation
Osborne plate
oscillating blade
oscillating gouge
oscillating microsaw
oscillating saw
oscillating sternotomy saw
Oscillo III plaster saw
O'Shaughnessy artery forceps
OSI Extremity elevator

Osler-Weber-Rendu disease
Osler-Weber-Rendu syndrome
Osler-Weber-Rendu telangiectasia
OsmoCyte Island wound dressing
OsmoCyte PCA pillow wound dressing
OsmoCyte pillow
osmolality equilibration
osmolality, fecal
osmolarity
Osmolite HN enteral feeding
osmotic agent
osmotically active particles
osmotic diarrhea
osmotic edema
osmotic fragility of red cells
osmotic laxative
osmotic pressure
osseous polyp
osseous tuberosity
Ossoff-Karlan microlaryngeal suction tube
Ostavir (tuvirumab) monoclonal antibody
osteoarticular graft
OsteoBiologics, Inc.
osteoblastic bony metastasis
osteocartilaginous graft
osteochondral graft
osteoclastic activity
osteoclast tension staple
osteogenic sarcoma
osteoid carcinoma
osteolytic activity
osteoma
Osteomark monoclonal antibody-based agent
Osteomark test
osteomyelitis
Osteone air drill
osteoperiosteal graft
osteophyte elevator
osteophyte nipper rongeur
osteophytes and skeletal abnormalities
osteoporosis
Osteoset bone graft substitute graft
osteotome
OST-577 human antihepatitis B antibody
ostial lesion
ostiomeatal stent
ostomate
ostomy (pl. ostomies) (see *colostomy; pouch; operation*)
ostomy appliance
ostomy bag
O'Sullivan-O'Connor abdominal retractor
O'Sullivan scoring system for dysphagia
OTC (over-the-counter) medications
otic obstruction
Otis urethrotome
OtoLam laser
OtoLam laser therapy
otologic drill
otorrhea, clear
O_2 (oxygen) toxicity
OTW (over the wire)
outer capsule
outer crossbar
outflow cannula
outflow, pancreatic duct
out-in-out technique suture
outlet constipation
outlet delay
outlet disorder of anorectum
outlet view
outpatient anesthesia
outpatient percutaneous liver biopsy
outpouching of mucosa
outpouching of testicular tissue
oval cherry-red raised lesion
oval-cup jaws
oval dissector
ovale malaria
oval-form colonic groove
OvaRex MAb
ovarian cancer
ovarian cyst

ovarian medulla
ovarian neoplasm
ovarian torsion
ovarian tumor
over-and-over suture
over-and-over whip suture
over-the-counter (OTC) medications
over-the-top position
overactivity, acquired benign adrenal
  androgenic
overbed table
overdistention of hollow viscus
overexpression, P53 protein
overhead film
overhead oblique view
overhead view
Overholt artery forceps
Overholt clip-applying forceps
Overholt thoracic forceps
overlap syndrome (connective tissue
  disease)
overlapping suture
overlay plate
overload, circulatory
overlying skin erythema
overlying structures
overnight basal acid output (BAO)
overnight dexamethasone suppression
  test
overnutrition
overproduction of normal adrenal
  hormones
oversewn, oversewing
overt colonic polyposis
Overton dowel graft
overventilation
overwhelming postsplenectomy sepsis
  (OPSS)
ovolactovegetarian diet
Ovum curette
Owen gauze
Owen gauze dressing
Owen silk suture
Owestry staple
owl incision technique reduction
  mammoplasty
oxaliplatin
oxaluria, enteric
oxamniquine
Oxandrin (oxandrolone)
oxandrolone
ox bile extract
Oxequip air
oxidation
oxidative stress
oxide radical
oxidized bile acid
Oximax pulse oximeter
oximeter
  MARSpo2 Tech pulse
  Masimo SET pulse
  Oximax pulse
  Oxi-Reader
  pulse
oximetry
Oxiplex
Oxi-Reader pulse oximeter
Oxo kitchen scissors
oxybuprocaine
Oxycel (oxidized cellulose) pad
Oxycel (oxidized cellulose) pledget
Oxycel (oxidized cellulose) strip
oxycodone HCl
oxycodone/oxycodone terephthalate/
  aspirin
OxyContin (oxycodone HCl)
oxygen bound to hemoglobin
oxygen-carrying capacity of blood
oxygen saturation
Oxygen Sensors (fuel cells)
oxygenated blood
oxygenation
oxygenator, Maxima Forté blood
Oxygent (emulsified perflubron) blood
  substitute
oxymetric data
oxymorphone HCl
oxyntic cell

oxyntic gland
oxyntic mucosa
oxyphenisatin, oxyphenisatin acetate
oxyphenonium
oxyphil cell hyperplasia

P, p

PA (posteroanterior) film
PA (posteroanterior) view
PA (pulmonary artery pressure)
PABA (p-aminobenzoic acid) test
Pace bipolar pacing catheter
pacemaker
  Enterra gastrointestinal
  gastric
  transvenous
pacemaker (gastric) cell
pacemaker (stomach) cell
pacemaker region, gastric
Pacesetter introducer
Pace ventricular needle
Pacifico-type suction tube
pack, packing (see also *bandage*)
  Adaptic
  Aquacel Hydrofiber
  Barrier
  ENTaxis nasal
  gauze
  iodoform gauze
  Kaltostat wound
  moist lap (laparotomy)
  Nu-Brede
  omental
  Pedi-Boro Soak Packs
  perihepatic

pack *(cont.)*
  petrolatum gauze
  Silverlon wound
  Sorbsan
  Tilley
  wound
packed cells, transfusion of (measured in units)
packed red blood cells
paclitaxel
$PaCO_2$
pad (see also *dressing*)
  abdominal (ABD)
  abdominal fat
  abdominal lap (laparotomy)
  ABS
  acetone prep
  alcohol prep
  Alpha Protech
  Alpha Protech Unreal Lambskin Soft Touch
  Aluma foam
  antimesenteric fat
  arch cookie
  axillary fat
  B-D Sensability Breast Self-Examination Aid
  calcium alginate

pad *(cont.)*
Carrington gel
CB GelPad hydrogel
circular
cookie
Curity ABD
Debrisan absorbent
Dynarex prep
electrode
Elta hydrogel
esophagogastric fat
fat
fibrocartilaginous
4 x 4
gauze
Gelfoam
hydrocolloid
Hydropad
impregnated
ischiorectal
Jack Frost Therapy Pack
J&J nonstick
J&J Surgipad
Johnson & Johnson Steri-Pad
Kaltostat Fortex
lap (laparotomy)
laparotomy (lap)
Medicell PVP foam
Medicell PVP HC
Medifil
Mesalt
"Mik" (Mikulicz)
M-Pact
MPM gel pad
navicular shoe cookie
Nutramax flexible strip
Oxycel
Paroplex
PDI electrode
PDI povidone iodine
Procare CPM
Smith & Nephew Transigel hydrogel
Starline nonadherent
Superstat hemostatic wound

pad *(cont.)*
SureFit electrosurgical grounding
SurePress absorbent
Surgicel strips
Surgipad Combine
Telfa adhesive
TID I combination
Triad PVP-1 prep
Tucks Pads
Weck laparotomy
paddle forceps
pad of fat, ischiorectal
Paecilomyces variotii
PAF (platelet activating factor)
PAF antagonist
Pafase (acetylhydrolase)
PAFD (percutaneous abscess and fluid drainage)
Pagedas retrieval pouch
Pagedas self-locking suture
Paget abscess
Paget carcinoma
Paget disease, extramammary
Paget disease of breast
Paget disease of perianal area
Paget quiet necrosis
pain (see also *tenderness*)
abdominal
back
boring
breast
burning
chest
colicky
constricting
cramping
crampy
cyclic
cyclical
dermatome
diffuse
diffuse abdominal
dull
dull right upper quadrant

pain *(cont.)*
- epicritic
- epigastric
- esophageal
- exacerbation of
- exquisite
- flank
- functional
- gallbladder
- gastrointestinal
- gnawing
- gynecologic
- headache
- hunger
- incapacitating
- intermittent
- intractable
- jaw
- knifelike
- lancinating
- left flank
- left lower quadrant
- left upper quadrant
- localized
- loin
- midline
- migrating
- motion
- musculoskeletal
- nagging
- nocturnal
- noncyclical
- onset of
- parietal (somatic)
- perirectal
- phantom breast
- phantom rectal
- pleuritic chest
- point of maximal
- poorly localized
- postlaparoscopic shoulder
- postoperative
- postprandial
- postural

pain *(cont.)*
- prolonged
- protopathic
- psychogenic
- radiating
- rebound
- rectal
- recurrent
- recurring
- referred
- referred periumbilical
- referred right subscapular
- refractory
- remission of
- retrosternal chest
- right flank
- right lower quadrant
- right-sided abdominal
- right upper quadrant
- severe
- sharp
- shoulder
- small of back
- somatic
- steady
- stomach
- subscapular
- substernal
- sudden onset of
- suprapubic
- tearing
- terrifying
- testicular
- unexplained abdominal
- unrelenting
- unrelieved
- unremitting
- vaginal
- visceral
- vise-like

pain abolished by breath-holding

pain accompanied by abdominal fullness

pain accompanied by nausea

pain accompanied by palpitation
pain accompanied by sensation of gas
pain accompanied by shortness of breath
pain accompanied by sweating
pain accompanied by weakness
pain aggravated by coughing
pain aggravated by deep breathing
pain aggravated by deep inspiration
pain and tenderness
PainBuster infusion pain management kit
pain continued unabated
pain control (see *anesthesia*)
pain following heavy meal
painful anesthesia
painful hepatomegaly
painful palpable gallbladder
painful swollen thyroid
pain in sternal articulations
pain indistinguishable from angina
pain induced with methacholine
painless breast mass
painless edema
painless indurated ulcer
painless jaundice
painless, large thyroid
painless lower GI bleeding
painless mammogram
painless pancreatitis
painless rectal bleeding
painless thyroiditis
pain "like being crushed under a heavy load"
pain "like being caught in a vise"
pain "like someone sitting on my chest"
pain migration
pain of gastrointestinal origin
pain of musculoskeletal origin
pain of psychogenic origin
pain on drinking cold liquid
pain on exposure to cold
pain on strong emotion
pain on swallowing
pain precipitated by emotional upset
pain precipitated by exertion
pain precipitated by strong emotion
pain radiating to back
pain radiating to epigastrium
pain radiating to jaw
pain radiating to left arm
pain radiating to neck
pain radiating to right arm
pain radiating to throat
pain rapidly extinguished by withdrawal of stimulus
pain relieved by antacids
pain relieved by belching
pain relieved by bowel movement
pain relieved by carotid massage
pain relieved by cimetidine
pain relieved by eating
pain relieved by food intake
pain relieved by leaning forward
pain relieved by passage of flatus
pain relieved by rest
pain reproduced by palpation
pain reproducible with moderate exercise
Painter colic
pain unaffected by position
pain unrelated to meals
pain unrelieved by nitroglycerin
pain when angry
pain when excited
pain with defecation
pair of pliers
PAIS (Psychosocial Adjustment to Illness Scale)
PAK (percutaneous access kit)
PAL (probe for aspiration and lavage)
Palacos cement adhesive
palate
palatopharyngeal fold
palatopharyngoplasty
palatoplasty
Palco EM-100 Oxylato
pale cell

pale skin
palliation of pain
palliation, surgical
palliation therapy
palliative care
palliative chemotherapy
palliative hepatojejunostomy
palliative operative procedure
palliative pain management
palliative resection
palliative surgery
palliative surgical procedure
palliative therapy
pallor
palmar erythema
palmar incision
palmar plate
Palmaz balloon-expandable stent
Palmaz Corinthian biliary stent
Palmaz Corinthian transhepatic biliary stent and delivery system
Palmaz-Schatz balloon-expandable stent
Palmaz-Schatz Crown balloon-expandable stent
Palmaz-Schatz Mini Crown stent
Palmaz-Schatz stent (PSS)
Palmer bone nail
palmitin test
palmoxirate sodium
palmoxiric acid
palm-to-axilla dressing
Palomar E2000 ruby laser
palonosetron hydrochloride
palpable adenopathy
palpable epigastric mass
palpable gallbladder
palpable mass
palpable mass after aspiration
palpable nodule
palpable, nontender, distended gallbladder
palpable pulse
palpable pyloric olive
palpable retroareolar mass
palpably enlarged gallbladder
Palpagraph breast tissue examination device
Palpagraph mammography device
palpation
palpitation
PALS tablets (chlorophyllin copper complex)
pamidronate disodium
Pamine (methscopolamine bromide)
P-aminosalicylic acid (PAS) hypothyroidism
Pamisyl (aminosalicylic acid)
pampiniform plexus
Panacryl absorbable suture
Panacryl braided synthetic absorbable suture
Panafil (papain; urea; chlorophyllin copper complex)
Panafil enzymatic debriding agent
Panafil White (papain; urea) ointment
Panalok RC absorbable soft tissue anchor
Panalok RC QuickAnchor Plus
Panalok suture anchor
pancake kidney
pancolitis
pancolonoscopy
pancopride
pancreas
  aberrant
  accessory
  anlage
  annular
  anterior surface of
  Aselli
  beta cells of the
  biopsy of
  blunt injury to
  body of
  burned-out
  cancer of
  Christmas tree appearance of
  congenital lipomatosis of

pancreas *(cont.)*
  degeneration of
  dorsal
  endocrine
  exocrine
  fibrofatty infiltration of
  head of
  heterotopic
  inferior surface of
  inflammation of
  lesser
  longitudinal filleting of the
  lower border of the
  neck of
  posterior surface of
  tail of
  uncinate process of
  ventral
  Willis
  Winslow
pancreas acinar cell growth
pancreas after kidney (PAK) transplantation
pancreas divisum
pancreas encircling the duodenum
pancreas transplant
Pancrease MT 20 (lipase; protease; amylase)
pancreatectomy (see *operation*)
  distal
  distal laparoscopic
  distal near-total
  distal subtotal
  donor
  en bloc distal
  laparoscopic distal
  left-to-right subtotal
  limited
  near-total
  partial
  proximal subtotal
  subtotal
  total
  transduodenal
  Whipple
pancreatic abscess
pancreatic acinar cells
pancreatic acinus atrophy
pancreatic adenoma
pancreatic allograft
pancreatic alpha$_2$ islet cell tumor
pancreatic amylase (P-type)
pancreatic ascites
pancreatic bed
pancreatic bud
pancreatic calculus
pancreatic cancer, exocrine
pancreatic carcinoma
pancreatic cholera
pancreatic cholera syndrome
pancreatic colic
pancreatic cutaneous fistula
pancreatic cyst
pancreatic cystic disease
pancreatic D cells
pancreatic diabetes
pancreatic divisum
pancreatic duct
  accessory
  duodenal end of dorsal
  duodenal end of main
  genu of
  main
  obstruction of
  proximal part of dorsal
pancreatic ductal adenocarcinoma
pancreatic ductal carcinoma
  iatrogenic
  traumatic
pancreatic duct disruption
pancreatic duct obstruction
pancreatic duct outflow
pancreatic duct sphincter (PDS)
pancreatic duct stent
pancreatic endocrine insufficiency
pancreatic endocrine tumor (PET) cell
pancreatic endoscopy
pancreatic endotherapy
pancreatic enteric fistula
pancreatic enzyme

pancreatic enzyme replacement
pancreatic enzyme therapy
pancreatic exocrine insufficiency
pancreatic exocrine secretions
pancreatic fibrosis
pancreatic fistula
pancreatic fluid
pancreatic function test (testing)
pancreatic gastrinoma (Zollinger-Ellison syndrome)
pancreatic gastrinoma and peptic ulcer disease
pancreatic glucagonoma tumor
pancreatic hamartoma
pancreatic head
pancreatic hormone
pancreatic infantilism
pancreatic insufficiency
pancreatic insulinoma
pancreatic islet
pancreatic islet cell
pancreatic islet cell markers
pancreatic islet cell transplantation
pancreatic islet cell tumor
pancreatic juice
pancreatic leak
pancreatic lipase
pancreatic malignancy
pancreatic necrosis
pancreatic non-beta islet cell tumor
pancreaticobiliary common channel
pancreaticobiliary diversion
pancreaticobiliary ductal junction
pancreaticobiliary sphincter
pancreaticobiliary tract
pancreatic obstruction
pancreaticocutaneous fistula
pancreaticocystostomy
pancreaticoduodenal artery
pancreaticoduodenectomy, Whipple
pancreaticoduodenostomy (see also *operation*)
  Child
  Dennis-Varco
pancreaticoduodenostomy *(cont.)*
  Waugh-Clagett
  Whipple
pancreaticogastrostomy
pancreaticohepatic syndrome
pancreaticojejunal anastomosis
pancreaticojejunostomy or pancreatojejunostomy (see also *operation*)
  Cattell-Warren
  caudal
  distal
  ductal
  duct-to-mucosa
  DuVal or Duval
  end-to-end intussuscepted
  end-to-end inverting
  end-to-side
  Frey
  invagination technique of
  isolated
  laparoscopic
  lateral
  longitudinal
  modified dunking
  Partington-Rochelle
  Puestow
  retrocolic end-to-end
  Roux-en-Y
  Roux loop
  side-to-side
  two-layer end-to-side
pancreaticolienal lymph node
pancreatic oncofetal antigen (POA) test
pancreaticopleural fistula
pancreaticosplenic gland
pancreaticosplenic lymph node
pancreaticosplenic omentum
pancreatic phlegmon
pancreatic pleural effusion
pancreatic polypeptide (PP)
pancreatic pseudocyst
pancreatic rest
pancreatic sepsis in acute pancreatitis
pancreatic steatorrhea

pancreatic stent therapy
pancreatic tissue
  ectopic
  heterotopic
pancreatic tumor
pancreatic tumor markers
pancreatic vein
Pancreatin 8X (pancreatin; lipase; protease; amylase)
pancreatitis
  acute
  acute biliary (ABP)
  acute gallstone
  acute hemorrhagic
  acute interstitial
  alcoholic
  apoplectic
  biliary
  calcareous
  calcifying
  centrilobar
  centrilobular
  chronic
  chronic alcoholic
  chronic calcific
  chronic calcifying
  chronic obstructive
  chronic relapsing
  diffuse
  familial
  focal
  fulminating
  gallstone
  groove
  hemorrhagic
  hemorrhagic necrotizing
  hereditary
  hormone-induced
  idiopathic
  infected necrotizing
  infectious
  interstitial
  Kasugai
  Marseille

pancreatitis *(cont.)*
  mumps
  necrotizing
  painless
  pentamidine-induced
  perilobar
  post-ERCP induced
  postoperative
  purulent
  Ranson
  recurrent
  recurring acute
  relapsing
  Santiani-Stone
  segmentary
  sterile necrotizing
  subacute
  suppurative
  unresolving
pancreatobiliary junction
pancreatoblastoma
pancreatoduodenal
pancreatoduodenectomy (see *operation*)
  conventional
  extended
  Kausch-Whipple
  partial
  pylorus-preserving (PPPD)
  radical
  subtotal
  two-step
  Whipple
pancreatogenous diarrhea
pancreatogram, pancreatography
  diagnostic
  endoscopic retrograde
  intraoperative
  magnetic resonance (MRP)
  retrograde
pancreatojejunostomy (see *pancreatico-jejunostomy*)
pancreatolithiasis
pancreatorrhaphy
pancreatoscope

pancreatoscopy
pancreatotomy
Pancrecarb MS-8 (lipase; protease; amylase)
pancrelipase
pancreoscopy, infragastric
pancreozymin-secretin test
Pancrezyme 4X (pancreatin; lipase; protease; amylase)
panculture
pancuronium bromide
pancystitis
pancytopenia
panduriform placenta
panel
  arthritis
  bleeding time coagulation
  chemistry
  clot retraction coagulation
  coagulation
  electrolyte
  enzyme
  fasting chemistry
  febrile agglutinin
  lipid
  liver
  NAP hepatitis B virus (HBV) quantitative
  partial thromboplastin time coagulation
  plasma assay coagulation
  platelet count coagulation
  prothrombin time coagulation
  rheumatoid (rheumatology)
  rheumatology
  SMA chemistry
  SMAC ("smack") chemistry
  test
  thyroid
  Triage *Clostridium difficile*
  Triage parasite
panel cell
panel coagulation
panendoscope (see *endoscope*)
panendoscopy
  fiberoptic
  lower
  upper
Paneth cell
Pan-HER
panhypopituitarism
panic attack
PanIN (pancreatic intraepithelial neoplasia)
panniculitis
  cytophagic histiocytic
  LE (lupus erythematosus)
  lobular
  nodular nonsuppurative
  relapsing febrile nodular nonsuppurative
  septal
  subacute nodular migratory
  Weber-Christian
panniculus adiposus
panniculus carnosus
panniculus, hanging
pannus formation
PanoGauze hydrogel-impregnated gauze
PanoPlex hydrogel dressing
panpiniform plexus
panproctocolectomy
Panretin (alitretinoin)
pantaloon embolism
pantaloon hernia
Pantoloc (pantoprazole)
Pantopaque contrast medium
Pantozol (pantoprazole)
pants-over-vest hernia repair
pants-over-vest herniorrhaphy
pants-over-vest repair
Panzer gallbladder scissors
PaO_2
PAP (prostatic acid phosphastase)
papable laryngeal fracture
papain
Papanicolaou (Pap)
Papanicolaou method

Papanicolaou smear
Papanicolaou test
Paparella angled ring curette
Paparella canal knife
Paparella drum elevator knife
Paparella duckbill elevator
Paparella fenestrometer
Paparella incudostapedial knife
Paparella mastoid curette
Paparella pick
Paparella retractor
Paparella sickle knife
Paparella straight needle
Paparella tissue press
papaya enzyme
PA–PCWP/CO x 80 (mean pulmonary artery pressure – pulmonary capillary wedge pressure/cardiac output x 80 = pulmonary vascular resistance)
paper drape
papilla (pl. papillae)
  acoustic
  anal
  bile
  circumvallate
  clavate
  conical
  dentinal
  dermal
  disinsertion of
  duodenal
  filiform
  foliate
  fungiform
  hypertrophic
  lingual
  major duodenal
  minor duodenal
  renal
  urethral
papilla of Vater
papillary adenocarcinoma
papillary adenoma
papillary carcinoma of thyroid gland
papillary cluster of cells
papillary cystadenocarcinoma
papillary cystic adenoma
papillary dermis
papillary gastric carcinoma
papillary hyperplasia of follicles
papillary hypertrophy of conjunctiva
papillary layer of dermis
papillary lesion
papillary muscle
papillary necrosis
papillary proliferation
papillary stenosis
papillary tumor
papillated surface
papillation
papillectomy
papillitis
  necrotizing
  necrotizing renal
papilloadenocystoma
papillocarcinoma
papilloma
  basal cell
  benign squamous
  choroid plexus
  cockscomb (also coxcomb)
  cutaneous
  duct
  fibroepithelial
  friable
  Hopmann
  intracanalicular
  intracystic
  intraductal
  inverted
  inverted ductal
  oral
  soft
  squamous
  transitional cell
  villous
  vocal cord
  warty

papilloma lactiferous duct
papilloma of bladder
papilloma of vocal cord
papillomavirus (also, papilloma virus)
papillomatosis
papillomatous benign tumor
papillotome
  Accuratome
  Apollo3 triple-lumen
  Bard high-flow
  bowed
  Cape Town steerable
  Classen-Demling
  Danish pattern
  double-lumen
  endoscopic
  Erlangen
  guidewire
  Howell rotatable
  Huibregtse
  Huibregtse-Katon
  Olympus needle-knife
  piggyback needle-knife
  precut
  ProForma
  shark fin
  single-lumen
  triple-lumen
  two-lumen
  Wilson-Cook
  Zimmon
papillotomy, endoscopic (EPT)
papillotomy transection of the sphincter of Oddi
Papineau graft
papovavirus
Pappenheimer body
Pap (Papanicolaou) smear
Pap test
papular lesion
papular mucinosis
papule
  fluid-filled
  Gottron
papule *(cont.)*
  lichenoid
  minute
  pearly penile
  pedunculated
  piezogenic
  pruritic urticarial (of pregnancy)
  rust-colored
  sessile
  split
  transitory
papulonecrotic lesion
PAR (postanesthesia recovery)
para-aortic lymph node
para-aortic node biopsy
para-aortic region
paracecal appendix
paracentesis, abdominal
paracentesis needle
paracentesis tray
paracetamol hepatotoxicity
Parachute corkscrew suture anchor
paracolic abscess
paracolic gutter
paracolic lymph node
paracolon bacillus
paracolostomy hernia
paracrine regulation pattern
paracystic pouch
paracytic
paradoxic increase
paradoxical movement
paraductal adenopathy
paraduodenal fold
paraduodenal fossa
paraesophageal hernia
paraesophageal herniation
paraesophageal hiatus hernia
paraesophageal varices
paraesophagogastric devascularization
paraffin cancer
paraffin tumor
parafollicular C cell
paraganglia

Paragon Champion stent system
Paragon CO_2 laser system
Paragon coronary stent
paraileostomal hernia
parainfluenza 2 virus
parainfluenza 3 virus
parainfluenza 4 virus
parallel to the tracheoesophageal groove
paralytic colonic or intestinal
  obstruction
paralytic ileus
parajejunal fossa
Paramax angled driver
paramedial incision
paramedian incision
parameters
  clinical
  clotting
paraneoplastic syndrome
parapatellar incision
parapharyngeal approach
pararectal abscess
pararectal pouch
pararectus incision
pararenal pseudocyst
parasite
  Enamoeba histolytica
  Giardia
  intestinal
  Isospora
parasitemia
parasitic abscess
parasitic cyst
parasitic disease
parasitic infection
parasitic infestation
Parasmillie double-bladed knife
parasternal gunshot wound
parasternal long-axis view
parasternal short-axis view
parasternal stab wound
parastomal hernia
parasympathomimetic drugs
parathyroid autotransplantation to
  forearm
parathyroid carcinoma
parathyroidectomy
  endoscopic
  incidental
  minimally invasive
  minimally invasive video-assisted
    (MIVAP)
  radioguided
  subtotal
parathyroid gland
parathyroiditis
parathyroid gland
parathyroid hormone analysis
parathyroid-hormone-related protein
  (PTHrp)
parathyroid hormone test
parathyroid hyperplasia
parathyroid tetany
parathyroid tissue placed in forearm
  muscles
parathyroid tumor
parathyroprival tetany
paratracheal node
paratyphoidal cholangiolitis
paraumbilical hernia
paraumbilical region
paravariceal sclerotherapy
paravertebral anesthesia
paravesical fossa
paravesical pouch
parchment induration
paregoric (PG)
Parell needle holder
parenchyma
  breast
  destruction of
  hepatic
  hepatic lobular
  heterogenous
  liver
  lung
  renal
  splenic
  thyroid

parenchymal cell
parenchymal damage
parenchymal destruction
parenchymal hemorrhage
parenchymal jaundice
parenchymal liver disease
parenchymal tissue
parenchymatous degeneration
parenchymatous goiter
parenchymatous inflammation
parenchymatous mastitis
parenchymatous myocarditis
parenchymatous nephritis
parenchymatous neuritis
parenchymatous pneumonia
parenchymography, endoscopic
retrograde (ERP)
parenchymous degeneration of liver
parenteral alimentation
parenteral antibiotic therapy
parenteral feeding
parenteral fluids
parenteral nutrition
Parepectolin (attapulgite)
paresis
paresthesias
Parfocal zoom
Parhad-Poppen arteriogram needle
Parham band circling needle
Parham-Martin fracture clamp
paricalcitol
parietal cell antibody
parietal cell index
parietal cell of fundus
parietal cell receptor
parietal cell vagotomy (PCV)
parietal fistula
parietal pain
parietal peritoneum
parietal (somatic) pain
parietal suture
Parietex composite mesh for hernia
surgery
parietomastoid suture
parieto-occipital suture
Paritene mesh graft for hernia surgery
park bench position
Parker-Kerr closed method of
end-to-end enteroenterostomy
Parker-Kerr enteroenterostomy
Parker-Kerr intestinal clamp
Parker knife
Parker retractor
Parkinson disease
Park posterior anal repair
Parks anal retractor
Parks anoscope
Parks fistulotomy
Parks hemorrhoidectomy
Parks ileal reservoir
Parks ileoanal anastomosis
Parks ileoanal reservoir
Parks ileostomy pouch
Parks partial sphincterotomy
Parks rectal retractor
Parks sphincterotomy retractor
Parks staged fistulotomy
Parks-TC needle holder
Parks transanal anastomosis
paromomycin sulfate
parotid abscess
parotid duct diversion, bilateral
(Wilke procedure)
parotid enlargement
parotid gland
paroxysmal motor disease
paroxysmal nocturnal hemoglobinuria
parrot clamp
parrot's beak clamp
Parsonnet clamp
partial adrenalectomy
partial bowel obstruction
partial colectomy
partial-curve blade
partial esophagectomy
partial fundoplication procedure
partial gastrectomy
partial hepatectomy

partial ileal bypass
partial lesion
partial lobectomy of liver
partial mastectomy
partial occluding clamp
partial occlusion clamp
partial pancreatectomy
partial pressure of oxygen
partial shunt
partial small bowel obstruction
partial thromboplastin (PTT)
partial thromboplastin time coagulation panel
partial thymectomy
partial transplantation
partially intrahepatic gallbladder
partially occluding vascular clamp
partially threaded pin
partially threaded rod
particle, Dane
particulate graft
Partipilo gastrostomy
partition, gastric
partitioning, gastric
Partsch chisel
Partsch gouge
parumbilical abscess
parvovirus B19, human
Pascal principle
PAS (P-aminosalicylic acid) hypothyroidism
PAS (periodic acid Schiff) stain
PAS (periodic acid Schiff) test
P.A.S. (peripheral access system)
P.A.S. Port catheter
P.A.S. Port Fluoro-Free catheter
passage
  biliary
  flatus
  hard stool
  stone
Passage catheter
passage of flatus per vagina
passage of gallstones
passage of perforated fluid
passage of stool
passage pressure
Passager introducing sheath
passive clot
passive congestion
passive congestion of stomach
passive congestive cirrhosis
passive cutaneous anaphylaxis
passive hyperemia
passive pneumonia
Passow chisel
patch
  Androderm testosterone transdermal
  bilayer
  BioGlue surgical
  Carrel
  circumferentially sutured onlay
  colic
  colonic
  Dacron
  Fluoropassiv
  fundic
  Graham
  Hemarrest
  Hemaseel HMN
  HRT (hormone replacement therapy)
  InterGard
  Kugel hernia
  Lichtenstein onlay
  Lyrelle
  mucosal
  Osteopatch
  Peyer
  pleural
  plug and
  preperitoneal
  RapiSeal
  Rutkow sutureless
  ScopeSeal endoscope
  seromuscular intestinal
  serosal
  vascularized gastric tissue
  white

patch and plug
patch-clamp
patch dressing
patch-reinforced mattress suture
patchy colonic ulceration
patchy intercellular edema
Patella disease (pyloric stenosis)
patellar clamp
patellar drill
patellar drill guide
patellar skyline view
patellar tendon graft
patency of common bile duct
patency, splenic vein
patent ductus arteriosus
patent ductus clamp
patent splenic and portal veins
Paterson-Brown-Kelly syndrome
Paterson-Kelly syndrome
Paterson rectal biopsy forceps
Patey modified radical mastectomy
Pathfinder catheter
Pathfinder irrigation device
Pathfinder microcatheter
Pathfinder mini microcatheter
Pathibamate
Pathilon (tridihexethyl chloride)
pathoanatomy
pathogenesis
pathogenic bacteria
pathogenic microorganism
pathogenic organism
  bacterium (pl. bacteria)
  fungus (pl. fungi)
  parasite (pl. parasites)
  virus (pl. viruses)
pathogenic pneumococci
pathognomic for hyperparathyroidism
pathognomonic feature
pathognomonic sign of a fistula
pathologic atrophy
pathologic diagnosis
pathologic fracture
pathologic nipple disease
pathologic reflux
pathological hypersecretory conditions
pathologist
pathology
  anatomic
  clinical
  forensic
  general
pathology report
pathophysiologic mechanism
pathophysiology
PathVysion HER-2 DNA probe kit
PATI (Penetrating Abdominal Trauma
  Index)
patient-controlled analgesia (PCA)
  pump
pattern
  abdominal wall venous
  adenoid
  airspace-filling
  airway
  alveolar
  anhaustral colonic gas
  ballerina-foot
  basket weave
  bowel gas
  branching
  breast reconstruction
  breathing
  butterfly
  cartwheel
  chromatin
  cobblestone
  cribriform
  elongate
  feathery
  fibrotic
  fleur de lis
  fold
  frondlike
  gas
  ground-glass
  haustral
  honeycomb

pattern *(cont.)*
- hourglass
- ineffective breathing
- interstitial
- irregular amputated mucosal
- juvenile
- lamellated
- layered
- lobular
- manometric
- micronodular fibrotic
- miliary
- mosaic
- mosaic duodenal mucosal
- mucosal
- mucosal guideline
- nonspecific gas
- nutmeg
- progestational
- proliferative
- railroad track
- rugal
- sawtooth
- signet ring
- speckled
- starry-sky
- stellate
- undifferentiated
- venous
- vesicular
- wax
- Wyse

Patterson trocar
patulous anus
patulous cardia
patulous hiatus
paucity of colon gas
paucity of fat
Paufique blade
Paufique knife
Paul-Miculicz resection
Paul-Mixter tube
Paulson knee retractor
Paulus plate
Pavlik bandage
Pavlov stomach
Pavulon (pancuronium bromide)
Paxene (paclitaxel)
Payne-DeWind jejunoileal bypass
Payr director
Payr forceps
Payr pyloric clamp
Pazo Hemorrhoid (ephedrine sulfate; zinc oxide)
PBC (primary biliary cirrhosis)
PBC-associated antibody
PBN catheter
PBTE (percutaneous transhepatic liver biopsy with tract embolization)
p.c. (L. *post cibum*, after meals)
PCA (prezatide copper acetate)
PCA cutting guide
PCA medullary guide
PCA (patient-controlled analgesia) pump
PCC (peripheral cholangiocarcinoma)
PCCL (percutaneous cholecysto-lithotomy)
PCI (pneumatosis cystoides intestinalis)
PCL (posterior collateral ligament) retractor
PCNA (proliferating cell nuclear antigen)
PCNL (percutaneous nephrosto-lithotomy)
pCO_2
PC Polygraf HR
PCPS (peroral cholangiopancrea-toscopy)
PCR (polymerase chain reaction)
PCS (postcholecystectomy syndrome)
PCT (porphyria cutanea tarda)
PCTCL (percutaneous transhepatic cholecystolithotomy)
PCV (parietal cell vagotomy)
PCWP (pulmonary capillary wedge pressure)
PDB (preperitoneal distention balloon)

PDB laparoscopic balloon system
PDC (peritoneal dialysis catheter)
PDS (pancreatic duct sphincter)
PDS (polydioxanone suture) pin
PDS (polydioxanone suture) II
  Endoloop suture
PDS Vicryl suture
PDT (photodynamic therapy) laser
PE (portal embolization)
peak and trough levels
PEAK channeled plate
peaked T waves
peak flow meter
peak inspiration
peak plasma concentration
peak pressure
peaks and troughs
peaks and valleys
peak secretory flow rate (PSFR)
Péan clamp
Péan forceps
peanut (small dissecting sponge)
peapod intervertebral disk forceps
peapod intervertebral disk rongeur
pearly white mass
Pease bone drill
pea soup stool
peau d'orange
PeBA C 4-mm anchor
PeBA RCR 5-mm anchor
PeBA S 2.8-mm anchor
PeBA suture anchor
PEBB (percutaneous excisional breast
  biopsy)
Peck-Joseph dissecting scissors
pectin
pectinate line
pectineal ridge
pectineus fascia
pectineus muscle
pectoral fascia
pectoral minor muscle
pectoral muscle
pectoralis fascia
pectoralis major muscle
pectoralis minor muscle
pedal edema, trace
pedal lymphangiography
Pederson vaginal speculum
Pedialyte (sodium, potassium, and
  chloride electrolytes) solution
Pedialyte RS (rehydrating solution)
  electrolyte solution
pediatric bulldog clamp
Pediatric Crohn's & Colitis
  Association, Inc.
pediatric Deaver retractor
pediatric endoscope
pediatric esophagoscope
pediatric Foley catheter
pediatric gastroscope
pediatric hernia
pediatric nasogastric feeding tube
pediatric ribbon retractor
pediatric scopes and instrumentation
pediatric vascular clamp
pediatric video optical intubation stylet
pediatric Y tube
Pedi-Boro Soak Packs (modified Burow
  solution)
pedicle
  inferior
  long splenic
  muscle
  omental
  vascular
  vertical
pedicle bone graft
pedicle clamp
pedicle graft
pedicle hook
pedicle plate
pedicle probe
pedicle technique reduction mammoplasty
pedicular rod
Pedi PEG tube
PediPort trocar

PedTE-Pak-4 (multiple trace elements)
Pedtrace-4 (multiple trace elements)
pedunculated mass of polyp
pedunculated papule
pedunculated polyp
pedunculation
peel-away introducer
PEEP (positive end-expiratory pressure)
Peers towel forceps
Peet splinter forceps
PEG (percutaneous endoscopic gastrostomy)
  PEG balloon
  PEG catheter
  PEG tube
PEG (polyethylene glycol)
  PEG-interferon alfa-2a
  PEG-interferon alfa-2b
  PEG-Intron (PEG-interferon alfa-2b)
  PEG-Intron A (interferon alfa-2b in polyethylene glycol carrier)
  PEG lavage
  PEG molecule
Pegasus Nd:YAG surgical laser
Pegasys (PEG-interferon alfa-2a)
peg-base plate
peg graft
pegvisomant
pegylated interferon
pegylated protein
pegylation
Peiper-Beyer laminectomy rongeur
PEJ (percutaneous endoscopic jejunostomy)
peliosis hepatis
pellegra skin changes
pelleted stools
pellet, radiopaque
Pelosi Illuminator device
Pelosi manipulator set
pelvic abscess
pelvic adhesion
pelvic brim
pelvic colon
pelvic exenteration
pelvic floor dysfunction
pelvic floor electromyography
pelvic floor function study
pelvic hematoma
pelvic infection
pelvic inflammatory disease (PID)
pelvic kidney
pelvic lymph node
pelvic peritoneum
pelvic plexus
pelvic sidewall
pelvimeter, Martin
pelvirectal abscess
pelvirectal achalasia
pelviscopy instrumentation
PEM (protein-energy malnutrition)
Pemberton sigmoid clamp
Pemberton spur-crushing clamp
pen
  Disetronic Insulin Pen
  Eckhoff mapping
  Humulin Pen
  Humulin R Pen
  Humalog Pen
  mapping
  Nibs mapping
  Novolin Pen
  Securline skin-marking
  Skin-Scribe skin-marking
pencil
  cautery
  electrocautery
  electrosurgical
pencil-like stool
PenduLaser 115 surgical laser system
pendulous pouch
penetrating abdominal trauma
Penetrating Abdominal Trauma Index (PATI)
penetrating atherosclerotic aortic ulcer
penetrating drill
penetrating injury

penetrating injury through the platysma
penetrating stab injury
penetrating trauma
penetrating ulcer
penetrating wound
Penfield dissector
Penfield elevator
Penfield retractor
Penfine needle
Penn fingernail drill
Pennington clamp
Pennington grasping forceps
Pennington rectal speculum
Pennington tissue forceps
Penn pouch for continent urinary diversion
Penn umbilical scissors
Penn wire-cutting scissors
Penrose drain
Penrose seton
pentagastrin gastric secretory test
pentagastrin infusion test
pentagastrin provocative test
pentagastrin-stimulated analysis test
pentagastrin-stimulated calcitonin concentration
pentagastrin stimulation
pentagastrin test
pentamidine-induced pancreatitis
Pentasa (mesalamine)
Pentax ECN-1530 choledochonephroscope
Pentax EC videoendoscope
Pentax EC-3430F videocolonoscope
Pentax EC-3430L videocolonoscope
Pentax EC-3440F videocolonoscope
Pentax EC-3440L videocolonoscope
Pentax EC-3830 videocolonoscope
Pentax EC-3830L videocolonoscope
Pentax EC-3830TL video colonoscope
Pentax EC-3840L videocolonoscope
Pentax EC-3840T videocolonoscope
Pentax ED-3430T videoduodenoscope
Pentax ED-3440T videoduodenoscope
Pentax EG videoendoscope
Pentax EG-1840 videogastroscope
Pentax EG-2530 gastroscope
Pentax EG-2540 videogastroscope
Pentax EG-2731 gastroscope
Pentax EG-2901 flexible gastroscope
Pentax EG-2930 gastroscope
Pentax EG-2940 videogastroscope
Pentax EG-3430 videogastroscope
Pentax EG-3440 videogastroscope
Pentax EG-3830T videogastroscope
Pentax EG-3840T videogastroscope
Pentax EndoNet endoscope
Pentax endoscopic camera
Pentax ES-3830 videosigmoidoscope
Pentax ES-3840 videosigmoidoscope
Pentax EUP-EC124 ultrasound gastroscope
Pentax FC endoscope
Pentax FC-38LV fiberoptic colonoscope
Pentax FC-38LX flexible colonoscope
Pentax FC-38LX flexible gastroscope
Pentax FC-38MV fiberoptic colonoscope
Pentax FCN-15H flexible choledochoscope
Pentax FD-32A side-viewing endoscope
Pentax FD-34V fiberoptic duodenoscope
Pentax FG-24V fiberoptic gastroscope
Pentax FG-29H flexible gastroscope
Pentax FG-29V fiberoptic gastroscope
Pentax FG-29X flexible gastroscope
Pentax FG-36UX echoendoscope
Pentax fiberoptic sigmoidoscope
Pentax flexible sigmoidoscope
Pentax FS-34A flexible sigmoidoscope
Pentax FS-34V fiberoptic sigmoidoscope
Pentax FS-38H flexible sigmoidoscope
Pentax-Hitachi FG32UA endosonographic system
Pentax side-viewing endoscope

Pentax SIG-E2 fiberoptic sigmoidoscope
Pentax videoendoscope
Pentax VSB-P2900 pediatric colonoscope
Pentax W fiberoptic endoscope
Pepcid AC (famotidine)
Pepcid RPD (famotidine)
PEPCK (phosphoenolpyruvate
carboxykinase) deficiency
Pepgen test
peppermint oil
pepsin
pepsinogen
Peptamen liquid diet
Peptavlon (pentagastrin)
peptic cell
peptic esophagitis
peptic stricture
peptic ulcer
peptic ulcer disease (PUD)
peptic ulceration
peptid bond hydrolysis
peptide bonds
peptide hormone
peptide, regulatory
Pepto-Bismol (bismuth subsalicylate)
Pepto Diarrhea Control (loperamide)
per anum intersphincteric rectal dissection and coloanal anastomosis
per os (p.o.)
per primam healing
per rectum
Perative formula
Perception 5000 PC-based ultrasound
scanner
Percival gastric balloon
Perclose suture device
Percor DL-II (dual-lumen) intra-aortic
balloon
Percor-Stat intra-aortic balloon
PercScope percutaneous diskectomy
endoscope
PercuCut cut-biopsy needle
Percuflex Plus biliary stent
PercuGuide
PercuPump disposable syringe and
injector
percussion hammer
percussion note
percussion tenderness
percutaneous ablation
percutaneous abscess and fluid drainage
(PAFD)
percutaneous access kit (PAK)
percutaneous appendectomy
percutaneous aspiration
percutaneous aspiration and drainage
percutaneous autogenous dowel bone
graft
percutaneous balloon dilation
percutaneous biopsy
percutaneous catheter
percutaneous catheter cecostomy
percutaneous catheterization (of the
portal vein)
percutaneous celiac nerve block
percutaneous cholecystolithotomy
(PCCL)
percutaneous cholecystostomy
percutaneous choledochoscopy
percutaneous closed-catheter drain
percutaneous cutting needle
percutaneous deflation of cecum
percutaneous deflation of sigmoid loop
percutaneous drain placement
percutaneous drainage
percutaneous drainage catheter
percutaneous drainage with CT
guidance
percutaneous drainage with ultrasound
guidance
percutaneous endoscopic gastrostomy
(PEG) tube
percutaneous endoscopic jejunostomy
(PEJ)
percutaneous ethanol injection (PEI)
percutaneous ethanol tumor injection

percutaneous excisional breast biopsy (PEBB)
percutaneous fibrin glue
percutaneous fine-needle biopsy
percutaneous gastroenterostomy (PGE)
percutaneous gastrostomy (PG) tube
percutaneous hepatic vein angioplasty (PHVA)
percutaneous jejunostomy tube
percutaneous lead introducer
percutaneous liver biopsy
percutaneous needle muscle biopsy
percutaneous nephrostolithotomy (PCNL)
percutaneous pin
percutaneous resection
percutaneous stent
percutaneous stone dissolution
percutaneous transfemoral dilatation
percutaneous transhepatic catheterization
percutaneous transhepatic biliary drainage (PTBD) catheter
percutaneous transhepatic cholangiogram (PTC)
percutaneous transhepatic cholangiography (PTC)
percutaneous transhepatic cholangioscopy (PTCS) tube stenting
percutaneous transhepatic cholangioscopy and lithotripsy for complicated hepatolithiasis
percutaneous transhepatic cholangioscopy tube stenting through a mature T-tube tract
percutaneous transhepatic cholecystolithotomy (PCTCL)
percutaneous transhepatic choledochoscopic electrohydraulic lithotripsy (PTCS-EHL) of common bile duct stones
percutaneous transhepatic decompression
percutaneous transhepatic liver biopsy with tract embolization (PTBE)
percutaneous transhepatic obliteration
percutaneous transhepatic pigtail catheter
Percy amputating saw
Percy amputation retractor
Percy intestinal forceps
Percy-Wolfson gallbladder retractor
perendoscopic biopsy specimen
Pereyra improved ligature cannula
PerFix Marlex mesh plug
PerFix plug and patch repair
PerFix Plus Plug polypropylene mesh
perflenapent
Perflex stainless steel stent and delivery system
perflisopent
perflubron
perflutren
perforate
perforated acid peptic ulcer
perforated acute appendicitis
perforated appendicitis
perforated appendix
perforated carcinoma
perforated cholecystitis
perforated colon
perforated gallbladder
perforated, Smillie
perforated ulcer
perforated viscus
perforating abscess
perforating aneurysm
perforating forceps
perforating injuries
perforating twist drill
perforating ulcer
perforating vessel
perforating wound
perforation
  bowel
  closure of
  colonic

perforation *(cont.)*
  duodenal
  endoscopic intraperitoneal
  extraperitoneal
  frank
  free
  gallbladder
  gastric
  gastrointestinal
  GI tract
  intestinal
  small bowel
  stomach
  subacute
  traumatic
  ulcer
  uterine
  vesiculocolic
perforation of bowel
perforation of diverticulum
perforation of stomach
perforator
perfusion
  altered tissue
  inadequate
  intraperitoneal hyperthermic (IPHP)
  peripheral
  portal venous liver
  remote access (RAP)
perfusion cannula
perfusion defect
periadrenal tissue
periampullary carcinoma
periampullary neoplasm
periampullary region
periampullary tumor
perianal abscess
perianal Bowen disease
perianal condyloma
perianal drainage
perianal hematoma
perianal hygiene
perianal reflex
perianal region
perianal skin
perianal skin tag
perianal soak
perianal wart
periaortic node
periappendiceal abscess
periappendiceal fluid
periappendiceal gas
periareolar augmentation mammoplasty
periareolar incision
pericardial effusion
pericardial effusion fluid
pericardial fluid
pericardial sac
pericardiocentesis
pericardiocentesis needle
pericardiophrenic artery
pericarditis
pericecal abscess
pericholangiolitic biliary cirrhosis
pericholangitis
pericholecystic abscess
pericholecystic adhesion
pericholecystic collection
pericholecystic edema
pericholecystic fluid
pericholedochal lymph node
perichondritis, auricular
Peri-Colace (casanthranol; docusate sodium)
pericolic abscess
pericolic membrane syndrome
pericolic phlegmon
pericolitis
pericolonic abscess
pericolonic fat
pericolostomy area
pericoronal tissues
pericostal suture
peridiverticular tissue
Peri-Dos (casanthranol; docusate sodium)
periductal fibrosis
peridural anesthesia

periesophageal abscess
periesophageal inflammation
Periflow peripheral balloon catheter
perihepatic abscess
perihepatic packing
perihepatic peritoneum
perihepatitis (Fitz-Hugh–Curtis syndrome)
perihepatitis, gonococcal
perihepatitis syndrome
peri-ileal periampullary duodenal tumor
perilobar pancreatitis
perilobular duct
perimolysis
perimylolysis
perineal descent
perineal ecchymosis
perineal nerve terminal motor latency
perineal rectosigmoidectomy
perineal sinus
perineovaginal fistula
perinephric tissue
perineural anesthesia
periodic abdominalgia
periodic acid Schiff (PAS) test
periodic familial peritonitis
periodic liver biopsy
periodic peritonitis syndrome
periodic vomiting
periodontal anesthesia
periodontal mucosal grafting
PerioGlas bone graft material graft
PerioLase laser
perioperative antibiotic
perioperative muscle strength
perioperative steroid replacement
perioperative vomiting
perioral numbness
perioral tingling
periorbital edema
periosteal elevator
periosteal release double-edge knife
periosteal sarcoma
peripancreatic area
peripancreatic drain
peripancreatic space
peripancreatic tumor
periperitoneal fat stripe
peripheral alimentation
peripheral autonomic neuropathy
peripheral blood
peripheral blood smear
peripheral cyanosis
peripheral edema
peripheral embolism
peripheral hepatic necrosis
peripheral intravenous access
peripheral intravenous alimentation
peripheral lesion
peripheral necrosis
peripheral neurologic disorder
peripheral neuropathy
peripheral perfusion
peripheral smear
peripheral wasting
periportal area
periportal cirrhosis
periportal fibrosis of liver
periportal hepatocyte
periportal sinusoidal dilatation
periprosthetic capsulectomy, breast
perirectal abscess
perirectal cellulitis
perirectal injection
perirectal lymph node
perirectal pain
perirenal tissue
perisigmoid colon
perisinusoidal fibrosis
perisinusoidal space
peristalsis
  absent
  decreased
  equivocal primary
  gastrointestinal
  impaired esophageal
  visible
peristaltic activity

peristaltic contraction
peristaltic dysfunction
peristaltic reflex
peristaltic rush
peristaltic wave
peristomal area
peristomal skin
Peri-Strips Dry surgical staple-line reinforcement
Peri-Strips Dry wound sealant
peritoneal adhesion
peritoneal abscess
peritoneal-atrial shunt
peritoneal attachment
peritoneal band
peritoneal biopsy needle
peritoneal catheter
peritoneal cavity
peritoneal contamination from bowel perforation
peritoneal cytology
peritoneal dialysis
peritoneal dialysis catheter (PDC)
peritoneal drain
peritoneal edge
peritoneal effusion
peritoneal effusion fluid
peritoneal exudation
peritoneal flap
peritoneal fluid
peritoneal fold
peritoneal friction rub
peritoneal hernia
peritoneal implant
peritoneal irritation
peritonealization
peritonealize
peritoneal lavage
peritoneal metastasis
peritoneal mouse
peritoneal reflection
peritoneal rupture
peritoneal sac
peritoneal scarring
peritoneal seeding
peritoneal sign
peritoneal soilage
peritoneal soiling
peritoneal space
peritoneal studding
peritoneal tap
peritoneal toilet
peritoneal traverse by missile
peritoneal trocar
peritoneal-venous shunt (PVS)
peritoneal washings
peritoneocaval shunt
peritoneocentesis
peritoneography
peritoneointestinal reflex
peritoneoscope
peritoneoscopy
peritoneovenous shunt (PVS)
peritoneum
  abdominal
  parietal
  pelvic
  perihepatic
  posterior parietal
  visceral
peritoneum identified with hemostats
peritoneum was reapproximated
peritonism
peritonitis
  bacterial
  benign paroxysmal
  bile
  biliary
  chemical
  chronic proliferative
  diffuse
  exudative
  fecal
  full-blown bacterial
  generalized
  gonococcal
  periodic familial
  pneumococcal

peritonitis *(cont.)*
  primary
  proliferative
  puerperal
  sclerosing encapsulated
  spontaneous
  spontaneous bacterial (SBP)
  starch
  subacute nonspecific
  suppurative
  syphilitic
  tuberculous
peritonize
periumbilical abscess
periumbilical lymph node
periumbilical mass
periumbilical region
periumbilical vein engorgement
perivascular goiter
perivenular fibrosis
perivenular or pericellular fibrosis
Perkins left retractor
Perkins otologic retractor
Perkins right retractor
PermaClip endoscopic clip applier
Perma-Flow coronary bypass graft
Perma-Hand braided silk suture
Perma-Hand silk suture
Perma-Hand suture
PermaMesh graft
PermaMesh suture
Perman cartilage forceps
permanent colostomy
permanent end colostomy
permanent hypoparathyroidism
permanent lead introducer
permanent loop ileostomy
permanent section
permanent stoma
permanent tracheostomy
Perma-Seal dialysis access graft
PermCath double-lumen ventricular access catheter
permeability, intestinal
Perneczky aneurysm clamp
pernicious anemia
pernicious malaria
pernicious vomiting of pregnancy
peroneus brevis graft
peroral bougienage
peroxidase oxidation of iodide
peroxidase stain
peroxisome
Perras breast prosthesis
Perras-Papillon breast prosthesis
Perry ileostomy bag
PerryMeter anal EMG sensor
persistence, viral
persistent acidosis
persistent bacteremia
persistent breast abnormality
persistent hyperparathyroidism
persistent loop of distended small bowel
persistent mass after aspiration
persistent nipple discharge
persistent oligoanuria
persistent pylorospasm
persistent viral hepatitis (PVH)
persistent viral hepatitis C (PVH-C)
persistent viral hepatitis non-A, non B (PVH-NAB)
persistently raised E2-antimitochondrial antibody (AMA)
persisting fibrosis and nodule formation
personality changes
Perthes reamer
Peruvian balsam
pes cavus
pes planum
pessary, vaginal
pesticide, hepatocarcinogenic
PET (positron emission tomography)
PET balloon
petechia (pl. petechiae)
petechial angioma
petelin dissector
Petit hernia
Petit triangle

petrobasilar suture
petrosal ACTH
petrosphenobasilar suture
petrospheno-occipital suture
petrosquamous suture
Pettenkofer test
Petz clamp
Peutz-Jeghers gastrointestinal polyposis
Peutz-Jeghers polyp
Peutz-Jeghers syndrome (PJS)
Peutz-Jeghers syndrome of familial
  gastrointestinal polyposis
Peutz-Touraine syndrome
pexiganan acetate
Peyer gland
Peyer patch
Pezzer catheter
Pezzer drain
Pfannenstiel incision
p53 adenoviral gene
p53 mutation
p53 protein overexpression
PFGE (pulsed-field gel electrophoresis)
PFR95 filter
PFTE (polyfluorotetraethylene) graft
PG (paregoric)
PG (percutaneous gastrostomy)
PGA synthetic absorbable suture
PGA II (polyglandular autoimmune
  syndrome, type 2)
PGC (proximal gastric vagotomy)
PGE (percutaneous gastroenterostomy)
PGG glucan
PGP nail
PgR (progesterone receptor)
PG-TXL (polyglutamic acid paclitaxel)
PGV (proximal gastric vagotomy)
pH probe
  esophageal
  intraesophageal
phagocytic stellate cell
phagocytosis
Phalen position
Phaneuf artery forceps
phantom breast pain
phantom breast sensation
Phantom 5 Plus balloon catheter
phantom rectal pain
pharyngeal flap
pharmacomechanical coupling
pharmacotherapy
Pharmasealt tray
pharyngeal constrictor muscle
pharyngeal manometry
pharyngeal musculature
pharyngeal orifice
pharyngeal pouch
pharyngeal pouch syndrome
pharyngeal swallow reflex
pharyngoconjunctival fever virus
pharyngoesophageal function
pharyngoesophageal repair
pharyngoesophageal segment
pharyngoesophageal sphincter
pharyngogastrostomy
pharyngoglottal adduction reflex
pharyngoscope
pharyngostomy (fistulization of
  pharynx)
pharyngo-UES (upper esophageal
  sphincter) contractile reflex
pharynx
phase
  convalescent, of hepatitis
  gastric, of acid secretion
  icteric, of hepatitis
  intestinal, of acid secretion
  intradeglutitive, of swallowing
  postdeglutitive, of swallowing
  posticteric, of hepatitis
  preicteric
  venous
phase-contrast microscope
phasic contractions
Phazyme (simethicone)
Phemister elevator
Phemister onlay bone graft
Phemister rasp

Phenergan Fortis (promethazine HCl)
phenobarbital
Phenolax (phenolphthalein)
phenolphthalein
phenoltetrachlorophthalein test
phenomenon
  common cavity
  dawn
  Jod-Basedow
  mask
  satellite
  yo-yo weight fluctuation
phenoxybenzamine therapy
phentermine
phenylbutazone-induced hypothyroidism
phenylethanolamine-N-methyltransferase
pheochromocytoma
  bladder
  disseminated
  extra-adrenal
  malignant
  remote
PHG (portal hypertensive gastropathy)
Phillips LaxCaps
Phillips' Milk of Magnesia (magnesium hydroxide)
Phillips' M-O
pHisoHex scrub
phlebitis of thoracoepigastric vein
phlegmon formation
phlegmonous change
phlegmonous colitis
phlegmonous gastritis
phlegmonous mass
phlegmon, subhepatic
Phoenix cranial drill
Phoenix ventriculostomy catheter
phosphasoda cathartic
phosphate-binding antacid
phosphate buffered saline
phosphate depletion
phosphate enema
phosphatidyl choline (PC)
phosphoenolpyruvate carboxykinase (PEPCK) deficiency
phospholipase A
phospholipid, serum
phospholipid signal pathway
phosphoric acid
phosphorus necrosis
phosphorylase deficiency glycogen storage disease
phosphorylase, liver
phosphosoda enema
photocoagulation
  hemorrhoid
  infrared
  laser
photodynamic therapy (PDT)
photodynamic therapy, Foscan (temoporfin, mTHPC)
Photofrin (porfimer)
photometer, reflectant spectral
photon-deficient lesion
Photon Radiosurgery System (PRS)
photon scan
PhotoPoint laser
PhotoPoint light-activated technique
photosensitivity
photosensitizer
photothermal laser ablation of Barrett esophagus
phrenicocolic ligament
phrenicoesophageal ligament
phrenoesophageal ligament
phrenoesophageal membrane
phrenofundal reflection
phrenogastric ligament
phrygian cap deformity
physic (noun)
physical diagnosis
Physick pouch
physiograph for esophageal manometry
physiological gut-loop herniation
physiological irrigating solution
physiologic dead space

physiologic jaundice
physiologic reflux test (PRT)
physiological irrigating solution
phytobezoar
pica
PIC (peripherally inserted) catheter
PICC (peripherally inserted central catheter)
Piccolo blood analyzer
Pichinde virus
Pick cell
Pick chisel
picket fence guide
pickup
  DeBakey
  rat-tooth
pickup forceps
picornavirus
Pico-ST II catheter
Pidcock check pin
Pidcock nail
piecemeal necrosis
piecemeal swallowing
Pierse micro dissecting forceps
Pierse tip forceps
Piezolith-EPL (extracorporeal piezo-electric lithotriptor)
pigeon-breeder's lung
piggybacking of I.V.
pigmentary cirrhosis
pigment cirrhosis
pigmented gallstone
pigmented liver
pigmented satellite lesion
pigment stone
pigskin graft
pigtail catheter
pigtail connector
pigtail stent
pile, sentinel
piles (hemorrhoids)
Piliel gel (hair regrowth) dressing
pill esophagitis
Pilling-Liston rongeur
Pilling rigid laparoscope
Pilling Weck Surgical
Pilling Weck Y-stent forceps
Pillo Pro dressing
pillow sign
pilonidal abscess
pilonidal cyst
pilonidal disease
pilonidal fistula
pilonidal sinus
Pilot drill
Pilot suture
Pilot suturing guide
pimagedine HCl
pin
  absorbable
  absorbable polyparadioxanone
  Acufex distractor
  alignment
  Allofix freeze-dried cortical bone
  Austin Moore
  ball guide
  ball-point guide
  ball-tip guide
  beaded hip
  beaded reamer guide
  Beath
  Bilos
  biodegradable
  Biofix system
  Böhler (Boehler)
  Bohlman
  breakaway
  Breck
  calcaneal
  calibrated
  Canakis
  Charnley
  clavicle
  closed
  collapsible
  Compere threaded
  Compton clavicle
  Conley

pin *(cont.)*
Crego-McCarroll
cross
Crowe pilot point on Steinmann
Davis
Day
Denham
DePuy
Dcycrle II
distractor
drawing
drill
Ender
Fahey-Compere
femoral guide
Fischer transfixing
Fisher half
fixation
Gardner skull clamp
Gingrass and Messer
Gouffon hip
guide
Hagie
half
halo
Hansen-Street
Hare
Hatcher
Haynes
Hessel-Nystrom
hip
hook
hook-end intramedullary
hydroxyapatite-coated
in situ
Intraflex intramedullary
intramedullary
Jones compression
Knowles
Krankendonk
Küntscher (Kuentscher)
LIH (Lars Ingvar Hansson) hook
locating
Lottes

pin *(cont.)*
marble bone
Mayfield skull clamp
Mayo sterilizing
McBride
metallic
Modny
Moore
Olds
open
Oris
OrthoSorb absorbable fixation
partially threaded
PDS (poly-p-dioxanone)
percutaneous
Pidcock check
poly-p-dioxanone (PDS)
polyparadioxanone, absorbable
precurved ball-tipped guide
Pritchard Mark II
rasp
resorbable
Rhinelander
Riordan
Roger Anderson
Rush
Schanz
Schneider
Schweitzer
self-broaching
Serrato forearm
Shriner
skeletal traction
skull
Smith-Petersen
smooth Steinmann
socket
Sofield
Stader
Steinmann
Street medullary
strut-type
tapered
threaded

pin *(cont.)*
  threaded Steinmann
  tibial drill
  titanium half
  traction
  transarticular
  transfixing
  transfixion
  Turner
  Tutofix cortical
  Varney
  Venable-Stuck
  Vom Saal
  Wagner closed
  wrench
  Zimmer
pinch-band forceps
pinchcock effect
pinchcock mechanism at esophago-gastric junction
pinch forceps
pin clamp
pin cutter
PI90 double-headed stapler
Pink Bismuth (bismuth subsalicylate)
pinked up (verb)
Pinn.ACL guide
pinpoint gastric mucosal defect bleeding
PinPoint stereotactic arm
pinpoint suction
pin-retained palatal prosthesis
pin retractor
Pin-Rid (pyrantel pamoate)
Pinto Cobra, The
Pinto loop underminer
pinworm (*Enterobius vermicularis*)
Pin-X (pyrantel pamoate)
pioglitazone hydrochloride
PIP (pressure inversion point) on esophageal manometry
pipe, food
pipestem cirrhosis
pipestem stool
Pipelle endometrial suction catheter
Piper obstetrical forceps
piperamide maleate
piperazine, piperazine calcium edetate, piperazine edetate calcium
PIPIDA scan
pi plate
pirenzepine HCl
piriform fossa
piriform sinus
piritrexim
piroglíride, piroglíride tartrate
PI surgical stapler
pit
  anal
  colonic
  gastric
  postanal
pitch worker's cancer
pitchfork retractor
Pitkin spinal needle
pit of stomach
Pitressin Synthetic (vasopressin)
pitting edema
Pittman IMA retractor
pituitary adenoma
pituitary cachexia
pituitary Cushing syndrome
pituitary dwarfism
pituitary enlargement
pituitary forceps
pituitary gland
pituitary hyperfunction
pituitary hypersecretion
pituitary insufficiency
pituitary irradiation
pituitary knife
pituitary mass
pituitary rongeur
pituitary scissors
pituitary secretion
pituitary suppression
pituitary tumor

pituitary tumor syndrome (acromegaly, galactorrhea, Cushing syndrome)
Pivanex
PIVKA-II levels
Pivotal coagulator
Pivotal dissector
Pivotal grasper
Pivotal scissors
Pixie fiberoptic scope
PiZZ $alpha_1$ antitrypsin deficiency
PJS (Peutz-Jeghers syndrome)
placement of intraperitoneal drain
placement of silastic ring band
placement, trocar
placental polyp
plain catgut suture
plain film of abdomen
plain gut
plain gut suture
plain pattern plate
plain splinter forceps
plain suture
plain tissue forceps
plain view
planar plate
planar view
plane (pl. planes)
  axial
  biparietal
  coronal
  fascial
  fat
  horizontal
  ischiorectal fossa
  pelvic
  sagittal
  subcostal
  subfascial
  supracrestal
  transumbilical
  transverse
  umbilical
  vertical
planing brush
planned pancreaticoduodenectomy
plantar axial view
plantar plate
plantar puncture wound
plantar flexion stress view
planus, lichen
plaquelike linear defect
Plasbumin-25 (human albumin)
plasma aldosterone
plasma assay coagulation panel
plasma basal and stimulated (with pentagastrin or calcium) calcitonin measurements
plasma carbon dioxide
plasma cell dyscrasia
plasma cell hepatitis
plasma cell mastitis
plasma clotting time
plasma coagulation time
plasma concentration
plasma electrolytes
plasma Endotoxin concentration
plasma expander
plasma, fresh frozen (FFP)
plasma gastrin level
plasma glucose level
plasma lipotropic hormone (LPH, lipotropin) concentration
Plasma-Lyte A pH 7.4
Plasma-Lyte 148 (combined electrolyte solution)
Plasmanate (plasma protein fraction)
plasma pH
plasmapheresis
Plasma-Plex (plasma protein fraction)
plasma pool
plasma protein fraction
plasma renin activity
Plasma Scalpel
Plasmatein (plasma protein fraction)
plasma total cortisol

plasma volume expander (see also *medications*)
  dextran 40 (10% LMD)
  dextran 40 (Rheomacrodex)
  Hespan (hetastarch)
  Hextend
  Rheomacrodex (dextran 40)
  10% LMD (dextran 40)
Plasmodium falciparum
Plasmodium malariae
plaster cast instruments
plaster knife
plaster of Paris (POP) bandage
plaster saw
plaster scissors
plaster shears
plastic clot
plastic drape
plastic nasopharyngeal airway
plastic-sheathed malleable aluminum stylet
plastic suture
plate
  acetabular reconstruction
  AcroMed VSP
  Aesculap ABC cervical
  alar
  anal
  anchor
  AO blade
  AO condylar blade
  AO contoured T
  AO hook
  AOI blade
  AO reconstruction
  AO semitubular
  AO small fragment
  Armstrong
  ASIF right-angle blade
  axial
  Badgley
  Bagby angled compression
  basal
  Batchelor

plate *(cont.)*
  biodegradable
  blade
  Blount blade
  bone
  bone flap fixation
  bony
  Bosworth spine
  Burns
  buttress
  Calandruccio side
  cap-and-anchor
  cartilaginous growth
  CASP (contoured anterior spinal)
  Caspar cervical
  cervical locking
  cloverleaf
  coaptation
  cobra-head
  Collison
  compression
  condylar
  conical tectal
  connecting
  Continuum total knee base
  contoured T-plate
  cortical
  cranial bone fixation
  cribriform
  C-shaped
  DCP (dynamic compression)
  deck
  DePuy
  Deyerle
  dorsal
  double-H
  Driessen hinged
  dual
  Duopress
  Dwyer-Hall
  dynamic compression (DCP)
  eccentric dynamic compression (EDCP)
  Eggers bone

plate *(cont.)*
- 11-hole
- Elliott femoral condyle blade
- end
- epiphyseal cartilage
- ethmovomerine
- E-Z Flap cranial bone
- femoral
- fibrocartilaginous
- fiducial
- five-hole (5-hole)
- fixed-angle blade
- flat
- flexor palmar
- foot
- Forte distal radius
- four-hole (4-hole)
- frontal
- fusion
- gait
- Gallannaugh bone
- growth
- Hagie sliding nail
- Haid cervical
- half-circle
- Hansen-Street
- Harlow
- Harm posterior cervical
- Harris
- heavy-duty femur
- heavy side
- Hicks lugged
- hilar
- Hoen skull
- Holt nail
- Howmedica Microfixation cranial
- H-shaped
- Hubbard
- interfragmentary
- intertrochanteric
- I plate of Yuan
- Jergesen I-beam
- Jergesen tapered
- Jewett nail overlay

plate *(cont.)*
- Jones compression
- Kaneda
- Kessel
- Laing
- Lane
- Lawson-Thornton
- LC-DCP
- Leibinger Micro Plus
- Leibinger Micro System cranial fixation
- Leibinger 3-D
- Letournel
- limiting
- liver cell
- localization-compression grid
- Lorenz cranial
- Louis
- low contact dynamic compression (LC-DCP)
- L-shaped
- Luhr micro
- Luhr Microfixation cranial
- Luhr mini
- Luhr pan
- Lundholm
- Luque-Galveston
- Luque II
- malleable
- Massie
- McBride
- McLaughlin intertrochanteric
- Mears sacroiliac
- Medoff sliding
- meningioma of the cribriform
- Meurig Williams
- micro
- microfixation
- Milch
- mini
- minifragment
- Moe intertrochanteric
- Moore sliding nail
- Moreira

plate *(cont.)*
Morscher cervical
Müller (Mueller) compression blade
nail
Neufeld
neutralization
Newman
Nicoll
occipitocervical
Ogden
orbital
Orozco cervical
orthotic
Osborne
overlay
palmar
Paulus
PEAK channeled
pedicle
peg-base
pi
plain pattern
planar
plantar
pterygoid
Pugh
pylon attachment
quadrangular positioning
quadrigeminal
reconstruction
resorbable
Richards-Hirschhorn
Richards side
roof
Rotator Cuff Buttress (RCB)
Roy-Camille cervical
Roy-Camille occipitocervical
Roy-Camille pedicle
Schweitzer spring
semitubular compression
Senn
serpentine
seven-hole (7-hole)
17-hole

plate *(cont.)*
Sherman bone
side
Simmons
six-hole (6-hole)
skull
slide
slotted femur
Smith-Petersen
Smith-Petersen intertrochanteric
SMO (supramalleolar orthosis)
spoon
stabilization
stainless steel
stainless steel preformed skull
steel sole
Steffee
Steffee pedicle
Steffee screw
stem base
Storz Microsystems cranial fixation
subchondral bone
supracondylar
Synthes cervical
Synthes dorsal distal radius
Synthes Microsystems cranial fixation
Synthes mini L-plate
Syracuse I
T
tantalum preformed skull
tarsal
T buttress
tectal
Temple University
tendon
Thornton nail
3-D (three-dimensional)
three-hole (3-hole)
titanium
toe
Townley tibial plateau
Townsend-Gilfillan
trial base

plate *(cont.)*
  T-shaped
  T-shaped AO
  tubular
  Tupman
  twisted
  two-hole (2-hole)
  UCP compression
  Uslenghi
  V blade
  Venable
  vertebral body
  Vitallium
  V nail
  volar
  VSP (variable screw placement)
  Wainwright
  Wenger
  Whitman
  Wilson
  wing
  Wright
  Wurzburg
  X-shaped
  Y bone
  Y-shaped
  Zimmer femoral condyle blade
  Zimmer side
  Zimmer Y
  Z-shaped
  Zuelzer hook
plate driver
plate-holding forceps
platelet activating factor (PAF)
platelet-activating factor acetylhydrolase, recombinant (rPAF-AH)
platelet activity
platelet count
platelet count coagulation panel
platelet-derived growth factor
platelet dysfunction
platelet plug
platelet-poor blood (PPB)
platelet storage
platelet trapping
platysma
PLE (protein-losing enteropathy)
pleating of small bowel
Pleatman sac
pledget dressing
pledgeted Ethibond suture
pledgeted mattress suture
pledget, Oxycel
Plenk-Matson rasp
pleomorphic destructive cholangitis
Plester self-retaining retractor
Plester suction tube
pleural biopsy needle
pleural effusion
pleural fluid
pleural metastasis
pleural patch
pleural space
pleural space flow of fluid
pleural tube
Pleur-evac suction tube
pleuritic chest pain
pleuropericardial effusion
pleuroperitoneal canal
pleuroperitoneal membrane
pleuropneumonia-like (PPLO) organism
plexus
  abdominal aortic
  Auerbach mesenteric
  biliary
  brachial
  choroid
  colic
  colonic myenteric
  cystic
  esophageal
  gastric
  gastroesophageal variceal
  hemorrhoidal
  hepatic
  ileocolic
  muscularis

plexus *(cont.)*
- myenteric
- nerve
- pampiniform
- pelvic
- prostatic venous
- rectal
- submucosal venous
- testicular pampiniform venous
- venous

pliable stent
plica (pl. plicae)
plicae circulares
plicae gastropancreaticae
plicate, plicated
plicating
plication
- Childs-Phillips bowel
- fundal
- intestinal
- Noble bowel
- Rehne-Delorme
- suture
- transgastric
- transmesenteric

plication of bowel
plication of fascia
plication of mesentery (mesenteropexy)
plication suture
pliers
- Compaction
- double-action wire-extraction
- flat-nose
- Howmedica Microfixation System
- Leibinger Micro System
- locking
- Luhr Microfixation System
- mesh
- needle-nose
- needle-nose locking
- pair of
- polypropylene mesh
- PowerGrip
- slip joint

pliers *(cont.)*
- Storz Microsystems
- Synthes Microsystems
- taper-nose
- wire-cutting

plug
- bile
- bone
- decannulation
- Gilbert free-formed umbrella-shaped
- Herniamesh surgical mesh
- Marlex PerFix
- meconium
- mucus
- patch and
- PerFix Marlex mesh
- platelet
- R-Med
- Rutkow sutureless plug and patch
- sutureless

plug effect of connector
plug and patch
plug-and-patch hernia repair
plugged liver biopsy
plug of tissue
Plum drug delivery pump
plume
- laser
- smoke

Plummer disease
Plummer esophageal dilator
Plummer-Vinson syndrome
plunging goiter
Plus Reusable Silicone Resuscitator
PMC (pseudomembranous colitis)
PMMA (polymethylmethacrylate) rod
PMN (polymorphonuclear leukocyte)
PMT biopsy needle
pneumatic bag
pneumatic bag esophageal dilatation
pneumatic balloon catheter dilation
pneumatic balloon dilator
pneumatic compression boot
pneumatic drill

pneumatosis coli
pneumatosis cystoides intestinalis (PCI)
pneumatosis intestinalis
pneumatosis of the bowel
pneumaturia
pneumobilia
pneumococcal peritonitis
pneumococcus vaccine
pneumocolon
Pneumocystis carinii (PCP)
pneumogastric
pneumogastrography
pneumoinsufflation needle
Pneumo-Needle reusable instrument
pneumonia
pneumoperitoneum, carbon dioxide
pneumoperitoneum needle
pneumoscrotum, ipsilateral
Pneumo Sleeve laparoscopic airlock
pneumothorax
Pneu-Stick needle
PNTML (pudendal nerve terminal
  motor latency) test
pO_2
p.o. (L. *per os*, by mouth, orally)
p.o. antibiotic
POA (pancreatic oncofetal antigen) test
pocket aneroid
pocketed calculus
pocket
  breast reconstruction
  fluid
  pus
  subcutaneous
point
  acupressure
  Addison
  bleeding
  blunt
  Boas
  Chauffard
  Crowe pilot
  Desjardins
  dorsal

point *(cont.)*
  drill
  Ethiguard blunt
  Hartmann
  Lane
  Lanz
  Mackenzie
  McBurney
  Munro
  pressure inversion (PIP)
  Ramond
  respiratory inversion
  Robson
  Sudeck
pointed awl
pointed-nose grasper
point-in-space stereotactic biopsy
point of attachment
point of maximal pain
point of respiratory reversal
  on esophageal manometry
Poirier gland
poison, poisoning
  acetaminophen
  bacterial food
  carbon tetrachloride
  caustic acid
  caustic alkali
  chloroform
  ethylene glycol
  food
  halothane
  salicylate
  salmonella food
  staphylococcal food
  toxic mushroom
Poison Control Center
Polaris 1.32 Nd:YAG laser
Polaris RF catheter
polarographic $P(ti)O_2$ catheter probe
Polaroid camera
Polaroid endocamera EC-3
Polaroid SX-70 with ACMI adapter
Polhemus-Schafer-Ivemark syndrome

Policot II sponge
polidocanol sclerosant
poliglacaprone absorbable suture material
polio
poliomyelitis virus
poliovirus
pollen, bee
Pollock grasper
Polocaine (mepivacaine)
poloxamer 188 (Flocor)
Polya anastomosis
Polya gastrectomy
Polya technique
polyarteritis nodosa
polybutester suture
polycystic chronic esophagitis
polycystic kidney
polycystic liver
polycystic liver disease
polycythemia vera
Polydek suture
Polyderm foam wound dressing
Polyderm hydrophilic polyurethane foam dressing
polydioxanone suture (PDS)
polydipsia
polydrug therapy
polyester mesh (Mersilene)
polyester mesh + silicone with memory, pre-shaped
polyester suture
polyester tripled hamstring graft
polyester-reinforced Dacron tape
polyester-reinforced silicon sheeting
polyethylene cannula
polyethylene glycol (PEG)
polyethylene glycol electrolyte solution
polyethylene tube
PolyFlo peripherally inserted central catheter (PICC)
polyfluorotetraethylene (PTFE) plastic graft material
PolyGIA stapler
polyglacine suture
polyglactin mesh dural graft
polyglactin rod
polyglactin suture material
polyglactin 370, polyglactin 910 absorbable suture material
polyglactin 910 mesh
polyglactin 910 suture
polyglandular autoimmune syndrome, type II (PGA II)
polyglandular deficiency syndrome, type II
polyglandular dysfunction
polyglutamic acid paclitaxel (PG-TXL)
polyglycolic acid mesh
polyglycolic acid suture material
polyglycolic suture
polyglycolide, self-reinforced rod
polyglyconate absorbable suture material
polyglyconate suture
PolyHeme (human hemoglobin cross-linked with glutaral) blood substitute
polylobar liver
PolyMem foam wound dressing
polymerase chain reaction (PCR)
polymerase technique
polymeric IgA antigen complex
polymethylmethacrylate-copolymer beads
polymicrobial bacteremia
polymorphic fungi
polymorphism
polymorphonuclear leukocyte (PMN)
polymorphonuclear leukocyte cell
polymyositis
polyneuropathy
  diabetic
  familial amyloid
polyoma virus
polyp
  adenomatous
  benign
  benign adenomatous

polyp *(cont.)*
- bleeding
- broad-based
- bronchial
- cardiac
- cellular
- cervical
- choanal
- colon
- colonic mucosubmucosal elongated
- colorectal
- cystic
- dental
- diffuse GI hamartoma
- duodenal
- endometrial
- fibrinous
- fibroepithelial
- fibrovascular
- gallbladder
- gastric
- gastrointestinal
- gelatinous
- hamartomatous gastric
- Hopmann
- hydatid
- hyperplastic gastric
- inflammatory fibroid
- juvenile
- laryngeal
- lipomatous
- lymphoid
- malignant
- metaplastic
- metastatic
- mucous
- multiple hamartomatous
- myomatous
- nasal
- neoplastic
- osseous
- pedunculated mass of
- Peutz-Jeghers
- placental

polyp *(cont.)*
- polypoid adenocarcinoma
- postinflammatory
- premalignant colonic
- pulp
- rectal
- regenerative
- retention
- sessile
- sigmoid
- single
- stalk of
- tubular
- tubulovillous
- uterine
- vascular
- villous

polyparadioxanone, absorbable pin
poly-p-dioxanone suture (PDS) pin
polypectomy
- colonoscopic
- electrosurgical snare
- endoscopic

polypectomy snare
polypectomy snare with banana plug connector
polypectomy snare with Olympus connector
polypeptide
- gastric inhibitory (GIP)
- glucose-dependent insulinotropic (GIP)
- islet amyloid (IAPP)
- pancreatic (PP)
- parathyroid-like
- vasoactive intestinal (VIP)

polypeptide antigen
polypeptide chain
polyp forceps
polyp grasper, four-pronged
polyp grasping forceps
polyphagia
polyp hook
polyphrenic gene

polyplastic cell
polypoid adenocarcinoma polyp
polypoidal tumor
polypoid carcinoma
polypoid lesion
polypoid lymphoid hyperplasia
polypoid lymphoma
polypoid mass
polypoid polyp
polypoid tissue
polyposis
  adenomatous
  diffuse mucosal
  familial
  familial adenomatous (FAP)
  familial colorectal
  familial gastrointestinal
  familial intestinal
  filiform
  gastric
  gastrointestinal
  hamartomatous intestinal
  hyperplastic
  intestinal
  juvenile
  melanoplakia-intestinal
  multiple familial
  multiple intestinal
  Peutz-Jeghers gastrointestinal
polyposis coli, familial
polypous gastritis
polypropylene mesh
polypropylene mesh/gelatin film graft
polypropylene mesh with memory
polypropylene suture
polyps and spots syndrome
polyps of hypertrophied mucosa
polyp snare technique
polyp stalk
polys (polymorphonuclear leukocytes)
Polyskin II dressing
Polysorb braided synthetic absorbable suture
polysplenia syndrome
Polystan catheter
polytetrafluoroethylene mesh graft
Polytrac Gomez retractor
polyurethane foam (PFD) dressing
polyvalent pneumococcal vaccine post-splenectomy
polyvinyl alcohol sponge
polyvinyl sponge graft
PolyWic wound filling material
Pondimin (fenfluramine)
Ponka anesthesia technique in herniorrhaphy
Ponka classification of groin hernias (types 1–2)
Ponka herniorrhaphy
Ponka technique for local anesthesia
Ponsky Endo-Sock retrieval bag
Ponsky "Pull" gastrostomy feeding device
Pontén-type tubed pedicle
Pontocaine HCl (tetracaine HCl)
pool, pooling
  abdominal
  bile acid
  blood
  gastric
  plasma
  vallecular
Poole abdominal suction tube
pooled plasma
Poole instrument
Poole suction
Poole suction tube
Poole tip
poorly defined vascular space
poorly differentiated adenocarcinoma
poorly differentiated adenoma
poorly differentiated carcinoma
poorly localized pain
poorly opsonized pathogen
poor operative candidate
poor prognosis
poor tissue turgor
poor uptake

poor visualization
POP (plaster of Paris) bandage
popliteal pulse
pop-off needle
pop-off suture
pop-off valve
Poppen-Blalock carotid clamp
Poppen-Blalock-Salibi clamp
Poppen forceps
Poppen-Gelpi laminectomy retractor
Poppen Gigli saw guide
Poppen intervertebral disk rongeur
Poppen saw
Poppen ventricular needle
population, viral
porcelain gallbladder
porcine dermal collagen graft
porcine islet preparation, encapsulated
porcine transmissible gastroenteritis
porcine xenograft
porfimer sodium
porfiromycin
porous polyethylene graft
porphyria
  acute
  acute intermittent (AIP)
  congenital erythropoietic
  hepatic
  hepatoerythropoietic (HEP)
porphyria cutanea tarda (PCT)
port
  endoscopic
  Fastrac gastrostomy access
  Hasson
  Import vascular-access port with BioGlide
  Port-A-Cath
  suction
  two-way laparoscopic
portable blood irradiator
portable film
portable insulin infusion pump
portable view
Port-A-Cath
portacaval anastomosis
portacaval H graft
portacaval shunt
Portagen diet
Portagen formula
porta hepatic lymph node
porta hepatis
portal and splenic veins
portal and systemic endotoxemia
portal azygous collateral
portal canal
portal cannula
portal catheter
portal circulation
portal cirrhosis
portal decompression
portal embolization (PE)
portal endotoxin
portal fibrosis
portal fibrosis of liver
portal fissure
portal hypertension from liver cirrhosis
portal hypertension-induced variceal bleeding
portal hypertension with severe hypersplenism
portal hypertensive gastropathy (PHG)
portal lobule
portal pressure
portal pyemia
portal pylethrombophlebitis
portal space
portal spread
portal systemic anastomosis
portal-systemic anastomotic area
portal-systemic collateral blood flow
portal-systemic collateral circulation
portal-systemic encephalopathy (PSE)
portal-systemic (or portosystemic) shunt
portal system of veins
portal thrombophlebitis
portal-to-portal bridging
portal-to-portal fibrosis
portal triad

portal vascular bed
portal vein
portal vein (end) to IVC (side)
portal vein gas
portal vein resection
portal vein thrombosis
portal venous hypertension
portal venous liver perfusion
portal venous pressure (PVP)
portal venous system thrombosis
portal vessel rupture
portal zone
portal zone granuloma
port closure needle
Porter duodenal forceps
Portex blue line intubation
Portnoy ventricular cannula
Portnoy ventricular catheter
portocaval shunt
portocaval synthetic H-graft
portoenterostomy, Kasai
portogram
portography, percutaneous transhepatic
portoportal anastomosis
portopulmonary shunt
portosystemic (or portal-systemic)
portosystemic anastomosis
portosystemic encephalopathy
portosystemic gradient
portosystemic shunt
portosystemic shunting
port site
port-site metastasis
port-site recurrence of tumor
POSICAM system
position
  abdominal brace
  antero-oblique
  barber chair
  bayonet fracture
  beach chair
  Bonner
  Bozeman
  Brickner

position *(cont.)*
  Buie
  calcaneal stance
  conjugate forward gaze
  decubitus
  dorsal
  dorsal lithotomy (*not* dorso-lithotomy)
  dorsal recumbent
  dorsal supine
  dorsosacral
  figure-4
  Fowler
  frog-leg
  full lateral
  Gaynor-Hart
  hook-lying
  horizontal
  infraumbilical
  intrinsic plus
  jackknife
  jet pilot
  Jones
  jumper's knee
  knee-chest
  knee-elbow
  kneeling
  Kraske jackknife
  lateral decubitus
  lateral park bench
  leapfrog
  left decubitus
  left lateral decubitus
  lithotomy
  lotus
  Mayo-Robson
  medial genicular
  modified dorsal lithotomy
  modified lithotomy
  near-anatomic
  neutral calcaneal stance
  neutral hip
  neutral spine
  normal anatomic

position *(cont.)*
occipitoanterior
occipitoposterior
occipitotransverse
opisthotonic
over-the-top
park bench
Phalen
prayer
prone
proximal bow
rectus
resting calcaneal stance
reverse Trendelenburg
right antero-oblique
right lateral decubitus
Robson
Rose
scissor-leg
semi-Fowler
semi-sitting
side-lying
Sims
sitting
ski
spinal fusion
static
stress tolerant
supine
three-quarters prone
Trendelenburg
W-sitting
positional stasis
positive bowel sounds
positive Chvostek sign
positive family history
positive inotropy
positive margin
positive Murphy sign
positive nodal metastasis
positive peritoneal space pressure
positive peritoneal tap
positive-pressure ventilation
positive surgical margins
positive test for occult blood
positive tetany
positive Trousseau sign
positron emission tomography (PET)
positron emission tomography with fluorodeoxyglucose
possible paracrine growth of adenocarcinoma of the stomach
postablative hypopituitarism
postablative hypothyroidism
postadenoidectomy
postage stamp-type skin graft
postanal pit
postanal repair
postanesthesia recovery room
postaugmentation mammoplasty bra
postaural regurgitation
post balloon angioplasty restenosis
postbulbar duodenal ulcer
postcholecystectomy flatulent dyspepsia
postcholecystectomy syndrome (PCS)
postcibal symptoms
postcoital bleeding
postcolonoscopy distention syndrome
postcricoid area
postcricoid web
postdeglutitive phase of swallowing
postemesis longitudinal tear
postemetic esophageal rupture
postendoscopic cholangitis
post-ERCP-induced pancreatitis
posterior abdominal wall
posterior choanal atresia
posterior colporrhaphy
posterior diaphragm
posterior diaphragmatic gastropexy
posterior extension of the lateral thyroid lobe
posterior fixation
posterior fossa-atrial shunt
posterior fossa retractor
posterior hemifundoplication
posterior hiatoplasty
posterior horn of the spinal cord

posterior incision
posterior inferior pancreaticoduodenal
  artery
posterior midline
posterior perforated duodenal ulcer into
  the pancreas
posterior rectopexy
posterior rectus fascia
posterior rectus sheath
posterior repair of the diaphragmatic
  hiatus
posterior sagittal and 3-flap anoplasty
posterior superior pancreaticoduodenal
  artery
posterior surface of pancreas
posterior surface of prostate
posterior triangle of the neck
posterolateral
posteromedial aspect of the thyroid
  gland
postevacuation film
postevacuation view
postfundoplication dysphagia
postfundoplication syndrome
postgastrectomy
postgastrectomy stasis
postgastrectomy syndrome
postgastric surgery syndrome
posthepatic cirrhosis
postherniorrhaphy neuropathy
posticteric phase of hepatitis
postinflammatory polyp
postinjury immunologic defect
postlaparoscopic shoulder pain
postlymphangiography abdomen
postmastectomy radiation therapy
postmenopausal
postmortem clot
postmortem knife
postmortem needle
  double-curve cutting-edge
  half-curved cutting-edge
postmyotomy reflux
postnecrotic cirrhosis
postnecrotic scar
postop (postoperative)
postoperative chemotherapy
postoperative abscess
postoperative adhesion
postoperative anesthesia
postoperative antibiotic
postoperative atelectasis
postoperative complications
postoperative diagnosis
postoperative ductal dilation
postoperative dysphagia
postoperative esophagitis
postoperative feeding schedule
postoperative hematoma
postoperative hemorrhage
postoperative hernia
postoperative hydrocele
postoperative hypocalcemia
postoperative ileus
postoperative incentive spirometry
postoperative infection
postoperative neuropathy
postoperative pain
postoperative pancreatitis
postoperative paraesophageal hiatus
  hernia
postoperative regimen for oral early
  feeding (PROEF)
postoperative residual stone
postoperative seroma
postoperative serum calcitonin level
postoperative "settling" of breast
  following reduction
postoperative T-tube cholangiography
postoperative view
postoperative vomiting
postpancreatectomy hyperglycemia
postpartum constipation
postpartum mastitis
postpartum period
postpartum pituitary necrosis
postpolio syndrome
postpolypectomy coagulation syndrome

postprandial abdominal discomfort
postprandial abdominal distention
postprandial antral hypomotility
postprandial blood glucose level
postprandial discomfort
postprandial distention
postprandial fullness
postprandial hypoglycemia
postprandially
postprandial pain
postprandial rise in peripheral glucose
postprandial vomiting
postpyloric feeding tube
postpyloric ulcer
postreduction ischemic necrosis
post-retching hematemesis
post-retching longitudinal tear
post-secretin challenge gastric level
post-shunt encephalopathy
postsplenectomy complications
postsplenectomy sepsis
postsurgical abdomen
postsurgical gastric stasis
postsurgical hypoglycemia
postsurgical hypothyroidism
postsurgical muscular or neurogenic
postsurgical nonabsorption syndrome
postsurgical recurrent ulcer
postsurgical stricture
post-transfusion hepatitis
post-transplant diabetes mellitus
post-transplant lymphoproliferative
disorder
post-transplantation lymphoproliferative
disorder (PTLD)
post-tussive vomiting
postural response of aldosterone
postvagotomy diarrhea
postvagotomy dysphagia
postvagotomy gastroparesis
postvagotomy syndrome
potassium (K)
potassium iodide
potassium supplement
potassium-titanyl-phosphate (KTP)
laser light therapy
potato liver
Pott abscess
Potter syndrome
Potts aortic clamp
Potts bronchus forceps
Potts bulldog forceps
Potts clamp
Potts-Cournand needle
Potts-DeMartel vascular scissors
Potts forceps
Potts needle
Potts-Nieder clamp
Potts patent ductus clamp
Potts rib shears
Potts right-angled scissors
Potts-Satinsky clamp
Potts 60° angled scissors
Potts-Smith aortic occlusion clamp
Potts-Smith dressing forceps
Potts-Smith tissue forceps
Potts-Smith vascular scissors
Potts tenotomy scissors
Potts thumb forceps
Potts tie suture
Potts vascular forceps
Potts-Yasargil scissors
pouch (see also *appliance; barrier; device*)
antral
apophyseal
Bard Extra Ileo B
Bard Integrale
blind
blind upper esophageal
branchial
Broca pudendal
celomic
closed-end ostomy
Coloplast Flange
coloplasty
continent ileal
ConvaTec Little One Sur-Fit

pouch *(cont.)*
- Cymed Micro Skin
- Dansac DuoSoft
- Dansac Karaya Seal
- Dansac Nova ostomy
- Dansac Standard Ileo
- deep perineal
- Denis Browne
- dilatation of the
- Douglas rectouterine
- drainable ostomy
- endodermal
- endorectal ileal
- esophageal
- fluid collection
- Fobi
- formation of intestinal
- fourth bronchial
- fourth pharyngeal
- gastric
- Graham omental
- Greez EZ Access drainage
- Hartmann
- haustral
- Heidenhain
- hepatorenal
- hernia
- Hollister First Choice
- Hollister Holligard
- Hollister Karaya 5 ostomy
- Hollister Karaya Seal
- Hollister Premium
- Hunt-Lawrence
- hypophysial
- ileal J
- ileal S
- ileal W
- ileoanal
- ileocecal
- Indiana
- jejunal
- J-shaped ileal
- Karaya ring ileostomy
- Kock ("coke")

pouch *(cont.)*
- lateral-lateral
- Mainz pouch urinary reservoir
- Marlen Gas Relief
- Marlen Odor-Ban
- Marlen Solo ileostomy
- Marlen Zip Klosed
- marsupial
- Morison
- Nu-Hope ileostomy
- Nu-Hope Nu-Self
- one-piece ostomy
- open-end ostomy
- ostomy
- Pagedas retrieval
- paracystic
- pararectal
- paravesical
- Parks ileostomy
- pendulous
- Penn
- pharyngeal
- Physick
- Prussak
- Rathke
- rectal
- rectouterine
- rectovaginal
- rectovaginouterine
- rectovesical
- Remedy
- renal
- Seessel (2 e's, 2 s's)
- S-shaped
- superficial inguinal
- superficial perineal
- Sur-Fit Mini
- terminal ileal
- third branchial
- third pharyngeal
- three-loop ileal
- two-loop J-shaped ileal
- two-piece ostomy
- UCLA

pouch *(cont.)*
  ultimobranchial
  United Bongort Lifestyle
  United Max-E
  United Surgical Bongort Lifestyle
  United Surgical Featherlite ileostomy
  United Surgical Shear Plus
  United Surgical Soft & Secure
  uterovesical
  vertical stapled small gastric
  vesicoureterine
  VPI nonadhesive
  water-filled
  Willis
  W-shaped
  Zenker
pouched ileostomy
pouchitis
pouchlike
pouch of Douglas
pouchography, evacuation
Poupart ligament shelving edge
povidone-iodine impregnated drape
powder (see also *enteral nutrition; feeding*; *medications*)
  absorbable dusting
  Accuprep HPF
  Amin-Aid
  Domeboro
  Helicosol lyophilized
  Hepatic-Aid
  hyCURE protein
  hydrophilic
  karaya
  Lonalac
  Multidex hydrophilic
  Precision Isotein HN
  Precision Isotonic
  Precision LR
  Seidlitz
  Sween Micro Guard
  Travasorb HN
  Vivonex elemental
  Vivonex HN
powdered bone graft
powder-free Latex exam gloves
PowerCut drill blade
PowerCut gold surgical system
PowerCut pneumatic power system
power-driven reamer
power-driven saw
power driver
power-drive staple
PowerGrip pliers
PowerGrip stent delivery system
PowerLink endoluminal graft
power magnification
power-mode color Doppler imaging
power oscillating saw
PowerPro
power rasp
power reamer
PowerSculpt cosmetic surgery system
power setting (for laser)
PowerVision ultrasound system
PPAF (progressive perivenular alcoholic fibrosis)
PP (pancreatic polypeptide) cell
PP-CAP IgA enzyme immunoassay
PPI treatment
PPMA (polymethylmethacrylate-copolymer) beads
PPoma
PPP (pituitary, pancreas, parathyroid tumors)
PPPD (pylorus-preserving pancreato-duodenectomy)
Prader-Willi syndrome
pramlintide acetate
Pramoxine HC (hydrocortisone acetate; pramoxine)
Prandase (acarbose)
Prandin (repaglinide)
Pratt bivalve retractor
Pratt crypt hook
Pratt proctoscope
Pratt rectal forceps
Pratt rectal hook
Pratt rectal probe

Pratt rectal scissors
Pratt rectal speculum
Pratt scissors
Pratt speculum
Pratt tumor forceps
prayer position
praziquantel
prazosin
PRBC transfusion
preampullary portion of bile duct
Pre-Attain
pre-bent nail
prebiopsy mammogram
precancerous lesion
PreCare Conceive nutritional supplement
Precedex (dexmedetomidine)
precipitating factor
precirrhosis
Precision Dynamics Corp.
Precision High Nitrogen
Precision HN (high nitrogen) powdered feeding
Precision Isotein HN powdered feeding
Precision Isotonic powdered feeding
Precision LR powdered feeding
precision-point conventional cutting
precision-point reverse cutting
Precision QID blood glucose monitor
Precision Therapy
precore-core promoter mutant infection
Precose (acarbose)
precursor lesion
precurved ball-tipped guide pin
precut foam bandage
Precut intermediate Hi-Lo tracheal tube with stylet
precut sphincterotome
precut sphincterotomy
prediabetes (diet-controlled gestational diabetes)
predigested protein formula
predisposing factor
prednisolone enema
prednisone
pre-eclampsia
pre-esophageal dysphagia
preexisting condition
preexisting infection
Prefil nebulizer
preformed prosthetic mesh
Pregestimil (enzymatically hydrolyzed protein formula)
pregnancy, ectopic
prehepatic
prehyoid gland
preicteric phase
preileal appendix
preinvasive carcinoma
preinvasive lesion
preliminary diagnosis
preliminary film
preliminary view
preload
premalignant colonic polyp
premalignant neoplasm
premalignant skin lesion
premalignant state
Premarin (conjugated estrogens)
prematurely closed suture
premenstrual edema
Premidex-Aldehyde
Premier Platinum HpSA test
Premilene suture
Premium Americot sponge
Premium Barrier for ostomy skin
Premium CEEA circular stapler
Premium dissecting knife
Premium Plus CEEA disposable stapler
premium-point reverse cutting suture
premium-point spatula suture
prenatal diagnosis
prenatal genetic diagnosis
preneoplastic intraductal lesion
preoperative antibiotic
preoperative assessment
preoperative chemotherapy
preoperative diagnosis

preoperative endoscopic biliary stenting
preoperative endoscopic drainage
preoperative esophageal manometry
preoperative localization
preoperative placement of needle
  localization wire
preoperative placement of radiologic
  marker
preoperative plasmapheresis
preoperative view
prep (bowel prep) (see *bowel prep; enema*)
prepapillary bile duct
Preparation H anorectal cream
Preparation H cleansing tissues
Preparation H Cooling Gel
Preparation H rectal suppositories
preparation, islet cell
prepared and draped in a sterile fashion
Prepcat (barium sulfate)
preperitoneal approach
preperitoneal compartment
preperitoneal distention balloon (PDB)
preperitoneal fat
preperitoneal fat on the cord structures
preperitoneal hernioplasty
preperitoneal patch and plug hernia
  repair technique
preperitoneal prosthetic mesh repair
  of hernia via laparoscopy
preperitoneal space
preplaced suture
Prep Mitt surgical adhesive mitt
Prepodyne solution
prepped and draped in a sterile fashion
prepped and draped in the usual sterile
  manner
prepyloric antrum
prepyloric atresia
prepyloric gastric ulcer
prepyloric sphincter
prepyloric ulcer
prereduction view
prerenal FENa
presacral anesthesia
presacral drainage
presacral edema
presacral rectopexy
presacral space
presacral tumor
presbyesophagus
Presbyterian Hospital staphylorrhaphy
  elevator
Presbyterian Hospital tubing clamp
Presbyterian tube-occluding clamp
presence of bile
preservation of vagal innervation
preserved dural homograft
presinusoidal intrahepatic portal hypertension
pressor support
pressure
  anal sphincter squeeze
  atmospheres of
  backup of portal
  bile duct
  biliary-duodenal
  blood
  central venous (CVP)
  choledochal basal
  continuous positive airway (CPAP)
  decreased blood
  diastolic blood
  direct
  duodenobiliary
  elevated portal
  end-expiratory
  esophageal peristaltic
  free hepatic venous
  gastric
  gastrosphincteric
  hepatic venous
  hepatic wedge
  increased gastric
  increased intra-abdominal
  increased intracranial
  increased intraluminal
  increased portal

pressure *(cont.)*
- indirect hepatic vein wedge
- intra-abdominal
- intra-anal
- intracranial
- intraductal
- intraesophageal peristaltic
- intragastric
- intraluminal esophageal
- Koala intrauterine
- left ventricular end diastolic (LVEDP)
- LES (lower esophageal sphincter)
- lower esophageal sphincter
- low urethral (LUP)
- maximum anal resting (MARP)
- mean arterial (MAP)
- mean end-expiratory
- needle
- negative inspiratory
- negative pleural space
- orthostatic blood
- osmotic
- passage
- peak
- portal
- portal venous (PVP)
- positive end-expiratory (PEEP)
- positive peritoneal space
- pulmonary artery (PA)
- pulmonary capillary wedge (PCWP)
- resting anal sphincter
- sinusoidal
- splanchnic
- squeeze
- systemic
- systolic blood
- UOS tonic
- wedged hepatic venous (WHVP)

pressure anesthesia
pressure dressing
pressure gauge
pressure inversion point (PIP)
pressure measurement of sphincter of Oddi
pressure necrosis
pressure needle
pressure-sensitive valve in shunt tube
pressure sore
pressure support (ventilatory)
pressure symptoms
Pressure Ulcer Scale for Healing (PUSH) tool
pressurized pulsatile irrigation system
Prestige Smart System (PSS) glucose monitor
prestomal ileitis
Preston ligamentum flavum forceps
presumptive diagnosis
preternatural anus
pretibial edema
pretibial myxedema
pretransplant crossmatch
PRE 2 suture
Prevacid (lansoprazole)
Prevacid triple therapy
Prevail gel
Prevalite (cholestyramine resin)
Prevatac (exisulind)
Prevenzyme
prevertebral fascia
Prevpac (lansoprazole; clarithromycin; amoxicillin)
PreVue *B. burgdorferi* antibody detection assay
prezatide copper acetate
Pribham suction tube
Price muscle biopsy clamp
Price-Thomas bronchial forceps
prickle cell carcinoma
priliximab
Prilosec (omeprazole)
Prima laser
Primaderm semipermeable foam dressing
Primapore absorptive wound dressing
primary adrenocortical insufficiency
primary anastomosis
primary benign liver tumor

primary bile duct cancer
primary biliary cirrhosis (PBC)
primary carcinoma
primary (preoperative) chemotherapy
primary closure
primary contraction
primary diffuse malignant peritoneal mesothelioma
primary direct linear closure
primary esophageal motility
primary GI tract lymphoma
primary hepatic carcinoma
primary hyperaldosteronism
primary hyperparathyroidism
primary hypersplenism
primary ileal villous atrophy (PIVA)
primary intestinal lymphangiectasia
primary intraosseous carcinoma
primary lesion
primary liver cancer
primary malignancy
primary peristaltic wave
primary peritonitis
primary pituitary pathology
primary reanastomosis
primary sclerosing cholangitis (PSC)
primary suture
primary thyroid hyperplasia
primary thyroid malignancy
primary tumor
Primer compression dressing or wrap
principal diagnosis
Pringle maneuver for clamping the hepatic pedicle
Pritchard lipiodol syringe
Pritchard Mark II pin
Pritchard syringe
p.r.n. (L. *pro re nata*, as needed)
p.r.n. antacid
PRN bandage
Pro-Banthine (propantheline bromide)
probe
  Acculite Contour Tip
  AccuProbe 600 cryotherapy probe

probe *(cont.)*
  Acufex
  angled
  Arthrocare Wand
  arthroscopic
  Barr D/E fistula
  Barr fistula
  Beckman 39042 pH
  BiCAP electrocoagulation
  BiLAP bipolar cutting and coagulating
  biliary balloon
  biplane sector
  bipolar
  bipolar cautery (BiCAP)
  blunt
  Bowman
  broach
  Brodie
  Buie rectal
  Bunnell dissecting
  Bunnell forwarding
  buttonhole
  Cameron-Miller monopolar
  Circon-ACMI electrohydraulic lithotriptor
  continuously perfused
  core
  Core suction/irrigation
  Dandy
  Desjardins gallstone
  dissecting
  double ended
  Earle rectal
  8-channel cross-sectional anal sphincter
  electrohydraulic
  electromagnetic focusing field (EFF)
  endoesophageal
  Endo-Flo
  endoscopic BiCAP
  endoscopic heat
  Endotrac
  esophageal temperature

probe *(cont.)*
- Fenger gallbladder
- Fisch rectal
- fistula
- Fluhrer rectal
- Fogarty biliary
- forwarding
- Frigitronics
- gallstone
- galvanic
- heater
- hemispherical contact
- high-frequency
- high-frequency miniprobe
- Hydromer coated bipolar coagulation
- Hydro-Temp
- intraosseous
- Jacobson
- Jacobson micro
- Jannetta
- J-hook ElectroProbe
- Jobson Horne
- Klear-Temp
- lacrimal duct
- laparoscopic Doppler
- Larry rectal
- laser
- laser Doppler
- Laserflo Doppler
- LDF (laser-Doppler flowmetry)
- malleable
- Maloney endo-otoprobe
- Mammotome
- Mayo common duct
- Mayo gall duct
- McCain TMJ
- Medi-Tech bipolar
- Medrad Mrinnervu (also MRinnervu) endorectal colon
- micro
- microballoon
- Microelectrode MI-506 small-caliber

probe *(cont.)*
- Mitek Vapor
- Mixter dilating
- Modulap
- Moynihan bile duct
- Moynihan gallstone
- multilumen
- needle electroprobe
- neo-therm
- Neurotrend
- Nucleotome aspiration
- Nucleotome Flex II cutting
- Ochsner flexible spiral gallstone
- Ochsner gall duct
- OCT surgical imaging
- Olympus heat
- Olympus RU-12M-R1 rectal
- Olympus RU-75M-R1 rectal
- Olympus UM-1W endoscopic
- Oratec electrocautery
- PathVysion HER-2 DNA probe kit
- pedicle
- pH
- polarographic P(ti)O_2 catheter
- Pratt rectal
- radiofrequency
- Radiometer GK2803C pH
- Sandhill P32 pH antimony
- silver
- simple suction
- skin temperature monitoring
- SmokEvac electrosurgical
- spatula electroprobe
- spear-ended
- Steffee
- StrykcFlow electrocautery
- suction irrigation
- Surgical Dynamics aspiration
- Surgiflex
- tactile
- telomere-specific
- TEMPprobe
- thermal
- tulip

probe *(cont.)*
  24-hour pH
  ultrasonic
  Valleix
  Vanguard splinter
  Verbatim balloon
  water
  Watson-Cheyne
  wire-guided
  Wound Stick
  Yankauer
probe dilator
probe for aspiration and lavage (PAL)
probes/grooved director
probe with eye
probiotic agent
procaine HCl
Pro-Cal-Sof (docusate sodium)
procedure (see *operation* for a quick-reference list of diagnostic, operative, and therapeutic procedures)
Proceed hemostatic surgical sealant
process (pl. processes)
  altered thought
  autoimmune
  AuTolo Cure Process
  chronic inflammatory
  energy-producing respiratory
  finger-like epithelial
  inflammatory
  metabolic
  Tutoplast
  uncinate
prochlorperazine
procidentia
  anal
  internal
  rectal
procidentia recti
Pro-Clude dressing
Pro-Clude transparent film wound dressing
procoagulants (PCA)
ProCross Rely over-the-wire balloon catheter
proctalgia fugax
proctectomy
  abdominoperineal
  intersphincteric
  Kraske transsacral
  laparoscopic
  mucosal
  partial
  perineal
  permanent
  radical
  restorative
  sphincter-preserving
  subtotal
  total
Procter-Livingstone endoprosthesis
proctitis
  acute
  diversion
  factitial
  gonorrheal
  nonspecific ulcerative
  radiation
  ulcerative
proctocolectomy
  laparoscopic total
  pan-
  primary
  restorative
  secondary stage
  single-stage total
  total
proctocolitis
  idiopathic
  radiation
  venereal
Proctocort (hydrocortisone)
ProctoCream-HC (hydrocortisone acetate)
Procto-Esthesia
ProctoFoam NS (pramoxine HCl)
proctogenous constipation

proctogram, proctography
  balloon
  evacuation
proctopexy, Orr-Loygue transabdominal
proctoplasty
proctorectoscopy
Proctor-Livingston tube
proctoscope (also *anoscope, endoscope, rectoscope, speculum*)
  ACMI
  Alan-Parks rectal speculum
  Arakawa
  Bensaude
  Blond
  Brinkerhoff
  disposable
  Enproct disposable
  Fansler
  Fansler-Ives anoscope
  front lifting hood rectoscope
  Gabriel
  Galencia disposable
  Heine
  Hirschman
  Jasan rigid
  Ives
  Ives-Fansler
  Karl Storz
  Kelly straight
  Kelly tapered
  KleenSpec disposable
  Medix
  Naunton Morgan
  Newman anoscope
  Pratt
  Ricord rectal speculum
  Romanoscope
  Roschke rectal speculum
  Sani-Scope
  Sapimed
  Sawyer rectal speculum
  Sklar
  slotted
  St. Mark's

proctoscope *(cont.)*
  Storz
  Strauss rectoscope
  Tuttle
  UniSpec disposable
  videorectoscope
  Welch anoscope
proctoscope and obturator
proctoscopy
proctosigmoiditis
proctosigmoidoscope
proctosigmoidoscopy
proctotomy
ProCyte transparent adhesive film dressing
Proderm Topical (castor oil; Peruvian balsam)
prodromal symptoms
prodrome
production
  catecholamine
  decreased pituitary
  digestion
  ectopic hormone
  endogenous inflammatory mediator
  exocrine
  excessive cortisol
  gastric acid
  gastrin-induced excessive gastric acid
  glucocorticoid
  increased gastric acid and pepsin
  metabolic energy
  pepsin
  suboptimal thyroid hormone
products of digestion
PROEF (postoperative regimen for oral early feeding)
proemial breast
Profiber enteral nutritional formula
profile
  adverse event
  ASTRA
  Contour Profile

profile *(cont.)*
  gut-hormone
  lipid
  liver function
  ultra-low
Pro-Flo XT catheter
Profore four-layer bandaging system
profound catabolic response
profound dehydration
profound malnutrition
profuse bleeding
profuse vomiting
progastrin
progeria
progestational pattern
progesterone-associated colitis
progesterone receptor (PgR)
progesterone-receptor analysis
progesterone-receptor-negative tumor
progesterone-receptor-positive tumor
progesterone-receptor status
prognosis
prognostic indicator
prognostic marker
Prognostic Nutritional Index (PNI)
prognostic value
Prograf (tacrolimus)
program, "Be In Charge" hepatitis
programmed cell death (apoptosis)
progressive abdominal distention
progressive ascites
progressive coagulopathy
progressive decline in mental status
progressive decompensation
progressive diet
progressive distention
progressive dysphagia
progressive emphysematous necrosis
progressive familial cirrhosis
progressive hypoxemia
progressively larger reamer
progressive obstruction
progressive perivenular alcoholic
  fibrosis
progressive suppurative cholangitis
progressive thinning of stool
PRO infusion catheter
proinsulin level
projectile vomiting
prokinetic agent
prokinetic drugs
prolactin deficiency
prolactin level
prolapse
  anal
  anorectal mucosal
  bladder
  hemorrhoidal
  intestinal
  massive genital
  rectal
  stomal
  uterine
  vaginal vault
prolapsed hemorrhoids
prolapsed stoma
prolapsed vaginal vault
prolapse gastropathy
prolapse with defecation
prolapsing internal hemorrhoids
ProLease drug delivery system
Prolene Hernia System (PHS) bilayer
  patch repair
Prolene mesh tape
Prolene polypropylene hernia mesh
Prolene polypropylene mesh
Prolene polypropylene suture
Prolene suture
Proleukin (aldesleukin)
proliferating cell nuclear antigen
  (PCNA)
proliferation
  bile duct
  cytotoxic lymphocytic
  ductal
  monoclonal B cell
  papillary
  vascular

proliferation of acini
proliferation signal inhibitor
proliferative hypertrophic gastritis
proliferative of undifferentiated cells
proliferative pattern
proliferative peritonitis
prolonged bleeding from wound
prolonged fasting
prolonged H_2-receptor blockade
prolonged ischemia
prolonged nausea or vomiting
prolonged pain
prolonged respiratory alkalosis
prolonged ventilatory support
prolonged vomiting
PROloop coagulator
PROloop electrosurgical device
promethazine HCl
Prometheus test
prominent thyroid nodule
promontory cartilage
promontory, sacral
Promycin (porfiromycin)
prone film
prone lateral view
prone position
prone view
pronounced leucocytosis
Pronova nonabsorbable suture
Pronova poly (hexafluoropropylene-
  VDF) suture
ProOsteon 500 bone graft substitute
ProOsteon 500 bone implant
propantheline bromide
Propel cannulated interference screw
properdin
properitoneal fat
properitoneal flank stripe (on x-ray)
properitoneal hernia
properitoneal space
prophylactic antibiotic
prophylactic cholecystectomy
prophylactic colectomy
prophylactic drain
prophylactic gastrojejunostomy
prophylactic intravenous antibiotic
prophylactic penicillin
prophylactic removal of uninvolved
  lymph node
prophylactic subcutaneous mastectomy
prophylactic thyroidectomy
prophylaxis
  antibiotic
  antimicrobial
  CMV
  long-term
Prophyllin (sodium propionate;
  chlorophyll derivatives)
Propimex-2
propiram
Proplast graft
propofol
propolis natural resin
Propper scalpel
propranolol
propylthiouracil (PTU)
Proscope
ProSobee liquid formula
ProSol 20% (amino acids) nutrition mix
Prosphyg sphygmomanometer
ProstaCoil self-expanding stent
prostaglandin E1 (PGE1)
prostaglandin E2 (PGE2)
Prostalase laser
Prostar percutaneous closure device
Prostar Plus percutaneous closure
  device
Prostar XL percutaneous closure
  device
ProstaScint (CYT-356 radiolabeled with
  ^{111}In) imaging agent
prostate
  adenocarcinoma of
  apex of
  ballotable
  high-riding
  inferolateral surfaces of
  lateral lobe of

prostate *(cont.)*
  lymph vessel of
  median lobe of
  posterior surface of
prostate cancer
prostate chip
prostatectomy
  laser
  Madigan
  perineal
  radical
  retropubic
  retropubic prevesical
  suprapubic prevesical
  transurethral
  transurethral balloon
  TULIP (transurethral laser-induced)
prostate enlargement
prostate gland
prostate-specific antigen (PSA)
prostatic abscess
prostatic acid phosphatase (PAP)
prostatic adenocarcinoma
prostatic calculus (pl. calculi)
prostatic capsule
prostatic carcinoma
prostatic concretion
prostatic cyst
prostatic duct
prostatic fluid
prostatic hyperplasia
prostatic malignancy
prostatic shaving
prostatic sinus
prostatic urethra
prostatic venous plexus
prostatitis
  acute
  acute bacterial
  allergic
  chronic
  chronic bacterial prostatitis (CBP)
  eosinophilic
  nonspecific granulomatous

prosthesis (see also *breast implant; endoprosthesis*; *implant*)
  Acticon neosphincter implantable
  Amoena breast
  Angelchik antireflux ring
  antireflux
  asymmetrical breast
  Becker breast
  Becker tissue expander/breast
  Belle-Amie breast
  bilioduodenal
  bladder neck support
  breast
  Charnley femoral
  CUI gel breast
  CUI saline breast
  delayed insertion of breast
  Discrene breast
  Dow Corning Silastic breast
  Dumon-Gilliard
  endoscopic
  endoscopic biliary endoprosthesis
  esophageal
  Gianturco expandable (self-expanding) metallic biliary
  GunSlinger shoulder orthosis
  Hartley breast
  HD II (or 2) total hip prosthesis
  Hemobahn endovascular
  iridium
  large-bore bile duct
  Leading Lady breast
  McGhan saline-filled
  Moore
  Nearly Me breast
  Perras breast
  Perras-Papillon breast
  pin-retained palatal
  Restore orthobiologic soft tissue implant
  silicone donut
  Spenco breast
  stent
  subpectoral breast

prosthesis *(cont.)*
  Surgitek
  Trulife silicone breast
  Wilson-Cook
  Yours Truly breast
prosthesis driver
prosthesis exchange
prosthesis sizer
prosthetic breast
prosthetic device
prosthetic femoral distal graft
prosthetic hook
prosthetic mesh
Prosthex sponge
Prostigmin
ProStream infusion wire
ProTack stapler
protamine zinc insulin
protease digestive enzyme
ProTec (isofylline)
Protect-a-Pass suture passer
protecting the spinal cord
Protectiv I.V. catheter safety system
Protector meniscus suture
Protect Point needle
protein
  anti-Tamm-Horsfall
  bacterial
  bacterial cellular
  bone morphogenic (BMP)
  BPI (bactericidal/permeability-increasing)
  cerebrospinal fluid (CSF)
  coagulated
  conserved helix-loop-helix ubiquitous kinase) (CHUK)
  copper-binding (CBP)
  cow's milk
  C-peptide
  C reactive (CRP)
  dietary
  Emdogain enamel matrix
  enamel matrix
  Endostatin

protein *(cont.)*
  endotoxin binding
  fluid
  fusion
  heat shock (HSP)
  high
  intracellular
  lipopolysaccharide-binding (LBP)
  mammastatin
  Ne-Osteo bone morphogenic (BMP)
  parathyroid hormone-related (PTHrp)
  pegylated
  plasma
  receptor
  serum
  therapeutic
  villin
proteinase enzyme
protein C activity
protein C deficiency
protein-energy malnutrition (PEM)
protein-losing enteropathy (PLE)
protein-losing gastropathy
protein pump inhibitor
protein-rich fluid
protein S antigen deficiency
protein S deficiency
Protek joint implant
Protenate (plasma protein fraction)
proteolytic enzyme
Proteus mirabilis
Proteus inconstans
Proteus morganii
Proteus vulgaris
Prothecan (PEG-captothecin)
prothrombin
prothrombin time (PT, pro time)
prothrombin time coagulation panel
prothrombotic disorder
prothrombotic state
pro time (prothrombin time)
protirelin

protocol
  chemotherapy
  Edmonton fresh islet
  Gerson therapy protocol
  Haemonetics red blood cell
    collection
  immunomodulatory
  immunosuppressive
  Nigro
  treatment
protocolectomy
Protocult stool sampling device
proton-density image
proton efflux rate
Protonix (pantoprazole)
proton magnetic resonance
  spectroscopy
proton permeability
proton pump inhibitor (PPI)
protopathic pain
protoporphyria, erythrohepatic
Protostat (metronidazole)
protozoal infection of bowel
Protractor retractor and wound
  protector
protruded gastric carcinoma
protruding fat
protrusion of mucosa
protuberant abdomen
proud graft
proudflesh
Providence Hospital artery forceps
Providencia alcalifaciens
Providencia rettgeri
Provir (sirirumab)
Provis cannula
provisional anatomic diagnosis
provocative test
proximal bile duct obstruction
proximal bow position
proximal clot
proximal diverting ostomy
proximal duct excision
proximal end of colon
proximal esophageal lumen
proximal esophagus
proximal gastrectomy
proximal gastric vagotomy (PGV)
proximal jejunum
proximal part of dorsal pancreatic duct
proximal saline injection
proximal splenorenal shunt
proximal to the ligament of Trietz
Proximate flexible linear stapler
Proximate ILS curved intraluminal
  stapler
Proximate linear cutter
Proximate skin staple
PRS (Photon Radiosurgery System)
PRT (physiologic reflux test)
Pruitt-Inahara shunt
Prulet (white phenolphthalein)
prune-belly abdomen
prune-belly syndrome
prune juice peritoneal fluid
pruning sign
pruritic urticarial papule
pruritus
pruritus ani
Prussak pouch
PSA 4000 anesthesia monitoring system
psammoma body
PSC (primary sclerosing cholangitis)
PSE (portal-systemic encephalopathy)
Pseudallescheria boydii
pseudoaneurysm
pseudobacillus
pseudobacterium
pseudocapsule of tumor
pseudochylous ascites
pseudocirrhosis, cholangiodysplastic
pseudocyst
  adrenal
  communicating
  pancreatic
  pararenal
  pulmonary
pseudocyst gastrostomy, pancreatic

pseudocyst of pancreas
pseudodiverticulum
pseudoductular transformation of hepatocyte
pseudohermaphroditism
pseudohyperparathyroidism
pseudohypoparathyroidism
pseudolymphoma, gastric
pseudomelanosis
pseudomembranous colitis (PMC)
pseudomembranous enterocolitis
pseudomembranous gastritis
pseudomembranous inflammation
pseudomembranous radiation gastritis
Pseudomonas-like bacteria
pseudomucinous cystadenocarcinoma
pseudomyxoma peritonei
pseudo-obstruction
  bowel
  chronic idiopathic intestinal (CIIP)
  chronic intestinal (CIP)
  colonic
  familial intestinal
  idiopathic intestinal
  intestinal
  nonfamilial intestinal
  Ogilvie
pseudo-obstructive syndrome
pseudopalisade formation
pseudopalisading
pseudoparenchyma
pseudopolyp
pseudopolyposis
pseudoprecocious puberty
pseudopseudohypoparathyroidism
pseudopyogenic granuloma
pseudorabies virus
pseudosac
pseudosacculation
pseudosarcoma
pseudostone
pseudoxanthoma elasticum
PSFR (peak secretory flow rate) test
p.s.i. or psi (pronounced "sigh") (pounds per square inch)
PSI-TEC aspirator
PSI-TEC system
PSI-TEC tubing
psoas abscess
psoas fascia
psoas gap
psoas hitch
psoas inflammation
psoas major muscle
psoas margin
psoas muscle
psoas muscle abscess
psoas shadow
psoas sign
psorelcosis
psorenteritis
PSS (Prestige Smart System) glucose monitor
PSS (progressive systemic sclerosis)
PST staging
psychogenic colic
psychogenic colitis
psychogenic vomiting
Psychosocial Adjustment to Illness Scale (PAIS)
psyllium hydrophilic mucilloid
PT (prothrombin time)
PTBD (percutaneous transhepatic biliary drainage) catheter
PTC (percutaneous transhepatic cholangiography)
PTCS tube
PTD (percutaneous transhepatic drainage)
p10 protein
pterygoid plate
PTFE (polytetrafluoroethylene) graft
PTH (parathyroid hormone) test
PTH assay
p30 protein
PTHrp (parathyroid-hormone-related protein)

PTLD (post-transplantation lymphoproliferative disorder)
ptosis, mammary
ptosis of breasts
ptosis of testicle
ptotic breasts
PT (prothrombin time)
PTT (partial thromboplastin time)
ptyocrinous cell
pubic hair line
pubic symphysis
pubic tubercle
pubocervical ligament`
pubococcygeal line
pubococcygeus muscle
puborectalis loop
puborectalis sling
PUD (peptic ulcer disease)
puddle sign
puddling on barium enema
Puddu view
pudendal anesthesia
pudendal artery
pudendal hernia
pudendal nerve terminal motor latency
(PNTML) test
Pudenz peritoneal catheter
Pudenz shunt
puerperal breast abscess
puerperal peritonitis
puerperal sepsis
puerperium
Puestow-Gillesby operation
Puestow pancreaticojejunostomy
Pugh-Child grading system for bleeding
esophageal varices
Pugh classification of Child liver
criteria
Pugh sliding nail
Puka chisel
pullout suture
pullout wire suture
pull-through procedure
abdominal
continuous

pull-through procedure *(cont.)*
Duhamel laparoscopic
endorectal
endorectal ileal
ileal
ileoanal
rapid (RPT)
sacroabdominoperineal
Soave endorectal
station (SPT)
Swenson abdominal
Pull-thru Network
pulmonary autograft (PA)
pulmonary cirrhosis
pulmonary congestion
pulmonary consolidation
pulmonary edema
pulmonary embolism
pulmonary embolus
pulmonary emphysema
pulmonary function
pulmonary gas exchange
pulmonary gases
pulmonary hypertension
pulmonary infarct
pulmonary infection
pulmonary orifice
pulmonary pseudocyst
pulmonary segment
pulmonary stenosis
pulmonary tissue–blood barrier
pulmonary venous blood
pulpar cell
pulpiform nucleus forceps
pulp polyp
pulp, splenic
Pulsalith lithotriptor
Pulsar CO_2 laser system
pulsatile abdominal mass
pulsatile mass in the neck
pulsation balloon
Pulsavac III wound debridement system
pulse (pl. pulses)
abdominal
brachial

pulse *(cont.)*
  carotid
  distal
  distal abdominal
  dorsalis pedis
  epigastric
  femoral
  jugular
  palpable
  popliteal
  posterior tibial
  radial
pulsed-dye laser therapy
pulsed-field gel electrophoresis (PFGE)
pulsed ultrasound
pulse inversion Harmonic imaging
PulseMaster laser
PulseMaster Nd:YAG laser
pulse oximeter, Masimo SET (signal
  extraction technology)
Pulse*Spray injector
pulsion diverticulum
Pulsolith (coumarin pulsed-dye laser)
Pulsolith laser
Pulsolith laser lithotriptor
pulsus paradoxus
Pulver-Taft fishmouth suture
Puma 2002
pump
  Abbott
  Autofuse Byron infiltration
  balloon
  Baxter mini-K thermia
  breast
  Colleague 3 (triple channel) infusion
  computerized peristaltic
  Curlin 2000 Plus infusion
  Dahedi 25 insulin
  D-Modem and insulin pump therapy
  Endolav lavage
  Felig insulin
  Harvard 2 dual syringe
  Harvard infusion
  Hemopump

pump *(cont.)*
  H-TRON plus V100 insulin infusion
  Infusaid hepatic
  Infusaid implantable drug infusion
  infusion
  insulin
  irrigation
  IsoMed implantable drug
  IVAC MedSystem III multichannel
    infusion
  IVAC Space·Saver volumetric
  IVAC volumetric infusion
  Klein
  laparoscopic irrigation
  McGaw volumetric
  McKinley EpM analgesic infusion
  Medex Protégé 3010 syringe infusion
  Medfusion 2001 syringe infusion
  MedSystem III infusion
  MultA
  patient-controlled analgesia (PCA)
  Plum drug delivery
  portable insulin infusion
  Seabrook
  Stat 2 Pumpette
  Storz high-flow insufflator
  V.A.C. Plus
punch
  Acufex rotary
  bone
  bone graft
  boxer's (fracture of the fifth
    metacarpal)
  Caspari suture
  cervical laminectomy
  Charnley femoral prosthesis neck
  cone skull
  cutaneous
  disk
  dural
  DyoVac suction
  Hajek-Koffler
  Hajek laminectomy
  Hardy sellar

punch *(cont.)*
    Hartmann tonsil
    Hirsch hypophyseal
    Hunstad
    Inner Dyne single-action single-tooth biopsy
    Inner Dyne spoon biopsy
    intervertebral disk
    Kerrison
    Keyes cutaneous
    Keyes dermal
    laminectomy
    Miltex
    Raney laminectomy
    Rhoton sellar
    rotary basket
    Rowe glenoid
    Sauerbruch-Frey bone
    Schlesinger
    Schmeden tonsil
    sellar
    skull
    suture
    tibial
    tubular
    window
    Yankauer
punch biopsy
punch-drunk syndrome of boxers
punched-out ulcer
punch forceps
punctate area
punctate hemorrhage
punctate keratotic lesion
punctate ulcer
Punctur-Guard needle
puncture aspiration of cyst of breast
puncture incision
puncture site for laparoscopy
puncture wound
pupil, blown
pure respiratory acidosis
pure respiratory alkalosis
pure tissue hernia repair
purgative
Purge (castor oil)
purging, self-induced
Puri-Clens wound cleanser
purified factor VIII concentrations
Puritan oxyadaptor
purple striae
purpura
    adult chronic immune thrombocytopenic
    Henoch-Schönlein
    hyperglobulinemic
    idiopathic thrombocytopenic (ITP)
    thrombotic thrombocytopenic (TTP)
purpuric bleeding
purpuric lesion
pursestring ligature
pursestring or purse-string suture
pursestringed (verb)
pursestring ligature
Purstring device
Pursuer CBD (common bile duct) basket
Pursuer CBD Helical or Mini-Helical stone basket
Purtilo syndrome
purulent debris
purulent discharge
purulent lesion
purulent material
purulent pancreatitis
pus-forming bacteria
push enteroscope
push enteroscopy
pusher (small dissecting sponge)
pusher catheter
pusher tube
push-pull ankle stress view
push-pull hip view
PUSH (Pressure Ulcer Scale for Healing) tool
pus, frank
pus smear
pus under pressure

Putti bone rasp
Putti bone raspatory
putty kidney
PVH (persistent viral hepatitis)
PVH-B (persistent viral hepatitis, type B)
PVH-NAB (persistent viral hepatitis, non-A, non-B)
PVP (portal venous pressure)
PVP-I Solution Skin Prep Trays
PVR (pulmonary vascular resistance)
PVS (peritoneovenous shunt)
PWB (Puno-Winter-Byrd) rod
pyeloileocutaneous anastomosis
pyelonephritic kidney
pyemia, portal
pylephlebitis
pylethrombophlebitis
pylon attachment plate
pylorectomy
  Billroth
  Kocher
Pylori-Check test kit (also, Pylori-Chek)
pyloric antrum
pyloric antrum cardiacum
pyloric artery
pyloric canal
pyloric channel
pyloric channel obstruction
pyloric channel ulcer
pyloric exclusion with gastro-jejunostomy
pyloric gland
pyloric lymph node
pyloric mucosa
pyloric orifice
pyloric outlet obstruction
pyloric ring
pyloric sphincter
pyloric spreader
pyloric stenosis
pyloric stricture
pyloric string sign
Pylorid (ranitidine bismuth citrate)
PyloriProbe assay
Pyloriset
PyloriTek *Helicobacter pylori* test
pyloroduodenal junction
pyloroduodenal obstruction
pyloromyotomy
  circumumbilical
  extramucosal
  Fredet-Ramstedt
  Kocher
  laparoscopic
  Ramstedt-Fredet
  surface umbilical
  umbilical
pyloroplasty
  double
  Finney
  Heineke-Mikulicz
  Jaboulay
  laparoscopic
  Mikulicz
  Ramstedt
  reconstructive
  transhiatal
  vagotomy and
  Weinberg modification of
  Yu
pylorospasm
pylorostenosis
pylorotomy
pylorus (pl. pylori), hypertrophic
pylorus-preserving modification
pylorus-preserving pancreatoduo-denectomy (PPPD)
pylorus-preserving resection
pylorus-preserving Whipple procedure
pylorus-sparing Whipple procedure
Pynchon suction tube
pyoderma gangrenosum
pyogenic abscess
pyogenic bacteria
pyogenic cholangitis
pyogenic infection

pyogenic liver
pyogenic liver abscess
pyogenic organism
pyogenic thyroiditis
pyopneumocholecystitis
pyopneumohepatitis
pyopneumoperitoneum
pyopneumoperitonitis
pyopneumothorax, subphrenic
pyostomatitis vegetans
pyramid tip
pyramidal lobe
pyramidal tip trocar
pyramidal trocar
pyrantel pamoate
Pyridium
pyridostigmine
pyriform (see *piriform*)
pyrogen-free heparin
pyroglycolic acid suture
pyrosis (heartburn)
Pyrost graft
pyrrole metabolism
pyruvate kinase deficiency
PYtest (^{14}C urea)
PZI (protamine zinc insulin)

Q, q

QALY (quality-adjusted life-year)
QHS (quantitative hepatobiliary
scintigraphy)
QLI (quality of life index)
QOL (quality of life)
QRS complex
Q-switched neodymium:YAG laser
Q-switched ruby laser
QT change
Quad-Lumen drain
quadrangular positioning plate
quadrant
left lower (LLQ)
left upper (LUQ)
right lower (RLQ)
right upper (RUQ)
quadrant of breast
lower inner
lower lateral
lower medial
lower outer
upper inner
upper lateral
upper medial
upper outer
quadrantectomy, axillary dissection, and
radiotherapy (QUART) for breast
cancer
quadrants, all four
quadrants of abdomen
left lower
left upper
right lower
right upper
quadrate lobe of liver
quadratus lumborum
quadrigeminal plate
Quadripolar cutting forceps
Quadripolar electrosurgical forceps
Quadripolarity
quadruple therapy (bismuth, ranitidine,
amoxicillin, and metronidazole)
QualiCode test
quality-adjusted life-year (QALY)
quality of life (QOL)
quality of life index (QLI)
Quantison imaging agent
quantitative fecal fat test
quantitative hepatobiliary scintigraphy
(QHS)
QUART (quadrantectomy, axillary
dissection, and radiotherapy)
for breast cancer
quartz rod and laser scalpel
Quarzan (clidinium bromide)
quasispecies distribution

queasiness
queasy
Quervain abdominal retractor
query
questionable calcifications
questionnaire, Rhodes Inventory of Nausea and Vomiting
Questran (cholestyramine)
Questran Light (cholestyramine resin)
Questus Leading Edge cutter
Questus Leading Edge grasper
Questus Leading Edge sheathed knife
Quick AC Enema Kit
Quick Bend flex clamp
QuickSilver hydrophilic-coated guide wire
Quick test
QuickVue one-step *H. pylori* test
QuickVue one-step influenza test
QuickVue UrinChek 10+ urine test strips
quiescent hepatitis
quiet bowel sounds
quiflapon sodium
Quilimmune-M vaccine
quilted suture
Quimby scissors
quinacrine HCl
Quincke edema
Quincke lumbar puncture needle
quinidine intoxication
Quinlan test
Quinton Mahurkar dual-lumen peritoneal catheter
Quinton suction biopsy instrument
Quinton tube
quotidian malaria

R, r

rabbit stools
rabeprazole sodium
rabies virus
Rabiner neurological hammer
Rabuteau test
raccoon eyes
race-track oval shaped polypropylene
 mesh graft with pocket
Rachitome
Racobalamin-57 radioactive agent
racquet-shaped incision
RAD Airway laryngeal blade
radial groove
Radial Jaw single-use biopsy forceps
Radial Osteo Compression (ROC)
 soft tissue anchor
radial scar
radial sclerosing lesion
radiating pain
radiation colitis
radiation enteritis
radiation esophagitis
radiation gastritis
radiation-induced colitis
radiation-induced ulceration
radiation, intestinal graft
radiation necrosis
radiation proctitis
radiation proctocolitis
radiation therapy
radical cholecystectomy
radical D2 gastrectomy
radical, free
radical mastectomy, including pectoral
 muscles, axillary and internal
 mammary lymph node (Urban
 operation)
radical mediastinal dissection
radical neck dissection
radical surgery
radicle
 biliary
 intrahepatic
 tertiary
radicular abscess
radioactive agent (see *imaging agent*)
radioactive-labeled marker
radioactive therapy
radiocholesterol analogue
radiocontrast agent
Radiofocus Glidewire
radiofrequency energy
radiofrequency probe
radiograph
radiographic imaging
radiographic procedure

radio-guided parathyroidectomy
radioimmunoassay (see *assay; test*)
radioimmunoluminography
radioiodine ablation
radioiodine-labeled metaiodobenzyl-guanidine (MIBG)
radioiodine scan
radioiodine uptake
radioisotope (see *imaging agent; medications*)
radioisotope bone scan
radioisotope scan
radioisotope scanning of the thyroid
radioisotope scintigraphy
radioisotope stent
radiolabeled peptide alpha-M2
radiolabeled RBC scan
radiologically proven arthritis
radiolucency
radiolucent filling defect
radiolucent gallstone
radiolucent stone
Radiometer GK2803C pH probe
radionuclide esophageal emptying time
radionuclide-labeled leukocytes
radionuclide-labeled platelets
radionuclide scan
radionuclide scanning
radionuclide uptake
radiopacity
radiopaque calculus
radiopaque contrast material
radiopaque density
radiopaque dye
radiopaque gallstone
radiopaque marker
radiopaque Ocrilon polyurethane
radiopaque stone
radiopaque suture
radiopaque Teflon biliary dilating catheter
radiopharmaceutical
radioresistant tumor
radioscintigraphy
radiosensitizer
  Broxine (broxuridine)
  Neomark (broxuridine)
radiotherapy
  adjuvant
  extended-field (EFRT)
  3-D conformal
radiotherapy-induced hypopituitarism
Radius coronary stent
Radius enteral feeding tube
radius of varices
Radolf forceps
RAE endotracheal tube
ragged red appearance
Ragnell-Davis retractor
Ragnell dissecting scissors
Ragnell handheld retractor
Ragnell retractor
railroad track pattern
railroad track scars
Raimondi hemostatic forceps
Raimondi peritoneal catheter
Raimondi scalp forceps
Raimondi spring catheter
Raimondi ventricular catheter
raised, slightly pigmented lesion
rake retractor
rake ulcer
Ralk hand drill
Ralks mallet
raltitrexed
Ramond point
ramoplanin
Rampley sponge-holding forceps
Ramsay tissue forceps
Ramstedt-Fredet pyloromyotomy
Ramstedt pyloroplasty
Randall stone forceps
Randall suction curette
randomized trial
random needle biopsy
random stool sample
Raney clamp
Raney clip

Raney clip-applying forceps
Raney coagulating forceps
Raney cranial drill
Raney hemostasis clip
Raney laminectomy punch
Raney laminectomy rongeur
Raney perforator drill
Raney rongeur forceps
Raney saw
Raney saw guide
Raney scalp clip-applying forceps
Ranfac cholangiographic catheter
Ranfac laparoscopic instruments
range, hepaptotoxic
ranitidine
Rankin clamp
Ranson criteria for acute pancreatitis
ranula
RAO (right anterior oblique) view
RAP (recurrent abdominal pain)
rapacuronium bromide
Rapamune (sirolimus)
rapamycin
raphe, anococcygeal
Rapicide disinfectant/sterilant
rapid-acting anesthetic
rapid emptying of dye
rapid enlargement
Rapide suture
Rapidgraft arterial vessel substitute graft
rapid premature sexual development
rapid pull-through (RPT) esophageal manometry technique
rapid relapse
rapid serum amylase test
rapid transit time
rapid uptake
rapid weight loss
RapiSeal patch
Raplon (rapacuronium bromide) anesthesia
Rappaport classification of gastric lymphoma

rasp, raspatory
  Acufex
  Acufex convex
  Alexander
  Alexander-Farabeuf
  angled
  Aufricht glabellar
  Austin Moore
  Babcock
  Bacon
  Bardeleben
  Black
  Bristow
  Brown
  carbon-tungsten
  Charnley
  convex
  Coryllos
  costal
  Cottle-MacKenty
  DePuy
  diamond
  Doyen costal
  Doyen rib
  Endotrac
  Epstein bone
  Farabeuf bone
  Farabeuf-Collin
  Farabeuf-Lambotte
  Filtzer interbody
  Fisher
  Fomon
  Forman nasal
  Gallagher
  glabellar
  Good
  Herczel rib
  Hylin
  interbody
  intramedullary
  Israel
  Jansen
  Joseph nasal

rasp *(cont.)*
  Key
  Kirmission periosteal
  Kleinert-Kutz
  Koenig
  Lambotte
  Langenbeck
  Lewis periosteal
  Mallory-Head
  Maltz
  Mathieu
  McCabe-Farrior
  McCabe perforation
  McKenty
  micro
  Miller
  Nicola
  Nicoll
  Olivecrona
  Phemister
  Plenk-Matson
  power
  Putti bone
  rib
  Rubin
  Schneider
  Schneider-Sauerbruch
  Seawell
  Sedillot
  Semb rib
  sympathetic
  Thompson
  Yasargil micro
  Zoellner
rasp pin
ratchet on demand
Rathke pouch
Rathke pouch cyst
ratio
  amylase to creatinine clearance
  antigen-antibody
  basal maximal acid output (BAO:MAO)
ratio *(cont.)*
  BCAA/AAA plasma
  effective thyroxine (ETR)
  Hybritech Tandem PSA (free PSA/total PSA)
  insulin:glucose
  lactulose/rhamnose permeability (L/R ratio)
  thyroid hormone-binding (THBR)
  thyroxine/TBG
Ratliff-Blake gallstone forceps
Ratliff-Mayo forceps
rat-tail appearance on pancreatogram
rat-tail sign
rat-tooth forceps
rat-tooth pickup
raw surface of liver bed
Ray-Cot sponge
rayon cotton ball
Raypaque sponge
Ray-Parsons-Sunday staphylorrhaphy elevator
Rayport dural dissector and knife
Rayport muscle biopsy clamp
Ray-Tec x-ray detectable sponge
Ray TFC device
Ray ventricular cannula
razor blade
RBC (red blood cell)
RBC casts
RBC smear
RCF (Ross carbohydrate-free) formula
RC Mini-Open lighted retractor
RCS (red color sign)
RCT (randomized controlled trials)
RDG (retrograde duodenogastroscopy)
RE (reflux esophagitis)
re-FRED the lens
Re-New forceps
Re-New laparoscopic scissors
Re-New laparoscopic surgical tip
Reabilan HN enteral nutritional therapy
reabsorbable suture

reabsorption of H_2O
reaction
  acute hypersensitivity
  antibody-mediated immune (type III)
  argentaffin
  cell-mediated immune
  delayed hypersensitivity
  glucose
  graft versus host
  hot-shot PCR (polymerase chain reaction)
  IgE-mediated immune (type I)
  intragraft PCR (polymerase chain reaction)
  insulin
  PCR (polymerase chain)
  reverse-transcriptase polymerase chain (RT-PCR)
  scar tissue
  Sgambati
  single and rapid polymerase chain reaction/restriction fragment length
  transfusion
reactive hypoglycemia
Read gouge
reagent strips
  Clinistix
  Diascan
  DiaScreen
  First Choice
  Glucofilm
  Glucometer Elite
  Glucometer Encore
  Glucostix
  One Touch
  Tes-Tape
Real coronary artery scissors
real-time electronic imager
real-time ultrasonography
reamer
  acetabular
  Anspach

reamer *(cont.)*
  Arthrex coring
  Aufranc
  Austin Moore
  ball
  barrel
  blunt tapered T-handled
  bone
  brace-type
  calcar
  Campbell
  cannulated Henderson
  chamfer
  Charnley
  Charnley deepening
  Charnley expanding
  Charnley taper
  Charnley trochanter
  Christmas tree
  congruous cup-shaped
  conical
  corrugated
  cup
  deepening
  DePuy
  expanding
  female
  femoral shaft
  fenestrated
  flexible medullary
  grater
  Gray
  grooving
  Hall Versipower
  handle-type
  Harris center-cutting acetabular
  hemispherical
  hollow mill
  Indiana
  Intracone intramedullary
  intramedullary
  Küntscher (Kuentscher) intramedullary
  male

reamer *(cont.)*
  Marin
  medullary canal
  MicroAire
  Mira
  Moore bone
  multisized
  Norton ball
  Perthes
  power
  power-driven
  progressively larger
  Richards
  rigid
  Rotalink flexible-shaft
  Rush awl
  self-centering
  Smith-Petersen
  spherical
  spiral cortical
  spiral trochanteric
  square
  starting
  step-cut
  straight
  Swanson
  tapered
  tapered hand
  T-handled
  triangular bone
  trochanteric
  Wagner acetabular
reaming awl
reanastomosis
reapproximate
reapproximating
Rebar microcatheter
Rebetol (ribavirin)
Rebetron (ribavirin/interferon alfa-2b)
rebiopsy
rebleed
rebound hypocalcemia
rebound pain
rebound sign
rebound tenderness on palpation
rebreathing anesthesia
Recamier curette
recanalization
recanalization reducible mass
recently healed surgical incision
receptor, insulin
receptor protein
receptor status
recess
  azygoesophageal
  cecal
  duodenal
  duodenojejunal
  hepatorenal
  ileocecal
  inferior duodenal
  inferior omental
  intersigmoid
  paracolic
  paraduodenal
  retrocecal
  retroduodenal
  splenic
  splenorenal
  subphrenic
  superior azygoesophageal
  superior duodenal
  superior ileocecal
  superior omental
recipient hepatectomy
recipient, organ
recipient site
reciprocating saw
Reclomide (metoclopramide HCl)
recombinant human thyroid-stimulating hormone (rhTSH)
recombinant human thyroid-stimulating hormone, thyrotropin alfa
recombinant immunoblot assay (RIBA)
Recombivax HB (hepatitis B virus vaccine, recombinant)

reconstruction (see also *breast reconstruction; operation*)
  biliary
  breast
  free flap breast
  full-thickness
  Kiricuta breast
  lateral transverse thigh flap on breast
  Lewis-Tanner subtotal esophagectomy and
  Roux-en-Y esophagojejunostomy
  Rubens flap
  "saddle bags" breast
  transverse rectus abdominis myocutaneous flap
reconstruction nail
reconstruction plate
reconstructive mammoplasty
reconstructive pyloroplasty
recording, esophageal pressure
recovery, organ
Rectacort (hydrocortisone acetate)
Rectagene (live yeast cell derivative; shark liver oil)
rectal abscess
rectal akinesia
rectal alimentation
rectal ampulla
rectal-anal inhibitory reflex
rectal anesthesia
rectal artery
rectal balloon
rectal biopsy forceps
rectal biopsy punch
rectal bleeding
rectal cancer
rectal cellulitis
rectal contrast medium
rectal dilator
rectal distention
rectal endoscopic ultrasonography (REU)
rectal evacuatory disorder
rectal examination
rectal fissure
rectal fistula
rectal fold
  inferior transverse
  superior transverse
rectal granuloma
rectal incontinence
rectal inhibitory reflex
rectal instruments
rectal intussusception
rectal linitis plastica (RLP)
rectal manometry
rectal mucosa
rectal mucosectomy
rectal multiplane transducer
rectal muscle cuff
rectal neovagina
rectal nerve
rectal occlusion clamp
rectal plexus
rectal polyp
rectal pouch
rectal probe
rectal procidentia
rectal prolapse
rectal prolapse repair
rectal reflex
rectal shelf
rectal sleeve advancement
rectal snare
rectal speculum (see *speculum; proctoscope*)
rectal sphincter
rectal stenosis
rectal stricture
rectal stump
rectal submucosal mass
rectal submuscula fluctuance
rectal trauma
rectal tube
rectal valve
rectal varices
rectal vault
rectal vein

rectangular awl
rectangular rod
rectocele
Rectolax (bisacodyl)
rectopexy
  abdominal
  anterior
  Ivalon sponge
  Marlex mesh abdominal
  posterior
  presacral
  Ripstein anterior sling
  Teflon sling
  Wells posterior
rectoproctoscope
rectoscope (see also *anoscope; endoscope*, *proctoscope; speculum*)
  Arakawa
  Blond
  Enproct disposable
  front lifting hood
  Galencia disposable
  Heine
  Ives
  Ives-Fansler
  KleenSpec disposable
  Medix
  pratt
  Romanoscope
  Sani-Scope
  Sapimed
  Sklar
  slotted
  Strauss
  UniSpec disposable
  video
rectosigmoid carcinoma
rectosigmoid colon
rectosigmoid function
rectosigmoid junction
rectosigmoid manometry
rectosigmoidectomy, perineal
rectosigmoidoscopy
rectourethral fistula
rectouterine fold
rectouterine pouch
rectovaginal fistula
rectovaginal pouch
rectovaginal septum
rectovaginopexy procedure
rectovaginouterine pouch
rectovesical fistula
rectovesical pouch
rectovesical septum
rectum, ampulla of
rectus abdominis flap
rectus abdominis muscle
rectus fascia
rectus muscle was divided
rectus muscle was separated
rectus position
rectus sheath
  anterior
  posterior
rectus sheath hematoma
rectus sheath incision
recumbent view
recurrent abdominal pain (RAP)
recurrent appendicitis
recurrent bleeding
recurrent bouts of vomiting
recurrent episodes of diverticulitis
recurrent hepatitis
recurrent hernia
recurrent inguinal hernia
recurrent laryngeal nerve injury
recurrent laryngeal nerve paralysis
recurrent lower GI bleeding
recurrent nerve
recurrent nerve injury
recurrent pain
recurrent pancreatitis
recurrent perirectal abscess
recurrent pyogenic cholangiohepatitis (RPC)
recurrent pyogenic cholangitis
recurrent stricture
recurrent ulcer

recurrent upper respiratory tract infection (RURTI)
recurrent volvulus
recurring acute pancreatitis
recurring hernia
recurring pain
red blood cell casts
red blood cells (RBCs), packed
red cell mass, increased
red cell membrane
red cell surface area
red color sign (RCS)
red light neon laser
red pulp of spleen
red Robinson catheter
red rubber catheter
red wale marking (RWM)
Reddick cystic duct cholangiogram catheter
Reddick grasper
Reddick Olsen forceps
Reddick-Saye screw
Reddick-Saye screw catheter
Reddick-Saye suture
Reddick-Saye suture grasper
reddish-brown tumor mass
reddish tumor
Redifurl TaperSeal IAB catheter
Redigrip pressure bandage
redness and inflammation
Redo intestinal clamp
Redon wound drainage needle
REDS (remote endoscopic digital spectroscopy)
reduced lactose diet
reduced liver transplant (RLT)
reduced-size liver transplant (RSLT)
reduce spontaneously
reduced transhepatic blood flow
reducer
  cannula
  Seal-Up II
  Versaport Plus
reducible hernia
Reducin (somatostatin)
reducing substances in stool
reducing substances test
reduction mammoplasty (see *mammoplasty*)
reduction mastopexy (see *mastopexy*)
redundant hernia sac
redundant loop of bowel
redundant sac tissue
redundant sigmoid
redundant sigmoid loop
redundant tissue
Redux (dexfenfluramine)
reentry
Reese osteotomy guide
Reese's Pinworm (pyrantel pamoate)
Rees-Martel flap forceps
Rees scissors
reexploration
ReFacto (factor VIII SQ, recombinant)
referred epigastric discomfort
referred hip pain
referred pain
referred pain from CO_2 on the diaphragm
referred pain to the tip of the shoulder
referred periumbilical pain
referred right subscapular pain
reflectance spectroscopy
reflectant spectral photometer
reflected portion of Poupart ligament
reflecting edge of ligament
reflection
  costopleural
  hepatoduodenal
  hepatoduodenal-peritoneal
  hepatoduodenoperitoneal
  lateral pleural
  mediastinodiaphragmatic pleural
  peritoneal
  phrenofundal
  sternal pleural
  vertebral pleural

reflex (pl. reflexes)
  abdominal
  abdominocardiac
  absent gag
  accommodation
  acquired
  anal
  arc
  cardiac
  cremasteric
  crossed
  Cushing
  deep tendon (DTRs)
  deglutition
  emetic
  epigastric
  esophagoglottal closure
  esophagosalivary
  gag
  gastrocolic
  gastroileac
  gastroileal
  gastropancreatic
  ileogastric
  intestinointestinal
  open loop
  orienting
  perianal
  peristaltic
  peritoneointestinal
  pharyngeal swallow
  pharyngo-UES (upper esophageal sphincter) contractile
  pharyngoglottal adduction
  rectal
  rectal inhibitory
  rectal-anal inhibitory
  renointestinal
  Rogers
  somatointestinal
  vasovagal
Reflex ELC clip applier
ReFlex wand
reflux
  abdominojugular
  acid
  bile
  cholangiovenous
  duodenobiliary
  duodenogastric (DGR)
  duodenopancreatic
  endoscopy-negative
  esophageal
  free
  gastroesophageal (GER)
  hepatojugular (HJ)
  high-volume
  intrarenal
  long-term duodenobiliary
  nasopharyngeal
  nocturnal gastric
  pathologic
  postmyotomy
  silent
  vesicoureteral
reflux bile gastritis
reflux esophagitis (RE)
reflux gastritis
refluxant
refluxed gastric contents
reflux of gastric contents
refractile material
refractory ascites
refractory bile duct stone
refractory bleeding
refractory constipation
refractory gastroesophageal reflux disease
refractory hepatic hydrothorax
refractory hyperplasia
refractory pain
refractory pancreatic fistula
refractory to conservative treatment
refractory to medical management
refractory to medical therapy
refractory to medication
refrigeration anesthesia

Regan isoenzyme
Regen Biologics, Inc.
regenerating hepatic nodule
regeneration, liver
regenerative polyp
regimen
  antireflux
  chemotherapy
  diabetic
  empiric antibiotic
  medical
  postoperative
  Prevacid triple therapy
  treatment
region
  abdominal
  anal
  ankle
  axillary
  Beckwith-Wiedemann chromosome
  buccal
  calcaneal
  centrilobular
  choledochal
  colonic crypt
  cricopharyngeal
  deltoid
  epigastric
  femoral
  floor of inguinal
  frontal
  gastric pacemaker
  gluteal
  hypochondriac
  hypogastric
  hypopharyngeal
  inguinal
  long segment
  lumbar
  noncutaneous
  pacemaker
  para-aortic
  paraumbilical
  periampullary
region *(cont.)*
  perianal
  periumbilical
  retroperitoneal
  scapular
  subdiaphragmatic perirenal
  suprapubic
  umbilical
  urogenital
regional anesthesia
regional anesthetic
regional colitis
regional enteritis
regional enterocolitis
regional ileitis (Crohn disease)
regional ileocolitis
regional lymph node metastasis
regional lymphatic drainage
Regional Organ Procurement Agency (ROPA)
regional osteopenia in anorexia nervosa
regional spread of infection
regional thoracic lymphadenectomy
registry
  Autologous Bone Marrow Transplant Registry (ABMTR)
  bone marrow transplant
  International Islet Transplant Registry (ITR)
  International Pancreas Transplant Registry
  Laparoscopic Bowel Registry
  organ donor
  tumor
Reglan (metoclopramide HCl)
Regnault type B mastopexy
Regranex (becaplermin) gel
regression, sacral
Regulace (docusate sodium)
regular diet
Regular Iletin II (insulin)
Regular Iletin II U-500 (concentrated) (insulin)
Regular Purified Pork Insulin

regulatory peptide
Regulax SS (docusate sodium)
Reguloid (psyllium hydrophilic mucilloid)
regurgitant esophagitis
regurgitant fraction
regurgitation
  acid
  chronic
  nocturnal
  postural
Regutol
rehabilitation, nutritional
reherniation
Rehfuss test
Rehfuss tube
Rehne abdominal retractor
Rehne-Delorme plication
Rehydralyte (electrolyte solution)
Reichert fiberoptic sigmoidoscope
Reichert flexible sigmoidoscope
Reichert FPS-3 fiberoptic sigmoidoscope
Reichert MH-1 flexible sigmoidoscope
Reichert MS-1 flexible sigmoidoscope
Reichert-Mundinger biopsy needle
Reichert SC-48 flexible sigmoidoscope
Reichmann syndrome
Reich-Nechtow forceps
REI rigid laparoscope
Reimann syndrome
reimplantation of parathyroid glands
Reiner bone rongeur
Reiner plaster knife
Reiner rongeur
reinforced tracheal tube
reinforcing suture
Reinhoff clamp
reinsertion
reinsulate "U" style handle
reintubation
Reitman-Frankel test for SGOT
Reitman-Frankel test for SGPT
rejection
  cardiac transplant
  cellular xenograft
  chronic graft
  graft
  hyperacute
  irreversible
  kidney transplant
  organ
  transplant
rejection response
relaparotomy
relapsing appendicitis
relapsing febrile nodular nonsuppurative panniculitis
relapsing malaria
relapsing pancreatitis
relative
  first-degree
  second-degree
relative contraindications
relative molecular mass
relax the conjoint tendon
relaxation of pylorus
relaxation suture
relaxing incision
Release-NF catheter
release of ACTH
release of exocrine products
Reliance urinary control insert catheter
ReliaSeal skin barrier adhesive
Relia-Vac drain
ReliefBand NST
relief of symptoms
relieved with antacids
relieved with food
relieving incision
Remegel
Remicade (infliximab)
remifentanil
Remington Hobbs diathermy forceps
remission of pain
remittent malaria

remnant of the omphalomesenteric duct
remote access perfusion (RAP) cannula catheter
remote endoscopic digital spectroscopy (REDS)
remote pheochromocytoma
removal of ectopic tissue
removal of extrahepatic duct
removal of foreign body
removal of intact mammary implant
removal with clear margins
remove the appendix from abdomen
Renacidin Irrigation (bladder) solution
renal artery stenosis
renal calculus
renal cell carcinoma
renal dose dopamine
renal edema
renal failure of unknown cause
renal function parameters
renal impression
renal impression on liver
renal lithiasis
renal medulla
renal obstruction
renal papilla
renal parenchymal disease
renal pouch
renal stone
renal threshold for calcium
renal transplant patient
renal tubular acidosis
renal tubular necrosis
renal vasodilation
Rendu-Osler-Weber disease
renin-angiotensin system
renin serum level
Reno-M contrast medium
Reno-M-Dip
Renografin contrast medium
renointestinal reflex
renovascular hypertension
rent (a tear or rupture)
Renu enteral feeding
REO (respiratory enteric orphan) virus
reoperation
reovirus
repaglinide
repair (see *operation*)
repeat endoscopic sclerotherapy
repeat mammogram
repeat thoracentesis
Repel abdominal film
Repela surgical glove
Repel bioresorbable barrier film
Repel-CV abdominal film
reperfusion
reperfusion syndrome
reperitonealization
reperitonealize
repetitive nerve stimulation
replacement, pancreatic enzyme
replantation bandage
Replete enteral nutritional therapy
Replicare dressing
Replicare paste dressing
RepliCare hydrocolloid dressing material
Repliderm collagen-based dressing
Repliderm wound dressing
Repliform graft
Replogle tube
reposable clip applier
reposable trumpet
Repose surgical system
repositionable
reprep
Res-Q-Vac hand-powered suction
rescue treatment
resectable
resected malignant breast tumor
resected segment
resected tissue
resection (see also *operation*)
  abdominoperineal (APR)
  anterior colon
  band and
  colosigmoid

resection *(cont.)*
  curative restorative
  distal
  distal pancreatic
  en bloc
  endometrial
  endoscopic mucosal (EMR)
  esophageal
  gastric
  Harmann
  hepatic
  ileal
  ileocolic
  interval (of redundant sigmoid)
  laparoscopic bowel
  liver
  localized
  Lortat-Jacob hepatic
  low anterior (LAR)
  lung
  lymph node
  Mason abdomino-transsphincteric
  Miles abdominoperineal
  mucosal sleeve
  nipple flap duct
  palliative
  Paul-Mikulicz
  percutaneous
  portal vein
  pylorus-preserving
  segmental colon
  sigmoid
  small bowel
  snare
  surgical
  transsphenoidal
  wedge
resection and colostomy
resection and primary anastomosis of bowel
resection knife
resection of involved segment
resection of lung tumor
resection of pancreatic tail
resection of pylorus
resection of tail of pancreas
resection with Roux-en-Y hepaticojejunostomy
resective colostomy
resectoscope (see *endoscope*)
reservoir (see also *pouch*)
  Camey
  colonic
  continent ileal
  decreased gastric
  double-barrel
  double J-shaped
  fecal
  gastric
  ileal
  ileoanal
  ileoperistaltic
  intra-abdominal ileal
  J ileal
  J-shaped
  J-Vac suction
  Kock ileal
  lateral internal pelvic
  LeBag ileocolic urinary reservoir
  Mainz pouch urinary reservoir
  Parks ileal
  Parks ileoanal
  shunt
  S ileal
  sigmoid colon
  S-shaped
  W-stapled urinary
residual abscess
residual barium
residual calculous material
residual capacity
residual carcinoma
residual flaccid paralysis
residual locoregional differentiated thyroid cancer
residual postoperative hepatolithiasis and intrahepatic strictures
residual stone

residual stool
residual thrombus
residual tumor
resin, bile-salt binding
resistance to portal flow
Resol electrolyte solution
resolution, fluoroscopic
Resolut barrier
Resolut surgical mesh
resorbable pin
resorbable plate
resorbable rod
resorcinol-induced hypothyroidism
Resource enteral feeding
Resource Plus enteral nutritional therapy
respiratory acidosis
respiratory alkalosis
respiratory distress syndrome
respiratory embarrassment
respiratory-esophageal fistula
respiratory inversion point
respiratory obstruction
respiratory quotient
respiratory syncytial virus (RSV)
respiratory virus
response
  biochemical
  end-of-treatment
  end-organ
  fibroblastic tissue
  gag
  gastrocolonic
  inflammatory
  immune
  inflammatory
  postural
  profound catabolic
  rejection
  sustained
  vagal efferent tonic
  vasovagal
  virologic
Response electrophysiology catheter
rest
  bowel
  pancreatic
resting anal sphincter pressure
resting and residual lower esophageal sphincter pressures
resting calcaneal stance position
Reston foam wound dressing
Reston hydrocolloid dressing material
Restore (psyllium hydrophilic mucilloid)
Restore orthobiologic soft tissue implant
restrictive bandage
restrictive pulmonary disease
resuscitation, massive fluid
resuscitative measures
resuscitator
RET gene test for familial medullary thyroid carcinoma
RET proto-oncogene
retained antrum syndrome
retained barium
retained calculus
retained gallstone
retained gastric antrum following incomplete antrectomy
retained suture
retching
retching without emesis
retention
  barium
  chronic stool
  gastric (GR)
  stool
  suture
  water
retention cyst
retention enema
retention esophagitis
retention jaundice
retention meal
retention polyp
retention suture

rete pegs
Rethi incision
reticular network
reticulocyte
reticulocytosis
reticuloendothelial organ
  liver
  lymphatics
  spleen
reticuloendothelial system
reticulum cell sarcoma
reticulum, sarcoplasmic
retinal edema
retinal tumor
retinoblastoma hereditary human
  carcinoma
retinoids
retracted stoma
retraction of clot
retraction of nipples
retraction of skin of breast
retraction suture
retractor
  Adson-Anderson cerebellar
  Adson brain
  Adson cerebellar
  Adson hemilaminectomy
  Adson Zenker artery forceps
  Airlift balloon
  Alan-Parks rectal
  Allison lung
  Allport
  Alm self-retaining
  Alm wound
  amputation
  anal
  Anderson-Adson scalp
  angled
  Ankeney sternal
  appendiceal
  Army-Navy
  Aronson esophageal
  atrial
  Aufranc cobra

retractor *(cont.)*
  automatic skin
  baby Balfour
  baby Balfour abdominal
  baby Deaver
  baby Gelpi
  baby Harrington
  baby Mollison
  baby Roux
  Badgley laminectomy
  Bailey-Gibbon rib contractor
  Balfour abdominal
  Balfour self-retaining
  Ballantine hemilaminectomy
  Bankart shoulder
  Barr rectal
  Beardsley esophageal
  Beckman
  Beckman-Adson laminectomy
  Beckman-Eaton laminectomy
  Beckman thyroid
  Beckman-Weitlaner laminectomy
  B.E. Glass abdominal
  Bennett bone
  Bennett self-retaining
  Bennett tibia
  bent malleable
  bent-tine, forklike
  Berens esophageal
  Berkeley-Bonney self-retaining
    3-blade abdominal
  Billingham-Bookwalter
  Billroth
  blade
  Blount anvil
  Blount hip
  Blount knee
  Bodnar
  bone
  Bookwalter
  Boyes-Goodfellow
  brachial plexus root
  brain
  Breisky

retractor *(cont.)*
Breisky-Navratil
Brooke-Bookwalter retractor
Buck-Gramcko
Budde-Greenberg-Sugita
Buie-Smith
bunion
Burford
Burford-Finochietto
Cairns
Cairns ribbon
Campbell nerve root
Canny Ryall
carotid
Carroll-Bennett
Carroll hand
centrum
cerebellar
cervical disk
Chandler knee
Charnley
Charnley horizontal
Charnley initial incision
Charnley knee
Charnley pin
Charnley retractor
Charnley self-retaining
Charnley vertical
Cherry brain
Cherry laminectomy
Christie gallbladder
Cloward blade
Cloward brain
Cloward cervical
Cloward-Cushing vein
Cloward dural
Cloward-Hoen hemilaminectomy
Cloward-Hoen laminectomy
Cloward lumbar lamina
Cloward nerve root
Cloward skin
Cloward small cervical
Cloward tissue
cobra

retractor *(cont.)*
Collin abdominal
Collis-Taylor
cone
cone laminectomy
cone scalp
Contour scalp
Cooley atrial
Cooley rib
Coryllos
Cottle
Crawford aortic
Crego
Crile
Crile thyroid
Crotti-Kocher thyroid
Crotti thyroid
Cuda
curved
Cushing
Czerny rectal
David Baker bleph
Davidson scapula
Davis
Davis brain
Davis ribbon
Deaver
DeBakey-Cooley
decompression
Delaginiere abdominal
Denis Browne abdominal
Desmarres lid
Doane knee
Dohn-Carton brain
Dott
double-ended right-angle
double-hook Lovejoy
Downey hemilaminectomy
Downing
Doyen abdominal
dural
Durham
D'Errico
D'Errico-Adson

retractor *(cont.)*
- East-West
- Eccentric "Y"
- Echols
- Elite Farley
- endaural
- EndoRetract
- Endotrac
- Enker brain
- eXpose
- Fahey
- fan
- Farabeuf
- Farr spring-wire
- Farr wire
- fat pad
- Favaloro sternal
- Fine cross action
- finger
- Finochietto
- Fisch
- flexible
- FlexPosure endoscopic
- Foerster abdominal ring
- Foss bifid gallbladder
- Foss biliary duct
- Franz abdominal
- Frazier laminectomy
- Frazier lighted brain
- Friedman perineal
- Fritsch abdominal
- Fujita snake
- Fujita suction
- Fukushima
- gallows-type
- Garrett
- GasFree Omni-Lift
- Gazayerli endoscopic
- Gelpi
- Gelpi pediatric
- Gelpi perineal
- Gelpi self-retaining
- Genz-Arm pneumatic
- Gibson-Balfour abdominal

retractor *(cont.)*
- Gifford mastoid
- Gilvernet
- Glaser automatic laminectomy
- Goelet
- goiter
- Goligher
- Gosset appendectomy
- Goulet
- Grant gallbladder
- Green
- Greenberg Universal
- Green thyroid
- Haight-Finochietto rib
- hand
- handheld
- Hands Free
- Hardy spinal
- Harrington
- Harrington splanchnic
- Hartzler rib
- Haverfield-Scoville hemilaminectomy
- Haynes
- Hays hand
- Heaney
- Heaney hysterectomy
- heavy-duty two-tooth
- Hedblom rib
- Heiss soft tissue
- hemilaminectomy
- Henley carotid
- Henner T-model endaural
- Henning
- Hertzler rib
- Hibbs
- Hill rectal
- Hill-Ferguson rectal
- Himmelstein sternal
- Hoen
- Hohmann
- Holscher
- Holzheimer
- horizontal

retractor *(cont.)*
House-Fisch dura
humeral head
humpback Weitlaner
Hupp trachea
Hurd tonsil dissector and pillar
IMA (inferior mesenteric artery)
Inge laminectomy
initial incision
insulated Foman ball
Israel
Jackson
Jannetta posterior fossa
Jansen
Jansen-Wagner
Jarit P.E.E.R.
Joe's hoe
Johns Hopkins gallbladder
Johnson
Joll thyroid
Jordan-Bookwalter
Kartush insulated
Kasdan
Kelly
Kelly abdominal
Kennerdell-Maroon orbital
Kilner
Kilner catspaw
Kilner cheek
Kilner insulated
Kirklin atrial
Kirschner abdominal
Kleinert-Ragdell
Klemme
Knighton
Kocher
Koerte rake
Kuz-Medics total knee
Lahey thyroid
Lahey tissue
lamina
laminectomy
Landon
Lange-Hohmann bone

retractor *(cont.)*
Langenbeck
Langenbeck-Kocher
LaparoLift Airlift balloon
laparoscopic
laser ball
lateral collateral ligament
leaflet
Leyla
LIMAvator chest wall
Little
Lloyd Davies pelvic
Lone Star
Love
Love nerve
Lowman hand
Luer
Luer trachea
Lukens trachea
lumbar lamina
Luongo
Magrina-Bookwalter
Maison
Malcolm-Lynn C-RXF cervical
retractor frame
Malcolm-Rand
Malis brain
malleable
malleable ribbon
Marberger hilar
Markham-Meyerding
Mark II
Mark II Chandler
Martin nerve root
Mason-Judd suprapubic
mastoid
Mathieu
Mayo abdominal
Mayo-Adams abdominal
Mayo-Adams appendectomy
Mayo-Collins
Mediflex-Gazayerli
meniscus
metacarpal

retractor *(cont.)*
Meyerding finger
Meyerding laminectomy
Meyerding self-retaining
Micro-Retractor
microretractor
Middeldorpf
Mikulicz abdominal
Mikulicz fiberoptic
Millan retropubic
Miller-Senn
mini Hohmann podiatric
mini Metzenbaum
mini Roux
Miskimon
Mollison
Moon rectal
Morris
Murphy
Murphy gallbladder
Myers knee
narrow blade
narrow neck mini-Hohmann
Navratil
Nelson rib
nerve root
Nevyas drape
Norfolk-Norwich
North-South
Oberhill laminectomy
Ochsner ribbon
Oettingen abdominal
Oldberg brain
Olivier
Ollier rake
Omni
Omni-Lift
Omni-Tract adjustable wishbone
ophthalmic
optical
orbital
O'Sullivan-O'Connor abdominal
Paparella
Parker

retractor *(cont.)*
Parks anal
Parks sphincterotomy
Paulson knee
pediatric ribbon
pediatric Deaver
Penfield
Percy amputation
Percy-Wolfson gallbladder
Perkins
Perkins left
Perkins otologic
Perkins right
pin
pitchfork
Pitie-Salpetriere saphenous vein hook
Pittman IMA
Plester self-retaining
Polytrac Gomez
Poppen-Gelpi laminectomy
posterior fossa
Pratt bivalve
Protractor wound
Quervain abdominal
Ragnell-Davis
Ragnell handheld
rake
RC Mini-Open lighted
Rehne abdominal
retropubic
rib
ribbon
Richards abdominal
Richardson abdominal
Richardson appendectomy
Richardson-Eastman
Rigby appendectomy
right-angle
ring abdominal
R-Med mini retractor
Robin-Masse abdominal
Robotrac passive retraction system
Rochard abdominal

retractor *(cont.)*
Rollet
Roos brachial plexus root
Rosenberg
Rosenkranz pediatric
Rosenkranz pediatric sternal
Rosenkranz universal malleable
Roux
Roux-Magnus
Rowe capsular
Rowe humeral head
S
Sachs vein
SaphLITE, SaphLITE II
Sauerbruch
Sawyer rectal
scalp
Schink
Schoenborn trachea
Schwartz laminectomy
Scoville
Scoville-Haverfield
Scoville-Richter
Seletz-Gelpi
self-retaining
Semb lung
Senn double-end
Senn-Green
Senn-Kanavel
Senn-Miller catspaw
Sewell
sharp
Sheldon hemilaminectomy
Sherwin knee
Simon abdominal
Sims
single-hook auto
SJM Rosenkranz pediatric
skid humeral head
skin (trachea)
small rake
Smillie knee
Smillie meniscus hook
Smith anal

retractor *(cont.)*
Smith-Buie rectal
Smith nerve root suction
Smith rectal
snake
Snitman endaural
Sofield
Space-OR flexible internal
Spacekeeper
splanchnic
spoon
spring-wire
Spurling nerve root
S-shaped
St. Mark's deep pelvic
Stack hand
staple-shaped
sternal
stiff ribbon
Stiwer
straight
Stryker illuminated
Stuck
suction
"sweetheart" (Harrington)
Sydney Hospital
Taylor self-retaining
Teflon-coated brain
Temple-Fay
tibial
Tiemann shoulder
toothed
tracheal
Travers
trigeminal nerve
Tuffier abdominal
Tuffier-Raney
Tupper
two-prong rake
U.S.
U.S.A.
U.S. Army
universal
University of Minnesota

retractor *(cont.)*
 Upper Hands self-retaining
 U-shaped
 vaginal-cervical Ahluwalia retractor-elevator (VCARE)
 Valin hemilaminectomy
 vein
 Verbrugge-Hohmann bone
 Versatrac lumbar
 vertebral body
 vertical
 vessel
 Volkmann rake
 Wagner
 Walker gallbladder
 Walton
 Walton ribbon
 Wassmund
 Weary nerve root
 Webb-Balfour abdominal
 Weinberg vagotomy
 Weitlaner
 Weitlaner-Beckman
 Wertheim
 Wesson perineal
 West
 Wilkinson abdominal
 Wilson gonad
 Wiltse-Bankart
 Wiltse-Gelpi
 Wink
 wishbone
 Wolfson gallbladder
 Wullstein
 Wylie splanchnic
 Xomed Kartush insulated
 Zenker
 Zinn
retriever
 Carroll tendon
 Soehendra stent
retrobulbar anesthesia
retrocecal abscess
retrocecal appendix
retrocecal recess
retrocecal tissue
retrocolic appendix
retrocolic choledochojejunostomy
retrocolic end-to-side choledochojejunostomy
retrocrural space
retroduodenal artery
retroduodenal fossa
retroduodenal recess
retroesophageal position
retroflexed scope
retroflexed view
retrogastric-retrocolic tunnel
retrogastric tunnel
retrograde adrenal venography
retrograde Beaver blade
retrograde blade
retrograde cannulation
retrograde fashion
retrograde femoral nail
retrograde flow (on barium enema)
retrograde grasping forceps, double-action
retrograde ileoscopy
retrograde intussusception
retrograde knife
retrograde peristalsis
retrograde sphincterotomy
retrograde urethrogram (RUG)
retrograde venography
retrohepatic vena cava
retroileal appendix
retromammary space view
retropancreatic tunnel
retroperitoneal abscess
retroperitoneal approach
retroperitoneal cavity
retroperitoneal drainage
retroperitoneal fibrosis
retroperitoneal fistula
retroperitoneal hemorrhage
retroperitoneal hernia
retroperitoneal-iliopsoas abscess

retroperitoneal injury
retroperitoneal mass lesion
retroperitoneal organ
retroperitoneal region
retroperitoneal sarcoma
retroperitoneal space
retroperitoneal varices
retroperitoneal veins
retroperitoneally
retroperitoneoscopy
retroperitoneum
retropharyngeal approach
retropharyngeal position
retropubic prostatectomy
retropubic retractor
retrorectal abscess
retrosternal chest pain
retrovascular goiter
retrovirus, human mammary tumor
Retter aneurysm needle
Retter knot tier and ligature carrier
return of bowel sounds
Retzius
  space of
  system of
  vein of
REU (rectal endoscopic ultra-sonography)
reusable cannula
reusable grasper
ReVele imaging agent
Reverdin abdominal spatula
Reverdin epidermal free graft
Reverdin suture needle
reverse cutting suture
reversed Mercedes Benz sign
reversed peristalsis
reverse sphincterotome
reverse T3 or rT3
reverse-transcriptase polymerase chain reaction (RT-PCR) analysis
reverse Trendelenburg position
Revised Trauma Score
RevitaLase erbium cosmetic laser
Rexam Medical Packaging
Rex-Cantli-Serege line
Reye syndrome
Reynold pentad (Charcot triad plus altered mental status and shock)
Reynolds dissecting scissors
Reynolds vascular clamp
Rezipas (aminosalicylic acid)
Rezulin (troglitazone)
Rezyme
RFLP (restriction fragment length polymorphism)
R.F. tissue ablation device
RGEA (right gastroepiploic artery)
rhabdoid suture
rhabdomyolysis
rhabdomyoma
rhabdomyosarcoma
rhabdovirus
Rheaban (activated attapulgite)
Rheinstadter curette
Rheomacrodex (dextran 40) plasma volume expander
rhesus rotavirus-tetravalent vaccine (RRV-TV)
rheumatic lesion
rheumatoid panel
rheumatology panel
Rhinelander pin
Rhinoline endoscopic system
RhoC gene
RhoC GTPase gene
rhodanine stain
Rhode Island dissector sponge
Rhodes Inventory of Nausea and Vomiting
Rhoton ball dissector
Rhoton bayonet scissors
Rhoton bipolar forceps
Rhoton cup forceps
Rhoton curet
Rhoton-Cushing forceps
Rhoton dissecting forceps
Rhoton elevator

Rhoton enucleator
Rhoton forceps
Rhoton fork
Rhoton hook
Rhoton loop curet
Rhoton-Merz suction tube
Rhoton micro curet
Rhoton micro dissector
Rhoton needle
Rhoton needle holder
Rhoton osteotome
Rhoton pituitary curet
Rhoton punch
Rhoton scissors
Rhoton sellar punch
Rhoton spatula dissector
Rhoton spoon curet
Rhoton suction tip
Rhoton-Tew bipolar forceps
rhTSH (recombinant human thyroid-stimulating hormone)
RHV (right hepatic vein)
RIA (radioimmunoassay)
rib contractor
rib elevator
rib forceps
rib hook
rib rasp
rib retractor
rib shears (see shears)
Riba 3.0 SIA reagent kit for hepatitis C
RIBA (recombinant immunoblot assay)
RIBA HCV 3.0 SIA (strip immunoblot assay)
ribavirin and interferon alfa-2b
Ribble bandage
ribbon, iridium
ribbon retractor
ribbon stools
ribonuclease
ribovirus
rice-flour breath test
rice-fruit diet
rice-water stool
Richard Allen clip applier
Richards abdominal retractor
Richards angle guide
Richards mallet
Richards reamer
Richards reconstruction nail
Richards side plate
Richards-Hirschhorn plate
Richardson abdominal retractor
Richardson appendectomy retractor
Richardson-Eastman retractor
Richardson retractor
Richardson rod
Richard Wolf instruments and devices
Riches artery forceps
Riches diathermy artery forceps
Richet bandage
Richet fascia umbilicus
Richmar external ultrasound unit
Richter-Heath clip-removing forceps
Richter hernia
Richter laminectomy punch forceps
Richter-Monroe line
rickets, celiac
rickettsial infection
Ricord rectal speculum
ridge extension
ridge, pectineal
Ridlon plaster knife
Riechmann rod
Riedel lobe
Riedel struma
Riedel thyroiditis
Riepe-Bard gastric balloon
Riester economy otoscope
rifaximin
Rift Valley fever virus
Rigby appendectomy retractor
Riger, classic triad of
right adrenalectomy
right and left lateral coronary ligament
right and left lobes of the liver
right-angle chest tube
right-angle clamp

right-angle clip applier
right-angle dental drill
right-angle dissector
right-angle hook
right-angle knife
right-angle retractor
right-angle scissors
right antero-oblique position
right atrial pressure
right auricular appendix
Right Clip
right-cutting knife
right colectomy with ileostomy
right colic artery
right colon
right colonic flexure
right costal margin
right gastric artery
right gastroepiploic artery (RGEA)
right gastroepiploic vein
right gutter
right hemicolectomy
right hepatic artery injury
right hepatic duct injury
right hepatic lobectomy
right ileal fossa
right iliac fossa
right lateral decubitus position
right lateral decubitus view
right lobe
right lobe cyst
right lobe of liver
right lobe of thyroid
right lower quadrant
right pleural effusion
right-sided abdominal pain
right-sided congestive heart failure
right-sided lesion
right-sided mass
right-sided nail
right subcostal incision
right subdiaphragmatic space
right subscapular pain
right subscapular region
right upper quadrant (RUQ)
right upper quadrant mass
right upper quadrant pain
rigid biopsy forceps
rigid cervical collar
rigid dressing
rigid endoscope
rigid endoscopic access
rigid esophagoscopy
rigidity
  abdominal
  board-like
  involuntary reflex
rigid-lens endoscope
rigid reamer
rigid scoop
rigid sigmoidoscope
Rigiflex balloon dilator
Rigiflex TTS balloon catheter
Rigler sign (on x-ray)
Rigler, triad of
RIGScan
RIGScan CR49
Riley-Day syndrome (familial
  dysautonomia)
rim of fascia
rim sign
ring
  abdominal
  anorectal
  apex of external
  crural
  distal esophageal
  esophageal A
  esophageal B
  esophageal contractile
  esophageal mucosal
  esophageal muscular
  external
  external inguinal
  hemorrhoidal O
  ilioinguinal
  iliopsoas
  inguinal

ring *(cont.)*
  internal
  internal abdominal
  internal inguinal
  intrahaustral contraction
  Kayser-Fleischer
  Ochsner
  pyloric
  Schatzki
  Silastic
  silicone elastomer
  sphincter contraction
  superficial inguinal
ring abdominal retractor
ring abscess
Ring catheter
ring-cutter blade
ring cutter, finger
Ringer lactate
ring forceps
ring insertion tool
ringlike contractions
Ring–McLean sump tube
ring of esophagus, A or B
ring retractor
ring-shaped cluster
ring-wall lesion
Riopan (magaldrate)
Riopan Plus 2
Riordan pin
Ripstein anterior sling rectopexy
Rish periosteal elevator
rising hematocrit
rising intracranial pressure
risk factor
risk marker
risk of perforation
Ritebite biopsy forceps
Ritter SpeedClave
Ritter UltraClave
Rivas vascular catheter
Riwolith Impalso Pressure Generator
Riza-Ribe grasper needle
RLP (rectal linitis plastica)
RLQ (right lower quadrant)
RLT (reduced liver transplant)
R-Med mini retractor
R-Med plug
RNA molecule
RNA polymerase, virally encoded
RNA tumor virus
RNA virus (ribovirus)
Ro-Bile
Robbers forceps
Robengatope radioactive agent
Robert Jones bulky soft dressing with
  Hemovac drainage
Robert Jones dressing
Robert Shaw bronchus tube
Roberts artery forceps
Roberts-Gill periosteal elevator
Robertson sign
Robertson suture
Roberts rib shears
Robin-Masse abdominal retractor
Robinson catheter, red rubber
Robinson-Kepler-Power water test
Robinul, Robinul Forte (glycopyrrolate)
robin's egg–blue gallbladder
robot
  AESOP 2000 and 3000
  ZEUS robotic system
robot-assisted procedure
robot neurosurgical microscope
robotic surgery device, AESOP
  (Automated Endoscopic System
  for Optimal Positioning)
robotics, SurgiScope
Robotrac passive retraction system
Robotrac retractor
Robson point
Robson position
ROC EZ anchor
ROC EZ suture anchor
ROC suture fastener
ROC XS suture anchor
ROC XS suture fastener
Rocaltrol (calcitriol)

ROCAP syringe
Rochard abdominal retractor
Rochester-Carmalt forceps
Rochester gallstone forceps
Rochester lamina elevator
Rochester-Mixter forceps
Rochester-Ochsner forceps
Rochester-Péan clamps
Rochester-Péan forceps
Rochester-Péan hemostats
Rochester spinal elevator
Rockey-Davis incision
rod
  absorbable
  acetabular cup detaching
  acetabular cup push (pushing)
  Acufex TAG
  alignment
  Alta tibial/humeral
  Amset R-F
  auto-reinforced polyglycolide
  bendable metallic
  Bickel intramedullary
  Biethium ostomy
  biodegradable
  C-D or CD (Cotrel-Dubousset)
  colostomy
  compression
  Dacron-impregnated silicone
  degradable polyglycolide
  distraction
  Edwards-Levine
  Edwards reverse ratchet
  Ender
  Fixateur Interne
  fluted medullary
  gram-negative
  grooved titanium
  Hall
  Harrington compression
  Harrington distraction
  Harris condylocephalic
  Hartshill rectangle
  hinge

rod *(cont.)*
  humeral
  Hunter Silastic
  Hunter tendon
  Ilizarov telescoping
  impactor
  Isola
  Jacobs distraction
  Kaneda
  Knodt compression
  knurled
  Kostuik
  Küntscher (Kuentscher) condylocephalic
  Luque
  Meckel
  Moe distraction
  Moe-modified Harrington
  Moss
  Mouradian
  Olerud PSF
  partially threaded
  pedicular
  PMMA (polymethylmethacrylate)
  polyglactin
  polyglycolide, self-reinforced
  PWB (Puno-Winter-Byrd)
  rectangular
  Reichmann
  resorbable
  Richardson
  Rogozinski spinal
  Rush
  Russell-Taylor reconstruction
  Sage
  Schanz
  Schmidt
  Schneider
  Seidel humeral
  Seidel intramedullary
  Selby I and II
  Serrato forearm
  Silastic
  silicone flexor

rod *(cont.)*
 Smith & Nephew Richards
 spinal
 Steffee pedicular
 Stenzel
 straight threaded
 Synthes
 telescopic
 telescoping medullary
 tendon
 threaded
 titanium alloy
 top-loading
 True/Fit femoral intramedullary
 TSRH (Texas Scottish Rite Hospital)
 U Luque vertebral
 Ultimax distal femoral intramedullary
 V-A alignment
 VDS (ventral derotating spinal) compression
 VSF (Vermont spinal fixator)
 Wiltse
 Wissinger
 Zickel
 Zielke
rod bender
rod clamp
rodent ulcer
Rodney Smith biliary stricture repair
Roeder loop
roentgen knife
roentgen knife stereotaxic radiosurgical device
roentgen radiosurgical knife
rofecoxib
Roger Anderson pin
Roger syndrome
Roger wire scissors
Rogers reflex
Rogers wire-cutting scissors
Rogozinski hook
Rogozinski spinal rod
Roho air-filled mattress
Rokitansky-Aschoff sinus
Rokitansky-Cushing ulcer
Rokitansky disease
Rokitansky diverticulum
Rolaids, Calcium Rich
roll (noun)
roller forceps
RollerLOOP cautery
Rollet retractor
rolling hiatal hernia
Rolyan Firm D-Ring wrist support
Rolyan Gel Shell splint
Romanoscope anoscope
Romano surgical curved drilling system
Rome I and II criteria for irritable bowel syndrome
rongeur (see also *forceps*)
 Adson cranial
 angled jaw
 angled pituitary
 angular bone
 Bacon
 Bacon bone
 Baer bone
 Bane-Hartmann bone
 Bane mastoid
 basket
 bayonet
 Bethune
 Beyer
 Beyer-Stille bone
 Blumenthal bone
 Böhler (Boehler) bone
 bone-nibbling
 Bruening-Citelli
 Bucy laminectomy
 Campbell
 cervical laminectomy
 Cherry-Kerrison laminectomy
 Cicherelli bone
 Cintor bone
 Cleveland bone
 Cloward-English laminectomy
 Cloward-Harper laminectomy

rongeur *(cont.)*
- Cloward intervertebral disk
- Cloward pituitary
- Codman-Kerrison laminectomy
- Codman-Leksell laminectomy
- Codman-Schlesinger cervical laminectomy
- Cohen
- Colclough-Scheicher laminectomy
- Corbett bone
- Cottle-Kazanjiann
- cranial
- curved bone
- Cushing
- Cushing cranial
- Cushing intervertebral disk
- Cushing pituitary
- Dahlgren cranial
- Dale first rib
- Dean bone
- Decker microsurgical
- Decker pituitary
- Defourmentel bone
- DeVilbiss cranial
- disk
- double-action
- down-biting
- duckbill
- Echlin bone
- Echlin duckbill
- Echlin laminectomy
- Echlin-Luer
- Ferris Smith intervertebral disk
- Ferris Smith-Kerrison laminectomy
- Ferris Smith laminectomy
- Ferris Smith pituitary jaw
- Ferris Smith-Spurling disk
- Fine-Kerrison cervical
- first rib
- Fisch bone
- FlexTip
- FlexTip intervertebral
- Friedman bone
- Frykholm bone

rongeur *(cont.)*
- Fulton laminectomy
- Geiger
- Giertz
- gooseneck
- Gruenwald neurosurgical
- Guleke bone
- Hajek antrum
- Hajek-Koffler laminectomy
- Hakansson bone
- Hartmann bone
- Hein
- Hoen intervertebral disk
- Hoen laminectomy
- Horsley bone
- Hudson cranial
- Husk bone
- intervertebral disk
- Jackson intervertebral disk
- Jansen
- Jarit-Kerrison laminectomy
- Jarit-Liston bone
- Jarit-Ruskin bone
- Kerrison
- Kerrison down-biting
- Kerrison laminectomy
- Kleinert-Kutz bone
- Kleinert-Kutz synovectomy
- laminectomy
- Lebsche
- Leksell laminectomy
- Leksell-Stille thoracic
- Lempert bone
- Liston bone
- Liston-Littauer bone
- Littauer-West
- Love-Gruenwald intervertebral disk
- Love-Gruenwald pituitary
- Love-Kerrison cervical
- Love-Kerrison laminectomy
- Luer bone
- Luer-Friedman bone
- Luer-Hartmann
- Malcolm-Lynn

rongeur *(cont.)*
- Markwalder bone
- Marquardt bone
- Mayfield
- McIndoe bone
- Mead
- Mead bone
- Micro-Kerrison
- microlaminectomy
- Midas-Rex
- Miltex-Kerrison cervical
- mini-Ruskin
- monster rongeur
- Montenovesi
- Mount laminectomy
- Müller (Mueller)
- Nicola pituitary
- Oldberg intervertebral disk
- Oldberg pituitary
- Olivecrona
- osteophyte nipper
- peapod intervertebral disk
- Peiper-Beyer laminectomy
- Pilling-Liston
- pituitary
- Poppen intervertebral disk
- Raney laminectomy
- Reiner bone
- Rottgen-Ruskin bone
- Ruskin bone
- Ruskin-Jansen bone
- Ruskin-Jay
- Ruskin-Liston bone
- Ruskin-Rowland bone
- Rust
- Sauerbruch-Coryllos
- Sauerbruch rib
- Sauerbruch-Stille
- Schell bone
- Schlesinger cervical
- Schlesinger intervertebral disk
- Schlesinger laminectomy
- Schlesinger pituitary

rongeur *(cont.)*
- Selverstone intervertebral disk
- Semb
- Semb-Stille bone
- Shearer
- single-action
- Smith-Petersen laminectomy
- Spence intervertebral disk
- Spurling intervertebral disk
- Spurling-Kerrison cervical
- Spurling-Kerrison laminectomy
- Spurling-Kerrison up-biting and down-biting
- Spurling pituitary
- Stellbrink synovectomy
- Stille-Horsley bone
- Stille-Leksell
- Stille-Liston bone
- Stille-Luer bone
- Stille-Luer duckbill
- Stille-Luer-Echlin
- Stille-Ruskin bone
- Stookey cranial
- straight bone
- straight pituitary
- Strully-Gigli
- Strully-Kerrison
- synovectomy
- Takahashi
- thoracic
- up-biting
- Urschel first rib
- Walton-Liston bone
- Walton-Ruskin bone
- Watson-Williams intervertebral disk
- Weil-Blakesley intervertebral disk
- Whitcomb-Kerrison laminectomy
- Wilde intervertebral disk
- Yasargil pituitary
- Zaufel-Jansen bone

rongeur forceps

roof of abdomen

roof plate

room
  insufflation tank
  laparoendoscopic
  postanesthesia recovery
room air
Roos brachial plexus root retractor
Roos first rib shears
Roosevelt clamp
root
  anatomical
  brachial plexus
  lung
  nerve
root needle
root of small bowel mesentery
root of sigmoid mesentery
ROPA (Regional Organ Procurement Agency)
ropivacaine
ropy bile
Roschke rectal speculum
Rosch-Uchida transjugular liver access needle-catheter
rose bengal sodium (^{131}I-labeled) hepatic function test
rose bengal test
Rose-Bradford kidney
rosebud sponge
Rosenbach sign
Rosenbach-Gmelin test
Rosenberg retractor
Rosen elevator
Rosen fenestrometer
Rosen incision knife
Rosenkranz deep retractor blade
Rosenkranz pediatric retractor system
Rosenkranz pediatric sternal retractor
Rosenkranz universal clamp
Rosenkranz universal malleable retractor
Rosenkranz wire-basket retractor
Rosen needle
Rosen separator
Rosen suction tube
Rosenthal test
Rose position
Rose retractor
rose-thorn ulcer
rosette appearance of anus
rosette Beaver blade
rosette blade
Rosetti stitch
Rosetti technique for Nissen fundoplication
Rosidal bandage
rosiglitazone maleate
Rosser crypt hook
Rossetti modification of Nissen fundoplication
rosuvastatin
Rotablator abrasive bur
ROTACS guidewire
Rotalink flexible-shaft reamer
Rotamune vaccine
rotary basket punch
rotary forceps
rotary gamma scalpel
rotary punch
rotary scissors
RotaShield vaccine (rotavirus, live)
rotating lock
rotating sphincterotome
rotating wheel, large
Rotator Cuff Buttress (RCB) plate
rotatory scissors
rotavirus antigen
rotavirus diarrhea
rotavirus DNA virus
rotavirus gastroenteritis, diarrhea
rotavirus in stool specimen
Rotazyme test
Rotex cutting biopsy needle
Rotex II biopsy needle
Roth Grip-Tip suture guide
Roth polyp retrieval net
Roth retrieval net
roticulating endograsper
roticulator, Endo Grasp

roticulator stapler
Rotor syndrome
Rotter lymph node
Rotter node
Rottgen-Ruskin bone rongeur
rotund abdomen
roughage
round cell infiltration
round cell sarcoma
round cup forceps
round ligament (ligamentum teres)
round nose grasper
round stick sponge
round-tapped periosteal elevator
round ulcer
roundworm (nematode)
Rous-associated virus (RAV)
Rous sarcoma virus (RSV)
Rousek extractor
route, enteral administration
route of spread
routine magnification view
Roux-en-Y (also Roux-Y)
Roux-en-Y anastomosis
Roux-en-Y biliary bypass with
antrectomy
Roux-en-Y chimney surgical technique
Roux-en-Y choledochojejunostomy
Roux-en-Y cystojejunostomy
Roux-en-Y distal jejunoileostomy
Roux-en-Y esophagojejunostomy
reconstruction
Roux-en-Y gastric bypass
Roux-en-Y gastroenterostomy
Roux-en-Y gastrojejunostomy
Roux-en-Y hepaticojejunostomy
Roux-en-Y jejunoileostomy
Roux-en-Y limb
Roux-en-Y limb to gastric pouch
Roux-en-Y loop
Roux-en-Y pancreaticojejunostomy
Roux-en-Y procedure with vagotomy
Roux limb
Roux-Magnus retractor
Roux retractor
Rovsing sign
Rowasa (mesalamine) enema
Rowe capsular retractor
Rowe disimpaction forceps
Rowe glenoid punch
Rowe glenoid-reaming forceps
Rowe-Harrison bone-holding forceps
Rowe humeral head retractor
Rowe-modified Harrison forceps
roxatidine, roxatidine acetate HCl
Roxicodone (oxycodone)
Roxin (roxatidine acetate HCl)
Roy-Camille cervical plate
Roy-Camille occipitocervical plate
Roy-Camille pedicle plate
Royl-Derm wound cleanser/dressing
rPAF-AH (platelet-activating factor
acetylhydrolase, recombinant)
RPC (recurrent pyogenic cholangio-
hepatitis)
RP-HPLC (reverse phase-high perform-
ance liquid chromatography)
RPR (rapid plasma reagin) test
RPT (rapid pull-through) technique
RQ (respiratory quotient)
RR (respiratory rate)
rRNA ribosomal RNA
RRV-TV (rhesus rotavirus-tetravalent)
vaccine
RSLT (reduced-size liver transplant)
RSP thermocoupler
RSP thermocouple sensor
rubber band hemorrhoidal ligator
rubber band hemorrhoidectomy
rubber band ligation of hemorrhoid
rubber band ligature
rubber band loader
rubber dam
rubber drain
rubber pickup
rubber seton
rubber-shod clamp
rubber tube

rubbery change
rubbery consistency
rubbery gray mass
rubbery nodule
rubbery texture
rubella virus
Ruben gouge
Rubens flap for breast reconstruction
Rubin rasp
Rubin-Quinton small bowel biopsy tube
Rubinstein-Taybi syndrome
Rubio-TC wire twister
rubitecan
Rubratope-57 radioactive agent
ructus
Rudd-Clinic hemorrhoidal forceps
Rudd-Clinic ligator
Rudd hemorrhoidal ligator
rudimentary lung
Ruel forceps
ruga (pl. rugae)
rugal folds
rugal pattern
rule, Goodsall
rule of nines (9's)
rule of tens (10's)
rule of two (2)
rule of two-thirds (2/3)
rule out sepsis
RuLox (aluminum hydroxide; magnesium hydroxide)
rumble (bowel sounds)
rumbling bowel sounds
Rumel artery forceps
Rumel thoracic clamp
Rumel tourniquet flex cannula
rumination
running lock suture
running suture
runny stools
runs (noun) (diarrhea)
runs an oblique course
runting syndrome

rupture
- aneurysm
- appendix
- bladder
- blunt
- complete
- congenital aneurysm
- cystic duct
- delayed splenic
- diaphragmatic
- duodenal
- ERCA-induced
- esophageal
- gastric
- hepatic
- hernia
- intramural esophageal
- intraperitoneal viscus
- large bladder
- Mallory-Weiss mucosal
- membrane
- mesenteric
- peritoneal
- portal vessel
- postemetic esophageal
- splenic
- splenic vessel
- spontaneous
- traumatic
- umbilical hernia

ruptured AAA (abdominal aortic aneurysm)
ruptured aneurysm
ruptured aortic atheromatous plaque
ruptured appendix
ruptured disk
ruptured duodenum following blunt abdominal trauma
ruptured ectopic pregnancy
ruptured fallopian tube
ruptured follicle
ruptured hernia
ruptured intraperitoneal viscus
ruptured membrane

ruptured perineum
ruptured spleen
RUQ (right upper quadrant)
Ruschelit PVC tracheostomy tube
Rush awl reamer
rushes (bowel sounds), peristaltic
Rush flexible medullary nail
Rush mallet
Rush pin
Rush rod
Ruskin antrum trocar needle
Ruskin bone-cutting forceps
Ruskin bone rongeur
Ruskin bone-splitting forceps
Ruskin-Jansen bone rongeur
Ruskin-Jay rongeur
Ruskin-Liston bone cutter
Ruskin-Liston bone-cutting forceps
Ruskin-Liston bone rongeur
Ruskin rongeur forceps
Ruskin-Rowland bone-cutting forceps
Ruskin-Rowland bone rongeur
Russe bone graft
Russell gastrostomy kit
Russell percutaneous endoscopic gastrostomy
Russell-Taylor (R-T) nail
Russell-Taylor interlocking medullary nail
Russell-Taylor reconstruction rod
Russian forceps
Russian tissue forceps
Rust amputation saw
rust-colored papule
Rust rongeur
Rutherford-Morrison tissue forceps
Rutkow and Robbins
Rutkow-Robbins-Gilbert classification of groin hernias (types 1–7)
Rutkow sutureless plug and patch
Rutzen ileostomy bag
Ruysch disease
RX Herculink 14 biliary stent system
RX Herculink 14 premounted stent system
Rydell nail
Ryder micro needle holder
Ryder needle
Ryder needle holder
Ryder-TC needle holder
Ryerson bone graft
Ryle tube

S, s

Saathoff test
Saber BT blunt-tip surgical trocar
saber-cut incision
Sable catheter
Sabreloc conventional spatula
Sabreloc spatula
Sabreloc spatula needle
Sabreloc suture
sac
  abdominal
  air
  anal
  aneurysmal
  aortic
  endolymphatic
  enterocele
  fluid-filled
  gestational
  greater peritoneal
  hernia
  indirect hernia
  lesser peritoneal
  pericardial
  peritoneal
  Pleatman
  redundant hernia
  wide-mouth
saccharin
sacciform kidney
saccular colon
sacculation
Sachs brain suction tube
Sachs dural hook
Sachs nerve separator and spatula
Sachs suction tube
Sachs vein retractor
Sacks-Vine feeding gastrostomy tube
Sacks-Vine PEG (percutaneous endoscopic gastrostomy) tube
sacral anesthesia
sacral fixation
sacral promontory
sacral regression
sacrifice of facial nerve
sacrifice of lateral cremasteric bundle
sacroabdominoperineal pull-through
sacrococcygeal teratoma
sacrocolposuspension
sacrofixation operation
sacrogenital fold
sacroperineal approach
sacrosidase enzyme replacement therapy
saddle anesthesia

saddle block anesthesia
saddle clamp
S-adenosyl-methionine (SAMe)
Sadowsky hook wire
Saf-Clens chronic wound cleanser
SafeTap tapered spinal needle
Safetrak epidural needle
Safety AV fistula needle
safety shield
safety-shielded trocar
Saf-Gel hydrogel dressing
Safil synthetic absorbable surgical suture
Saf-T E-Z translucent needle shield
sage-grain stools
Sage rod
SAGES (Society of American Gastrointestinal Endoscopic Surgeons)
Sage triangular nail
sagittal cranial suture
sagittal plane
sagittal septum of rectus sheath
sagittal surgical saw
sagittal ultrasonography
sago-grain stool
sago liver
Sahli biopsy and aspiration needle
Sahli glutoid test
Sahli-Nencki test
Saint triad
SAL (suction-assisted lipectomy)
SAL (suction-assisted lipoplasty)
salazosulfapyridine
Salem duodenal sump tube
Salenius meniscus knife
Salibi carotid artery clamp
salicylate abuse
salicylate poisoning
salicylazosulfapyridine
saline breast implant
saline cleansing enema
saline continence test
saline drop test
saline flows freely
saline flush
saline infusion
Salinem infection
saline-moistened sponge
saline, normal
saline solution
saline test
Salinetrode electrode
Salisbury common cold virus
saliva aspiration
salivary amylase (S-type)
salivary calculus
salivary gland tumor
salivary gland virus
salivary stone
salivary tumor
Salkowski and Schipper test
Salkowski-Schipper test
salmon-patch hemorrhage
salmon-pink epithelium
Salmonella and *Campylobacter*-specific mass spectrometry
Salmonella colitis
Salmonella food poisoning
Salmonella osteomyelitis
salmonellosis
Salofalk (mesalamine)
Salomon test
salt and pepper duodenal erosion
salts, bile
Sal-Tropine (atropine sulfate)
salvage cytology
salvage surgery
SAMBA (simultaneous areolar mastopexy and breast augmentation)
SAMe (S-adenosyl-methionine)
sample, endoscopic tissue
SampleMaster biopsy needle
sampling of lymph node
Sampson medullary nail
Samuels forceps
sandbag
Sand gland

Sandhill P32 pH antimony probe
Sandifer syndrome
Sandimmune (cyclosporine)
Sandostatin
Sandostatin LAR Depot (octreotide acetate)
Sandoz suction/feeding tube
sandpaper gallbladder
sandwich radioimmunoassay
sandwiched iliac bone graft
sandy material
SangCya (cyclosporine; alcohol)
Sanger-Brown syndrome
sanguineous fluid
sanguineous infiltration
sanguinopurulent
sanguinoseropurulent
sanguinoserous
Sani-Scope anoscope
Sani-Supp (glycerin)
Santiani-Stone classification of pancreatitis
santonin test
Santorini, duct of
SaO_2 (oxygen saturation)
saphenofemoral junction
saphenous varix
saphenous vein extracranial-intracranial bypass graft
SaphFinder surgical balloon dissector
SaphLITE/SaphLITE II retractor system
SAPHtrak balloon dissector
Sapimed anoscope
Sapimed rectoscope
saponification of fat
Saratoga (zinc oxide; boric acid; eucalyptol)
sarcoepiplocele
sarcoid of Boeck
sarcoidosis, hepatic
sarcoma
    Abernethy
    alveolar soft-part
sarcoma *(cont.)*
    ameloblastic
    angiolithic
    botryoid
    endometrial stromal
    Ewing
    fascicular
    gastric Kaposi
    giant cell
    giant cell monstrocellular
    granulocytic
    hemangioendothelial
    immunoblastic
    intracolonic Kaposi
    Ito cell
    Jensen
    juxtacortical osteogenic
    Kaposi
    Kupffer cell
    leukocytic
    lipoblastic
    lymphatic
    medullary
    mixed cell
    multiple idiopathic hemorrhagic
    myelogenic
    myeloid
    neurogenic
    osteogenic
    periosteal
    reticulum cell
    retroperitoneal
    round cell
    Rous
    soft tissue
    spindle cell
    synovial
    telangiectatic osteogenic
    vasoablative endothelial (VABES)
sarcoma of retroperitoneal
sarcomatoid degeneration
sarcoplasmic material
sarcoplasmic reticulum
sargramostim

Sarmiento nail
Sarns electric saw
Sarns intracardiac suction tube
Sarot artery forceps
Sarot bronchus clamp
Sarot needle
Sarot needle holder
Sarot-TC needle holder
SART (standard acid reflux test)
satchel drape
satellite lesion
satellite metastasis
satellite nodule
satellite phenomenon
satellite structure
satellite virus
Satietrol Complete
satiety, early
SatinCrescent knife
SatinShortcut knife
Satinsky aortic clamp
Satinsky scissors
Satinsky vascular clamp
Satinsky vena cava clamp
Satin-Slip stylet
Satric-500
Satterlee amputating saw
Satterlee bone saw
satumomab pendetide
satumomab pendetide monoclonal antibody
saturated blood
saturation index (SI) of bile
saturation, oxygen
saturnine colic
saucerize
saucer-shaped excavation
Sauerbruch-Britsch rib shears
Sauerbruch-Coryllos rongeur
Sauerbruch-Frey bone punch
Sauerbruch-Frey rib shears
Sauerbruch retractor
Sauerbruch rib elevator
Sauerbruch rib forceps
Sauerbruch rib shears
Sauerbruch rongeur
Sauerbruch-Stille rongeur
Saundby test for blood in stool
Saunders disease
Saunders-Paparella stapes hook
Saunders-Paparella straight needle
Saunders-Paparella window rasp
Sauvage graft
Savage suture
Savary bougie
Savary-Gilliard dilator
Savary-Miller grading scale
Savary tapered thermoplastic dilator
saw
  Accutom low-speed diamond
  Adams
  Adson wire
  Aesculap
  air-powered
  amputating
  Bailey-Gigli
  Bailey wire
  bayonet
  Beaver
  Bier amputation
  Bishop
  bone
  bow-type
  Brun metacarpal
  cast
  Charriere amputating
  Charriere bone
  circular
  Cottle
  counter rotating
  craniotomy
  crosscut
  Cushing
  Davis
  Davis guide for Gigli
  DeMartel wire
  electric cast
  end-cutting reciprocating

saw *(cont.)*
Engel plaster
fenestration
Gigli
Gigli wire
Hall air-driven oscillating
Hall Micro E oscillating
Hall Micro E reciprocating
Hall Micro E sagittal
Hall sternal
Hall Versipower oscillating
Hall Versipower reciprocating
Herbert
Langenbeck metacarpal
Lebsche wire
Luck-Bishop bone
metacarpal
micro sagittal
MicroAire oscillating
micro oscillating
Midas Rex craniotomy
Mueller (Müller)
Olivecrona-Gigli
Orthair oscillating
oscillating
oscillating sternotomy
Oscillo III plaster
Percy amputating
plaster
Poppen
power oscillating
power-driven
Raney
reciprocating motor
reciprocating
Rust amputation
sagittal surgical
Sarns electric
Satterlee amputating
single-blade
Skilsaw
sternotomy
straight oscillating
Strully-Gigli

saw *(cont.)*
Stryker
twin-blade oscillating
Tyler-Gigli
Weiss amputation
Wigmore plaster
wire
Zimmer oscillating
SAWA shoulder brace
saw blade
sawcut
saw guide
Adson
Bailey Gigli
Blair
Cushing
Cushing-Gigli
Davis
Gigli
Lebsche
Poppen Gigli
Raney
saw handle, Strully Gigli
Sawtell artery forceps
Sawtell tonsil hemostatic forceps
sawtooth appearance sign
sawtooth configuration
sawtooth irregularity of bowel contour
sawtooth pattern
Sawyer rectal retractor
Sawyer rectal speculum
SAXX renal stent
Sayre bandage
Sayre periosteal elevator
SB, S-B (Sengstaken-Blakemore) tube
SBE (small bowel enteroscopy)
SBGM (self blood glucose monitoring)
SBO (small bowel obstruction)
SBP (spontaneous bacterial peritonitis)
SCA-EX ShortCutter catheter
scab, chronic
scale (see *classification*)
scale, Detecto weight
scale of 1 to 10

scaling dermatitis
scaling rash
scalloped bowel lumen (on x-ray)
scalp clip forceps
scalpel
- Barron
- Harmonic ultrasound
- LaserSonics Nd:YAG LaserBlade
- Plasma Scalpel
- Propper
- quartz
- rotary gamma
- Shaw electrical
- Shaw I and Shaw II hemostatic
- Smart Scalpel
- Surgiblade
- Ultracision Harmonic

scalpel blade
scalpel handle
scalp flap forceps
scalp infection
scalp marker staple
scalp needle
scalp retractor
scaly skin lesion
scan (see also *imaging*)
- bone
- CAT
- computed tomography (CT)
- computerized tomographic (CT)
- contrast-enhanced
- CT (computerized tomographic)
- dimethyl iminodiacetic acid
- DISIDA
- dual-phase spiral CT
- gallbladder
- gallium-67
- gastric emptying
- hepatobiliary
- HIDA
- HIDA/PRIDA
- indium 64-labeled white blood cell
- liver-spleen
- MAAP

scan *(cont.)*
- magnetic resonance imaging (MRI)
- Meckel
- non-contrast-enhanced
- nuclear bleeding
- nuclear medicine
- PIPIDA
- radioisotope
- radionuclide
- rose bengal sodium ^{131}I-labeled biliary
- SPECT
- sulfur colloid liver
- tagged red blood cell bleeding
- TcHIDA
- technetium ^{99m}Tc IDA scan
- technetium-labeled red blood cell
- technetium-labeled sulfur colloid
- thyroid
- ultrasound
- unenhanced

scan-directed biopsy
Scanlan loupe
scanner (see also *device; system*)
- Aquilion CT
- Bak-Pac portable ultrasound
- Bruel-Kjaer ultrasound
- FONAR-360 MRI
- LDS
- Longport digital
- Perception 5000 PC-based ultrasound
- Softscan laser
- T-Scan 2000 transpectral impedance

scanning electron microscopy
scant amount of tissue
scaphoid abdomen
scaphoid shoe cookie (pad)
scaphoid stomach
scapular lymph node
scapular region
scar, scarring
- burn
- calcified

scar *(cont.)*
  central
  duodenal
  excised
  flank
  incisional
  inframammary
  keloid
  peritoneal
  postnecrotic
  radial
  railroad track
  surgical
  tissue
  traumatic
  zipper
scar carcinoma
Scar Care dressing
scar formation
ScarGuard
scarification test
scarified duodenum
scar revision
scar tissue, enveloping
scar tissue reaction
scar tissue replacing normal esophageal lining
Scarlet Red ointment dressing
Scarpa fascia
Scarpa triangle
scarred down by gallstones
scarring
  duodenal
  peritoneal
  postnecrotic
scatoma
S-CCK-PZ (secretin, cholecystokinin, pancreozymin)
SCCS (simethicone-coated cellulose suspension)
S cell
SCFA (short chain fatty acid)
Schanz dressing
Schanz pin
Schanz rod
Scharff microbipolar and suction forceps
Schatzki ring
Schaumann body
Schaumann disease
Scheicker laminectomy punch forceps
Scheie ophthalmic cautery
Schell bone rongeur
Schiff test
Schilling test
Schimmelbusch bladder syringe
Schindler esophagoscope
Schindler peritoneal forceps
Schindler semiflexible gastroscope
Schink retractor
schistosomal bladder carcinoma
schistosomal liver disease
schistosomiasis
Schlein clamp
Schlesinger cervical punch forceps
Schlesinger cervical rongeur
Schlesinger intervertebral disk rongeur
Schlesinger laminectomy rongeur
Schlesinger pituitary rongeur
Schlesinger punch
Schlesinger rongeur forceps
Schmeden tonsil punch
Schmid-Fraccaro syndrome
Schmidt rod
Schmidt syndrome
Schmieden dural scissors
Schneider medullary nail
Schneider pin
Schneider rasp
Schneider rod
Schneider-Sauerbruch rasp
schneiderian carcinoma
Schnidt clamp
Schnidt artery forceps
Schnidt gall duct forceps
Schnidt thoracic forceps
Schnidt tonsil hemostat
Schoelly laparoscope

Schoemaker anastomosis
Schoemaker gland scissors
Schoenberg intestinal forceps
Schoenborn trachea retractor
Schoenrock inserter
Schrader air
Schrader Endo-Flo
Schroeder tenaculum forceps
Schubert biopsy forceps
Schuchart rib shears
Schuknecht suction tip
Schuknecht wire-cutting scissors
Schüller (Schueller) view
Schumacher biopsy forceps
Schumacher rib shears
Schumacher scissors
Schumaker aortic clamp
Schwachman-Bodian syndrome
Schwachman-Diamond syndrome
Schwann cell lipidosis
Schwann cell tube
schwannoma
Schwartz clamp
Schwartz clip-applying forceps
Schwartz laminectomy retractor
Schwartz micro clip
Schwartz-Pregenzer urethropexy
Schwartz temporary clamp-applying forceps
Schwartz temporary intracranial artery clamp
Schwartze chisel
Schwarz test
Schweitzer pin
Schweitzer spring plate
sciatic hernia
SCID (severe combined immuno-deficiency)
Sci-Med Express Monorail balloon
scintigraphic balloon
scintigraphic study
scintigraphy (see *imaging*)
  hepatobiliary
  quantitative hepatobiliary (QHS)
  radioistope
scintimammography (SMM)
scintiscan (see *imaging*)
  biliary
  gastroesophageal
scirrhous adenocarcinoma
scirrhous cancer
scirrhous carcinoma of breast
scirrhous lesion
scirrhous tumor
scissor dissection
scissor leg
scissors (see also *shears*)
  Abel
  Acme
  Acufex
  Adson ganglion
  Adson-Toennis
  alligator
  arthroscopic
  Aufricht dissecting
  Babcock wire-cutting
  Babcock wire
  baby Metzenbaum dissecting
  baby Reynolds dissecting
  bandage
  bandage and utility
  Bantam wire-cutting
  Barnes perineorrhaphy
  bayonet-shaped
  Beall circumflex artery
  Beebe wire-cutting
  Bellucci alligator
  bipolar cautery
  bladder
  blunt-tipped iris
  Bonn
  bowel
  Bowman
  brain
  Braun episiotomy
  Braun-Stadler
  bronchoesophageal
  Brook stitch
  Buck

scissors *(cont.)*
Buie rectal
Busch suture
Busch umbilical
cartilage
Castanares facelift
Castroviejo
Church
circumflex
coronary artery
Crafoord thoracic
crown and collar
CTS Harvester bipolar
curved
curved dissecting
curved double-action Metzenbaum
curved Mayo
curved unipolar
cuticle
Dandy neurosurgical
Dandy trigeminal nerve
Dean dissecting
Deaver
DeBakey dissecting
DeBakey endarterectomy
DeBakey valve
Decker alligator
Decker micro
Decker microsurgical
DeMartel neurosurgical
DeMartel vascular
diathermy
Diethrich coronary
Diethrich-Hegemann
Diethrich valve
Diethrich vascular
dissecting
Don Duralap
Don peritoneal
Doyen abdominal
Dubois
Duffield
dural
Duralap Metzenbaum

scissors *(cont.)*
Electroscope disposable laparo-
scopic
embryotomy
endarterectomy
Endo Shears
ENT (ear, nose, and throat)
enterotomy
enucleation
episiotomy
Esmarch plaster
Evershears and Evershears II bipolar
facelift
Ferguson
Finochietto-Metzenbaum
Finochietto thoracic
Fiskars Softouch
fistula
F. L. Fischer microsurgical
neurectomy bayonet
Forman rhinoplasty
Frazier dural
Friedland
Fukushima-Giannotta
Giertz-Stille
gland
Glassman dissecting
Goldman dissecting
Goligher abdominal
Gorney
Gradle
Haimovici arteriotomy
Halsey nail
Harrington
Harrington-Mayo thoracic
Harvey suture
Harvey wire-cutting
Haynes
Heath ligature
Heath suture
Hercules plaster and bandage
hook
hook, single-action
Howell coronary

scissors *(cont.)*
- iris
- Jacobson microneurosurgical
- Jameson
- Jannetta-Kurze dissecting
- Jorgenson
- Joseph dissecting
- Joseph nasal
- Kahn dissecting
- Kantrowitz vascular
- Karmody venous
- Kaye-TC
- Kelly dissecting
- Kelly fistula
- Kelly-Locklin
- Kilner dissecting
- Kitner dissecting
- Kleencut
- Knapp
- Knowles bandage
- Koenig nail-splitting
- Kreuscher
- Kurze dissecting
- Lahey
- LaparoSonic coagulating
- LaserScissors
- Lawson Tait perineorrhaphy
- ligature
- Lincoln
- Lincoln-Metzenbaum
- Lister
- Lister bandage
- Littauer stitch
- Little dissecting
- Litwak mitral valve
- Lloyd Davies
- Luque rod
- Malis bipolar cautery
- Malis neurological
- Martin
- Martin cartilage
- Martin stitch
- Mayo dissecting
- Mayo dressing

scissors *(cont.)*
- Mayo-Harrington
- Mayo-Lexer
- Mayo-Noble
- Mayo-Stille
- Mayo straight dissecting
- McCain TMJ
- McIndoe
- Medco Lister bandage
- Medi plaster
- meniscectomy
- meniscus
- Metzenbaum dissecting
- Metzenbaum-TC
- micro
- microneurosurgical
- Micro-One
- Micro-Two
- microscopic
- microsurgery or microsurgical
- microvascular
- Miller rectal
- Mills arteriotomy
- Mills vascular
- moleskin
- monopolar
- MPC scissors
- nail
- nail-splitting
- Nelson
- neurological or neurosurgical
- Nicola
- Northbent stitch
- Noyes iris
- Noyes microscopic
- nurses
- Nu-Tip disposable
- O'Brien
- Olivecrona dural
- Olivecrona trigeminal
- operating
- Ormon rectal
- Oxo kitchen
- Panzer gallbladder

scissors *(cont.)*
- Peck-Joseph dissecting
- Penn umbilical
- Penn wire-cutting
- pituitary
- Pivotal
- plaster
- Potts-DeMartel vascular
- Potts right-angled
- Potts 60° angled
- Potts-Smith
- Potts-Smith vascular
- Potts tenotomy
- Potts-Yasargil
- Pratt rectal
- Quimby
- Ragnell dissecting
- Re-New laparoscopic
- Real coronary artery
- Rees
- Reynolds
- Rhoton bayonet
- right-angle
- Rogers wire-cutting
- rotary
- rotatory
- Satinsky
- Schmieden
- Schmieden dural
- Schoemaker gland
- Schuknecht wire-cutting
- Schumacher
- Seutin plaster
- Shea
- Shortbent stitch
- Siebold abdominal
- Sims abdominal
- Sistrunk dissecting
- Slip-N-Snip
- Smillie meniscus
- Smith
- Smith bandage
- Smith wire-cutting
- Snowden-Pencer

scissors *(cont.)*
- Spay
- Spencer
- Spencer stitch
- spring-handled
- Stevens tenotomy
- Stille-Mayo
- stitch
- Stiwer
- Storz wire-cutting
- strabismus
- straight
- straight dissecting
- straight double-action
- straight double-action monopolar
- straight micro
- Strully dissecting
- Strully dural
- Strully neurological
- Supercut dissecting
- surgical
- suture
- Sweet esophageal
- Sweet pituitary
- Tagit antibacterial
- Take-Apart
- Taylor brain
- Taylor dural
- tenotomy
- Tessier undermining
- thoracic
- Thorek-Feldman gallbladder
- Thorek gallbladder
- Tindall
- Toennis dissecting
- trigeminal
- Turner Warwick diathermy
- Twisk
- umbilical cord
- valve
- Vannas micro
- Vantage iris
- Vantage Knowles bandage
- Vantage Lister bandage

scissors *(cont.)*
Vantage Metzenbaum
Vantage operating
Vantage Spencer stitch
Vantage strabismus
Vezien abdominal
Waldmann
Walton
Webster meniscectomy
Weck microsuture cutting
Wertheim
Westcott dissecting
Westscott
Wiet otologic
Willauer abdominal
Willauer thoracic
Wilmer dissecting
wire
wire-cutting
Yankauer
Yasargil bayonet
Yasargil micro
Z-Scissors
scissors dissection
scissors-excision hemorrhoidectomy
scissors sharpener, Miltex
Scivoletto test
SCLC (small cell lung carcinoma)
sclera (pl. sclerae)
anicteric
icteric
nonicteric
scleral icterus
scleroderma bowel disease
scleroderma-like esophagus
scleroderma of esophagus
scleroderma, systemic
ScleroLaser laser
Scleromate sclerosant
ScleroPlus HP laser
sclerosant
absolute alcohol
bucrylate
ethanolamine oleate
sclerosant *(cont.)*
morrhuate
polidocanol
Scleromate
sodium tetradecyl sulfate
Sotradecol
thrombin-Keflin-sotredochal
sclerosing adenosis of breast
sclerosing agent
sclerosing cholangitis
sclerosing encapsulating peritonitis
sclerosing hemangioma
sclerosing hepatic carcinoma (SHC)
sclerosing inflammation
sclerosing solution
sclerosing therapy
sclerosing well-differentiated carcinoma
sclerosis
central hyaline
endoscopic injection
esophageal variceal
gastric
hepatic
hepatoportal
laser
variceal
Sclerosol intrapleural aerosol
sclerotherapist
sclerotherapy
emergent endoscopic
endoscopic
esophageal variceal
fiberoptic injection (FIS)
hemorrhoidal
injection
intravariceal
paravariceal
sclerotherapy needle
sclerotic kidney
sclerotic stomach
SCNB (stereotactic core needle biopsy)
scolex (pl. scoleces)
scoliocide

scoop
  abdominal
  common duct
  Desjardins gall stone
  Desjardins gallbladder
  Ferguson gallstone
  gallbladder
  Klebanoff gallstone
  Luer-Koerte gallstone
  malleable
  Mayo common duct
  Mayo gallstone
  Moore gallstone
  Moynihan gallstone
  rigid
  Volkman
SCOOP 1 catheter
SCOOP 2 catheter
scope (see *endoscope*)
ScopeSeal endoscope patch
Scopinaro pancreaticobiliary bypass
score (also see *classification*)
  Beppu
  "bother"
  Braden
  Champion Trauma Score (CTS)
  Colon Injury (CIS)
  Demeester
  fecal incontinence
  Gleason
  Injury Severity
  KESS constipation
  Knodell periportal inflammation
  Revised Trauma
scoring incision in surgery
scorpion bite
Scotchcast 2 casting tape
Scott attic cannula
Scott jejunoileal bypass
Scott-McCracken periosteal elevator
Scott nasal suction tube
Scott silicone ventricular catheter
Scott ventricular cannula
scout film
Scoville blade
Scoville brain clip-applying forceps
Scoville brain spatula forceps
Scoville cervical disk retractor
Scoville-Haverfield hemilaminectomy retractor
Scoville hemilaminectomy retractor
Scoville nerve root hook
Scoville nerve root retractor
Scoville retractor
Scoville-Richter laminectomy retractor
Scoville ventricular needle
screw
  Barouk micro
  Doyen myoma
  Guardsman femoral
  Herbert bone
  Herbert-Whipple bone
  Howmedica Universal compression
  In-Fast bone
  Jeter lag
  KLS Centre-Drive
  lag
  Lindorf lag
  Magerl
  Propel cannulated interference
  Reddick-Saye
screw-holding forceps
scrotal ecchymosis
scrotal hernia
scrotum
Scudder forceps
Scudder intestinal clamp
Scudder intestinal forceps
scultetus bandage
scultetus binder
scybalous stools
SDI (Surgical Dynamics, Inc)
S*D*sorb meniscal stapler
sea anemone ulcer
sea-blue histiocyte syndrome
Seabrook pump
seabuckthorn seed oil
Sea-Clens wound cleanser

seal
  AccuPort
  Karaya 5
  optimal tracheal
  orbital reducer
sealant (see also *adhesive*)
  CoSeal surgical sealant
  CoStasis
  fibrin
  FloSeal matrix hemostatic
  FocalSeal
  FocalSeal-L
  FocalSeal-S
  Hemaseel APR fibrin
  Hemaseel HMN biological tissue glue
  HemaSyst
  Peri-Strips Dry
  Peri-Strips wound
  Proceed hemostatic
  Tisseel fibrin
  TraumaSeal
  VITEX fibrin
Seal-Up II reducer
seasick
seasickness
SeaSorb alginate wound dressing
seatbelt neck injury
seating chisel
Seawell rasp
sebaceous carcinoma
sebaceous cyst
Sebileau periosteal elevator
seborrheic keratosis
sebum
secondary adhesion
secondary adrenocortical insufficiency
secondary bacterial infection
secondary biliary cirrhosis
secondary biliary fibrosis
secondary biseptal cirrhosis
secondary cholangitis
secondary closure
secondary contraction
secondary hepatic cancer
secondary hyperaldosteronism
secondary hyperparathyroidism
secondary hypersplenism
secondary hypothyroidism
secondary infection
secondary jejunal ulcer
secondary lesion
secondary local ischemia
secondary malabsorption
secondary nontropical sprue
secondary peristaltic wave
secondary suture
secondary thyroid hyperplasia
second cyst recurrence
second degree hemorrhoid
second-look laparotomy
second-look operation
Secretin Ferring (secretin)
secretin-pancreozymin test
secretin provocation testing for gastrinoma
secretin-stimulated MRCP
secretin stimulation test
secretion
  basal acid
  exocrine
  gastric
  gastric acid
  ileal
  massive acid
  pituitary
  serous
  thin
  thyrocalcitonin
  watery
secretory diarrhea
section
  abdominal
  cross-
  deep
  fresh frozen
  frozen
  permanent

section *(cont.)*
  serial
  serosal
  serous fluid
  step
  transverse
  ultrathin
sectioning a block of tissue
sectioning of tissue specimen
Secu ("C-Q") clip
SecureLife skin barrier
securing hemostasis
securing the airway
Securline skin-marking pen
Sedan-Vallicioni cannula
sedation (see *medications*)
Sedillot periosteal elevator
Sedillot raspatory
seed, seeding
  iridium
  peritoneal
Seessel pouch
segment
  aganglionic
  apical
  apicoposterior
  bronchopulmonary
  cardiac
  colorectal
  fixed
  flail
  hepatic
  liver
  necrotic
  pharyngoesophageal
  pulmonary
  resected
  short
  ST
  stenotic
  strictured
  vaterian
segmental anesthesia
segmental appendicitis
segmental bowel infarction
segmental bowel transplantation
segmental change (on x-ray)
segmental colon resection
segmental enteritis
segmental epidural block
segmental graft
segmental ileitis
segmental lesion
segmental mastectomy
segmental osteotomy
segmental reduction and split graft techniques
segmental resection of bowel
segmentary pancreatitis
segmentectomy of liver
segmentectomy VIII (according to Couinaud classification)
Segura CBD (common bile duct) basket
Segura stone basket
SeHCAT (selenium-labeled hemocholic acid conjugated with taurine) test
Sehrt clamp
Seidel humeral locking nail
Seidel humeral rod
Seidel intramedullary rod
Seidlitz powder
Seitzinger tripolar cutting forceps
seizing forceps
seizures
Selby II hook
Selby II rod
SelCID (selective cytokine inhibitory drug)
Seldinger gastrostomy needle
Seldinger needle
Seldinger technique for cystic duct catheterization
Selecta 7000 laser
Select GT blood glucose monitor
selection injection of contrast material
selective angiography
selective cannulation
selective catheterization

selective cytokine inhibitory drug (SelCID)
selective mesenteric angiography
selective proximal vagotomy (SPV)
selective sampling
selective serotonin 5-HT (hydroxytryptamine) blocker
selective serotonin reuptake inhibitor (SSRI)
selective splenic arteriogram
selective vagotomy
selective venous sampling for gastrin
selective visceral hypersensitivity
Selector ultrasonic aspirator
selenium-75 (^{75}Se) radioisotope
selenomethionine (^{75}Se) pancreatic function test
selenomethionine radioactive agent (^{75}Se)
Seletz-Gelpi laminectomy retractor
Seletz nonrigid ventricular catheter
self-adhering bandage
self-aspirating cut-biopsy needle
self blood glucose monitoring (SBGM)
self-broaching nail
self-broaching pin
self-centering bone-holding forceps
self-centering reamer
self-esteem disturbance
self-examination
self-expanding metallic wall stent
self-expanding metal stent
self-induced vomiting
self-limited
self-locking nail
self-positioning balloon
self-retaining clamp
self-retaining laryngoscope
self-retaining retractor
self-retaining table-mounted retractor system
self-splint when coughing
sella punch forceps
Sellheim elevating spoon
Sellors rib contractor
Selman clamp
Selman vessel forceps
Selverstone carotid artery clamp
Selverstone cordotomy hook
Selverstone intervertebral disk rongeur
Selverstone rongeur forceps
semantic conditioning
Semb bone forceps
Semb ligature carrier
Semb lung retractor
Semb rib forceps
Semb rib rasp
Semb rib shears
Semb rongeur
Semb-Stille bone rongeur
semiclosed anesthesia
semielemental diet
semiflexible endoscope
semiformed stools
semi-Fowler position
semifundoplication (Toupet)
semi-invasive portal decompression
semilunar cartilage knife
semilunar fold
semilunar hiatus
semilunar incision
semilunar line
semilunar-shaped fold
seminal fluid
semiopen anesthesia
semirigid endoscope
semirigid sigmoidoscope
semisitting position
semisolid material
semisolid sebaceous debris
semisolid stools
semitendinosus graft
semitubular compression plate
Semken bipolar forceps
Semken delicate forceps
Semken tissue forceps
Semliki Forest virus
Semm biopsy suction curette

Semm rigid laparoscope
Semm-Wisap laparoscope
SEMS (self-expanding microporous stent [aneurysm])
Sendai virus
Senexon (senna concentrate)
Sengstaken balloon esophageal dilatation
Sengstaken-Blakemore (S-B) tamponade balloon
Sengstaken-Blakemore (S-B) tube
Senn double-end retractor
Senn-Green retractor
Senn-Kanavel retractor
Senn-Miller catspaw retractor
Senn plate
Senn retractor
senna concentrate
Senna-Gen (senoside)
Senning bulldog clamp
Senographe 2000D digital mammography imaging system
Senokot (senna concentrate)
SenoScan mammography
senosides
Sensability breast examination sheet
Sensability lubricated plastic sheet for breast self-examination
sensation
  burning
  foreign body
  globus
  phantom breast
sensation deficit
sensor
  anal EMG PerryMeter
  BIS Sensor
  BreastAlert differential temperature (DTS)
  gastrotonometer electronic
  globus
  Mon-a-therm skin temperature
  Optical
  Oxygen
sensor *(cont.)*
  PerryMeter anal EMG
  RSP thermocouple
  side-hole
  sleeve
  snaptrace silver chloride
  TAB thermocouple
  temperature
  thermistor
  Vasotrax blood pressure/heart rate
Sensorcaine MPF (bupivacaine)
sensorium change
sensory innervation
Sensory Threshold Tester
Sensostrip
sentinel blood clot
sentinel fold
sentinel gland
sentinel loop of small bowel
sentinel lymph node (SLN)
sentinel node
sentinel pile (hemorrhoid)
sentinel skin paddle graft
sentinel tag
Sepacell RZ-2000 leukoreduction device
separator, Benson pylorus
Sepracoat coating solution
Seprafilm bioresorbable membrane
Seprafilm tissue barrier
Sepragel bioresorbable gel
Sepramesh biosurgical composite mesh graft
Sepramesh prosthetic surgical mesh
Sepramesh suture
SEPS (subfascial endoscopic perforator surgery)
sepsis
  catheter
  gram-negative
  incarcerated
  intestinal
  intra-abdominal (IAS)
  intravenous line

sepsis *(cont.)*
  oral
  overwhelming postsplenectomy
    (OPSS)
  postsplenectomy
  puerperal
  Staphylococcus
sepsis syndrome
septal cirrhosis, diffuse
septal elevator
septal forceps
septal mucosa
septal panniculitis
septal tissue
septal wall
septectomy, transampullary
septic cholangitis
septicemia, transient
septic necrosis
septicopyemia
  cryptogenic
  metastatic
  spontaneous
septic shock
septic syndrome
septic wound
Septopal beads
septum, interhaustral
sequela (pl. sequelae)
sequence technique
sequential clamp and suture technique
sequential clamp, cut, and tie technique
sequestered foreign material
sequestrant, bile acid
sequestration, fluid
sequestration of circulating red cells
sequestration of medications
sequestration of platelets
sequestration, splenic
sequestrectomy
sequestrum forceps
Sequoia ultrasound system
Seracult Plus test
Seracult test
serendipity view
SergiScope (robotic microscope)
serial cardiac isoenzymes
serial cardiograms
serial cholangiograms
serial CK enzyme study (also CPK)
serial dilutions
serial hemoglobins
serial insulin measurements
serial lesions
serial liver biopsies
serial observations
serial sections
serially clamped, cut, and ligated
serially sectioned
series, gastrointestinal
sermorelin acetate
seroculture
serocystic
serofibrinous inflammation
serofibrinous pleurisy
serological muscle enzymes
serologic cross-reactivity
serologic markers for hepatitis
serologic testing
Seroma-Cath catheter
Seroma-Cath wound drainage system
seroma, postoperative
seromuscular intestinal patch graft
seromuscular layer
seromuscular stitch
seromuscular suture
seromuscular-to-edge suture
seroprevalence
serosa of GI tract
serosal involvement
serosal patch repair
serosal section
serosal surface
serosal tear
serosal transducers and manometry
serosanguineous discharge
serosanguineous fluid
serosanguinopurulent

serositis
serotinin degradation
serotonergic drug
serotonin antagonist
serous abscess
serous adenocarcinoma
serous atrophy
serous cystadenocarcinoma
serous cystadenoma
serous cystoma
serous diarrhea
serous effusion
serous exudate
serous fluid
serous gland of tongue
serous infiltration
serous inflammation
serous membrane
serous secretion
serpentine appendix
serpentine incision
serpentine plate
serpiginous ulcer
serpiginous ulceration
serrated forceps
serrated jaws
serrated suture
Serratia liquefaciens
Serratia marcescens
Serrato forearm pin
Serrato forearm rod
serratus anterior muscle
serrefine clamp (see *clamp; forceps; hemostat*)
serrefine, Dieffenbach
serum alanine aminotransferase (ALT)
serum ammonia
serum ammonia level
serum amylase
serum aspartate aminotransferase (AST)
serum bile acid
serum bilirubin
serum calcium
serum calcium level
serum carcinoembryonic antigen concentration
serum ceruloplasmin
serum cholesterol
serum complement level
serum concentrations of carbohydrate antigen
serum cortisol
serum creatinine, serum urea, creatinine clearance, urine volume, sodium excretion/UNaV)
serum DHEA level
serum globulin concentration
serum glucose value
serum HCV-specific antibody
serum hepatitis (SH) antigen
serum IgA antiendomysium antibody
serum interleukin
serum iron
serum lactate dehydrogenase (LDH)
serum lactic acid level
serum lipase
serum lipid
serum liver enzyme
serum magnesium
serum marker
serum parathormone level
serum potassium
serum protein
serum PTH
serum sodium
serum thyrocalcitonin level
serum total bilirubin
serum transaminase level
serum triglycerides
Serutan laxative (psyllium)
sessile adenoma
sessile lesion
sessile nodular carcinoma
sessile papule
sessile polyp
sestamibi scan
Sethotope radioactive agent

seton
  anal
  Penrose
  rubber
  silk
seton needle
seton placement
seton suture
seton wound
setophobia
SET three-lumen thrombectomy catheter
Seutin plaster scissors
Seutin plaster shears
seven-hole (7-hole) plate
severe acidosis
severe cardiac decompensation
severe hemorrhage
severe hypermetabolic state
severe hypersplenism
severe hypocalcemia
severe pain
severe salt-losing state
severe sunburn
severe thrombocytopenia
Sevrain cranial clamp
Sewall brain clip forceps
Sewall clip-applying forceps
Sewell retractor
sewing machine technique
sex chromatin mass
sex steroid
sexual precosity
sexual transmission
sexually transmitted disease
S-flap incision
Sgambati reaction or test for peritonitis
SGOT (serum glutamic-oxaloacetic transaminase) (now *AST*)
SGPT (serum glutamic-pyruvic transaminase) (now *ALT*)
shadowing, acoustic
shaking chill
shaking sound
Shaldon catheter
shallow mucosal ulcer
sham feeding test
sham therapy
Shambaugh-Derlacki duckbill elevator
Shambaugh fistula hook
Shambaugh irrigator
Shambaugh microscopic hook
Shambaugh narrow elevator
Shambaugh palpating needle
Shardle towel clip
shark liver oil
sharp and blunt dissection
sharp dissection
sharp hook
sharp knife
sharp retractor
sharp spoon
sharp versus dull
Sharplan SilkTouch flashscan surgical laser
Sharplan SilkTouch laser system
shave biopsy
shaver burr and cutter
Shaw aneurysm needle
Shaw catheter
Shaw electrical scalpel
Shaw II Teflon-coated hemostatic scalpel
SHC (sclerosing hepatic carcinoma)
Shea alligator forceps
Shea drill
Shea scissors
Shearer rongeur
shears (also see *scissors*)
  Bacon thoracic
  Baer rib
  Bethune-Coryllos rib
  Bethune rib
  biarticular bone
  Boehler plaster
  Brunner rib
  Bruns
  Bruns plaster

shears *(cont.)*
- cloth
- Collins rib
- Cooley rib
- Coryllos rib
- Endo Shears
- Esmarch plaster
- first rib
- Giertz-shoemaker rib
- Gluck rib
- Hercules plaster
- Horsley-Stille rib
- Ice hair trimming
- LaparoSonic coagulating
- Lefferts rib
- Liston-Key-Horsley rib
- Lorenz
- Medicut
- plaster
- Potts rib
- rib
- Roberts rib
- Roos first rib
- Sauerbruch-Britsch rib
- Sauerbruch-Frey rib
- Sauerbruch rib
- Schuchart rib
- Schumacher rib
- Semb rib
- Seutin plaster
- Shoemaker rib
- Stille-Giertz rib
- Stille plaster
- Stille rib
- subclavian peel-away
- utility
- Vantage first aid

sheath
- anterior rectus
- carotid
- coaxial
- cremasteric
- ERA resectoscope
- femoral

sheath *(cont.)*
- fibrous
- Hyfrecator pencil
- introducer
- Microgyn resectoscope
- muscle
- musculoaponeurotic
- Passager introducing
- posterior rectus
- rectus
- Slide-On EndoSheath
- sliding
- SLS (Spectranetics laser sheath)
- subclavian peel-away

sheath ligament
sheath of muscle
Sheehan chisel
Sheehan gouge
Sheehan syndrome
Sheehy round knife
SheerVision loupe
sheeting, Silastic
Sheffield hand elevator
Sheldon hemilaminectomy retractor
Sheldon-Spatz vertebral arteriogram needle

shelf
- Blumer rectal
- intraluminal
- mesocolic
- rectal

shelled out
shellfish, contaminated
shell out a cyst
shelving edge of Poupart ligament
Sheridan ET A6579CO2 Uncuffed
Sher-I-Temp skin temp sensor (Kendall)
Sherlock threaded suture anchor
Sherman bone plate
Sherpa guiding catheter
Sherwin knee retractor
Sherwood intrascopic suction/irrigation system (for laparoscopic procedure)

shield
  corneal
  eye
  Fuller rectal
  laparoscope
  laser guard
  safety
  Saf-T E-Z translucent needle
  Slim Stem scleral
  Sutcliffe Boey laser
shifting dullness on percussion
shift of intravascular fluid volume into peritoneal space
shift to the left on WBC count
shift to the right on WBC count
Shiley tracheal tube
Shiley tracheotomy tube
Shiner tube
shiny mass
Shirley wound drain
shirt-stud abscess
shock
  anaphylactic
  bacterial
  electrical
  endotoxic
  hemorrhagic
  hypoglycemic
  hypovolemic
  insulin
  septic
  toxic
shock absorption
shock kidney
shock liver
shock lung
shock syndrome, toxic
shock with bleeding
shocks given on lithotripsy
shoe cookie (pad)
shoelace technique for delayed primary closure of fasciotomy
shoe of the hook
Shoemaker intestinal clamp
Shoemaker rib shears
Shohl solution
short angled curette
short axis parasternal view
short axis view
Shortbent stitch scissors
short-bowel syndrome
short chain fatty acids (SCFA)
ShortCut knife
shorter halflife
short esophagus
short gastric artery
short gastric vein
short gastric vessel (SGV)
short gastrics from the spleen
short gut syndrome
shorthand vertical mattress stitch
short length hepatic vein stenosis (SLHVS)
short limb Roux-en-Y gastroenterostomy
short loose 360° fundoplication
short right-angle dissector
short-scar procedure in breast reduction
short-scar tumescent reduction mammoplasty
short segment Barrett esophagus (SSBE)
short spatula electrode
short-term treatment
short vessel graft
shotgun pellet embolism
shotty breast
shotty lymph node
Shouldice herniorrhaphy
Shouldice operation for hernia repair
Shriner pin
shrinking liver volume
shrunken liver
shrunken lung
shunt
  Allen-Brown vascular access
  atriocaval
  barium sulfate impregnated

shunt *(cont.)*
biliopancreatic
Cordis-Hakim
CSF (cerebrospinal fluid)
cysto-atrial
cystoperitoneal
Denver hydrocephalus
Denver peritoneal venous
distal splenorenal (DSR)
Drapanas
DVP flush
end-to-side portacaval
end-to-side splenorenal
endarterectomy
endolymphatic
esophageal
FloCoil
gastric venacaval
Gott
Hakim-Cortis ventriculoperitoneal
hermetic external
Heyer-Schulte neurosurgical
high-pressure
Hyde
infant
intrahepatic transjugular portosystemic
intrapulmonary
Javid
Kasai peritoneal venous shunt
LeVeen peritoneal
Linton
low pressure
lumbar arachnoid peritoneal
lumbar thecoperitoneal
lumboperitoneal (LP)
medium pressure
mesocaval H-graft
mesocaval interposition
mesocaval shunt (MCS)
migration of
modified Blalock-Taussig (MBTS)
Ommaya ventriculoperitoneal
one-piece

shunt *(cont.)*
peritoneal-atrial
peritoneal-venous
peritoneocaval
peritoneovenous (PVS)
portacaval
portal-systemic
portopulmonary
portosystemic
portosystemic shunting
posterior atrial fossa
proximal splenorenal
Pruitt-Inahara
Pudenz
side-to-side portacaval
silicone elastomer
small bowel
Spetzler lumboperitoneal
splenorenal
subdural-to-peritoneal
Sundt loop
surgical
surgical portosystemic
thecoperitoneal
transjugular intrahepatic portosystemic (TIPS or TIPSS)
T-tube
UNI-SHUNT hydrocephalus
ventriculoperitoneal
ventriculoatrial (VA)
ventriculojugular (VJ)
ventriculoperitoneal (VP)
ventriculosubarachnoid (VS)
ventriculovenous
Warren splenorenal

shunt failure, intermittent
shunt fraction
shunt function, cerebrospinal fluid
shunting of cerebrospinal fluid
shunting procedure
shunt malfunction
shunt patency test
shunt-related metastasis
shunt reservoir

shunt reversal
shunt revision
shunt syndrome
shunt tap
shunt tube
shunt valve
Shur-Clens wound cleanser
Shutt Mantis retrograde forceps
Shy-Drager syndrome
SI (International System of Units)
SI (saturation index) of bile
SI (sucrose-isomaltose)
SIA (strip immunoblot assay)
SIADH (syndrome of inappropriate antidiuretic hormone)
sialodochoplasty
sialography
sialolithotomy
sialorrhea
SIBS (surgical isolation bubble system)
sibutramine HCl
sickle cell anemia
sickle cell crisis
sickle cell disease
sickle knife
sickle-shape Beaver blade
sickle-shape blade
side-aspirating biopsy needle
side-biting clamp
side cutter
side-cutting spatulated needle
side effects of chemotherapy
side-hole recording site
side-hole sensor
side, ipsilateral
side-lying position
side-opening hook
side plate
sideropenic dysphagia
siderotic splenomegaly
side-to-side anastomosis
side-to-side anastomosis choledocho-choledochostomy
side-to-side anastomosis with small bowel
side-to-side portacaval shunt
side-viewing endoscope
sidewall of the bowel
sidewall, pelvic
SIDS (sudden infant death syndrome)
Siebold abdominal scissors
Siegel-Cattan-Mamou syndrome
Sieman irrigation injection needle
sieving of solid food
Siewerling-Creutzfeldt disease
SIF10 Olympus enteroscope
Siffert method
sigmaS serum tumor marker for breast cancer
sigmoidal artery
sigmoid anastomosis clamp
sigmoid artery
sigmoid carcinoma
sigmoid colectomy
sigmoid colon
sigmoid colon involvement
sigmoid colon reservoir
sigmoid colon twisted in counterclockwise direction (sigmoid volvulus)
sigmoid colon volvulus
sigmoid colostomy
sigmoid curve
sigmoid diverticulitis
sigmoidectomy, hand-assisted
sigmoid-end colostomy
sigmoid flexure
sigmoid fold
sigmoiditis
  allergic
  dietetic
  infectious
sigmoid fossa
sigmoid kidney
sigmoid loop
sigmoid loop rod colostomy
sigmoid mesocolon

sigmoid notch of radius
sigmoid, redundant
sigmoid sinus
sigmoid volvulus
sigmoidoscope
  ACMI flexible
  ACMI TX flexible
  adult
  fiberoptic
  flexible
  Fujinon EVS-E flexible
  Fujinon flexible
  Fujinon PRO-PC flexible
  Fujinon SIG-E2 flexible
  Fujinon SIG-EK flexible
  Fujinon SIG-ET flexible
  Fujinon SIG-PC flexible
  Heine
  Jasan flexible fiberoptic
  Lloyd Davies
  MIS Source
  Olympus CF-100S flexible
  Olympus CF-10L flexible
  Olympus CF-1TS2 flexible
  Olympus CF-P10S flexible
  Olympus CF-Q160L/I/S video
  Olympus CF-V10S
  Olympus CPF-P10-S
  Olympus fiberoptic
  Olympus flexible
  Olympus OSF-2 flexible
  Olympus OSF-235 flexible
  Pentax ES-3830 video
  Pentax ES-3840 video
  Pentax fiberoptic
  Pentax flexible
  Pentax FS flexible
  Pentax FS-34A flexible
  Pentax FS-34A flexible
  Pentax FS-34V fiberoptic
  Pentax FS-38H flexible
  Pentax SIG-E2 fiberoptic
  Reichert fiberoptic
  Reichert flexible

sigmoidoscope *(cont.)*
  Reichert MH-1 flexible
  Reichert SC-48 flexible
  rigid
  semirigid
  St. Mark's
  Welch Allyn flexible
  Welch Allyn video
sigmoidoscopic decompression of volvulus
sigmoidoscopic reduction of volvulus
sigmoidoscopy (see *operation*)
sigmoidoscopy table
sigmoidovesical fistula
sign
  Aaron
  accordion
  Ballance
  barber pole (on x-ray)
  Battle
  beading
  blue dot sign
  Blumberg (of peritonitis)
  Boas
  Boas gastric ulcer
  bowler hat
  Boyce
  Branham
  Carnett
  chain-of-lakes
  Chilaiditi
  Christmas tree
  Chvostek
  classic coffee bean
  cobblestoning
  coffee bean
  Cole
  colon cutoff
  comblike redness
  Courvoisier
  Cruveilhier
  Cullen
  Dance
  double-bubble

sign *(cont.)*
- "double duct"
- Federici
- fifth vital (pain)
- flapping tremor
- Fox
- Gilbert
- Grey Turner
- Grocco
- guarding
- hamburger
- Hamman
- Henning
- Horn
- Howship-Romberg
- iliopsoas
- inverted loop
- inverted V
- Kantor
- Kehr
- Klemm
- Kussmaul
- Lennhoff
- Leser-Trelat
- linguine
- liver flap
- lollipop tree (on x-ray)
- McBurney
- McCort
- meniscus
- moulage
- Murphy
- obturator
- omega
- pathognomonic (of a fistula)
- peritoneal
- pillow
- pruning
- psoas
- puddle
- pyloric string
- rat-tail
- RCS (red color)
- rebound

sign *(cont.)*
- red color (RCS)
- reversed Mercedes Benz
- Rigler
- Robertson
- Rosenbach
- Rovighi
- Rovsing
- sawtooth appearance
- Sister Mary Joseph
- stable vital
- Strauss
- string
- Sumner
- Terry fingernail
- tethered-bowel
- thumbprinting
- Trimadeau
- Troisier node
- Trousseau
- Turner

SignaDress hydrocolloid dressing material
Signa Special Procedures (SP) system
signet ring appearance
signet ring carcinoma
signet ring cell
signet ring cell carcinoma
signet ring pattern
signet ring type of gastric carcinoma
significant comorbid disease
significant long-term weight loss
signs and symptoms
signs of infection
signs of serosal involvement
Silace-C (docusate sodium)
Silastic catheter
Silastic collar-reinforced stoma
Silastic drip drain
Silastic ring
Silastic rod
Silastic sheeting
Silastic silo reduction of gastroschisis
Silastic stent

Silastic tape dressing
Silastic tube
Silberg graft passer
S ileal reservoir
S incision
silent abdomen
silent gallstone
silent reflux
silent thyroiditis
Silhouette laser system
silicone breast implant
silicone carving block
silicone catheter
silicone donut prosthesis
silicone elastomer band
silicone elastomer ring
silicone elastomer ring vertical gastroplasty (SRVG)
silicone elastomer shunt
silicone flexor rod
silicone gel implant
silicone implant
silicone ring
silicone rubber Dacron-cuffed catheter
siliconized silk
silicon-velvet composite graft
Silkam suture
silk glove sign
Silk guidewire
Silk Laser aesthetic carbon dioxide laser for skin resurfacing
silk ligature
silk mesh gauze dressing
silk pop-off suture
silk seton
silk suture
Silk Touch laser skin resurfacing laser
silk traction suture
silo-filler's lung
Silon tent for gastroschisis
Silon wound dressing
Siltex silicone gel breast implant
Silvadene (silver sulfadiazine)
SilverBullet electrode
silver cell
silver filigree
silver finisher's lung
silver-fork deformity
Silverlon wound packing strips
Silverman-Boeker needle
Silverman needle
silver nitrate
silver probe
silver stools
silver sulfadiazine (SSD, SSD AF)
SIM (small intestine mesentery)
Simaal Gel 2 (aluminum hydroxide; magnesium hydroxide; simethicone)
simaldrate
Simeco
simethicone
simethicone-coated cellulose suspension (SCCS)
Similac with iron formula
Simmonds disease
Simmons chisel
Simmons plate
Simon abdominal retractor
Simonsen technique for large rectovaginal fistula repair
Simplate bleeding time (BT)
simple cyst
simple goiter
simple liver amebic abscess
simple mastectomy
simple mechanical obstruction
simple obesity
Simple Suction Probe cannula
simple suture
Simplex adhesive
Simpson atherectomy catheter
Simpson forceps
Simpson-Luikart forceps
Simpson peripheral AtheroCath catheter
Simpson-Smith rectal suction tube
Sims abdominal scissors
Sims connector
Sims curette

Sims irrigation nozzle
Sims Portex
Sims position
Sims rectal speculum
Sims retractor
Sims uterine scissors
Sims vaginal speculum
Simulect (basiliximab) monoclonal antibody
SIMV (synchronous IMV)
sincalide
single-action jaws
single-action monopolar hook scissors
single-action rongeur
single and rapid polymerase chain reaction/restriction fragment length polymorphism (PCR/RFLP)
single-armed suture
SingleBAR electrode
single-blade saw
single cannula tracheal tube
single-chain intracellular precursor
single-contrast barium
single clamp
single fiber electromyography electrode
single-hook auto retractor
single-layer continuous closure
single-lumen papillotome
single onlay cortical bone graft
single-patient use (SPU) instrument
single pedicle flap
single pedicle TRAM flap
single photon emission tomography (SPECT)
single polyp
single-port, double-puncture laparoscopy
single-port laparoscopy
single-post Mayo stand
single-puncture laparoscope
single-stripe colitis (SSC)
single-use cannula
Singley intestinal forceps
Singley-Tuttle tissue forceps
singultus (hiccups)
sinogram
sinus
  anal
  medullary
  perineal
  pilonidal
  piriform
  Rokitansky-Aschoff
  sigmoid
  thyroglossal duct
sinus dressing
sinus tract
sinusitis
sinusoidal congestion
sinusoidal fibrosis
sinusoidal lymphocytes
sinusoidal pressure
sinusoid, hepatic
Sipple syndrome (MEA type II)
Sippy diet
Sippy esophageal dilator
sirolimus
SIRS (systemic inflammatory response syndrome)
SIRS/sepsis (systemic inflammatory response syndrome)
SIS wound dressing
Sisson fracture reducing elevator
Sister Mary Joseph lymph node
Sister Mary Joseph node
Sister Mary Joseph sign
Sistrunk dissecting scissors
site
  exit
  hormone receptor
  incision
  port
  puncture
  recipient
  side-hole recording
  stoma
  surgical
  trocar

SiteGuard MVP transparent adhesive film dressing
site of phagocytosis
Site ~ Rite 3 ultrasound system
SiteSelect percutaneous breast biopsy system
SITEtrac endoscope
situs inversus
situs inversus viscerum
sitz bath
Sitzmarks radiopaque marker
six-hole (6-hole) plate
six-strand suture
six-wire basket
SJM Rosenkranz pediatric retractor
Sjögren syndrome
skate-flap technique of nipple reconstruction
skeletal hyperostosis
skeletal metastasis
skeletal muscle cell
skeletal traction pin
skeletonize (verb)
skeletonized
Skene tenaculum forceps
skid humeral head retractor
ski-jump view
Skil saw
skin
  anicteric
  Composite Cultured Skin (CCS)
  dimpling of
  dusky
  fair
  hyperpigmentation of
  icteric
  jaundiced
  nonicteric
  pale
  perianal
  peristomal
  scaly
skin adhesive (see *adhesives*)
skin approximation
skin blade
skin blade knife
skin change
skin cleanser (see *cleanser; medications*)
skin clip
skin crease incision
skin defect
skin edema
skin flap
skinfold thickness
skinfold thickness test
skin glue
skin graft (see also *graft*)
  Braun
  Douglas
  Dragstedt
  Esser
  free
  full-thickness
  Krause-Wolfe
  Ollier-Thiersch
  pedicle
  postage-stamp type
  split-thickness
skin graft material
skin hook
skin incision
skin induration
skin infection
skin knife
skin lesion
Skinlight erbium YAG laser
skin line
Skinmarker and Ruler markers
skin markings of lymphedema (peau d'orange)
Skinmate marker
skin necrosis
skin preparation
skin replacement (see *skin substitute*)
skin retraction
skin staple
skin stapling

skin stone
skin striae
skin substitute (also see *graft*)
  Biobrane adhesive
  Biobrane glove
  Biobrane/HF
  Dermagraft-TC
  TransCyte
skin suture
skin tag
skin temperature monitoring probe
skin turgor, decreased
skin ulcer
Skin retractor (trachea)
Skin Skribe skin marker in surgery
skinny Chiba needle
skinny needle
skinny needle technique
Skinny dilatation catheter
Skinscan laser surgery device
SkinTegrity hydrogel dressing
Skinvisible hypoallergenic hand lotion
skip area
skip lesion (of Crohn disease)
ski position
Sklar disposable anoscope
skull bone graft
skull clamp
skull film
skull pin
skull plate
skull punch
skull punch forceps
Skylight system
skyline view
slave balloon
SLE (systemic lupus erythematosus)
SLE-like syndrome
sleep apnea
sleeve
  Dent
  laparoscopic
  laparoscopic trocar
  Pneumo Sleeve
  Williams overtube
sleeve of laparoscope
sleeve sensor
SLHVS (short-length hepatic vein stenosis)
Slick endotracheal styler
Slide-On EndoSheath
slide plate
slide, ThinPrep
sliding barrel hook
sliding clamp
sliding component
sliding esophageal hiatal hernia
sliding hernia
sliding hiatal hernia
sliding inlay graft
sliding sheath
Slim Fit Flex Camp
Slim Stem scleral shield
sling
  fascial
  Hemi Sling
  puborectalis
  SurgiSis sling/mesh
sling and swathe bandage
sling muscle fibers
Slinky catheter
slip joint pliers
slipknot
Slip-N-Snip scissors
slipped Nissen fundoplication
slit/cut mesh graft
slitlike defect
Slocum meniscal clamp
Slocum nail
slotted anoscope
slotted cannula
slotted femur plate
slotted hammer
slotted mallet
slotted needle
slotted speculum
sloughing of mucosa
slough of nipple
slough of skin

slow bleed
slow colonic transit
slow-growing skin mass
slowing of gastric emptying
slow intermittent blood loss
slowly enlarging mass
slow virus
SLP1000 (super long-pulse) diode laser system
SLS (Spectranetics laser sheath)
SLS Chromos 694 long-pulse ruby laser system
sludge
  bile
  biliary
  blood
  gallbladder
sludged blood
slurry of stool
slush machine
slush machine drape
SMA (smooth muscle antibody)
SMA (superior mesenteric artery)
SMA chemistry panel
SMA formula
SMAC ("smack") panel
small accessory vein
small aperture
small bowel
small bowel congenital abnormality
small bowel contrast study
small bowel enema
small bowel enteroscopy (SBE)
small bowel fistula
small bowel follow-through
small bowel infarct
small bowel injury
small bowel meal
small bowel mesentery
small bowel mucosa
small bowel obstruction (SBO)
small bowel perforation
small bowel plus liver transplantation
small bowel resection
small bowel series
small bowel shunt
small bowel transit time
small bowel transplantation
small bowel tube
small-caliber esophagogastroduodenoscopy
small-caliber stools
small cell anaplastic carcinoma
small cell carcinoma
small cell lung carcinoma (SCLC)
small cell tumor
small-droplet fatty liver
small egress cannula
small fibroadenoma
small granule cell
small hernia defect
small inferior artery to the thyroid
small intestine
small intestine bacterial overgrowth (SIBO)
small intestine dysmotility
small intestine endoscopy
small intestine enteroscopy
small intestine gland
small intestine leiomyosarcoma
small intestine malignant lymphoma
small intestine transit time
small lymphocytic lymphoma
small noncleaved cell lymphoma
small of back pain
small rake retractor
small round cell carcinoma
small round cell infiltrate
small-stomach syndrome
small to intermediate lymphoid cells
small vessel to the splenic pulp
small window
S.M.A.R.T. (shape memory alloy recoverable technology) biliary stent
SmartDose prefilled infusion system
smart loop coagulator
SmartNail
SmartNeedle

Smart Scalpel
SMAS (superior mesenteric artery syndrome)
Smead-Jones closure
smear (see also *stain, test*)
- AFB (acid-fast bacillus)
- air-dried
- alimentary tract
- bacteriologic
- blood
- bronchoscopic
- cul-de-sac
- cytologic
- eosinophil
- fast
- feces
- fungal
- KOH
- lower respiratory tract
- malaria
- nasal
- oral
- Pap (Papanicolaou)
- peripheral
- peripheral blood
- potassium hydroxide (KOH)
- pus
- sputum
- stool
- Tzanck
- urine
- wet

Smedberg hand drill
Smedberg twist drill
SMF (streptozocin, mitomycin C, and 5-FU) chemotherapy protocol
Smiley-Williams arteriogram needle
smile incision
smiling incision
Smillie-Beaver knife
Smillie cartilage chisel
Smillie cartilage knife
Smillie hook
Smillie knee retractor
Smillie meniscotomy chisel
Smillie meniscus hook retractor
Smillie meniscus knife
Smillie meniscus scissors
Smillie nail
Smillie perforator
Smith & Nephew Richards rod
Smith & Nephew video camera system
Smith anal retractor
Smith automatic perforator drill
Smith bandage scissors
Smith bone clamp
Smith-Buie rectal retractor
Smith-Buie rectal speculum
Smith cartilage knife
Smith cranial drill
Smith nerve root suction retractor
Smith-Petersen chisel
Smith-Petersen curved gouge
Smith-Petersen femoral neck nail
Smith-Petersen gooseneck gouge
Smith-Petersen intertrochanteric plate
Smith-Petersen laminectomy rongeur
Smith-Petersen pin
Smith-Petersen plate
Smith-Petersen reamer
Smith-Petersen straight gouge
Smith-Petersen transarticular nail
Smith rectal retractor
Smith scissors
Smith test
Smith wire-cutting scissors
Smithwick button hook
Smithwick clip-applying forceps
Smithwick hook
Smithwick nerve hook
Smithwick nerve hook and dissector
Smithwick sympathectomy hook
SMM (scintimammography)
SMO (supramalleolar orthosis) plate
smoke eliminator, Core laparoscopic
smoke evacuation unit
smoke plume
smoker's lung

SmokEvac electrosurgical probe
SmokEvac trumpet-valve smoke evacuator
smoking
smooth diet
smooth goiter
smooth muscle
smooth muscle antibody (SMA)
smooth muscle motility disorder
smooth Steinmann pin
smooth-tipped jeweler's forceps
smooth tissue forceps
smooth tongue
SMV (superior mesenteric vein)
SMX/TMP (sulfamethoxazole and trimethoprim)
snake retractor
Snap Kover
snapper plunger lock
snaptrace silver chloride sensor
snap-twist plunger lock
snare
  Carr-Locke
  diathermy rectal
  Douglas rectal
  electrosurgical
  endoscopic
  Eve tonsil
  Frankfeldt rectal
  Frankfeldt rectal diathermy
  Krause nasal
  long-nose retriever
  Nakao I and II
  Norwood rectal
  Olympus disposable
  polypectomy
  rectal
  Tydings tonsil-seizing
  Weston rectal
  Wilson-Cook polypectomy
snare cautery
snared
snare loop biopsy
snare resection (band and snare)
snare technique
snare wires
Snitman endaural retractor
Snowden-Pencer forceps
Snowden-Pencer scissors
snuffbox, anatomical
Snugs bandage
Snugs dressing
Soaker Catheter
soapsuds enema (SSE)
Soave abdominal pull-through operation
Soave endorectal pull-through operation
social drinker
Society of American Gastrointestinal Endoscopic Surgeons (SAGES)
Society of Laparoendoscopic Surgeons
socket pin
SOD (sebaceous cysts, osteomas, desmoid tumors)
SOD (sphincter of Oddi dysfunction)
sodium (Na)
sodium amidotrizoate
sodium bicarbonate
sodium citrate
sodium diatrizoate with Menoquinon
sodium/H_2O retention
sodium iodine (^{131}I)
sodium iodine (^{123}I) thyroid function test
sodium iodine (^{125}I) thyroid function test
sodium iodipamide
sodium iopamide contrast medium
sodium iopodate
sodium iothalamate
sodium ioxaglate
sodium ipodate
sodium lactate, compound solution of
sodium loading
sodium metrizoate
sodium morrhuate
sodium nitroprusside (SNP)
sodium oxybate
sodium perborate

sodium phosphate
sodium restriction
sodium stibogluconate
sodium tetradecyl (STD) sulfate
sodium tetradecyl sulfate sclerosant
sodium tyropanoate
Soehendra dilator
Soehendra stent retriever
Sof-Band bulky bandage dressing
Sofield pin
Sofield retractor
Sof-Kling dressing
Sofpulse pulsed magnetic energy device
Sofrature gauze
Sof-Rol dressing
Sofsilk braided silk suture
Sofsilk nonabsorbable silk suture
SofSilk suture
SofSorb absorptive dressing
soft abdomen
Sof-Tact glucose monitor
soft bland diet
soft bulky dressing
Softcat chromic suture
Softcat plain suture
SoftCloth absorptive dressing
SoftFlex computer glove
soft food dysphagia
soft goiter
Soft Guard XL Skin Barrier for ostomy skin
Softgut surgical chromic suture
soft laser
SoftLight laser
Soft N Dry Merocel sponge
soft palate
soft papilloma
Softscan laser mammography system
Softscan laser scanner
soft spleen
soft stool
Soft Thoracoport obturator
soft tissue
soft tissue abscess
soft tissue mass
soft tissue necrosis
soft tissue sarcoma
soft tissue shaving cannula (liposhaver)
soft tissue stranding
Soft Torque uterine catheter
Soft-Vu Omni flush catheter
Sof-Wick drain sponge
Sof-Wick dressing
Sof-Wick lap pad
Sof-Wick sponge dressing
solid bolus challenge
solid crystals
solid food dysphagia
Solidifier fluid solidification system, The
solid mass
solid organ transplant
solid organ transplantation
solid sphere test
solid state esophageal manometry catheter
solitary adenoma
solitary benign adenoma
solitary gland of large intestine
solitary lactiferous duct
solitary lesion
solitary lymph node
solitary myeloma
solitary nodule
solitary rectal ulcer syndrome (SRUS)
solitary thyroid nodule
solitary tumor
solitary ulcer syndrome
Solo catheter with Pro/Pel coating catheter
SoloPass catheter
SoloPass stent/catheter
Solo-Prep topical scrub
Solos cystoscope
Solos endoscope
SoloSite hydrogel dressing
SoloSite wound gel
Solos rigid laparoscope

Solu-Biloptin contrast medium
solubilization
soluble antigen
soluble bacterial exotoxin
soluble CD-14 concentration
solution (also see *medications*)
  Aminofusin L Forte amino acid
  antibiotic
  balanced electrolyte
  Belzer
  Bicarbolyte bacteriostatic
  Bouin fixative
  Collins (for liver transplant)
  CytoLyt
  electrolyte-polyethylene glycol lavage
  Elliott's B
  Euro-Collins
  FreAmine amino acid
  FRED (fog reduction elimination device)
  FRED Lite alcohol-free
  gentamicin
  GoLytely
  HepatAmine amino acid
  iced lactated Ringer
  lactated Ringer
  Liposyn II fat emulsion
  Lugol
  lymph node-revealing solution (LNRS)
  Lytren electrolyte
  Mefoxin-saline
  Monsel hemostatic
  normal saline
  Pedialyte electrolyte
  Resol electrolyte
  Ringer lactate
  sclerosant
  sclerosing
  Sepracoat coating
  Soyalac fat emulsion
  Sporox II
  Synthamin amino acid
solution *(cont.)*
  Travamulsion fat emulsion
  tumoricidal
  University of Wisconsin
  UW (University of Wisconsin)
  Vamin amino acid
  warm saline
Soluvit
Solvang graft
somatic death
somatic neuromuscular action
somatic neuropathy
somatic pain
somatic sensitivity
somatointestinal reflex
SomatoKine (IGF-BP3 complex)
somatostatin (SS)
somatostatin analog
somatostatin therapy
somatostatinoma syndrome
somatropin and glutamine
somatropin
Somavert (pegvisomant)
Somer forceps
Somogyi unit (to measure amylase)
Sonablate 200 tissue ablator
Sonazoid ultrasound imaging agent
Sonde enteroscope
Sones catheter
Sones woven Dacron catheter
Sonnenberg classification of erosive esophagitis
SonoCT Real-Time Compound Imaging
sonogram, fatty meal (FMS)
sonographer
sonographic guidance
sonography, endoscopic
Sonolith 3000 lithotriptor
Sonolith 4000+ lithotriptor
Sonolith Praktis lithotriptor
Sonoprobe SP-501 system for endoscopic procedures
Sonopsy 3-D ultrasound breast biopsy system

SonoRx (simethicone-coated cellulose)
SonoSite 180 handheld ultrasound
SonoSurg ultrasonic cutting and coagulation
Sonotron radiofrequency device
Soprano cryoablation system
Sorb-It sponge
SorbaView composite wound dressing
sorbitol
Sorbsam topical wound dressing
Sorbsan wound packing pads (calcium alginate fiber)
Sorbsan topical wound dressing
Sorenson Laboratories
Soto-Hall bone graft
Soto USCI balloon
Sotradecol (sodium tetradecyl sulfate)
Sotradecol sclerosant
sound (see also *bowel sounds*)
  absent bowel
  auscultation of bowel
  bladder
  bowel
  Clutton bladder
  common duct
  esophageal
  hypoactive
  Klebanoff common duct
  Kocher bronchocele
  LeFort urethral
  shaking
  succussion
  unguided
  unilateral breath
  urethral
  uterine
  Van Buren urethral
sour brash
sour stomach
Souttar tube
Sovereign multifire clip applicator
Soyalac fat emulsion solution
soy-based formula
space
  anatomical dead
  Bogros
  dead
  Disse
  extracellular
  extraperitoneal
  fourth intercostal
  indirect
  intercostal
  intracellular
  Kiernan
  left diaphragmatic
  Lesgaft
  masticator
  mechanically dead
  Meckel
  peripancreatic
  perisinusoidal
  peritoneal
  physiologic dead
  pleural
  preperitoneal
  presacral
  properitoneal
  retrocrural
  retromammary
  retroperitoneal
  Retzius
  right subdiaphramatic
  subdiaphragmatic
  subhepatic
  submandibular
  submental
  subperitoneal
  subumbilical
  suprahepatic
  supralevator
  thenar
  third
  Traube semilunar
  vascular
Spacekeeper retractor
Spacemaker (and II) balloon dissector

Spacemaker VBD-300 dissector
space-occupying disease
space-occupying lesion
space of Bogros
space of Retzius
Space-OR flexible internal retractor
SpaceSEAL cannula
Spachmann tube
span
  digit
  levator
  liver
Spand-Gel dressing
Sparkles (sodium bicarbonate; citric acid; simethicone)
spasm
  anal
  bladder
  diffuse esophageal (DES)
  esophageal
spasmodic colic
spasmodic stricture
Spasmolin (atropine sulfate; scopolamine hydrobromide; hyoscyamine hydrobromide; phenobarbital)
Spasmophen
spastic colon
spastic constipation
spastic esophagus
spastic ileus
Spastosed (calcium carbonate; magnesium carbonate)
spatula
  bladder
  bow-shaped
  Davis
  distal
  Haberer abdominal
  Kocher bladder
  micropoint
  Reverdin abdominal
  Sabreloc conventional
  Sachs nerve
  spoon-shaped

spatula *(cont.)*
  Tuffier abdominal
  Ultima
spatula electroprobe
spatula electrode
spatula forceps
spatula One-Piece cannula
spatula-tip Toomey syringe cannula
Spay scissors
Speare dural hook
specialized columnar cells
specialized intestinal metaplasia
specialized tissue-aspirating resectoscope (STAR)
specific gravity
specific, layered infiltration
specimen knife
specimen retrieval bag
  Endo Catch
  Endobag laparoscopic
  EndoMate endoscopic
specimen, yarn-collected
speckled appearance
speckled pattern
SPECT (single photon emission computerized tomography) scan
Spectranetics laser sheath (SLS) laser
SpectraScience biopsy forceps
SpectraScience Optical Biopsy system
SpectraScience reusable biopsy forceps
spectrometry, *Salmonella* and *Campylobacter*-specific mass
spectroscopy
  fluorescence
  light-scattering
  reflectance
Spectrum adjustable breast implant
speculum
  Alan-Parks rectal
  Auvard
  Barr rectal
  Barr-Shuford rectal
  Beckman nasal
  Bensaude rectal

speculum *(cont.)*
beveled
Bodenhammer rectal
Brewer
Brinkerhoff rectal
Chelsea Eaton anal
Cook rectal
Cusco vaginal
Cusco "Swiss pattern" vaginal
Czerny rectal
David rectal
Fansler
Ferguson-Moon
Fergusson
Gabriel rectal
Graves
Graves vaginal
Halle infant
Hartmann nasal
Hinkle-James rectal
Hirschman
House stapes
Kelly rectal
Killian rectal
Killian septum
KleenSpec disposable
Kogan
Kogan-Burke
Kristeller
Martin-Davis rectal
Mathews rectal
Mathier trivalve rectal
Mathieu rectal
Miltex
Naunton Morgan rectal
Parks rectal
Pederson
Pennington rectal
Pratt rectal
rectal
Ricord rectal
Roschke rectal
Sawyer rectal

speculum *(cont.)*
Sims rectal
slotted
Smith-Buie rectal
SRT (smoke-retrieval tube) vaginal
vantage Graves vaginal
Vernon-David rectal
Vienna nasal
Speedy balloon catheter
Spence intervertebral disk rongeur
Spence rongeur forceps
Spence, tail of
Spencer disease
Spencer scissors
Spencer stitch scissors
Spencer Wells artery forceps
Spenco breast prosthesis
Sperma-Tex preshaped mesh graft
spermatic cord
spermatic vessel
Spetzler lumboperitoneal shunt
Spexil (trospectomycin)
sphenoethmoidal suture
spheno-occipital suture
spheno-orbital suture
sphenoparietal suture
sphenopetrosal suture
sphenosquamous suture
sphenotemporal suture
sphenovomerine suture
spherical lesion
spherical neoplasm
spherical reamer
spherocytosis
spheroplast, mycobacterial
sphincter
anal
anorectal
antral
artificial
basal
bicanalicular
biliary
Boyden

sphincter *(cont.)*
  canalicular
  cardiac (stomach)
  cardioesophageal
  choledochal
  colic
  cricopharyngeal
  duodenal
  duodenojejunal
  esophageal
  external anal
  external rectal
  extrinsic
  first duodenal
  gastroesophageal
  Giordano
  hyperactive
  hypertensive lower esophageal
  Hyrtl
  incompetent
  inferior esophageal
  inguinal
  internal anal (IAS)
  internal rectal
  lower esophageal (LES)
  Lütkens (Luetkens)
  mechanically defective
  Nélaton
  Oddi
  O'Beirne
  pancreatic duct
  pancreaticobiliary
  pharyngoesophageal
  prepyloric
  pyloric
  rectal
  upper esophageal (UES)
sphincteral achalasia
sphincter atony
sphincter contraction ring
sphincter dysfunction
sphincterectomy
sphincteric mechanism
sphincter of anal canal, involuntary
sphincter of bile duct
sphincter of hepatopancreatic ampulla
sphincter of Oddi dysfunction (SOD)
sphincter of Oddi manometry
sphincter of Oddi pressure measurement
sphincter of Oddi spasm
sphincteroplasty
  anal
  transduodenal
sphincteroscope
sphincterotome
  balloon
  basket
  Demling-Classen
  hybrid
  needle-knife
  Olympus
  precut
  reverse
  rotating
  Wilson-Cook (modified) wire-guided
sphincterotomy (see also *operations*)
  biliary
  Doubilet
  endoscopic (ES)
  internal
  lateral internal
  Mulholland
  Parks
  Parks partial
  precut
  retrograde
  transduodenal
  "zipper"
sphincterotomy basket
sphincterotomy of papilla
sphincterotomy with stone extraction
sphincter-saving operation
sphincter tone
sphincter urethral muscle
sphingomyelin accumulation in liver and spleen

sphygmomanometer
  analog
  Diagnostix
  digital
  Multikuf
  Prosphyg
  Tycos aneroid
SPI-Argent II peritoneal dialysis catheter
spica bandage
spiculated mass
spiculations on colon
spicule in profile
spicy food
spider angioma (pl. angiomata; angiomas)
spider nevus (pl. nevi)
spider telangiectasia
spider-web clot
Spiess 25 4 mm rigid laparoscope
Spiess endoscope
spigelian fascia
spigelian hernia
spigelian hernia belt
Spigelian line
spike a fever
spike-burst electrical activity
spike burst on electromyogram of colon
spike, fever
spiking fever
spillage of tumor cells
spilled gallstones
spinach stool
spinal afferent
spinal anesthesia
spinal cord injury, concomitant
spinal cord removal instrument
spinal drain
spinal elevator
spinal epidural abscess (SEA)
spinal fluid
spinal fusion gouge
spinal fusion position
spinal headache
spinal immobilization
spinal medulla
spinal needle
spinal perforating forceps
spinal retractor blade
spinal rod
spinal stenosis
spindle cell carcinoma
spindle cell sarcoma
spindle cell thymoma
spindle colonic groove
spindle-shaped incision
spine, anterior superior iliac
SpineCATH intradiscal catheter
Spinelli biopsy needle
SpineScope percutaneous endoscope
spinocan spinal needle
spiral bandage
spiral basket forceps
spiral computed tomography
spiral cortical reamer
spiral CT
spiral drill
spiral fold
spiraling of rectal mucosa
spiral-shaped bacteria
spiral trochanteric reamer
spiral valve of Heister
SpiraStent ureteral stent
spirit lamp
spirochetal jaundice
spirochetosis, Lancereaux-Mathieu-Weil
SpiroFlo bioabsorbable prostate stent
spirometry, incentive
spironolactone
Spiros inhaler
Spivack valve
splanchnic anesthesia
splanchnic AV fistula
splanchnic nerve
splanchnic pressure
splanchnic retractor
splanchnic vasoconstriction

splanchnic vein
splanchnicectomy, intraoperative
 chemical
splash, succussion
S-plasty
splayed cranial suture
spleen
 accessory
 blunt rupture of
 deep purple
 drifting
 ectopic
 enlarged
 floating
 function of
 hyperfunctioning
 inflammation
 long axis of
 marginal zone of
 migrating
 missed accessory
 red pulp of
 ruptured
 sago
 soft
 spontaneous rupture of
 systopic
 tickle of
 wandering
 white pulp of
spleen index
spleen injury
spleen laceration
spleen tip
splenectomy
 en bloc
 incidental
 urgent
splenic abscess
splenic agenesis syndrome
splenic anemia
splenic artery
splenic artery aneurysm
splenic artery embolization
splenic atrophy
splenic AV fistula
splenic blood flow
splenic capsule
splenic cell
splenic congestion
splenic cyst
splenic dullness
splenic engorgement
splenic enlargement
splenic flexure of colon
splenic flexure syndrome
splenic flexure volvulus
splenic hilar adenopathy
splenic hilar lymph node
splenic hilum
splenic hyperplasia
splenic hypertrophy
splenic laceration
splenic notch
splenic parenchyma
splenic ptosis
splenic-renal angle
splenic rupture, delayed
splenic salvage operation with wrapping
 Vicryl mesh
splenic sequestration
splenic tissue
splenic trauma
splenic tumor
splenic vein
splenic vein (SV) and superior mesenteric vein (SMV) thrombosis
splenic vein deformity
splenic vein occlusion
splenic vein patency
splenic vein stenosis
splenic vein stent
splenic vein thrombosis
splenic venography with pressure
 measurement
splenic vessel
splenic vessel rupture
splenitis, acute septic

splenium
splenobronchial fistula
splenocolic ligament
splenogastric omentum
splenoid gland
splenomegalic cirrhosis
splenomegaly
  chronic congestive
  congenital
  congestive
  Egyptian
  fibrocongestive
  Gaucher
  hemolytic
  infectious
  infective
  myelophthisic
  siderotic
  spodogenous
splenoportal hypertension
splenoportography, magnetic resonance
splenoptosis
splenorenal anastomosis
splenorenal angle
splenorenal ligament
splenorenal recess
splenorenal shunt
splenorenal vein anastomosis
splenorenal venous operation
splenorrhaphy
splenosis, thoracic
splinter forceps
splinting of abdomen
splinting of incision with pillow
split calvarial bone graft
split ileostomy
split incision
split overtube
split-sheath catheter
split-thickness skin graft
SPN (support parenteral nutrition)
spodogenous splenomegaly
SpO_2 finger probe for pulse oximetry

sponge
  absorbable
  absorbable collagen
  absorbable gelatin
  Actifoam
  autocount
  Avitene Ultrafoam collagen hemostatic
  bronchial
  butterfly
  cherry
  cherry dissector
  cherry endosponge
  cherry-pit
  Col-R-Sponge
  corneal shield
  cylindrical
  Delicot
  diamond knife
  dissecting
  dissector
  ear packing
  ear wick
  Eder rectal
  eye spear
  eye wick
  fibrin
  flat stick
  4 x 4
  gauze
  gelatin
  Helistat absorbable collagen hemostatic
  impregnated
  Incert
  Incert bioabsorbable implantable
  instrument wipe
  Ivalon
  K-dissector
  Kerlix disposable laparotomy
  Kittner
  Kling
  Krimpt
  K-Sponge

sponge *(cont.)*
  lap (laparotomy)
  Lapwall laparotomy
  Merocel
  moist
  nasal
  nasal dressing
  NeuroCol
  Non-Stix
  Optipore wound-cleaning
  peanut
  Policot II
  polyvinyl alcohol
  Premium Americot
  Prosthex
  Ray-Cot
  Ray-Tec x-ray detectable
  Raypaque
  Rhode Island dissector
  rosebud
  round stick
  saline-moistened
  Sof-Wick drain
  Soft N Dry Merocel
  Sorb-It
  stick
  Surgifoam absorbable gelatin
  triangle
  Ultracot
  Unicot
  Vistec x-ray detectable
  Weck-cel
sponge and needle counts
sponge clamp
sponge count
sponge counter bag
sponge curafoam
sponge dissection
sponge dissector (dissecting sponge)
sponge forceps
sponge holder
sponge-holding forceps
sponge kidney
sponge-on-a-stick
sponge stick
sponge-stick packet
sponge traction
spontaneous bacterial peritonitis (SBP)
spontaneous lateral ventral hernia
spontaneously reduce
spontaneous nipple discharge
spontaneous rupture
spontaneous rupture of liver from subcapsular hematoma
spontaneous rupture of spleen
spontaneous septicopyemia
spontaneous thrombosis
spontaneous ventrolateral hernia
spoon
  elevating
  gall duct
  hernia
  Mayo common duct
  Sellheim elevating
  sharp
  single action
  Volkmann pancreatic calculus
spoon blade
spoon clamp
spoon electrode
spoon forceps
spoon-grasping forceps, spring-loaded, spoon plate
spoon retractor
spoon-shaped spatula
sporadic goiter
sporadic porphyria cutanea tarda
sporadic tumors
Sporanox (itraconazole)
Sporidin-G (*Cryptosporidium parvum* bovine colostrum IgG concentrate)
Sporox II solution
spot
  cold
  DeMorgan
  epigastric
  hematocystic (HCS)
  hot

spot film
spot view
S pouch, ileal
spout, ileal
Sprague Rappaport stethoscope
Spratt curet
SprayGel Adhesion Barrier System
spreader
  Benson pylorus
  bladder neck
  cast
  Finochietto rib
  Hennig cast
  Mayo-Adams
  Millin bladder neck
  pyloric
  rib
  Tuffier rib
spreader graft
spreading forceps
spread suture
Spring Clip surgical stapler
Spring Grip surgical stapler
spring-handled scissors
spring hook
spring-loaded nail
spring-loaded, retractable blunt inner protective tube
spring-wire retractor
Sprinz-Dubin syndrome
Sprinz-Nelson syndrome
Sprotte needle
sprue
  celiac
  collagenous
  nontropical
  secondary nontropical
  tropical
S/P (status post) surgical blade
SPT (station pull-through) technique
S-P-T (thyroid, desiccated porcine)
SP-303, SP-501 Sonoprobe endoscopy system
SPTL-1b vascular lesion laser
SPU (single-patient use) instrument
spud and needle
spud dissector
spur-crushing clamp
Spurling intervertebral disk rongeur
Spurling-Kerrison cervical rongeur
Spurling-Kerrison laminectomy rongeur
Spurling-Kerrison rongeur forceps
Spurling-Kerrison up-biting and down-biting rongeur
Spurling nerve root retractor
Spurling pituitary rongeur
spurting blood
sputum smear
SPV (selective proximal vagotomy)
Spyglass angiography catheter
Spyrogel hydrogel wound and burn dressing
SQS-20 subcuticular skin stapler
squamocolumnar junction
squamocolumnar mucosal junction
squamosomastoid suture
squamosoparietal suture
squamososphenoid suture
squamous anal intraepithelial lesion
squamous carcinoma
squamous carcinoma in situ
squamous cell carcinoma (SCC)
squamous cell carcinoma antigen
squamous cell carcinoma of the esophagus
squamous intraepithelial lesion
squamous island
squamous lining
squamous metaplasia
squamous papilloma
squamous suture
square hollow chisel
square knot
square-L electrode
square reamer
square-shaped awl
squeeze pressure profile of anal sphincter

squeeze, sphincteric
Squirt wound irrigator
S retractor
SRH (stigmata of recent hemorrhage)
SRMD (stress-related mucosal disease)
S-ROM total hip system
SRT (smoke removal tube) vaginal speculum
SRUS (solitary rectal ulcer syndrome)
SRVG (silicone elastomer ring vertical gastroplasty)
SS (somatostatin)
Ssabanejew-Frank gastrostomy
SSBE (short segment Barrett esophagus)
SSC (single-stripe colitis)
SSD, SSD AF (silver sulfadiazine)
SSE (soapsuds enema)
S-shaped brain retractor
S-shaped ileal pouch
S-shaped incision
S-shaped reservoir
S660 small vessel stent
SSRI (selective serotonin reuptake inhibitor)
stabilization plate
stabilizer, Octopus tissue
stabilizing staple
stable diabetes mellitus
stable vital signs
stab incision
stab wound
stab wound incision
Stack autoperfusion balloon
Stack hand retractor
Stader pin
stage A Hodgkin disease
stage B Hodgkin disease
stage, Hinchey diverticulitis
stage I or II medullary carcinoma
staghorn calculus
staghorn stone
staging (see *classification*)
staging and defining arterial and venous involvement
staging celiotomy
staging laparotomy
staging neoplasm
staging of cancer, surgical
staging of cervical carcinoma
staging of malignancy
staging of malignant melanoma
staging operation
stagnant bile
stagnant loop syndrome
stagnation of blood
Stahl clip applier
stain (see also *dye*)
    anti-Schiff
    esterase
    Gram
    hematoxylin and eosin (H&E)
    indigo carmine
    Lugol solution
    methylene blue
    oil-red-O
    PAS
    peroxidase
    rhodanine
    Sudan
    toluidine blue
    Wright
    Ziehl-Neelsen
stainless steel clamp
stainless steel mesh
stainless steel plate
stainless steel preformed skull plate
stainless steel staple
stainless steel surgical blade
stainless steel suture
stainless steel wire
stainless steel wire suture
stairstep air-fluid levels
stale fish syndrome
stalk of polyp
Stamey-Malecot catheter

Stamm gastrostomy
Stamm tube
standard acid reflux test (SART)
standard Allis grasping forceps, 16 mm jaw-length, double-action
standard Bassini inguinal hernia repair
standard bunny kit
standard dissecting knife
standard endoscopic forceps
standard grasper
standard incision
standard Kocher incision
standard One-Piece cannula
standard Whipple pancreaticoduodenectomy
standard with flex tube
standing dorsoplantar view
standing lateral view
standing weightbearing view
stannous pyrophosphate
stannous sulfur colloid
staphylococcal (staph)
staphylococcal food poisoning
staphylococcal sepsis
staphylococcus colitis
Staphylococcus aureus
staphylorrhaphy elevator
staple
  automatic
  barb
  barbed
  Blount
  bone
  Coventry
  Day
  Downing
  duToit
  endostaple
  epiphyseal
  Hernandez-Ros bone
  Howmedica Vitallium
  Johannesberg
  Lactomer absorbable subcuticular skin
staple *(cont.)*
  metallic
  Mitek
  O'Brien
  osteoclast tension
  Owestry
  power-drive
  Proximate
  scalp marker
  skin
  stabilizing
  stainless steel
  Stone four-point
  surgical
  suture
  tabletop Stone
  TA-30 4.5 mm
  titanium
  Vitallium
  Wilberg bone
  Zimaloy
staple and transect the appendix at the base
stapled hemorrhoidectomy
stapled-off ileum
staple driver
staple extractor
staple-ligated
staple line dehiscence
staple line is inspected for hemostasis
staple mesh to abdominal wall over the hernia site
stapler (see also *suture*)
  Auto Suture
  Auto Suture Multifire Endo GIA 30
  Auto Suture One-Shot
  Auto Suture Premium CEEA
  Auto Suture Premium TA-55 surgical
  Auto Suture surgical
  Auto Suture SurgiStitch
  CEEA (curved end-to-end)
  CEEA 21 or 25
  CEEA circular

stapler *(cont.)*
- circular
- Cobe
- curved circular
- DePalma
- double-headed PI90
- EEA (end-to-end anastomosis)
- EEA Auto Suture
- Endoclip II surgical
- Endo Close surgical
- Endo GIA surgical
- Endo GIA II
- Endo Hernia
- Endo Hernia surgical
- Endo Hernia Universal
- Endopath EMS hernia
- Endopath ES reusable endoscopic
- Endopath EZ45 No Knife endoscopic linear
- Endopath linear cutter
- Endopath multifeed
- Endopath no-knife
- Endo Stitch
- endoscopic articulating (EAS)
- endoscopic multifeed (EMS) TA-90
- GIA (gastrointestinal anastomosis) surgical
- hemoclip
- ILS (intraluminal stapler) surgical
- In-Tac bone anchor
- LDS surgical
- linear
- Multifire Endo GIA
- Multifire Endo Hernia
- Multifire GIA surgical
- Multifire TA surgical
- Multifire VersaTack
- No Knife
- Origin Tacker
- PI surgical
- PolyGIA
- Premium CEEA circular
- Premium Plus CEEA disposable stapler

stapler *(cont.)*
- ProTack
- Proximate flexible linear
- Proximate ILS curved intraluminal
- Proximate linear cutter
- Roticulator
- S*D* sorb
- Spring Clip
- Spring Grip surgical
- SQS-20 subcuticular skin
- stainless steel
- Surgeons Choice
- Surgigrip
- Surgineedle surgical
- TA-30 Auto Suture
- TA-55 Auto Suture
- TA90-BN
- 3M
- TL-90
- VCS Clip adapter
- VersaTack
- Visistat

stapler-facilitated rectal eversion
staple-shaped retractor
staple the mesoappendix
staple the overlying peritoneum shut
stapling device
stapling esophagodiverticulostomy by endoscopy
stapling, gastric
stapling off of small gastric pouch
STAR (specialized tissue-aspirating resectoscope)
STAR (study of tamoxifen and raloxifene)
StarBAR electrode
STAR excimer laser system
starch bandage
starch blocker
starch peritonitis
Starck dilator
Starion thermal cautery hook
Starline select instruments
Starlix (nateglinide)

starry-sky pattern
starting reamer
starvation acidosis
stasis
  antral
  bile
  bile duct
  biliary
  esophageal
  fecal
  gallbladder
  gastric
  gastrointestinal
  ileal
  intestinal
  liver
  postgastrectomy
  postsurgical gastric
  venous
stasis cirrhosis
stasis dermatitis
stasis esophagitis
stasis gallbladder
stasis liver
stasis ulcer
Stata software analysis
Statak suture
State end-to-end anastomosis
Statham P23 strain gauge
static locking nail system
static position
stationary angle guide
stationary grasper
station pull-through esophageal
  manometry technique
STATLase-SDL diode endoscopic laser
StatLock Universal Plus
Stat*Simple test
STAT2 Pumpette extension set
STAT2 Pumpette primary set I.V. (IV)
  gravity flow controller
status
  ECOG performance
  hemodynamic
status *(cont.)*
  hydration
  intravascular volume
  mental
  nodal
  nutritional
  progesterone-receptor
  receptor
status post (S/P)
stay suture
STC (slow transit constipation)
steady manual pressure
steady pain
steakhouse syndrome
steamy appearance
steatohepatitis
steatorrhea
  idiopathic
  pancreatic
  tropical
steatosis
  drug-induced
  toxic
Stecher arachnoid knife
steel sole plate
Steelex suture
steep LAO (left anterior oblique) view
steerable guidewire system
Steffee pedicle plate
Steffee pedicular rod
Steffee plate
Steffee probe
Steffee screw plate
Steinbach mallet
Stein-Leventhal syndrome
Steinhauser bone clamp
Steinmann extension nail
Steinmann intestinal forceps
Steinmann pin
Steinmann tendon forceps
Steis needle
stellate cell
stellate mass
stellate pattern

Stellbrink synovectomy rongeur
stem base plate
stem cell autograft
stenosis
  ampullary
  anal
  antral
  aortic valve
  arterial
  benign papillary
  bowel
  bronchial
  cardiac valvular
  cervical
  choledochoduodenal junctional
  congenital hypertrophic pyloric
  congenital pyloric
  discrete
  esophageal
  hiatal
  hypertrophic pyloric
  inflamed (of sigmoid colon)
  intestinal
  left-sided segmental portal
  mitral
  papillary
  pulmonary
  pyloric
  rectal
  short length hepatic vein (SLHVS)
  spinal
  stomal
stenosis of anastomosis
stenosis of breast duct
stenosis of esophageal hiatus
stenosis of pouch
stenosis of renal artery
stenotic lesion
stenotic segment
Stenotrophomonas maltophilia
stent
  Acculink self-expanding
  ACS Multi-Link OTW Duet
  ACS RX Multi-Link

stent *(cont.)*
  Amsterdam
  Anaconda
  Anastaflo
  AneuRX
  AngioStent balloon-expandable
  autologous vein-covered
  balloon-expandable
  Bard Memotherm colorectal
  Bard XT bifurcated
  beStent
  beStent Rival
  biliary
  BioSorb resorbable urology
  Biostent
  Bx Velocity
  Bx Velocity coronary artery
  Bx Velocity sirolimus-coated
  carboplatin-coated plastic biliary
  Champion nitinol
  choledochal
  colorectal
  Cook Oasis biliary
  coronary
  CrossFlex LC
  CrossFlex TMLC coronary
  crutched stick-type biliary duct
  Czaja-McCaffrey rigid
  double pigtail
  DoubleStent biliary endoprosthesis
  Dynalink self-expanding biliary
  EES (expandable esophageal)
  endobiliary
  ENDOcare nitinol
  EndoCoil biliary
  EndoCoil esophageal
  endoscopic biliary
  endovascular
  Enforcer SDS
  EsophaCoil self-expanding
    esophageal
  esophageal
  esophageal Z-Stent with Dua
    antireflux valve

stent *(cont.)*
- expandable metal
- Firlit drip
- flexible
- Flexima biliary
- French
- GFX 2
- Gianturco expandable (self-expanding) metallic biliary
- Gianturco-Rösch Z-stent
- Gianturco-Roubin flexible coil
- GR II
- Harrell Y
- Hemobahn
- Hepamed-coated Wiktor
- Herculink 14 biliary
- HIPS (heparin infusion prior to stenting)
- Hood stoma
- Horizon
- INR neurological
- InStent self-expanding
- IntraStent DoubleStrut biliary endoprosthesis
- IntraStent DoubleStrut XS
- IntraStent LP biliary
- intravascular
- INX stainless steel
- iridium-192-loaded
- IRIS coronary
- IsoStent radioisotope
- Lubri-Flex
- Megalink biliary
- Memotherm biliary
- Memotherm colorectal
- Memotherm Flexx biliary
- Memotherm nitinol
- Memotherm nitinol self-expanding
- Merogel
- Microvasive Rapid Exchange biliary system
- Mini Crown
- MPD (main pancreatic duct)
- Multi-Flex

stent *(cont.)*
- Multi-Link Tetra
- neurovascular
- NexStent carotid
- NIR ON Ranger
- NIR Primo Monorail
- Niroyal Elite Monorail
- Niroyal Monorail
- nitinol
- Olympus biliary
- OmniStent
- ostiomeatal
- Palmaz
- Palmaz balloon-expandable
- Palmaz Corinthian
- Palmaz Corinthian transhepatic biliary
- Palmaz-Schatz
- Palmaz-Schatz balloon-expandable
- Palmaz-Schatz Crown
- Palmaz-Schatz Crown balloon-expandable
- Palmaz-Schatz Mini Crown
- Palmaz-Schatz (PSS)
- Palmaz vascular
- pancreatic
- pancreatic duct
- Paragon Champion
- Paragon coronary
- Percuflex Plus
- percutaneous
- Perflex
- Perflex stainless steel
- pigtail
- Pilling Weck Y-stent forceps
- pliable
- PowerGrip
- preoperative endoscopic biliary
- ProstaCoil self-expanding
- radioisotope
- Radius
- RX Herculink
- RX Herculink 14 biliary
- RX Herculink 14 pre-mounted

stent *(cont.)*
- S.M.A.R.T. (shape memory alloy recoverable technology) biliary
- S660 small vessel
- SAXX renal
- self-expanding metal
- self-expanding metallic wall
- self-expanding microporous (SEMS)
- SEMS (self-expanding microporous)
- Silastic
- SMART biliary
- SoloPass
- SpiraStent ureteral
- SpiroFlo bioabsorbable prostate
- splenic vein
- straight
- Strecker
- Supra G
- Symphony
- Symphony nitinol
- Talent LPS
- transhepatic biliary
- T-tube
- T–Y
- Ultraflex Diamond biliary
- Ultraflex
- Uni-trac
- UroCoil self-expanding
- UroLume
- U-tube
- Vistaflex biliary
- Wallstent
- Wiktor
- Wiktor GX Hepamed
- Wilson-Cook French
- X-Trode
- XT
- Z

stent-assisted angioplasty
stent dressing
stenting, endobiliary
stent placement
stent remover, Carr-Locke
stent retriever, Soehendra
Stenver view
Stenzel rod
step-cut reamer
step-down effect
step drill
Step minimally invasive surgical access device
step-on can
step section
stercolith, appendiceal
stercoraceous vomiting
stercoral appendicitis
stercoral diarrhea
stercoral ulcer
stercoral ulceration
StereoEndoscope
StereoGuide stereotactic needle core biopsy
StereoScope camera head
stereotactic aspiration biopsy
stereotactic biopsy needle
stereotactic brain biopsy
stereotactic breast biopsy
stereotactic core needle biopsy (SCNB)
stereotactic laser microsurgery
stereotactic (or stereotaxic) operating microscope
stereotactic transsphenoidal hypophysectomy
stereotaxic endoscope
stereotaxically guided interstitial laser therapy
Stericare glycerine hydrogel dressing
Steri-Drape plastic incise drape
sterile drape
sterile dressing
sterilely prepared and draped
sterilely prepped and draped
sterile necrotizing pancreatitis
sterile pancreatic necrosis
sterile paper drape
steri-stripped incision
Steri-Strips dressing
Steri-Strips suture

sternal pleural reflection
sternal retractor
sternal split approach
sternal-splitting incision
sternal wire suture
Sternberg-Reed cell
sternocleidomastoid muscle or forearm autograft of parathyroid gland
sternocostal hiatus
sternotomy incision
sternotomy saw
steroid
  contraceptive
  nonabsorbable
steroid-dependent patient
steroid foam enema
steroid synthesis inhibition
steroid taper
Sterrad sterilization system
Stethodop, Adscope
stethoscope
  Bowles
  DeLee-Hillis
  Littmann Cardiology III
  Littmann Classic II S.E.
  Littmann Master Cardiology
  Littmann Master Classic II
  Littre hernia
  Mon-a-therm esophageal
  Sprague Rappaport
Stetten intestinal clamp
Stevens-Johnson syndrome
Stevenson alligator forceps
Stevenson grasping forceps
Stevens tenotomy scissors
Stewart crypt hook
St. George hemorrhoid-seizing forceps
stick sponge
stick-tie
Stieglitz splinter forceps
Stifcore aspiration needle
stiff ribbon retractor
stigmata of recent hemorrhage (SRH)
Stiles seizing forceps
Stiles tissue-grasping forceps
still camera
Stille-Barraya intestinal forceps
Stille bone chisel
Stille bone drill
Stille bone gouge
Stille cranial drill
Stille-Crawford clamp
Stille elevator
Stille gallstone forceps
Stille-Giertz rib shears
Stille hand drill
Stille-Horsley bone forceps
Stille-Horsley bone rongeur
Stille-Leksell rongeur
Stille-Liston bone cutter
Stille-Liston bone rongeur
Stille-Liston bone-cutting forceps
Stille-Luer bone rongeur
Stille-Luer duckbill rongeur
Stille-Luer-Echlin rongeur
Stille-Luer rongeur
Stille-Luer rongeur forceps
Stille-Mayo scissors
Stille plaster shears
Stille rib shears
Stille-Ruskin bone rongeur
Stille-Sherman bone drill
Stille vessel clamp
Stimson dressing
stimulant laxative
stimulated gastric secretion test
stimulation (also see *test*)
  cholecystokinin
  endogenous
  excess TSH
  faucial thermal-tactile
  gastrin
  LARSI
  long-acting thyroid (LAT)
  nerve
  nerve root
  pentagastrin
  repetitive nerve

stone *(cont.)*
- opaque
- pigmented
- postoperative residual
- radiolucent
- radiopaque
- refractory bile duct
- renal
- residual
- salivary
- skin
- staghorn
- struvite
- tear
- ultrasound disruption of
- ureteric
- urinary
- vein
- womb

stone analysis
stone basket (dislodger)
Stone clamp applicator
stone extraction
Stone four-point staple
stone fragmentation
stone-grasping forceps
Stone-Holcombe intestinal clamp
stone-holding basket forceps
stone impaction
Stone intestinal clamp
stonelike calculus
stonelike mass
stone mole
Stookey cranial rongeur
stool (pl. stools)
- abdominal
- acholic
- bacteria in
- bilious
- black tarry
- bloody
- brown
- bulky
- caddy (dark, sandy mud)

stool *(cont.)*
- caliber of
- clay-colored
- Clinitest-negative
- Clinitest-positive
- color and caliber
- consistency of
- continent of
- currant jelly
- dark
- dark green
- diarrhea
- elimination of
- excess fluid loss in
- fatty
- flattened
- floating
- foamy
- formed
- foul-smelling
- frank blood in
- frequency of
- Gram stain of
- green
- gross blood in
- guaiac-negative
- guaiac-positive
- hard
- heme-negative
- heme-positive
- huge
- impacted
- lienteric
- light gray
- liquid
- loose
- mahogany-colored
- malodorous
- maroon-colored
- melenic (not melanotic)
- mucoid
- mucous
- mushy
- nonbloody

stool *(cont.)*
- occult blood in
- oily
- pale
- pea soup
- pelleted
- pencil-like
- pipestem
- progressive thinning of
- rabbit
- reducing substance in
- residual
- retention of
- ribbon
- rice-water
- runny
- sago-grain
- scybalous
- semiformed
- semisolid
- silver
- slurry of
- soft
- spinach
- tarry black
- undigested food in
- unformed
- watery
- white fatty
- Wright stain of

stool color
stool consistency
stool culture
stool cytoxin test
stool electrolyte test
stool for occult blood
stool for ova and parasites (O&P)
stool guaiac
stool guaiac negative
stool guaiac positive
stool incontinence
stooling
stool osmotic gap test
stool smear
stool softener
stool specimen
stool urobilinogen
Stoppa posterior approach
Stoppa-Rives giant prosthetic repair of the visceral sac
storage disease
store (pl. stores)
- glycogen
- hepatic glycogen
- hepatic iron
- iron
- liver iron

storm
- thyroid
- thyrotoxic

Storz 26033 AP 0° 10 mm rigid laparoscope
Storz 26033 BP 0° 10 mm rigid laparoscope
Storz 9050B AutoexposureColor endoscopic camera
Storz AP 26003 0° 10 mm rigid laparoscope
Storz bronchoscope
Storz camera
Storz cholangiograsper
Storz cystoscope
Storz dolphin-nose grasper
Storz endoscope
Storz esophagoscope
Storz high-flow insufflator pump
Storz high insufflator
Storz high-speed insufflator
Storz Hopkins laparoscope
Storz hysteroscope
Storz KSA-2S SuperCam endoscopic camera
Storz laparoscope
Storz laparoscopic telescope
Storz laparoscopic video camera
Storz LaproFlator
Storz Microsystems cranial fixation plate

Storz Microsystems microplate
Storz Microsystems plate-holding
forceps
Storz Microsystems pliers
Storz minilaparoscope
Storz OR1 electronic endoscopy system
Storz printer
Storz proctoscope
Storz resectoscope
Storz rigid laparoscope
Storz videoscope
Storz wire-cutting scissors
Storz 0° 10 mm telescope
Stovkis test
strabismus scissors
straight biopsy cup forceps
straight bone rongeur
straight chain fatty acid
straight chest tube
straight chisel
straight clamp
straight Crile forceps
straight cutting needle
straight dissecting scissors
straight dissector
straight double-action monopolar
scissors
straight dura hook
straight-end cup forceps
straight forceps
straight gouge
straight incision
straight Kelly forceps
straight knife
straight micro grasper
straight micro scissors
straight oscillating saw
straight periosteal elevator
straight pituitary rongeur
straight reamer
straight retractor
straight scissors
straight stent
straight taper point
straight threaded rod
strain-gauge manometry
straining at defecation
straining at stool
stranding
fascial
mesenteric
mesenteric fat (on CT scan)
soft tissue
strangulated bowel
strangulated bowel obstruction
strangulated hemorrhoid
strangulated hernia
strangulated paraesophageal hernia
strangulated viscus
strangulation, intestinal
strangulation necrosis
strangulation obstruction
strangulation of hernia
strangulation of inguinal hernia
strap muscles
Strassburg test
StrataSorb composite wound dressing
stratified clot
Stratis II MRI system
Stratte needle
Stratte-TC needle holder
Strauss rectoscope
Strauss sign
strawberry gallbladder
strawberry hemangioma
strawberry nevus
straw-colored ascites
straw-colored fluid
streaking
Strecker stent
Street medullary pin
Street nail
Strelinger colon clamp
strep (streptococcus)
anhemolytic
beta hemolytic
group B (GBS)
hemolytic
nonhemolytic

streptavidin-polyperoxidase
Streptococcus viridans
streptozocin, mitomycin C, and 5-FU (SMF) chemotherapy protocol
streptozotocin
stress Broden view
stress eversion view
stress film
stress gastritis
stress incontinence
stress-induced gastritis
stress-induced organ dysfunction
stress, intra-abdominal sheer
stress inversion view
stress reduction with regional anesthesia
stress-related mucosal disease (SRMD)
Stresstein (multiple branched-chain amino acids)
Stresstein liquid feeding
stress tolerant position
stress ulcer
stress ulceration
stress view
Stretta device for delivery of radio-frequency energy
stria (pl. striae)
striae distensae
striated muscle
Strickland suture
Strickland suture technique
stricture
  anal
  annular esophageal
  antral
  benign biliary
  bile duct
  biliary
  chronic (of the small bowel)
  cicatricial
  contractile
  cricopharyngeal
  division of
  esophageal
  gastric outlet

stricture *(cont.)*
  hilar
  intrahepatic
  irritable
  longitudinal esophageal
  peptic
  pharyngeal
  postsurgical
  pyloric
  rectal
  recurrent
  spasmodic
  ureteral
strictured segment
stricture formation
stricturoplasty
stridor
strike-through
string cell carcinoma
string guideline
string-of-beads appearance
string sign in terminal ileum
string test
strip
  bovine pericardium
  Chin-Up Strip
  glucose monitoring test
  Gore-Tex
  Oxycel
  reagent
  Steri-Strips
  tricortical iliac
strip biopsy
strip biopsy method
stripe, properitoneal flank
strip immunoblot assay (SIA)
stripper
  Matson rib
  Mayo external vein
  Meyer vein
  Nabatoff vein
strobe flash endoscopic light source
stroke
Stromagen

stromal fibrosis
stromal hemorrhage
stromal necrosis
Stromectol (ivermectin)
Strong Iodine (iodine; potassium
  iodide)
strongyloidiasis
structural aberration
structural homology
structural lesion
Strully dissecting scissors
Strully dural
Strully dural hook
Strully-Gigli rongeur
Strully-Gigli saw
Strully-Kerrison rongeur
Strully neurological scissors
Strully scissors
struma fibrosa
struma lymphomatosis
struma nodosa
strut bone graft
strut template
strut-type pin
struvite stone
StrykeFlow electrocautery probe
StrykeFlow suction irrigator
Stryker cartilage knife
Stryker endoscopy video camera system
Stryker illuminated retractor
Stryker laparoscope
Stryker microdebrider
Stryker microsurgery drill
Stryker notch view
Stryker saw
Stryker stent
Stryker 380-10, 0° 10 mm rigid
  laparoscope
Stryker 380-11, 0° 10 mm rigid
  laparoscope
Stryker 380-12, 30° 10 mm rigid
  laparoscope
Stryker 590 color endoscopic camera
Stryker trumpet valve
Stryker wedge suture anchor
ST segment
STSG (split-thickness skin graft)
Stuck laminectomy retractor
Stucker bile duct dilator
studding
  omental
  peritoneal
study (see also *test*)
  APC (adenoma prevention with
    celecoxib) study
  coagulation
  colonic transit
  contrast
  Early Treatment Diabetic
    Retinopathy Study
  enema contrast
  esophageal motility
  fecal fat
  gastric motility
  gastrografin contrast
  HALT-C (hepatitis C antiviral
    long-term treatment to prevent
    cirrhosis)
  kinetic gallbladder
  manometric
  marker transit
  mecholyl
  noninvasive localization
  nuclear technetium-99
  nuclear-tagged red blood cell
    bleeding
  pelvic floor function
  serial CK enzyme
  small bowel contrast study
  upper GI contrast
  videoendoscopic swallowing (VESS)
stump
  appendiceal
  blind
  cervical
  distal cremasteric
  distal artery
  duodenal

stump *(cont.)*
  gastric
  limb
  rectal
stump ligation
St. Vincent tube occluding clamp
stylet
  intubation
  malleable aluminum
  pediatric video optical intubation
  plastic-sheathed malleable
    aluminum
  Satin-slip
  TFX Medical catheter
  video optical intubation
Stylet internal esophageal MRI coil
S-type amylase (salivary)
Stypven time test
subacute appendicitis
subacute granulomatous thyroiditis
subacute hepatic necrosis
subacute hepatitis
subacute inflammation
subacute necrosis
subacute necrotizing encephalomyopathy
subacute nodular migratory panniculitis
subacute nonspecific peritonitis
subacute obstruction
subacute pancreatitis
subacute perforation
subacute thyroiditis
subannular mattress suture
subaponeurotic abscess
subarachnoid anesthesia
subarachnoid block
subarachnoid catheter
subarachnoid hemorrhage
subareolar duct, dilation of the
subcapsular hematoma
subcarinal node
subcecal appendix
subcholangiopancreatoscope
subchondral bone plate
subchondral drill
subclavian catheter
subclavian-external carotid artery graft
subclinical hepatitis
subclinical infection
subclavian line
subclavian peel-away sheath
subclavian vein
subcostal incision
subcostal margin
subcostal plane
subcu (subcutaneous)
subcutaneous breast implant
subcutaneous catheter tunnel
subcutaneous emphysema
subcutaneous fat
subcutaneous fat necrosis
subcutaneous gas
subcutaneous inflammation
subcutaneous injection artifact
subcutaneous layer
subcutaneous mastectomy
subcutaneous nodule
subcutaneous pannus
subcutaneous structure
subcutaneous suture
subcutaneous tissue
subcutaneous tissue flap
subcutaneous tunnel
subcutaneous ulcer
subcutaneous ventricular reservoir
  catheter
subcutaneous wound
subcuticular layer
subcuticular suture
subdiaphragmatic abscess
subdiaphragmatic diverticulum
subdiaphragmatic perirenal region
subdural abscess
subdural drainage catheter
subdural effusion
subdural hematoma
subdural hemorrhage
subdural-to-peritoneal shunt

subendoscope
subfascial bleeder
subfascial endoscopic perforator surgery (SEPS)
subfascial hematoma
subgaleal abscess
subglandular augmentation mammoplasty
subglottic airway
subhepatic abscess
subhepatic area
subhepatic cecum
subhepatic phlegmon
subhepatic space
subhepatic space fluid
subjective dysphagia
submandibular space
submassive hepatic necrosis
submassive necrosis
submental space
submental vertex view
Sub-Microinfusion catheter
submucosa
submucosal abscess
submucosal carcinoma of the thoracic esophagus
submucosal development
submucosal dissection
submucosal esophageal venous plexus
submucosal fluctuance
submucosal hematoma
submucosal hemorrhage
submucosal saline injection technique
submucosal thickening
submucosal tumor
submucosal tunnel technique
submucosal venous plexus
submuscular breast implant
subnormal serum calcium concentration
suboptimal film
suboptimal thyroid hormone production
subperiosteal abscess
subperiosteal bone resorption
subperitoneal appendicitis
subperitoneal space
subphrenic abscess
Subramanian clamp
subsequent hernia formation
subsequent reanastomosis
subsequent T-tube track ductal dilatation and postoperative choledochoscopy
subserosal hemorrhage
subserosal layer
subserosal needle catheter jejunostomy
subserosal tumor
subsigmoid fossa
substernal extension from an enlarged thyroid
substernal gland
substernal goiter
substernal pain
substernal thyroid gland
substituted benzimidazole
subtotal colectomy
subtotal gastrectomy
subtotal lesion
subtotal pancreatectomy
subtotal parathyroidectomy
subtotal thyroidectomy
subtraction film
subumbilical incision
subumbilical space
subungual abscess
subungual melanoma
subvesical duct
subxiphoid trocar
subxiphoid view
subxiphoid window
succinylacetone
succussion sound
succussion splash (over the stomach)
sucker, sump
sucking chest wound
sucralfate
sucrose intolerance, congenital
sucrose-isomaltose (SI) deficiency

sucrose-isomaltose malabsorption,
  congenital
suction (see also *tube*)
  bulb
  closed
  continuous NG
  DeLee
  Endo-AID suction irrigation
  flexible dental
  FlowGun
  Gomco
  lavage and
  low intermittent
  mucosal resection
  nasogastric (NG)
  nasogastric tube (NTS)
  pinpoint
  Poole
  Res-Q-Vac hand-powered
  suctioned
  Wangensteen
suction-assisted lipoplasty (SAL)
suction biopsy
Suction Buster catheter
suction cannula
suction cap method of endoscopic
suction-coagulator, Cameron-Miller
suction-coagulator with valves
suction cup, endoscopic
suction drain
suction handle
  Medi-Vac Flexi-Clear
  Medi-Vac Yankauer
suction irrigation electrode (SIE)
suction irrigation probe
suction/irrigation system, Sherwood
  intrascopic
suction-irrigator, House-Radpour
suction-ligator
suction liner
  Medi-Vac CRD
  Medi-Vac Flex Advantage
suction lipectomy
suction port
suction retractor
suction tip
suction tube
Sudan stain
sudden cardiac death
sudden infant death syndrome (SIDS)
sudden onset of pain
Sudeck point
suffocative goiter
sugar-icing liver
Sugita right-angle aneurysm clamp
Sugiura esophageal variceal transection
sulciolar gastric mucosa
sulcus, inframammary
Sulfalax Calcium (docusate sodium)
Sulfamylon (mafenide acetate)
sulfasalazine
sulfasalazine enema
sulfasalidine (Azulfidine; Azulfidine
  EN-tabs)
sulfate (SO_4^{2-})
sulfobromophthalein sodium test
sulfonamide
sulfonylurea
sulfur colloid liver scan
Sumner sign
sump (see *drain; tub*e)
sump drain
sump nasogastric tube
sump sucker
sump syndrome
sun exposure
Sunday staphylorrhaphy elevator
Sundt loop shunt
sunrise view
sunset view
SuperAnchor suture anchor
Superblade blade
SuperChar
Supercut dissecting scissors
superficial abscess
superficial basal epithelial membrane
  (SBEM)
superficial circumflex iliac artery

superficial gastric carcinoma
superficial gastritis
superficial infection of the breast
superficial inguinal lymph node
superficial inguinal pouch
superficial inguinal ring
superficial layer, fatty
superficial necrosis
superficial perineal pouch
superficial spreading melanoma
Superglue (cyanoacrylate) tissue
adhesive
superior border of pancreas
superior duodenal fold
superior duodenal recess
superior hemorrhoidal artery (superior
rectal)
superior hemorrhoidal vein
superior laryngeal nerve
superior laryngeal nerve injury
superior mesenteric arteriogram
superior mesenteric artery (SMA)
superior mesenteric artery syndrome
(SMAS)
superior mesenteric artery thrombosis
superior mesenteric vein
superior pancreaticoduodenal artery
superior parathyroid gland
superior pedicle technique reduction
mammoplasty
superior pharyngeal wall
superior pole of the thyroid
superior pubic ligament
superior rectus suture
superior thoracic aperture
superior thoracic artery
superior thyroid artery
superior thyroid vein
superior transverse rectal fold
superior vena cava
supernumerary breast nipple
supernumerary kidney
superselective vagotomy
Super Seracult test
Superstat hemostatic wound pad
SuperStitch
Super-supraglottic swallow
supervaterian duodenum
supervised community abstinence
superwet reduction mammoplasty
supine abdominal film
supine film
supine full view
supine position
supine position driver
supine view
supplement (see also *feeding*)
caloric
Casec calcium
food
Gluco-Pro nutritional
Travasorb MCT
support
arm
BiPAP S/T-D 30 ventilatory
BiPAP S/T-D ventilatory
bladder neck
breast
cervical
compression
nutritional
pressor
pressure
prolonged ventilatory
ventilating
wrist
support parenteral nutrition (SPN)
suppository
suppressed thyrotropin level
suppressing dose of dexamethasone
suppression
acid
dexamethasone
pituitary
thyroid
TSH (thyroid-stimulating hormone)
suppression of thyroid nodule

suppressor T cell
suppuration
suppurative appendicitis
suppurative appendix
suppurative cholangitis
suppurative cholecystitis
suppurative choledochitis
suppurative infection
suppurative pancreatitis
suppurative peritonitis
suppurative thyroiditis
supraceliac aorta
supraceliac aortic cross-clamp
supraclavicular block anesthesia
supraclavicular lymphadenopathy
supraclavicular lymph node
supracolic compartment
supracondylar plate
supracrestal plane
supraduodenal approach
Supra G coronary stent
suprahepatic abscess
suprahepatic caval cuff
suprahepatic space
suprahepatic vena cava
suprahyoid neck dissection
supralevator abscess
supralevator space
Supramid Extra suture material
supramylohyoid
supranuclear lesion
suprapatellar cannula
suprapubic pain
suprapubic region
suprapubic trocar
suprarenal aortic cross-clamp
suprarenal impression
suprasphincteric fistula
suprasternal notch view
supraumbilical DPL
supravaterian duodenum
Supreme electrophysiology catheter
Supreme II blood glucose meter
sural nerve biopsy
suramin sodium
SureBite biopsy forceps
Sure-Closure skin-stretching system graft
SureCuff catheter
SureCuff tissue in-growth cuff
SureFit electrosurgical grounding pad
Sure-Flex dilatation catheter
SureLac (lactose enzyme)
SurePress compression dressing
Sureshot metal sheathed injection needle
SureSite transparent adhesive film dressing
SureStep glucose monitor
SureStep Pro blood glucose monitor
Suretac suture
surface (see *facies*)
surface electrode
surface elevation
surface epithelium
surface of gland
surface of liver bed
surface umbilical pyloromyotomy
Surfak (docusate calcium)
Surfit adhesive
Sur-Fit AutoLock ostomy device
Sur-Fit Mini Pouch (ostomy)
Sur-Fit Natura ostomy device
Sur-Fit Pouch Cover
Sur-Fit Stoma Cap
Surgalloy needle
Surgenomic endoscope
surgeon square knot
Surgeons Choice stapler
surgeon's knot
surgery (see *operation*)
  antireflux
  bariatric
  complication of
  debulking
  definitive
  emergent
  exploratory

surgery *(cont.)*
 flexible endoscopic
 HALS (hand-assisted laparoscopic surgery)
 keyhole
 laparoscopic
 minimally invasive
 salvage
Surgiblade sterile scalpel blade
surgical abdomen
surgical airway
surgical anesthesia
surgical approach for drainage
surgical catgut
surgical clipper
surgical complication
surgical cricothyroidotomy
surgical debridement
surgical decompression
surgical drainage
Surgical Dynamics aspiration probe
surgical emphysema
surgical excision
surgical exploration
surgical field
surgical gut
surgical gut suture
 chromic
 plain
surgical herniorrhaphy
surgical intervention
surgical isolation bubble system (SIBS)
surgical laparoscopy
surgically bypassed from fecal stream
surgically correctable hypertension
surgically implanted hemodialysis catheter (SIHC)
surgical margins
surgical mesh
surgical microinstruments
Surgical No Bounce mallet
surgical palliation
surgical portosystemic shunting
surgical reinforcement material, Enteryx biopolymer
surgical resection with wide margins
surgical scar
surgical scissors with TC blades
surgical scrub (see *cleanser*)
surgical sealant (see *adhesive*; *glue; hemostat; medications*)
surgical shunt
Surgical Simplex P adhesive
surgical site infection
surgical solution
surgical splenectomy
surgical staging of cancer
surgical stainless steel suture
surgical stapling
surgical steel skin clip
surgical therapy
surgical treatment of morbid obesity
surgical ulcer
surgical vagotomy
surgical wrap
Surgicel fibrillar absorbable hemostat
Surgicel gauze
Surgicel Nu-Knit absorbable hemostat
Surgicel Nu-Knit hemostatic agent
Surgicel pads (cellulose, oxidized)
Surgicel strips
Surgiclip
Surgidac braided coated polyester Dacron suture
Surgidac braided polyester suture
Surgidac suture material
Surgidyne
Surgiflex Wave suction/irrigation system
Surgifoam absorbable gelatin sponge
Surgigrip stapler
Surgigut chromic suture
Surgigut plain suture
Surgi-Kleen skin cleanser
Surgilase CO_2 laser
Surgilase Nd:YAG laser
Surgilase 150 laser
SurgiLav irrigation instrument

SurgiLav Plus
SurgiLav Plus hydrodebridement system
Surgilene suture
Surgilon suture
Surg-I-Loop
Surgi-Mark
Surgimotor
Surgineedle surgical stapler
Surgipeel cover
Surgiport 10-11 trocar
Surgiport trocar
Surgi-Prep depilatory
Surgi–Prep (Betadine, povidone-iodine)
Surgi-Press pressure infuser
Surgipro mesh graft
Surgipro mesh suture
Surgipro monofilament polypropylene suture
Surgipro polypropylene mesh
Surgipro Prolene mesh graft
SurgiScope endoscope
SurgiScope robotic surgery system
SurgiSis sling/mesh graft
Surgispike
Surgi-Start Kit single-basin set
Surgitech laparoscope
Surgitie ligating loop suture
Surgivac drain
Surgiview laparoscope
Surgiview multiuse disposable laparoscope
Surgiwand suction device
Surgiwand II
surreptitious administration of insulin
surreptitious vomiting
surrounding breast stroma
surrounding fatty tissue
surveillance, endoscopic
Surveillance, Epidemiology, and End Results (SEER) database
survey, Third National Health and Nutrition Examination Survey (NHANES III)
survival benefits
survival
  disease-free
  five-year cancer
  graft
  long-term
  median length of
  overall
  patient
Susano (atropine sulfate; scopolamine hydrobromide; hyoscyamine hydrobromide; phenobarbital)
suspensory breast ligament
suspensory muscle of duodenum
suspicion of cancer
suspicious calcification
suspicious lesion
suspicious tissue
Sustacal enteral nutritional therapy
Sustacal HC (high-calorie) liquid feeding
Sustacal HN (high-nitrogen) liquid feeding
Sustacal Pudding
Sustagen enteral nutritional therapy
Sustagen liquid feeding
sustained response
Sutcliffe Boey laser shield
sutilains enzymes
Sutralon suture
SutraSilk suture
Suturamid suture material
suture (also called *stitch*, *suture material; staple*)
  Aberdeen knot
  absorbable
  Acier stainless steel
  Acufex bioabsorbable Suretac
  Ailee
  Albert
  alternating blue and white mattress
  anchoring
  angle
  apical
  Appolito

suture *(cont.)*
- approximation
- ArthroSew
- atraumatic
- atraumatic chromic
- Auto Suture
- Auto Suture ABBI system
- Auto Suture One-Shot anastomotic device
- Auto Suture Soft Thoracoport
- Auto Suture SurgiStitch
- Auto Suture universal retractor base
- Bard endoscopic suturing
- baseball stitch
- basilar
- basting
- Becker
- Bell
- bioabsorbable
- BioSorb
- Biosyn monofilament synthetic absorbable
- Biosyn synthetic monofilament
- biparietal
- black
- blue and white
- blunt-point
- bolster
- Bondek absorbable
- Bone Bullet
- braided
- braided Ethibond
- braided Mersilene
- braided Nurolon
- braided silk
- Bralon braided nylon
- bregmatomastoid
- bridging
- bridle
- bunching
- bundle
- Bunnell crisscross
- Bunnell wire pullout
- buried

suture *(cont.)*
- buried interrupted
- buried-knot
- Capio CL suture-capturing device
- cardinal
- cardiovascular silk
- catgut
- cerclage
- chain
- chromic
- chromic catgut
- chromic gut
- chromic interrupted
- circular
- circular wire
- circumferential
- Closer
- clove-hitch
- coapting
- coated
- coated Vicryl
- coated Vicryl Rapide
- collagen
- colposuspension
- compression stay
- Connell
- continuous
- continuous running
- convertible slip knot
- Corkscrew suture anchor
- coronal
- cosmetic conventional cutting
- cosmetic reverse cutting
- cotton
- coupled
- cranial
- crisscross
- crossed-swords technique
- cruciate four-strand
- Cushing
- Cutalon nylon polyamide surgical
- Czerny
- Czerny-Lembert
- Dacron

suture *(cont.)*
- Dacron-bolstered
- Dafilon surgical
- Dagrofil
- deep
- deep retention
- Deklene II
- Deknatel
- delayed closure of
- dentate
- Dermabond
- dermal
- Dermalene
- Dermalon
- Dexon
- Dexon Plus
- Dexon II
- DG Softgut
- diastasis of
- Donati
- double-armed (DAS)
- doubly ligated
- dural tack-up
- dural tenting
- dural traction
- Endoknot
- Endoloop
- Endo Stitch
- Endosuture
- end-to-end
- end-to-side
- EPTFE (expanded polytetra-fluoroethylene) vascular
- Ethibond
- Ethibond Excel polyester
- Ethicon
- Ethicon Excel
- Ethiflex
- Ethilon
- Ethilon monofilament nylon
- Ethilon nylon
- ethmoidolacrimal
- ethmoidomaxillary
- everting

suture *(cont.)*
- everting mattress
- Excel polyester
- extracorporeal knot
- fascial
- fast absorbing surgical gut (plain)
- FASTak suture anchor
- figure-of-8
- fine
- fisherman's knot
- fishmouth
- flat
- Flexon steel
- four-strand
- four-strand Savage
- Frater
- frontal
- frontolacrimal
- frontomaxillary
- frontonasal
- frontoparietal
- frontosphenoid
- frontozygomatic
- funicular
- furrier
- Gambee
- Gely
- GI (gastrointestinal)
- Giampapa
- gift wrap technique
- Gillies
- Gillies horizontal dermal
- granny knot
- grasping loop
- Gregory stay
- Gruber
- Gussenbauer
- gut
- Halsted
- Harpoon suture anchor
- Hawkeye
- heavy monofilament
- heavy silk
- heavy wire

suture *(cont.)*
helical
hemostatic
Herculon suture
hexafluoropropylene-VDF
horizontal
horizontal mattress
Horsley
imbricating
In-Tac
intermittent
interparietal
interrupted
interrupted near-far, far-near suture
interrupted pledgeted
intracuticular
intradermal
intraluminal occluding
inverted
inverting
Investa
jugal
Kelly plication
Kessler
Krackow
Krause
lambdoid
lambdoidal cranial
laparoscopic extracorporeal knot
Lapra-Ty absorbable
lashing
Le Dentu
leg of
Lembert
Linatrix
lock-stitch
locked
locking
locking loop
longitudinal
loop
loop mattress
Lukens PGA synthetic absorbable
Maciol laparoscopic

suture *(cont.)*
magnetic controlled suturing (MCS)
mamillary
mattress
Maxon
Maxon polyglyconate monofilament
McLaughlin modification of Bunnell pullout
Mersilene
Mersilene braided nonabsorbable
Mersilene polyester fiber
Mersilk braided silk
metopic cranial
MetraTie knot pusher
Micrins microsurgical
Miralene
Mitek
Mitek Mini GII
modified Kessler
Monocryl
monofilament
monofilament absorbable
monofilament nylon
monofilament polypropylene
monofilament stainless steel
Monosof monofilament nylon
multifilament
multiple-strand
Multitak
muscle-to-bone
myodesis
near-far
nerve
nonabsorbable
nonabsorbable blue monofilament
nonabsorbable dark blue braided stainless steel
nonabsorbable green and white braided
nonabsorbable green braided Ethibond
nonabsorbable white braided
noneverting
nonfusion of cranial

suture *(cont.)*
- nonmutagenic surgical
- Novafil
- Nurolon
- Nurolon braided nylon
- nylon
- occipital
- occipitomastoid
- occipitoparietal
- occipitosphenoid
- orienting
- out-in-out technique
- over-and-over
- over-and-over whip
- overlapping
- Owen silk
- Pagedas self-locking
- Panacryl
- Panacryl absorbable
- parietal
- parietomastoid
- parieto-occipital
- patch-reinforced mattress
- PDS (polydioxanone suture) II Endoloop suture
- PDS II (polydioxanone)
- PDS Vicryl
- pericostal
- Perma-Hand braided silk
- Perma-Hand silk
- PermaMesh
- petrobasilar
- petrosphenobasilar
- petrospheno-occipital
- petrosquamous
- PGA synthetic absorbable
- Pilot
- plain
- plain catgut
- plain gut
- plastic
- pledgeted
- pledgeted Ethibond
- pledgeted mattress

suture *(cont.)*
- plication
- poliglacaprone absorbable
- polybutester
- Polydek
- polydioxanone (PDS)
- polyester
- polyglacine
- polyglactin 370 absorbable
- polyglactin 910 absorbable
- polyglycolic acid
- polyglyconate absorbable
- PolySorb
- pop-off
- Potts tie
- PRE 2
- prematurely closed
- Premilene
- premium point reverse cutting
- premium point spatula
- preplaced
- primary
- Prolene
- Prolene polypropylene
- Pronova
- Pronova nonabsorbable
- Pronova Poly
- Protector meniscus
- P-3
- pullout
- pullout wire
- Pulver-Taft fishmouth
- pursestring or purse-string
- pyroglycolic acid
- quilted
- radiopaque
- Rapide
- reabsorbable
- Reddick-Saye
- reinforcing
- relaxation
- retention
- retraction
- reverse cutting

suture *(cont.)*
- rhabdoid
- Richardson angle
- Robertson
- Roth Grip-Tip suture guide
- running
- running interlocking
- running lock
- running locking
- Sabreloc (spatula needle)
- Safil synthetic absorbable surgical
- sagittal cranial
- Savage
- secondary
- Sepramesh
- seromuscular
- seromuscular-to-edge
- serrated
- seton
- shorthand vertical mattress stitch
- silk
- Silkam
- silk pop-off
- silk traction
- simple
- single-armed
- six-strand
- skin
- slipknot
- Sofsilk braided silk
- Sofsilk nonabsorbable silk
- Softcat chromic
- Softcat plain
- Softgut surgical chromic suture
- sphenoethmoidal
- spheno-occipital
- spheno-orbital
- sphenoparietal
- sphenopetrosal
- sphenosquamous
- sphenotemporal
- sphenovomerine
- splayed cranial
- spread

suture *(cont.)*
- squamosomastoid
- squamosoparietal
- squamososphenoid
- squamous
- stainless steel wire
- staple
- Statak
- stay
- Steelex
- Steri-Strips
- sternal wire
- stick-tie (suture ligature or transfixion suture)
- stitch
- Strickland
- subannular mattress
- subcutaneous
- subcuticular
- superior rectus
- SuperStitch
- Supramid
- Supramid Extra
- Suretac
- surgical catgut
- surgical gut
- surgical linen
- surgical silk
- surgical stainless steel
- Surgidac braided coated polyester Dacron
- Surgigut chromic
- Surgigut plain
- Surgilene
- Surgilon
- Surgipro mesh
- Surgipro monofilament polypropylene
- Surgitie ligating loop
- Sutralon
- SutraSilk
- Suturamid
- Suture Clinch
- Sutured-Clip

suture *(cont.)*
Suture Lok
Sutureloop
Sutureloop colposuspension
swaged-on
synthetic
Synthofil
tack
taper point
tapercutting
Teflon
Teflon-coated Dacron
Teflon-pledgeted
Teflon-pledgeted mattress
temporal
tenting
Tevdek
The Closer
Thiersch
three-strand
through-and-through
through-and-through continuous
through-the-wall mattress
Ti-Cron (also Tycron)
tight
Tom Jones closure suture
traction
transfixion
transition
transosseous
transverse
Trumbull
twisted
two-strand
Tycron (also Ti-Cron)
U double-barrel
umbilical tape
undyed
undyed braided polyglycolic acid
undyed Vicryl
Vascufil
vertical
vertical mattress
Vicryl

suture *(cont.)*
Vicryl Rapide synthetic absorbable
whipstitch
white
white silk
wing
wire
wire pullout
X-PRESS
Z
Zimmer Statak
suture abscess
suture anchor (see *anchor*)
Suture Assistant endoscopic suturing device
Suture Assistant knot-tying device
suture bite
suture bridge fixation
suture button
Suture Clinch fastener
Suture Clinch suture
suturectomy
Sutured-Clip clip
Sutured-Clip suture
suture displacement
suture "ears"
suture fastener
ROC
ROC XS
Suture Clinch
suture forceps
suture grasper
suture guide
Investa
Pilot
suture hook
suture isometry
suture joint
sutureless closure
sutureless electrode lead
sutureless myocardial electrode
suture ligated
suture ligature
suture limb

suture line
suture line dehiscence
suture line leak
Suture Lok ligator
Suture Lok suture
Sutureloop colposuspension suture
Sutureloop needle/suture
suture needle
suture passer
  Bone Bridge
  Carter-Thomason
  MetraPass
  Protect-a-Pass
suture punch
suture-release needle
suture Roticulator
suture scissors
Suture-Self dressing
Suture Strip Plus
Suture Strip Plus stretch wound closure strip
suture sundries
Suture/VesiBand organizer
suture-welding device
suturing, endoscopic
SV (stroke volume)
Sven-Johansson driver
Sven-Johansson extractor
Sven-Johansson femoral neck nail
SVR (systemic vascular resistance)
SVR/BSA (systemic vascular resistance/ body surface area = systemic vascular resistance index)
SVRI (systemic vascular resistance index)
swab, Frankfeldt rectal
swaged
swaged needle
swaged-on needle
swaged-on suture
swallow
  barium
  dry
  Gastrografin

swallow *(cont.)*
  ice-water
  pain on
  piecemeal
  video barium
  water
  water-soluble contrast esophageal
  wet
swallowed air
swallowing center
swallowing mechanism
swallowing, piecemeal
swallowing therapy
swamp cancer
Swan aortic clamp
Swan-Ganz catheter
Swan-Ganz waveform
swan-neck catheter
swan-neck chisel
swan-neck gouge
Swann-Morton surgical blade
Swanson elevator
Swanson lunate awl
Swanson mallet
Swanson reamer
Swanson scaphoid awl
Swartz SL Series Fast-Cath introducer catheter
Swedish needle
Swedish pattern dissector
Sween-A-Peel Skin Barrier
Sween Cream for ostomy skin
Sween Micro Guard Cream
Sween Micro Guard Powder
Sween Prep skin prep dressing
sweep, duodenal
Sweet clip applying forceps
Sweet esophageal scissors
Sweetheart clamp
Sweet pituitary scissors
swelling, glandular
Swenson abdominal pull-through procedure
swimmer's view

Swiss celia and suture forceps
Swiss jewelers forceps
Swiss lithoclast
Swiss lithoclast lithotriptor
Swiss-pattern blade breaker
swivel clamp
swivel knife
SYBIOL (synthetic bio-liver) device
Sydney Hospital retractor
Syllact (psyllium seed husks)
Syme aneurysm needle
Symlin (pramlintide acetate)
symmetric chest expansion
symmetrical breast prosthesis
sympathectomy hook
sympathetic ganglion
sympathetic nervous system
sympathetic nervous system symptom
sympathetics
sympathomimetic drug
Symphony nitinol stent (extremities/ biliary)
symptom
  compressive
  dyspeptic
  obstructive
  postcibal
  pressure
  prodromal
  relief of
  sympathetic nervous system
symptomatic attack
symptomatic esophagitis
symptomatic gallstone
symptomatic hyperglycemia
symptomatic hyperparathyroidism
symptomatic hypocalcemia
symptomatology
Symptom Distress Scale
symptoms of sympathetic discharge
synchronized videofluoroscopy and manometry
syncopal episode
syncope
syncytial knot formation
syndromatic hepatic ductular hypoplasia
syndrome (see also *disease*)
  Aagenaes (cholestasis-lymphedema)
  Aarskog
  abdominal muscle deficiency
  ablepharon-macrostomia
  absent abdominal muscle
  Achard-Thiers
  acquired immunodeficiency (AIDS)
  ACTH deficiency
  adrenogenital
  afferent loop
  AIDS (acquired immunodeficiency)
  Alagille
  albatross
  Albright
  Algid malaria
  alpha chain
  Alstrom
  anorexia-cachexia
  anterior abdominal wall
  APECED (autoimmune polyendocrinopathy; candidiasis; ectodermal dysplasia)
  apple-peel syndrome
  Arias
  Armenian
  Asherson
  asplenia
  bacterial overgrowth
  Banti
  Barrett
  Bartter
  basal cell nevus
  Bassen-Kornzweig
  Bearn-Kunkel-Slater
  Beckwith
  Beckwith-Wiedemann
  Bedford
  Behçet
  Bernard-Sergent
  Bessauds-Hilmand-Augier
  Biörck
  blind (stagnant) loop

syndrome *(cont.)*
- Bloodgood
- Bloom
- blue diaper
- blue rubber bleb nevus
- Boerhaave
- Bouveret
- Bowen
- Brachmann-de Lange
- Brandt
- Brennemann
- Budd
- Budd-Chiari
- buried bumper
- Burnett
- burning vulvar syndrome
- café coronary
- Canada-Cronkhite
- carbohydrate-deficient glycoprotein, type 1a
- carcinoid
- carnitine-deficiency
- Caroli
- Carpenter
- Carter-Horsley-Hughes
- cast
- cat-eye
- caudal regression
- celiac artery compression
- cerebrohepatorenal
- CHARGE (coloboma, heart, atresia of the choanae, retardation of growth and development, genital and urinary anomalies, and ear anomalies [also tracheoesophageal fistula])
- Chiari-Budd
- Chilaiditi
- cholestasis-lymphedema
- cholestatic
- chronic fatigue and immune dysfunction (CFIDS)
- chronic intestinal pseudo-obstruction
- Clarke-Hadefield

syndrome *(cont.)*
- Cohen
- colonic solitary ulcer
- complex regional pain (CRPS)
- Conn
- Cornelia de Lange
- Courvoisier-Terrier
- couvade
- CREST
- Crigler-Najjar
- Cronkhite-Canada
- CRPS (complex regional pain)
- Cruveilhier-Baumgarten
- Cushing
- cyclic vomiting
- Danbolt-Closs
- Dejerine-Sottas
- descending perineum
- diencephalic
- DiGeorge
- DIMOAD (diabetes insipidus, diabetes mellitus, optic atrophy and deafness)
- Down
- Drummond
- Dubin-Johnson
- Dubin-Sprinz
- dumping
- Eagle-Barrett
- ectopic ACTH
- Ehlers-Danlos
- eosinophilic gastroenteritis
- euthyroid sick (ESS)
- exomphalos-macroglossia-gigantism
- familial polyposis
- Felty
- fibrocystic breast
- fish-odor
- Fitz-Hugh–Curtis (perihepatitis)
- Flood
- flulike
- Forbes-Albright
- Fröhlich (Froehlich)
- full-blown

syndrome *(cont.)*
functional bowel
gallstone ileus
Gardner
gas-bloat
gastrocardiac
gastroesophageal laceration-hemorrhage
gastrointestinal dysmotility
gastrojejunal loop obstruction
gay bowel
Gee-Herter-Heubner
Gianotti-Crosti
Gilbert
glucagonoma
Goldberg-Maxwell
Gopalan
gourmand
Guillain-Barré
Hadefield-Clarke
Hanot-Chauffard
Heerferdt-Waldenstrom
HELLP (hemolysis with a micro-angiopathic blood smear, elevated liver enzymes, and low platelet count)
hemolytic-uremic (HUS)
hepatopulmonary
hepatorenal (HRS)
hereditary MEA
Hermansky-Pudlak
Howel-Evans
Hutchinson-Weber-Peutz
hypoglycosylation, type 1a
impaired regeneration (IRS)
inhibitory
inspissated bile
inspissated sump
insulin-resistance
intestinal polyposis-cutaneous pigmentation
irritable bowel (IBS)
Ivemark
Jegher

syndrome *(cont.)*
jejunal
Kelly-Paterson
Kimmelstiel-Wilson
kinky hair
Klinefelter
Koenig (König)
Kunkel
Ladd
Laubry-Soulle
Laurence-Moon-Bardet-Biedl
leaky gut
lentigo-polypose-digestive
levator ani
Lloyd
locker room
Lofgren
loin pain hematuria (LPHS)
Lucey-Driscoll
lupus-like
Lyell
lymphadenopathy (LAS)
lymphoproliferative
Lynch I
Lynch II
malabsorption
malignant B cell
Mallory-Weiss
MEA (multiple endocrine adenomatosis)
meconium plug
Meigs
MEN I (multiple endocrine neoplasia I)
mesenteric artery
milk-alkali
Mirizzi
Mosse
mucosal neuroma (MEA type III)
multiorgan dysfunction syndrome (MODS)
multiple endocrine deficiency, type II
multiple hamartoma

syndrome *(cont.)*
- Munchausen
- non-Lynch
- obesity hypoventilation (OHS)
- Obinsky
- Ogilvie
- Oldfield
- Osler-Weber-Rendu
- overlap (connective tissue disease)
- pancreatic cholera
- pancreaticohepatic
- paraneoplastic
- Paterson-Brown-Kelly
- Paterson-Kelly
- pericolic membrane
- perihepatitis
- periodic peritonitis
- Peutz-Jeghers (PJS)
- Peutz-Jeghers familial gastro-intestinal polyposis
- Peutz-Touraine
- pharyngeal pouch
- pituitary Cushing
- pituitary tumor
- Plummer-Vinson
- Polhemus-Schafer-Ivemark
- polyglandular autoimmune (PGA II)
- polyglandular deficiency, type II
- polyps and spots
- polysplenia
- postcholecystectomy (PCS)
- postcolonoscopy distention
- postfundoplication
- postgastrectomy
- postgastric surgery
- postpolio
- postpolypectomy coagulation
- postsurgical nonabsorption
- postvagotomy
- Potter
- Prader-Willi
- prune-belly
- pseudo-obstructive
- Purtilo

syndrome *(cont.)*
- Reichmann
- Reimann
- reperfusion
- respiratory distress
- retained antrum
- Reye
- Riley-Day (familial dysautonomia)
- Roger
- Rotor
- Rubinstein-Taybi
- runting
- Sandifer
- Sanger-Brown
- Schmid-Fraccaro
- Schmidt
- Schwachman
- Schwachman-Bodian
- Schwachman-Diamond
- sea-blue histiocyte
- sepsis
- Sheehan
- short-bowel
- short-gut
- Shy-Drager
- Siegel-Cattan, Mamou
- Sipple (MEA type II)
- Sjögren (Sjoegren)
- SLE-like
- small stomach
- solitary rectal ulcer (SRUS)
- solitary ulcer
- somatostatinoma
- splenic agenesis
- splenic flexure
- Sprinz-Dubin
- Sprinz-Nelson
- stagnant loop
- stale fish
- steakhouse
- Stein-Leventhal
- Stevens-Johnson
- sump
- superior mesenteric artery (SMAS)

syndrome *(cont.)*
- systemic inflammatory response (SIRS)
- Takahara
- terminal reservoir
- TORCH (toxoplasmosis; other agents; rubella; cytomegalovirus; herpes simplex)
- Torres
- Townes Brooks
- toxic shock (TSS)
- Turcot
- Turner
- type I hepatorenal
- type II hepatorenal
- VACTERL (vertebral anomalies; anal atresia; congenital cardiac disease; tracheoesophageal fistula; renal anomalies; radial dysplasia; and other limb defects) syndrome
- Verner-Morrison
- Vinson
- vulvar vestibulitis
- Waldenstrom macroglobulinemia
- wasting
- Waterhouse-Friderichsen
- watery diarrhea
- Watson-Alagille
- WDHA (watery diarrhea, hypokalemia, achlorhydria)
- Weil
- Welt
- Wermer (MEA type I)
- Werner
- Wernicke-Korsakoff
- Wiedemann-Beckwith
- Wiscott-Aldrich
- Wolfram
- X-linked lymphoproliferative (XLP)
- ZE
- Zellweger
- Zieve
- Zollinger-Ellison (ZES)

syndrome of inappropriate antidiuretic hormone (SIADH)
syndrome of inappropriate secretion of antidiuretic hormone [ADH]
Synercid (quinupristin/dalfopristin)
Synergraft
Synergy ultrasound system
syngeneic transplant
Synovator arthroscopic blade
synovectomy blade
synovectomy rongeur
synovial biopsy
synovial fluid
Synsorb Cd
Synsorb-PK (8-methoxycarbonyloctyl oligosaccharides)
Syntel latex-free embolectomy catheter
Synthaderm dressing
Synthaderm occlusive wound dressing
Synthamin amino acid solution
Synthes cervical plate
Synthes dorsal distal radius plate
Synthes drill
Synthes Microsystems cranial fixation plate
Synthes Microsystems microplate
Synthes Microsystems pliers
Synthes Microsystems plate-holding forceps
Synthes mini L-plate
Synthes rod
Synthes transbuccal trocar
Synthes wire guide
synthesis, impaired lecithin
synthetic ^{13}C-urea lyophilized powder
synthetic cortisol
synthetic mesh
synthetic mesocaval H-graft
synthetic suture
Synthofil suture
Synthroid (levothyroxine sodium)
syphilis
syphilitic cirrhosis
syphilitic necrosis

syphilitic peritonitis
Syracuse I plate
syringe
  Asepto irrigation
  aspiration
  Autoblock safety
  CoverTip safety
  Daxor quantitative injection syringe kit
  EasySafe disposable
  ENSI syringe
  Humalog Pen
  Humulin Pen
  Inject-Ease 100
  Lewy Teflon glycerine mixture
  Luer-Lok
  Medex Protégé 3010 infusion pump
  monojet Toomey
  Omnican Piston
  Pritchard
  Pritchard lipiodol
  ROCAP
  Schimmelbusch bladder
  Ultraject prefilled
  Uni-Matic infiltration
Syringe Avitene dressing
Syringe Avitene endoscopic delivery system
system (see also *device*)
  Aastrom CPS (cell-production)
  ABBI (advanced breast biopsy instrumentation)
  Ablatherm HIFU (high-intensity focused ultrasound)
  ADICOL insulin delivery
  AeroView optical intubation
  AERx diabetes management
  AERx pain management
  AESOP (Automated Endoscopic System for Optimal Positioning)
  AESOP 2000; 3000 endoscope
  Airis II open MRI
  Alexa 1000 noninvasive breast lesion diagnostic

system *(cont.)*
  AlgoMed drug infusion
  alimentary
  Allon
  Anaconda device and delivery
  AngioStent balloon-expandable stent and delivery
  Aspen ultrasound
  Atlas 2.0 diagnostic ultrasound
  AU5 system, ultrasound
  Aurora diode laser
  Aurora MR breast imaging
  AutoSonix
  Auto Suture ABBI
  autotransfusion
  Autovac autotransfusion
  Autovac LF autotransfusion
  Bard Composix mesh graft material
  Bard endoscopic suturing
  BAT (B-mode acquisition and targeting)
  Beacon Technology (BTS)
  Beamer injection stent
  BiCAP hemostatic
  Biofield diagnostic
  BioLogic-DT (now Liver Dialysis Unit)
  BioLogic-HT (now ThermoChem-HT)
  BiPAP S/T-D 30 ventilatory support
  BI-RADS (Breast Imaging Reporting and Data System)
  B-mode acquisition and targeting (BAT)
  BSD-2000
  CathTrack catheter locator
  CDIS (controlled distention irrigation system)
  CDI 2000 blood gas monitoring
  Cell Recovery (CRS)
  Cell Saver Haemolite autotransfusion
  Cenflex central monitoring
  Centauri Er:YAG laser

system *(cont.)*
CFC BioScanner
closed
closed drainage
Coaguloop
CollectFirst autotransfusion
Colormate TLc BiliTest
Computerized Thermal Imaging
Core Entree Plus laparoscopic trocar and cannula
CRYOcare
CRYOguide
CSM Stretta
CycloTech cyclosporine delivery
da Vinci surgical
DBx diagnostic
DermaLase Er,Cr:YSGG laser
DermaScan
Dialock hemodialysis access
DOBI (Dynamic Optical Breast Imaging)
EDC endoscopic imaging
800 series KTP/YAG surgical laser
EndoALPHA integrated endosurgical
EndoCinch suturing
EndoMed laparoscopic
E-Z Tac soft tissue reattachment
F.A.S.T. 1 (First Access for Shock and Trauma)
FemRx Soprano cryotherapy
Flo-Stat fluid management
Fluid Alarm System (FAS) glove integrity
FluoroNav virtual fluoroscopy
GE Senographe 2001 digital mammography
GITS (gastrointestinal therapeutic)
Given Diagnostic Imaging
GliaSite implantable radiation therapy
Guidant Origin
GVHD (graft-versus-host disease) grading

system *(cont.)*
HDI 3000 ultrasound
Hemasure r/LS red blood cell filtration
Hemopure
Hercules Nd:YAG laser
Hinchey diverticulitis grading/staging
Illumina PROSeries laparoscopy
Intercept Platelet
intermittent open
Intuitive
IRMA blood analysis
Irrijet DS debridement and irrigation
Isolex 300i stem cell selection
IsoMed constant-flow infusion
IVAC SmartSite needleless
Kaplan PenduLaser 115 surgical laser
KOH colpotomizer
KTP/YAG surgical laser
LAGB gastric banding
Laparolife gasless laparoscopy
Lap-Band adjustable gastric banding (LAGB)
LifeShirt monitoring
Liver Dialysis Unit
LORAD StereoGuide stereotactic breast biopsy
LSTAT (life support trauma and transport)
Luxtec fiberoptic
lyophilized liposomal delivery
Lyra laser
Mammex TR mammography
Mammotest breast biopsy
Mammotest Plus breast biopsy
MCAS (modular clip application)
medicated urethral system for erection (MUSE)
Medstone STS-T transportable lithotripsy
MIBB breast biopsy
Multitak suture

system *(cont.)*
Navion BioNavigation
Navitrack
NeoCure cryoablation
Octopus2 tissue-stabilization
Olympus CV-1 endoscopic
Olympus CV-100 endoscopic
On-Q pain management
Opdima digital mammography
Optical Biopsy
Optical Tracking System (OTS)
Optistar MR contrast delivery
ORI electronic endoscopy
Origin distention balloon
Palpagraph breast examination
PDB laparoscopic balloon
Photon radiosurgery
Photon Radiosurgery System (PRS)
portal venous
POSICAM
PowerCut gold surgical
PowerCut pneumatic power
PowerSculpt cosmetic surgery
pressurized pulsatile irrigation
Profore four-layer bandaging
ProLease drug delivery
Protectiv I.V. catheter safety
PRS (Photon Radiosurgery System)
PSA 4000 anesthesia monitoring
Pulsavac III wound debridement
Repose surgical
Retzius
Romano surgical curved drilling
Senographe 2000D digital mammography imaging
Sherwood intrascopic suction/irrigation system for laparoscopic procedures
SiteSelect breast biopsy
SJM Rosenkranz pediatric retractor
SmartDose prefilled infusion
Softscan laser mammography
Sonoprobe SP-501 system for endoscopic procedures

system *(cont.)*
Soprano cryoablation
SpectraScience Optical Biopsy
Squirt wound irrigation
Storz OR1 electronic endoscopy
Sure-Closure skin-stretching
surgical isolation bubble (SIBS)
SurgiLav Plus hydrodebridement
Ternamian EndoTIP
ThermoChem-HT (formerly BioLogic-HT system)
Thermo-STAT
Thora-Klex chest drainage
3DC endoscopic imaging
TLc.BiliTest
TraumaJet wound debridement
videoendoscope
Xillix LIFE-GI fluorescence endoscopy
Xillix LIFE-Lung GI fluorescence endoscopy
XPS Sculpture System
Zone Specific II meniscal repair
systemic carnitine deficiency
systemic circulation
systemic effects carcinoma
systemic fungal infection
systemic glucocorticosteroids (GCS)
systemic infection
systemic inflammation
systemic inflammatory response syndrome (SIRS)
systemic lesion
systemic disseminated lupus erythematosus
systemic lupus erythematosus (SLE)
diffuse
focal
systemic mast cell disease
systemic mastocytosis
systemic mercury intoxication
systemic necrotizing arteritis
systemic pressure
systemic scleroderma

systemic therapy
system of Retzius
systolic blood pressure
systolic pressure gradient
systolic spleen
Szabo-Berci needle driver
Szabo test

T, t

TAB (tumescent absorbent bandage)
Tabb double-ended flap knife
Tabb elevator
Tabb myringoplasty knife
Tabb pick knife
TAB thermocouple sensor
Tabb 3 mm ruler
TAB wound dressing
table
  Maquet endoscopy
  sigmoidoscopy
tabletop Stone staple
TAC (total abdominal colectomy)
TACE (transcatheter arterial chemoembolization)
tachyarrhythmias
tachycardia
tachygastria
Tacit threaded anchor
tack
tacked behind the uterus
tacked down
tacker, Origin
tack suture
tack-up
tacrolimus
Tactilaze angioplasty laser catheter
tactile anesthesia
tactile probe
TAE (total abdominal evisceration)
taenia (also tenia) strip of soft tissue
Taenia (genus of tapeworm)
Taenia saginata
Taenia solium
taeniacide
tag
  edematous
  external skin
  hemorrhoidal
  perianal skin
  sentinel
  tonsil
Tagamet HB (cimetidine)
tagged ligament
tagged RBC study
tagged red blood cell bleeding scan
TAG suture anchor
tail, axillary
tail of breast
tail of breast tissue
tail of pancreas
tail of Spence
Tait graft
Takahara syndrome
Takahashi forceps
Takahashi rongeur

Take-Apart elevator
Take-Apart knife
Take-Apart nerve hook
Take-Apart handle
Take-Apart scissors and forceps
takedown of adhesions
takedown of colostomy
taking down of adhesions
Talent endoluminal stent-graft system
  (AAA repair)
talking digital thermometer
tamoxifen, tamoxifen citrate
tamponade
  balloon
  cardiac
  esophagogastric
  ferromagnetic
tamponade with viable omentum
tampon tube
tandem lesion
tangential incision
tangential scapular view
tangential view
tangential wound
Tangier disease
tangle of hemorrhoidal veins
Tanner operation
tantalum gauze
tantalum gauze mesh
tantalum preformed skull plate
tap
  abdominal
  clear
  peritoneal
  positive peritoneal
  shunt
  spinal
tap-water enema
Tapazole (methimazole)
tape
  adhesive
  appy (appendectomy)
  braided
  Cath-Secure hypoallergenic tape

tape *(cont.)*
  circular
  compression
  Dacron
  elastic
  Elastikon elastic
  Hypafix nonwoven tape
  hypoallergenic
  Hy-Tape
  lap (laparotomy)
  MaxCast
  Mersilene
  Microfoam surgical tape
  Montgomery
  paper
  polyester-reinforced Dacron
  Prolene mesh
  Scotchcast 2 casting
  Shur-Strip (Deknatel)
  Silastic
  sterile wound closure tape
  Transpore surgical
  TSH-01 transdermal tape
  umbilical
  vascular
  white cotton umbilical
tape ligature
tapercut
tapercutting suture
tapered hand reamer
tapered Maryland dissector
tapered needle
tapered pin
tapered reamer
tapered right-angle dissector
tapered rubber bougie
taper-jaw forceps
taper-nose pliers
taper point needle
taper point suture
Tapertome sphincterotome
TAPET (tumor amplified protein
  expression therapy)
tapeworm (cestode)

TAPP (transabdominal preperitoneal) hernia repair
TAPP (transabdominal preperitoneal) laparoscopic hernioplasty
tar cancer
tardive dyskinesia
target cell
targeted brain biopsy
targeted cryoablation device
Targeted Ablation Therapy
target lesion
target organ complications of type 1 diabetes
target organ deterioration of diabetes
Targis microwave catheter-based system
tarry black stools
tarsal plate
taurolidine
Taut cystic duct catheter
taxanes, taxoids
Taxol (paclitaxel)
Taxotere (docetaxel)
Taylor brain scissors
Taylor delicate forceps
Taylor dressing forceps
Taylor dural scissors
Taylor gastric balloon
Taylor percussion hammer
Taylor scissors
Taylor self-retaining spinal retractor
Taylor spinal retractor blade
Tazocin
tazofelone
TBZ (thiabendazole)
^{99m}Tc (see *technetium*)
T cell
T cell lymphoma
TCA (trihydrocoprostanic acid)
TCD/CBDE (transcystic duct/common bile duct exploration)
TcHIDA scan
TC (tungsten carbide) needle holder
TCR (T cell receptor)
TD glucose monitoring system
TDMS (Trex digital mammography system)
TDT (transmission disequilibrium test)
Teale forceps
tear (rupture)
  capsular
  diastatic serosal
  esophageal
  flap
  gastric
  liver
  Mallory-Weiss
  Mallory-Weiss mucosal
  mesenteric
  micro
  post-emesis longitudinal
  post-retching longitudinal
  serosal
teardrop breast prosthesis
teardrop radiographic appearance of cecal bascule
tearing pain
tear of liver and capsule
tear stone
tear-tip cover
teasing needle
Tebamide (trimethobenzamide HCl)
technetium-99m (^{99m}Tc)
  ^{99m}Tc albumin colloid
  ^{99m}Tc albumin microspheres
  ^{99m}Tc arcitumomab
  ^{99m}Tc DISIDA
  ^{99m}Tc disofenin
  ^{99m}Tc DMSA
  ^{99m}Tc DTPA aerosol
  ^{99m}Tc GHP
  ^{99m}Tc HDP
  ^{99m}Tc HIDA
  ^{99m}Tc IDA scan
  ^{99m}Tc lidofenin
  ^{99m}Tc MAA (macroaggregated albumin)
  ^{99m}Tc MDP
  ^{99m}Tc medronate

technetium-99m *(cont.)*
- ^{99m}Tc murine MAb to human alfa-fetoprotein (AFP)
- ^{99m}Tc pentetic acid
- ^{99m}Tc pertechnetate
- ^{99m}Tc PIPIDA
- ^{99m}Tc polyphosphate
- ^{99m}Tc PYP (pyrophosphate)
- ^{99m}Tc SC (sulfur colloid)
- ^{99m}Tc sestamibi
- ^{99m}Tc sodium pertechnetate
- ^{99m}Tc solesomab monoclonal antibody
- ^{99m}Tc SPP (stannous pyrophosphate)

technetium-labeled autologous red blood cell scan

technetium-labeled red blood cell scan

technetium-labeled stannous methylene disphosphonate

Techni-Care surgical scrub

technique (see also *method*; *operation*)
- autosuture
- bipolar surgical
- Burhenne
- clamp, cut, and tie
- continuous pull-through
- cross-sectional imaging
- EMR (endoscopic mucosal resection) suction cap method
- endoscopic reversal
- endoscopic sewing machine
- extraction balloon
- finger-fracture
- Giampap suture
- Hofmeister
- J needle
- Karydakis
- microsurgical
- modified Delphi
- modified tumescent
- PhotoPoint light-activated
- Polya
- polyp snare

technique *(cont.)*
- preperitoneal patch and plug hernia repair
- rapid pull-through esophageal manometry
- Rosetti
- RPT (rapid pull-through)
- sequential clamp and suture
- Simonsen
- snare
- SPT (station pull-through)
- station pull-through esophageal manometry
- Thermal Quenching cooling
- three-trocar cholecystectomy
- tip deflection
- transabdominal preperitoneal approach
- transanal double-stapling
- transduodenal drainage
- transgastric drainage
- transpapillary drainage
- Traverso-Longmire
- tumescent
- Turnbull
- Vayre suturing
- vertical pedicle in breast reduction

technology
- antisense
- Beacon
- Coblation
- FACT (Focal Angioplasty Catheter)
- islet separation
- LAST (large-area sensing)
- Masimo SET (signal extraction)
- MCAT (modular coded aperture)
- SET (signal extraction)
- S.M.A.R.T. (shape memory alloy recoverable)
- USS-Trex Universal advanced radiology
- XenoMouse

Technomed Sonolith 3000 lithotriptor

Technos ultrasound system
Tee connector
TEF (tracheoesophageal fistula)
TefGen-guided tissue membrane
Teflon-coated brain retractor
Teflon-coated Dacron suture
Teflon-coated driver
Teflon-coated guidewire
Teflon-coated hollow-bore needle
Teflon drain, nasobiliary
Teflon ERCP catheter
Teflon insulated coating
Teflon nasobiliary tube
Teflon-pledgeted mattress suture
Teflon sling rectopexy
Teflon sling repair
Teflon suture
Teflon tube
Tegaderm HP transparent dressing
Tegaderm transparent dressing
Tegagel hydrogel dressing and sheet
Tegagen HG alginate wound dressing
Tegagen HI alginate wound dressing
Tegapore contact-layer wound dressing
tegaserod
Tegasorb hydrocolloid dressing
Tegtmeier elevator
telangiectasia
  blanching spider
  gastrointestinal
  hereditary hemorrhagic (HHT)
  Osler-Weber-Rendu
  spider
telangiectatic angioma
telangiectatic lesion
telangiectatic osteogenic sarcoma
telangiectatic vessel
Telecam DX
Telecam SL
TeleMed reusable biopsy forceps
telemetry, multiple parameter (MPT)
Telepaque (topanoic acid)
Telepaque contrast medium
telescope (also see *endoscope; laparoscope*)
  Hopkins II
  Hopkins II forward oblique
  Storz laparoscopic
  Storz 0° 10 mm
  Wolff
telescope bridge
telescopic rod
telescopic wire guide
telescoping medullary rod
telescoping nail
Teletrast absorbable surgical gauze
television monitor
Telfa gauze dressing
Telfa gel
telithromycin
telomerase transcription
telomere-specific probe
TEM (transanal endoscopic microsurgery)
Temnolaparoscopy device
temperature sensor
Temperlite saw blade
Temple-Fay laminectomy retractor
Temple University nail
Temple University plate
Tempo (aluminum hydroxide; magnesium hydroxide; calcium carbonate; simethicone)
temporal artery biopsy
temporal fascia graft
temporal suture
temporary colostomy
temporary end colostomy
temporary enteroscope
temporary fecal diversion
temporary hypoparathyroidism
temporary loop ileostomy
temporary ostomy
temporary pacing wire
TEMPprobes
tenaculum (see *forceps*)
tenaculum-reducing forceps

Tenckhoff peritoneal catheter
Tenckhoff peritoneal dialysis catheter
tender epigastrium
tender liver
Tender Tykes digital pacifier
  thermometer
tenderness
  breast
  cervical motion
  costovertebral angle (CVA)
  cyclic
  diffuse abdominal
  epigastric
  exquisite
  focal
  hepatic
  liver
  localizing
  percussion
  rebound
tenderness and induration
tendon forceps
tendon gouge
tendon-holding forceps
tendon hook
tendon-passing forceps
tendon-passing needle
tendon plate
tendon-pulling forceps
tendon-retrieving forceps
tendon rod
tendon-seizing forceps
tendon-tunneling forceps
tenesmus, rectal
tenia (see *taenia*)
Ten-K
Tennis Racquet catheter
tennis-racquet-type closure
tenotomy knife
tenotomy scissors
TENS unit
tense ascites
tensilon testing
Tensilon test
tension-eliminating repair
tension-free anastomosis
tension-free hernia repair
tension-free hernioplasty
tension-free Nissen fundoplication
tension-free prosthetic repairs
tension-free technique
tension pneumothorax
tent, Silon
tentative diagnosis
tenting, baseline
tenting suture
Tenzel elevator
TEP (totally extraperitoneal) hernia
  repair
TEP (totally extraperitoneal) laparoscopic hernioplasty
TEP (tracheoesophageal puncture)
Tepanil
terahertz wave
teratogenicity
teratoma, sacrococcygeal
terlipressin
terminal bile duct
terminal colostomy
terminal duct carcinoma
terminal hemorrhagic enteropathy
terminal ileal disease
terminal ileal Paneth cell
terminal ileal pouch
terminal ileitis
terminal ileostomy
terminal ileum
terminal infection
terminal inferior vena cava thrombosis
terminal reservoir syndrome
termite forceps
Ternamian EndoTIP system
terrifying pain
Terry fingernail sign
Terry-Mayo needle
Terry nail
tertian malaria
tertiary contractions

tertiary hyperparathyroidism
Terumo guidewire
Tesamone (testosterone)
Teslac (testolactone)
Teslascan (mangafodipir trisodium)
Tessier undermining scissors
test (see also *assay*)
  acid clearance (ACT)
  acid perfusion
  acid reflux
  acidification of stool
  ACS:180 BR breast cancer screening
  Actalyke activated clotting time (ACT)
  Adenovirus EIA
  alanine aminotransaminase (ALT) (formerly SGPT) liver function
  AlaSTAT latex allergy
  Alatest Latex-specific IgE allergen
  Alexagram breast lesion diagnostic
  alpha-2 antiplasmin functional assay
  ALT (alanine aminotransferase) (newer name for SGPT)
  aminopyrine breath
  ammonia N 13
  antiendomysial antibody
  Anti-Pr-3 ELISA autoimmune
  arclofenin (hepatic function)
  argentaffin reaction
  AST (serum aspartate aminotransferase) (formerly SGOT)
  ASTRA profile
  Bactigen Salmonella-Shigella
  Baermann
  balloon expulsion
  Bard BTA
  basal secretory flow rate (BSFR)
  B-D Easy A1c
  bentiromide
  bentonite flocculation
  Bernstein esophageal acid infusion
  betazole stimulation
  BTA stat (bladder tumor assay)

test *(cont.)*
  BTA TRAK bladder tumor
  bile acid breath
  bile acid tolerance
  bile solubility
  BiliChek bilirubin
  binder
  Bioclot protein S assay
  Bio-Enzabead
  Biofield diagnostic system
  Biosafe PSA4
  BladderScan
  bladder tumor assay (BTA)
  blood urea level
  Boas gastric ulcer
  bolus challenge
  Bonney stress incontinence
  Bourne
  Bozicevich
  BRACAnalysis genetic susceptibility
  breath hydrogen
  BSP (bromosulfophthalein)
  BTA stat urine
  "cake mix" kit for hematopoietic progenitor assay
  cancelling A's (mental test for hepatic encephalopathy)
  C&S (culture and sensitivity)
  CA 19-9 (carbohydrate antigen)
  Captopril
  carcinoembryonic antigen (CEA)
  CARDS O.S. mono
  Casoni skin
  C-cholyl-glycine breath excretion
  CEA (carcinoembryonic antigen
  cephalin-cholesterol flocculation
  C-glycocholic acid breath
  chew-and-spit
  cholecystokinin
  Cholestech L.D.X.
  CholesTrak
  Cholestron, Cholestron PRO
  Chymex (bentiromide)
  C lactose

test *(cont.)*
- Clinitest stool
- CLOtest
- coagulation study
- Colaris
- ColoCare
- colonic transit
- Colopath
- Colormate TLc BiliTest
- ColoScreen Self-Test
- ColoScreen Slide
- copper-binding protein
- cornflake esophageal motility
- CSF glutamine
- culture and sensitivity (C&S)
- ^{14}C urea
- D-xylose absorption
- deferoxamine mesylate infusion
- dexamethasone suppression
- Diagnex Blue gastric acid
- DNA flow cytometry
- drop
- duodenal string
- Easy A1C
- E-cadherin expression test for classification of breast carcinoma
- edrophonium
- EIA-2 (enzyme-linked immunoassay)
- Einhorn string
- ELISA titer
- ELISA-3 titer
- Elucigene
- Emit 2000 cyclosporine specific assay
- EndoCab ELISA
- endogenous TSH stimulation
- Entero-Test
- Entero-Test Pediatric
- *Escherichia coli* O157:H7 assay
- esophageal acid infusion
- esophageal function
- esophageal manometry
- esophageal motility study

test *(cont.)*
- esophageal pH
- EZ Detect colorectal screening
- Ez-HBT
- fasting gastric bile acid
- FastPack system
- FDL (fluorescein dilaurate)
- fecal alpha$_1$-antitrypsin
- fecal fat study
- fecal leukocyte count
- fecal occult blood (FEOT)
- Fisher exact
- Fishman-Doubilet
- 5-HT (5-hydroxytryptamine)
- FlexPack HP
- FLU OIA assay
- flutamine
- Fouchet
- Francis
- free thyroxine (FT_4)
- free thyroxine index (FT_4I)
- FTI (free thyroxine index)
- gastric acid
- gastric analysis
- gastric bile acid
- gastric content
- gastric emptying
- gastric function
- gastric motility study
- gastric secretion rate
- gastrin
- gastrin-secretin stimulation
- gastrin stimulation
- Gastroccult
- Gastro-Test
- GGT (gamma-glutamyl transferase)
- Gluco-Protein
- Gluco-Protein OTC self-test
- glucose tolerance
- Gluzinski
- Glycacor
- Glycosal diabetes
- glycyltryptophan
- Gmelin

test *(cont.)*
graded esophageal balloon distention
Graham
Gram stain of stool
Grassi
Great Smokies intestinal permeability
Gross
guaiac
guaiac occult blood
Guenzberg
Hamel
Hanger
Harrison spot
hatching
Hay
H_2 breath
Helicobacter pylori breath
Helisal rapid blood
Hema-Check
Hematest
HemDetect three-field occult blood
HemeSelect reagent and collection kit
Hemoccult
Hemoccult SENSA
Hemoccult II
Hemochron high-dose thrombin time (HiTT)
HemoQuant fecal occult blood
Heprofile ELISA (enzyme-linked immunosorbent assay)
HercepTest
Herp-Check
Herzberg
high-dose dexamethasone suppression
Histalog stimulation
histamine
Hollander
Home Access Hepatitis C Check
Horizons C-13 urea breath for *H. pylori*

test *(cont.)*
hot-shot PCR (polymerase chain reaction)
Huppert
Hybrid Capture CMV DNA
Hybrid Capture cytomegalovirus DNA
Hybrid Capture HPV DNA
Hybritech Tandem PSA ratio (free PSA/total PSA) (PSA, prostate-specific antigen)
hydrochloric acid
hydrogen breath
^{131}I uptake (thyroid function)
iliopsoas
IMAGN 2000 cellular analysis
ImmunoCard STAT! Rotavirus
indium-labeled (^{111}In) autologous leukocyte
indocyanine green
INFORM HER-2/neu breast cancer
Innofluor FPIA (fluorescence-polarization immunoassay) assay
insulin tolerance
!nSure fecal occult blood
intraductal secretin (IDST)
intraesophageal acid
intraesophageal pH
intragraft polymerase chain reaction (PCR) assay
intraluminal pH electrode
intraoperative endoscopic Congo red (IECRT)
IOS immunoassay system
iprofenin
IRMA blood analysis system
IRMA-M
IRMA SL
Isletest and Isletest-ICA
Isletest-GAD
Jacoby
Javorski
Jolles
Kapsinow

test *(cont.)*
Kashiwado
Kato
Kelling
Kinberg
Kleihauer-Betke
Kleihauer-Betke acid elution
Krokiewicz
lactose breath
lactose breath hydrogen
lactulose-mannitol
LAP (leucine aminopeptidase)
latex fixation
LDH (serum lactate dehydrogenase)
Leo
leuvine aminopeptidase
levulose
LFTs (liver function tests)
LHMT (low-range heparin management)
Ligat
lipase
lipid profile
litmus milk
liver function (LFT)
long-acting thyroid-stimulating hormone (LATS)
low-dose dexamethasone suppression
low-range heparin management test (LHMT)
Lundh
Lüttke (Luettke)
Machado-Guerreiro
MacLean
magnetic susceptibility
Maly
Mann-Whitney U (data analysis)
manometric
Marechal-Rosen
marker transit study
Masset test for bile pigments in urine

test *(cont.)*
Matritech NMP22
MATRIX assay
McNemar ascites
McNemar test for ascites
measurement
mebrofenin hepatobiliary function
mecholyl
methyl red
Mitscherlich
Mohr
Moynihan
Myers and Fine
Mylius
N High Sensitivity CRP (C-reactive protein)
Nakayama
NAP hepatitis B virus (HBV) quantitative panel
Nardi test (morphine-prostigmine)
NBT-PABA
Neomark-BU (broxuridine)
NeoTect
Neukomm
nitrogen partition
NuMA
O&P (ova and parasites)
OncoChek immunoassay
OnCyte assay
optimized serum pancreolauryl test
overnight dexamethasone suppression
PABA (p-aminobenzoic acid)
palmitin
Pap (Papanicolaou)
parathyroid hormone (PTH)
PAS (periodic acid-Schiff)
PathVysion HER-2 DNA probe kit
peak secretory flow rate (PSFR)
pentagastrin
pentagastrin gastric secretory
pentagastrin infusion
pentagastrin provocative
pentagastrin stimulated analysis

test *(cont.)*
Pepgen
perineal nerve terminal motor latency
periodic acid-Schiff (PAS)
Pettenkofer
phenoltetrachlorophthalein
physiologic reflux (PRT)
PIVKA-II level
PNTML (pudendal nerve terminal motor latency)
POA (pancreatic oncofetal antigen)
PP-CAP IgA enzyme immunoassay
Premier Platinum HpSA
PreVue *B. burgdorferi* antibody detection assay
Prometheus
prostate-specific antigen (PSA)
Protocult
provocative
pudendal nerve terminal motor latency (PNTML)
Pylori-Chek
PyloriProbe
Pyloriset
PyloriTek *Helicobacter pylori*
PYtest
QualiCode
quantitative fecal fat
Quick
QuickVue one-step *H. pylori*
QuickVue one-step influenza
Quinlan
Rabuteau
radioimmunoassay (RIA) CA27.29 antigen
rapid serum amylase
recombinant immunoblot assay (RIBA)
reducing substances
Rehfuss
Reitman-Frankel
RET gene familial medullary thyroid carcinoma

test *(cont.)*
Rhodes Inventory of Nausea and Vomiting
Riba 3.0 SIA reagent kit for hepatitis C
RIBA (recombinant immunoblot assay)
RIBA HCV 3.0 SIA (strip immunoblot assay)
rice-flour breath
Robinson-Kepler-Power water
rose bengal
rose bengal sodium (^{131}I-labeled) hepatic function
Rosenbach-Gmelin
Rosenthal
Rotazyme
Saathoff
Sahli glutoid
Sahli-Nencki
saline
saline continence
Salkowski and Schipper
Salomon
sandwich radioimmunoassay
santonin
SART (standard acid reflux)
Saundby
S-CCK-Pz (secretin, cholecystokinin, pancreatozymin)
Schiff
Schilling
Schwarz
Scivoletto
secretin-CCK stimulation
secretin-pancreozymin
secretin provocation
secretin stimulation
SeHCAT (selenium-labeled homocholic acid conjugated taurine)
^{75}Se-labeled bile acid
selenomethionine (^{75}Se) pancreatic function
Seracult

test *(cont.)*
Seracult Plus
serum amylase
serum complement level
serum DHEA level
serum glucose value
serum iron
serum protein
serum transaminase level
72-hour fecal fat
Sgambati reaction for peritonitis
SGOT (now *AST*)
SGPT (now *ALT*)
sham feeding
shunt patency
SIA (strip immunoblot assay)
Smith
sodium iodide (^{123}I or ^{125}I) thyroid function
solid sphere
squeeze pressure profile of anal sphincter
standard acid reflux (SART)
Stat*Simple
stimulated gastric secretion
Stokvis
Stoll
stool cytotoxin
stool electrolyte
stool osmolality
stool osmotic gap
Strassburg
string
strip immunoblot assay (SIA)
Stypven time
sulfobromophthalein sodium
Super Seracult
Szabo
Tensilon
thallium treadmill exercise
thyroid antibody
thyroid function (TFT)
thyroid hemagglutination
thyroid microsomal antibody

test *(cont.)*
thyroid-stimulating hormone (TSH)
thyroid suppression
thyroid uptake of radioactive iodine
thyrotropin-releasing hormone (TRH) stimulation
thyroxine ratio, effective (ETR)
thyroxine/TBG ratio
thyroxine-binding globulin (TBG)
TIBC (total iron-binding capacity)
tilt
TMT (trail making)
Topfer
Torquay
total fecal weight
total iron-binding capacity (TIBC)
total serum T_4 (total serum thyroxine)
total thyroxine
trail making (TMT)
transferrin
transmucosal electrical potential
Triage *Clostridium difficile* panel
Triage parasite panel
triceps skinfold thickness
Trinity adenovirus EIA
Trousseau
Truquant BR radioimmunoassay (RIA)
TSH immunoassay
24-hour ambulatory pH
24-hour gastric acidity
two-stage triolein
Tyson
UBT (urea breath test) for *Helicobacter pylori*
Udranszky
Uffelmann
Ultzmann
Uni-Gold *H. pylori*
urea breath (UBT)
urease breath
URINELISA for *Helicobacter pylori*
UriSite microalbumin/creatinine urine

test *(cont.)*
- Uri-Test
- van den Bergh
- van Jaksch
- Velogene rapid VRE assay
- Virgo antimitochondrial antibody kit
- vitamin B_{12} absorption
- Voges-Proskauer
- V-scan
- Wagner
- water-gurgle
- water recovery
- water-sipping
- water-soluble contrast esophageal swallow
- WEST (Weinstein Enhanced Sensory Test) for diabetic neuropathy
- Whipple triad
- Winckler
- Witz
- Woldman
- Wolff-Junghans
- xylose tolerance
- Zappacosta
- ZstatFlu
- zylose absorption

Tes-Tape reagent strip
test breakfast
test dinner
testicular appendage
testicular artery
testicular atrophy
testicular pain
testicular pampiniform venous plexus
testicular torsion
testicular tumor
testicular vessel
testing fluid
testing hepatitis
testis
- descent of
- free-floating

testis appendix
test meal
testolactone
testosterone
test panel
Testred (methyltestosterone)
tetanus-prone wound
tetany
- hypocalcemic
- parathyroid
- parathyroprival

tethered-bowel sign
tetracaine HCl
tetracycline
tetradecyl sulfate
tetrahydrocannabinol (THC)
tetraiodothyronine (T_4)
tetralogy of Fallot
Tevdek pledgeted suture
Tevdek suture
T-fastener gastropexy
TFE polymer pledget
TFT (thyroid function test)
TFX Medical catheter stylet
Tg bandage
TGF (tissue growth factor)
thalassemia major
Thal esophageal stricture repair
Thal esophagogastrostomy
Thal fundic patch operation
thalidomide
thallium treadmill exercise test
thallium-201 (^{201}Tl)
Thal-Nissen fundoplasty
Thalomid (thalidomide)
Thal repair of esophageal stricture
Thal stricturoplasty
Thatcher forceps
Thatcher nail
THBR (thyroid hormone binding ratio)
THC (tetrahydrocannabinol)
THC (thulium, holmium, chromium): YAG laser
THC (transhepatic cholangiography)
THE (transhepatic embolization)

The Bandeau postaugmentation bra
thecal abscess
thecal sac
thecoperitoneal shunt
Theiler virus
thenar space abscess
theophylline level
theophylline olamine enema
theophylline toxicity
The Pinto Cobra
Thera-Boot compression dressing
theraccine, Theratope-STn
Theradigm-HBV (hepatitis B virus)
Theragyn
Theralax
therapeutic anesthesia
therapeutic endoscopy
therapeutic intervention
therapeutic malaria
therapeutic protein
therapeutic transjugular procedure
therapist
  enterostomal
  occupational
  physical
  respiratory
  stoma
therapy
  ablative
  ablative laser
  adjuvant
  adjuvant systemic
  androgen
  anticholinergic
  antigastrin
  antilymphocyte induction
  antimicrobial
  antireflux
  antisecretory drug
  anti-TNF
  antiviral
  beta blockade
  breast-conserving
  CadPlan cancer planning

therapy *(cont.)*
  combined modality
  conservative
  curative
  decompression
  diet
  diuretic
  electrolyte
  electrosurgical
  empirical
  endocrine
  endoscopic injection (EIT)
  enteral nutritional (EN)
  enterostomal
  enzyme replacement
  extracorporeal shock-wave (ESWT)
  gamma brachytherapy
  gene
  Gerson
  Hemopure (hemoglobin glutamer-250 [bovine]) oxygen
  herbal
  hormonal
  hormone replacement (HRT)
  highly active antiretroviral (HAART)
  induction
  instillation
  interferon-ribavirin
  intralesional
  intravenous
  lamivudine
  laser
  life-long suppressive
  long-term thyroxine
  low-intensity laser (LILT)
  medical
  mono-
  multiagent
  multimodal
  multipolar electrocoagulation (MECT; MPEC)
  neoadjuvant hormonal (NHT)
  nonoperative
  nutritional

therapy *(cont.)*
  palliation
  palliative
  pancreatic enzyme replacement
  parenteral
  pharmacotherapy
  photodynamic (PDT)
  polydrug
  postmastectomy radiation
  Precision Therapy
  Prevacid triple
  pulsed-dye laser
  pump
  radiation
  radioactive
  sclerosing
  sham
  steroid
  suppressive
  surgical
  swallowing
  systemic
  Targeted Ablation Therapy
  TheraSphere radiation
  tumor amplified protein expression (TAPET)
  tumor necrosis (TNT)
TheraSeed palladium-103 implants
TheraSphere radiation therapy
Theratope vaccine
Theratope-STn
Therevac-Plus (docusate sodium; benzocaine)
Therevac-SB (docusate sodium)
Therex (huHMFG1) human monoclonal antibody
Thermacare warm air blower
Thermachoice uterine balloon therapy system
Therma Jaw (or Thermajaw) hot urologic forceps
thermal ablation
thermal anesthesia
thermal necrosis
thermal probe
Thermal Quenching cooling technique for laser treatment
thermal stimulation technique
Thermazene (silver sulfadiazine)
thermistor sensor
ThermoChem-HT lavage system (formerly BioLogic-HT system)
thermodilution
thermodilution catheter
thermometer
  IVAC Core·Check
  IVAC electronic
  talking digital
  Tender Tykes digital
Thermoplas sheet
Thermo-STAT system
TherOx 0.014 infusion guidewire
The Solidifier fluid solidification system
The Viewing Wand (surgical digitizer)
The Wand
thiabendazole (TBZ)
thiazolidinedione
thick adhesion
thick bile
thickened gallbladder wall
thickened material
thickened polypropylene thread
thickened wall
thickening
  asymmetric mural
  breast
  gallbladder wall
  haustral fold
  mediastinal
  mucosal
  multiple inflammatory fibrous
  mural
  submucosal
thickening in breast
thickening of gallbladder wall
thickening of haustral fold
thicker hepatic parenchyma
thickness, skinfold

thick-walled gallbladder
Thiersch anal incontinence operation
Thiersch graft
Thiersch medium split free graft
Thiersch suture
Thiersch thin split free graft
Thiersch wire
thiethylperazine
thin adhesion
THI needle
thin-needle percutaneous cholangiogram
ThinPrep slide
thin secretion
THINSite dressing
THINSite with BioFilm hydrogel
topical wound dressing
thin-walled gallbladder
Thioplex (thiotepa)
thiosalan
thiotepa
third branchial pouch
third-degree hemorrhoid
third pharyngeal pouch
Third National Health and Nutrition
Examination Survey (NHANES III)
third space fluid loss
thizide diuretics
THL (Transvaginal Hydro Laparoscopy)
system
Thomas Allis forceps
Thomas extrapolated bar graft
Thomas walking calipers
thombophilia
thombotic thrombocytopenic purpura
(TTP)
Thompson carotid artery clamp
Thompson rasp
Thomson Walker clamp
Thomson Walker-TC needle holder
thoracentesis
thoracentesis fluid
thoracentesis needle
thoracic aorta
thoracic arch aortogram
thoracic cavity
thoracic duct
thoracic duct injury
thoracic great vessel injury
thoracic great vessel
thoracic inlet
thoracic kidney
thoracic rongeur
thoracic scissors
thoracic splenosis
thoracic stomach
thoracic wall, abdominal
Thoracic instruments
thoracoabdominal esophagectomy
thoracoabdominal esophagogastrectomy
thoracoabdominal incision
thoracoacromial artery
thoracodorsal nerve
thoracophrenolaparotomy
Thoracoport
thoracoscopic esophagomyotomy
thoracoscopic repair of diaphragmatic
defect
thoracoscopic surgery
thoracoscopy cannula
thoracoscopy trocar
Thora-Klex chest drainage system
Thora-Klex chest tube
Thoralon biomaterial graft
Thora-Port
thorascopic esophagomyotomy
thorax
Thorek dissecting scissors
Thorek-Feldman gallbladder scissors
Thorek gallbladder forceps
Thorek gallbladder scissors
Thorek-Mixter gallbladder forceps
Thorek scissors
Thornton nail
Thornton nail plate
Thornwald antrum perforator and
irrigator
Thorotrast contrast exposure

Thorotrast contrast medium
threaded pin
threaded rod
threaded Steinmann pin
threadworm
three-armed basket forceps
three-edge cutting forceps
three-hole (3-hole) plate
three-in-one device
three-loop ileal pouch
three-nail forceps
three-point skull clamp
three-prong fork
three-pronged grasping forceps
three-quadrant hemorrhoidectomy
three-quarters prone position
Three-Spring Reservoir Wound Suction
  Drainage Kit
three-strand semintendinosus tendon
  graft
three-strand suture
three-way stopcock
thresher's lung
Thrombin-JMI (thrombin)
thrombin-Keflin-sotredochal sclerosant
thrombocytopenia associated with drug
  abuse
thrombocytopenia purpura
thrombocytosis
Thrombogen topical thrombin
thrombophlebitis of superficial breast
  vein
thrombophlebitis, portal
thrombosed external hemorrhoid
thrombosis
  arterial
  bland
  deep venous (DVT)
  diffuse microvascular
  extensive portal vein
  hepatic artery (HAT)
  indolent
  mesenteric
thrombosis *(cont.)*
  nonocclusive mesenteric
  portal vein
  splenic vein
  spontaneous
  superior mesenteric artery
  venous
thrombosis of hepatic vein
thrombosis of portal vein
Thrombostat (thrombin)
thrombotic mesenteric infarction
thrombotic occlusion of stent shunt
thrombotic thrombocytopenic purpura
thromboulcerative colitis
thromboxanes
thrombus, residual
through-and-through continuous suture
through-and-through incision
through-and-through injury
through-and-through laceration
through-and-through suture
through-the-scope (TTS) dilator
through-the-scope mechanical lithotripsy
through-the-wall mattress suture
thrush, oral
thumb-control suction tube
thumb forceps
thumb handle
thumbprinting of mucosa
thumbprinting sign
thymalfasin
thymectomy
  complete
  partial
  total
thymic anlage
thymic-dependent portion of the
  immune system
thymic hypoplasia (DiGeorge syndrome)
thymic tumor
Thymitaq (nolatrexed dihydrochloride)

thymoma
  epithelial cell
  lymphoid cell
  malignant
  mixed cell
  spindle cell
thymosin alpha 1
thymus-derived (T) lymphocyte
thymus, enlarged
thymus gland
Thypinone (protirelin)
Thyrar (thyroid, desiccated bovine)
Thyrel-TRH (protirelin)
Thyro-Block (potassium iodide)
thyrocalcitonemia
thyrocalcitonin assay
thyrocalcitonin secretion
thyrocervical angiography
thyrocervical trunk
Thyrogen (thyrotropin alfa)
thyroglobulin antibody
thyroglossal cyst
thyroglossal duct
thyroglossal duct cyst
thyroglossal duct sinus
thyroglossal fistula
thyroid
  aberrant
  accessory
  benign inflammatory
  C cells of
  desiccated
  desiccated bovine
  desiccated porcine
  ectopic
  fibrosis of
  glottic
  intrathoracic
  lingual
  long-standing stimulation of
  multicentric
  nodular
  overactive
  retrosternal
thyroid *(cont.)*
  substernal
  suprahyoid
  underactive
thyroid ablation
thyroid adenoma
thyroid antibody
thyroid antibody test
thyroid autoantibody
thyroid-binding globulin
thyroid cancer
  anaplastic carcinoma
  biologically active
  differentiated
  follicular carcinoma
  medullary (MTC)
  papillary carcinoma
thyroid capsulitis
thyroid carcinoma
thyroid "C" cells
thyroid crisis
thyroid cystadenoma
thyroid disease
thyroidectomy
  bilateral
  complete
  endoscopic
  Kocher collar
  near-total
  prophylactic
  subtotal
  total
  unilateral
thyroid function test (TFT)
thyroid gland
thyroid goiter
thyroid hemagglutination test
thyroid hormone (TH)
thyroid hormone binding ratio (THBR)
thyroid hormone replacement
thyroid infarction
thyroid instruments
thyroid irradiation
thyroid isthmus

thyroiditis
  adult pyogenic
  acute suppurative
  atrophic
  autoimmune
  chronic
  chronic fibrous
  chronic lymphocytic
  de Quervain
  fibrous
  giant cell
  granulomatous
  Hashimoto
  iatrogenic
  invasive
  ligneous
  nonsuppurative
  painless
  postpartum
  pyogenic
  radiation
  Riedel
  silent
  subacute
  subacute granulomatous
  suppurative
  viral
  vital
  woody
thyroid lobe appendage
thyroid lobectomy
thyroid mapping
thyroid microsomal antibody (MSA)
thyroid migration
thyroid neoplasm
thyroid nodule
thyroid panel
thyroid parenchyma
thyroid scan
thyroid-stimulating hormone (TSH) test
thyroid storm
Thyroid Strong (thyroid, desiccated)
thyroid suppression test
thyroid tumor
thyroid ultrasonography
thyroid ultrasound
thyroid uptake of radioactive iodine test
Thyrolar (liotrix)
thyromedan HCl
thyrothymic ligament
thyrotoxic crisis
thyrotoxic myopathy
thyrotoxicosis
  factitious
  neonatal
thyrotoxicosis without hyperthyroidism
thyrotoxic storm
thyrotrophic hormone
thyrotrophin
thyrotropic-releasing hormone
thyrotropin alfa
thyrotropin-releasing hormone (TRH)
  stimulation test
thyrotropin, suppressed
thyroxin-binding globulin capacity
thyroxine-binding globulin (TBG) test
thyroxine ^{125}I
thyroxine ^{131}I
thyroxine ratio, effective (ETR) test
thyroxine/TBG ratio test
Thytropar (thyrotropin)
tiabendazole
TIBC (total iron-binding capacity) test
tibial cutter guide
tibial cutting guide
tibial drill guide
tibial drill pin
tibial punch
tibial retractor
tick-borne virus
tickle of pancreas
tickle of spleen
ticklish
Ticlid (ticlopidine)
ticlopidine
Ticon (trimethobenzamide HCl)
Ti-Cron suture (also Tycron)
tidal volume

tie
  free
  ligature
  stick
  suture
Tielle absorptive dressing
Tielle hydropolymer foam dressing
Tielle Plus absorbent adhesive dressing with a multilayer structure
Tiemann catheter
Tiemann Meals tenolysis knife
Tiemann nail
Tiemann shoulder retractor
tie on a passer
tie-over bolus dressing
Tigan (trimethobenzamide hydrochloride)
tight abdomen
tight adhesion
tight defect
tight lesion
tight suture
tigroid appearance
tigroid mass
Tilley dressing and packing forceps
tilt test
time
  Actalyke activated clotting
  activated clotting (ACT)
  activated coagulation
  activated
  activated thromboplastin
  bleeding (BT)
  clotting
  coagulation
  dextrinizing
  Duke bleeding
  emptying
  esophageal
  esophageal transit
  gastric transit
  Ivy bleeding
  Lee-White clotting
  mean transit
time *(cont.)*
  Mielke bleeding
  partial thromboplastin (PTT)
  plasma clotting
  prothrombin (PT)
  radionuclide
  radionuclide esophageal emptying
  rapid transit
  Simplate bleeding
  small bowel transit
  small intestine transit
  tincture of
times three or x 3 ("The patient was oriented x 3.")
Tinckler rectal suction tube
tincture of benzoin
tincture of opium
tincture of time
Tindall scissors
tinkling bowel sounds
tinzaparin sodium
tip
  baby Tischler biopsy
  catheter
  integral
  Kevorkian biopsy
  Krause biopsy
  Micro-Probe
  Murphy
  Poole
  pyramid
  Re-new laparoscopic surgical
  Rhoton suction
  Schuknecht
  scissors
  spleen
  suction
  Tischler biopsy
tip deflection technique
Tip-it instrument guard
TIPS, TIPSS (transjugular intrahepatic portosystemic shunt) procedure (also portacaval shunt)
Tip-To-Tip radiopaque line

Tip-Trol handle
tirolimus
Tischler biopsy tip
Tischler cervical biopsy punch forceps
Tischler-Morgan biopsy forceps
Tisseel fibrin sealant
Tisseel "surgical glue"
Tissomat application device
Tissucol fibrin-collagen hemostatic material
Tissucol fibrin glue
tissue
- acinar
- adipose
- analogous
- areolar
- autogenous
- bites of
- cicatricial
- connective
- cortical
- dead pancreatic
- debridement
- dense breast
- ectopic pancreatic
- enveloping scar
- extirpation of
- extraperitoneal
- fatty
- fibroadipose
- fibrofatty
- fibroglandular
- fibrous
- fibrous stromal
- fragmented
- friable
- functioning thyroid
- granulation
- gut-associated lymphoid (GALT)
- heterotopic pancreatic
- infected
- lipomatous-like
- morcellation of
- necrosis of

tissue *(cont.)*
- necrotic
- nodal
- nonviable
- parenchymal
- periadrenal
- pericoronal
- peridiverticular
- perinephric
- perirenal
- plug of
- polypoid
- redundant
- resected
- retrocecal
- scar
- septal
- soft
- splenic
- subcutaneous
- surrounding fatty
- suspicious
- tail of breast
- thyroid
- vascularized gastric

tissue adhesive (see *adhesive*)
tissue and cuticle nipper
tissue approximation
tissue catabolism
tissue debridement
- fibrinolysin and desoxyribonuclease
- papain
- sutilains

tissue engineering
tissue equivalent material
tissue extraction
tissue expander
- AccuSpan
- Becker
- Cox-Uphoff International (CUI)
- Heyer-Schulte
- T-Span

tissue-fixed macrophage
tissue forceps

tissue growth factor (TGF)
tissue hypoxia
tissue invasion
tissue irrigation
tissue ischemia
tissue level of porphyrins
TissueLink Monopolar Floating Ball
tissue marker, MicroMark
tissue-mesh interface
tissue occlusion clamp
tissue penetration
tissue perfusion
tissue-selective estrogens
tissue-sparing technique
tissue vascularity
Tis-U-Trap endometrial suction catheter
titanium alloy rod
titanium half pin
titanium microsurgical bipolar forceps
titanium microsurgical needle holder
titanium nail
titanium plate
titanium staple
Titralac (calcium carbonate)
TLc.BiliTest system
TL-90 (Ethicon) stapler
TME (total mesorectal excision)
TMT (trail-making test)
TNB (transthoracic needle biopsy)
TNB (Tru-Cut needle biopsy)
TNF-alpha (tumor necrosis factor-alpha) level
TNFa, IL-1b, IL-6, IL-10, KC, MCP-1, MIP-2, and RANTES (inflammatory cytokines)
TNM classification of carcinoma
TNM classification of malignant tumors (T represents size of tumor, N clinical status of node, and M metastases)
  M0 No distant metastases
  M1 Distant metastases present
  MX Distant metastases not assessed

TNM classification *(cont.)*
  N0 Regional lymph node not involved
  N1 Regional lymph node involved
  NX Regional lymph node not assessed
  Stage I, T1-2, N0, M0—No extension or node involvement
  Stage II, T3, N0, M0—Advanced extension, unresectable
  Stage III, T1-3, N1, M0—Node involvement
  Stage IV, T1-3, N0-1, M1—Distant metastases present
  T1 Direct extension of primary tumor
  T2 Direct extension of primary tumor to specific organs
  T3 Direct advanced extension of tumor, unresectable
TNT (tumor necrosis therapy) staging system
to-and-fro anesthesia
Todd cirrhosis
Todd-Wells guide
Toennis-Adson dissecting scissors
Toennis dissecting scissors
Toennis dura hook
Toennis dura knife
Toennis tumor forceps
toe plate
toe-to-groin modified Jones dressing
toe ulcer
togavirus
Toggelite
toilet, peritoneal
Toilinox (stainless steel)
tolazamide
tolbutamide-induced cholestasis
tolbutamide sodium
tolbutamide stimulation test
Toldt, white line of

tolerance, activity
tolerance induction to islet allotransplantation
Tolerex enteral nutritional therapy
Tolinase (tolazamide)
tolrestat
toluidine blue stain
Tom Jones closure suture
Tomac nonconductive breathing
Tomocat (barium sulfate)
tomographic view
tomography (see *imaging*)
Tomudex (raltitrexed)
Tonalin (conjugated linoleic acid)
tongs, Gardner-Wells
tongue
  adder's
  bald
  base of
  beefy
  black hairy
  coated
  cobblestone
  flat
  furry
  raspberry
  smooth
tongue base
tongue blade
tongue pulsive force
tonic contraction
Tonopaque (barium sulfate)
tonsillar crypt
tonsillar forceps
tonsillar pillar
tonsil forceps
tonsil knife
tonsil scissors
tonsil sponge
tonsil sucker
tonsil tag excision
Toomey irrigating syringe
toothed Adson tissue forceps
toothed retractor
toothed tissue forceps
TOPA (topical oropharyngeal anesthesia)
topanoic acid (Telepaque)
Topaz CO_2 laser
Topel knot
Töpfer test
topical agent
topical anesthesia (see *anesthesia*)
topical anesthetic
topical bovine thrombin
topical hemostatic agent
topical nitrate
topical pharyngeal anaesthesia
topical podopyllin
topical steroid
top-loading rod
topogram, topography
  balloon
  scintigraphic balloon
toposcopic catheter
Torbot faceplate
TORCH (toxoplasmosis; other agents; rubella; cytomegalovirus; herpes simplex) syndrome
Torcon NB selective angiographic catheter
Torecan
toremifene citrate
Torquay test
torrential bleeding
Torres syndrome
torsion
  biliary tract
  intestinal
  large-bowel
  testicular
  ovarian
torsion forceps
torsion of cyst or fallopian tube
torsion of splenic vein
torso crease
tortuous bile duct
tortuous esophagus

tortuous lesion
Toshiba EccoCee ultrasound system
Toshiba 270 ultrasound system
Toshiba videoendoscope
tositumomab
total abdominal colectomy (TAC)
total abdominal evisceration (TAE) organ harvesting technique
total bilateral vagotomy
total bile acid
total bilirubin
total blood loss
total body sodium deficit
total colectomy
total esophagectomy
total fecal weight test
total food intolerance
total fundic wrap (Nissen-Rossetti)
total gastrectomy
total gastric wrap
total gastrin
total hepatectomy
total intravenous anesthesia
total iron-binding capacity (TIBC)
total left lobectomy of liver
total lesion
total lobectomy
total mastectomy
total mesorectal excision (TME)
total necrosis
total pancreatectomy
total pancreatectomy with lymphadenectomy
total parathyroidectomy
total parenteral alimentation
total parenteral nutrition (TPN)
total protein
total protocolectomy and ileostomy
total right lobectomy of liver
total sac excision
total serum T_3 (total serum triiodothyronine) test
total serum T_4 (total serum thyroxine) test
total shunt
total spinal anesthesia
total thoracic esophagectomy
total thymectomy
total thyroidectomy
total thyroxine test
total villous atrophy
totally (or total) extraperitoneal laparoscopic hernioplasty
totally intrahepatic gallbladder
Toti trephine drill
Toupet fundoplasty
Toupet fundoplication
Toupet hemifundoplication
Tourguide guiding catheter
Tourni-cot tourniquet
towel clamp
towel clip
Tower sterile packaging
Townes Brooks syndrome
Townley femur calipers
Townley tibial plateau plate
Townsend-Gilfillan plate
Townsend handle
toxemia, hepatic
toxic (diffuse) goiter
toxic atrophy
toxic cirrhosis
toxic colitis
toxic diarrhea
toxic diffuse goiter
toxic dilatation
toxic dilation of colon
toxic drug concentration in blood and tissues
toxic gastritis
toxic gastroenteritis
toxic goiter
toxic granulation
toxic granule
toxic hepatitis
toxic inflammation
toxic insult
toxic irrigant

toxicity
  drug
  gastrointestinal
  GI
  hepatic
  oxygen (O_2)
  theophylline
toxic level
toxic megacolon
toxic multinodular goiter
toxic mushroom poisoning
toxic myocarditis
toxic nephrosis
toxic neuritis
toxic nodular goiter
toxic or inflammatory myopathy or dysfunctional neuromuscular transmission
toxic pneumonia
toxic shock syndrome (TSS)
toxic steatosis
toxic substances test on venous blood
toxic thyroid state
toxic uninodular goiter
toxic vacuolization
toxigenic bacteria
toxin exposure
toxoplasmosis hepatitis
TPN (total parenteral nutrition)
TPN with lipids
TQa (transcutaneous access flow) device
trabecula (pl. trabeculae)
trabecular artery
trabecular carcinoma of skin
trabecular cirrhosis
trace edema
trace mineral
trace pedal edema
Tracer blood glucose monitor
Tracer hybrid wire guide for endoscopic surgery
tracheal blade
tracheal hook
tracheal retractor
tracheobronchial mucosal necrosis
tracheoesophageal (TE)
tracheoesophageal fistula (TEF)
tracheoesophageal junction
tracheoesophageal puncture (TEP)
tracheomalacia
tracheostomy tube
Trachlight
Tracker-10 catheter
Tracker-18 Soft Stream catheter
Tracrium (atracurium besylate)
tract
  alimentary
  biliary
  digestive
  fistulous
  gastrointestinal (GI)
  hepatic outflow
  ileal inflow
  iliopubic
  intestinal
  intramural fistulous
  lower gastrointestinal
  mature T-tube
  pancreaticobiliary
  pyramidal
  reproductive
  respiratory
  sinus
  upper gastrointestinal (UGI)
  urinary
traction anchor
traction diverticulum
traction hook
traction pin
traction suture
trail-making test (TMT)
TrakBack ultrasound catheter
TRAM (transverse rectus abdominis myocutaneous) flap
Tramex polypropylene mesh
transabdominal preperitoneal laparoscopic hernioplasty

transabdominal repair
transabdominal retroperitoneal node dissection
transabdominal sonography
transaminase, hepatic
transampullary septectomy
transanal approach
transanal deflation of sigmoid volvulus
transanal double-stapling technique
transanal endoscopic microsurgery (TEM)
transanal pouch advancement
transarterial chemoembolization (TACE)
transarticular pin
transaxillary subpectoral mammoplasty
transcatheter arterial chemoemboliza- tion (TACE)
transcatheter variceal embolization
transcatheter vessel embolization
transcellular fluid
transcervical route
transcoccygeal approach
transcorpus impalement
transcription factor
transcutaneous electrical nerve stimulation
transcystic common bile duct exploration
transcystic duct/common bile duct exploration (TCD/CBDE)
TransCyte skin substitute graft
transdermal anesthesia
Transderm Scop
transducer
  abdominal
  rectal
  rectal multiplane
  volume displacement
transducer fitting
transduodenal drainage technique
transduodenal endoscopic decompres- sion
transduodenal sphincteroplasty
transduodenal sphincterotomy
Transeal transparent adhesive film dressing
transect
transected stomach
transected vertical gastric bypass with Silastic ring band and gastrostomy
transection
transection of esophagus
transectomy of vagus nerves, truncal
Transelast bandage
transendoscopic catheter placement
transendoscopic electrocoagulation
transendoscopic tube
transesophageal endoscopy
transesophageal ligation of varices
transfemoral liver biopsy
transfer
  free flap
  free jejunum
  microsurgical free tissue
  microvascular flap
  nuclear
transference of muscle and blood supply
  latissimus dorsi flap
  rectus abdominis flap
transferrin saturation, percent
transfixing pin
transfixion pin
transfixion suture
transformation, malignant
transfuse
transfusion
  autologous
  donor-specific (DST)
  incompatible blood
  intraoperative autologous (IOT)
  massive blood
  multiple
transfusion hepatitis
transfusion malaria
transfusion of incompatible blood
transfusion of packed cells

transfusion reaction
transgastric drainage technique
transgastric ligation
transgastric plication
transgenic manipulation for organ transplantation
transglutaminase antibody
transhepatic biliary stent
transhepatic catheterization
transhepatic cholangiogram (THC)
transhepatic embolization (THE)
transhepatic portal and splenic venography
transhepatic portal venography
transhepatic tube
transhiatal blunt esophagectomy
transhiatal esophagectomy
transhiatal pyloroplasty
transient bacteremia
transient gastroparesis
transient hyperthyroidism
transient septicemia
TransiGel hydrogel-impregnated gauze
transillumination
transition suture
transitional cell carcinoma
transitional cell papilloma
transitory neonatal hypoparathyroidism
transitory papule
transjugular access catheter
transjugular balloon angioplasty
transjugular intrahepatic portal shunt procedure (TIPS)
transjugular intrahepatic portosystemic shunt (TIPS or TIPSS)
transjugular liver biopsy
transluminal extraction (TEC) catheter
transmesenteric plication
transmissible gastroenteritis of swine
transmissible infectious disease
transmission
  fecal
  fecal-oral
  horizontal

transmission *(cont.)*
  neuromuscular
  oral
  sexual
transmucosal electrical potential
transmucosal fentanyl citrate oral
transmural closure
transmural colitis
transmural extension
transmural fibrosis
transmural ileocolitis
transmural inflammation
transmural involvement
transmural lesion
transnasal bile duct catheterization
transnasal biopsy
transnasal videoendoscope
transomental posterior gastroenterostomy
transoral endoscopy
Transorbent multilayer dressing
Transorb MCT supplement
transosseous suture
transpapillary biopsy
transpapillary drainage technique
transpapillary endoscopic cholecystotomy
transparent adhesive film dressing
transparent cap-fitted endoscope
transparent dressing
transperineal ultrasonography
transperitoneal aortic access
transplant (see also *transplantation*)
  adult-to-adult living donor liver
  autologous bone marrow (ABMT)
  auxiliary
  bone marrow (BMT)
  cadaveric
  combined kidney and pancreas (CKPT)
  embryonic cell islet
  heart
  hepatic
  intestinal

transplant *(cont.)*
 kidney
 liver
 living-donor
 living-related
 lung
 multivisceral
 orthotopic liver (OLT)
 pancreas
 partial
 reduced-size liver (RSLT)
 rejection of
 renal
 solid organ
 syngeneic
transplantation (see also *transplant*)
 allogeneic
 bone marrow (BMT)
 combined liver and intestinal
 embryonic cell
 heterotopic
 human cell
 human islet
 intestinal
 islet
 islet-cell
 isolated pancreas
 kidney-pancreas
 liver
 multivisceral
 orthotopic
 orthotopic liver (OLT)
 pancreas
 pancreas after kidney (PAK)
 pancreatic islet cell
 segmental bowel
 small bowel
 small bowel plus liver
 solid organ
Transplantation Society
transplanted stamp graft
transplant candidate
transplant rejection
Transplatin (oxaliplatin)
Transpore surgical tape
transposition, gastric
transposition of anoperineal fistula
transposition of anovestibular fistula
transposition of great arteries
transpyloric line
transpyloric tube
transrectal drainage
transrectal drainage of pelvic abscess
transsacral approach
TransScan TS2000 electrical impedance breast scanning system
transseptal needle
transsphenoidal bipolar forceps
transsphenoidal hook
transsphenoidal removal of pituitary adenoma
transsphenoidal resection of tumor
transsphincteric anal fistula
transthoracic (transpleural or transparietal) and subcostal liver biopsy
transthoracic approach
transthoracic diaphragmatic hernia
transthoracic Nissen fundoplication
transthoracic resection of esophageal carcinoma
transtracheal oxygen catheter
transudative ascites
transumbilical breast augmentation (TUBA)
transumbilical augmentation mammoplasty
transumbilical plane
transurethral balloon Laserthermia prostatectomy
transurethral laser-induced prostatectomy (TULIP)
transvenous catheterization
transvenous (transjugular) liver biopsy
transversalis fascia
transverse abdominal muscle
transverse colectomy
transverse colon
transverse colostomy

transverse hook
transverse incision
transverse-loop rod colostomy
transverse mesocolon
transverse orientation
transverse plane
transverse process hook
transverse rectus abdominis myocutaneous (TRAM) flap for breast reconstruction
transverse section
transverse suture
transverse wedge excision
transversostomy
transversotomy
transversus abdominis aponeurosis
transversus abdominis muscle
transversus aponeurosis
transversus arch
trap, DeLee suction
trastuzumab (anti-HER2 humanized monoclonal antibody)
Traube neurological percussion hammer
Traube semilunar space
Traum-Aid HBC enteral feeding
trauma
  autoerotic rectal
  blunt
  blunt abdominal
  foreign body
  head
  homosexual rectal
  iatrogenic
  intraoperative
  liver
  massive splenic
  penetrating
  penetrating abdominal
  rectal
  splenic
TraumaCal (multiple branched-chain amino acids) enteral nutritional therapy
TraumaCal enteral feeding
TraumaJet wound debridement system
TraumaSeal sealant
traumatic anesthesia
traumatic appendicitis
traumatic extraperitoneal perforation of duodenal diverticulum
traumatic hernia
traumatic hyphema
traumatic lesion
traumatic placement of nasogastric tube
traumatic rupture
traumatic scar
traumatic tissue grab
traumatopneic wound
trauma zones (I, II, III)
Trautman Locktite prosthetic hook
Trautmann chisel
Travamulsion fat emulsion solution
Travasol in Dextrose
Travasol with electrolytes
Travasorb HN (high nitrogen) powdered feeding
Travasorb MCT (medium chain triglyceride)
Travasorb MCT enteral nutritional therapy
Travasorb MCT food supplement
Travasorb MCT liquid feeding
Travasorb STD enteral nutritional therapy
Travasorb STD liquid feeding
traveler's diarrhea
"traveling volvulus"
Travers retractor
traverse, peritoneal
traverse the internal ring
traversing the center
Traverso-Longmire technique
Treace drill
treatment algorithm
treatment modality
treatment protocol

tree
  biliary
  hepatobiliary
trefoil balloon
trefoil deformity
Treitz fossa
Treitz hernia
Treitz, ligament of
Trelex mesh graft
Trelex polypropylene mesh
trematode (fluke)
tremors of the hands and tongue
tremulousness
Trendelenburg position
trephine drill
trephine, Galt cranial
Treponema pallidum
tretromolar trigone
Trex digital mammography system (TDMS)
TRH (thyrotropin-releasing hormone)
Triacana (tiratricol; levothyroxine sodium)
triad
  Beck
  Charcot
  Dieulafoy
  fragile histidine (FHIT)
  hepatic
  portal
  Rigler
  Saint
  Whipple
triad of liver disease, arterial hypoxemia, and intrapulmonary vascular dilatation
triad of Rigler
Triage *Clostridium difficile* panel
Triage parasite panel
trial
  Breast Cancer Prevention Trial
  ADOPT (a diabetes outcome progression)
  clinical (phases 1–3)
trial *(cont.)*
  DPT–1 (diabetes prevention trial type 1)
  randomized (RT)
  randomized double-blind
  6C (cooperative colorectal cancer combination chemotherapy
  clinical)
trial base plate
triangle
  Calot
  cardiohepatic
  Charcot
  cystohepatic
  digastric
  gastrinoma
  Grynfeltt
  Henke
  Hesselbach
  iliofemoral
  inferior lumbar
  inguinal
  Keith abdominal
  Labbe
  Lesgaft
  Livingston
  lumbocostoabdominal
  mesenteric
  Petit
  posterior neck
  Scarpa
triangle sponge
triangular bone reamer
triangular ligament of liver
triangular medullary nail
Triban (trimethobenzamide HCl; benzocaine)
Tricam SL/IPM
triceps skinfold thickness
trichinosis
trichobezoar
trichocyst
trichomonal colitis
trichomoniasis, intestinal

Trichosporon beigelii
trichosporosis
Trichuris trichiura
Tricodur Epi (elbow) compression
 support bandage
Tricodur Omos (shoulder) compression
 support bandage
Tricodur Talus (ankle) compression
 support bandage
Tricofix bandage
tricortical bone graft
tricortical ilial strip graft
tricuspid orifice
tridihexethyl chloride
Tridrate bowel prep
Tridrate Bowel Evacuant Kit
trifid stomach
triflange nail
triflanged Lottes nail
trigeminal nerve retractor
trigeminal scissors
triglycerides
 long chain (LCT)
 medium chain (MCT)
 serum
triglyceride enzyme deficiency
trihydrocoprostanic acid (TCA)
trilostane
Trilucent breast implant
Trimadeau sign
Trimax fabric
Trimazide (trimethobenzamide HCl)
trimethoprim-sulfamethoxazole
trimethylaminuria (fish-odor syndrome)
trimmer, Little
Trinity adenovirus EIA test kit
Trinkle drill
trioiodothyronine (T_3)
triple antibiotics
triple-lumen catheter
triple-lumen papillotome
triple-lumen Sengstaken-Blakemore
 tube
triple-lumen tube
Triptone (dimenhydrinate)
triradial resector blade
trisegmentectomy of liver
Tri-State Hospital Supply Corp.
Tritec (ranitidine bismuth citrate)
tri-wing anoscope
Trizivir
Trizyme (amylase; protease; cellulase)
Trocan disposable CO_2 trocar and
 cannula
trocar
 abdominal
 accessory
 ascites
 blunt
 Bluntport
 Bluntport laparoscopic
 camera
 Coakley antrum
 conical
 Cooper Surgical
 Core audible
 Core Entree Plus
 Core Entree II
 Core shielded laparoscopic
 Davidson thoracic
 DeRoyal
 dilating tip
 Don Congreve
 Duke
 Endopath laparoscopic
 Endopath TriStar
 Entree Plus
 Entree II
 Entree thoracoscopy
 Ethicon Endo-Surgery
 Ethicon Surgiport
 gallbladder
 Hasson
 Hunt-Reich
 Hurwitz thoracic
 hydrocele
 Iotec
 Landau

trocar *(cont.)*
- laparoscopic
- Nelson thoracic
- New Eder Corporation
- Ochsner gallbladder
- Origin
- Patterson
- PediPort
- peritoneal
- pyramidal
- pyramidal tip
- Saber BT blunt-tip surgical
- safety-shielded
- Step minimally invasive surgical
- subxiphoid
- suprapubic
- Surgiport
- Synthes transbuccal
- Ternamian EndoTIP system
- thoracoscopy
- Trocan disposable CO_2
- TroGARD Finesse
- umbilical
- VanAlyea antrum
- VersaPort
- Visiport optical
- Wangsteen
- Wolf
- Yankauer

trocar cannula
trocar hernia
trocar placement
trocar site tumor implant
trocar tent
trocar wound-site complication
trocar and sheath
trochanter, greater
trochanter-holding clamp
trochanter reamer
Troeltsch dressing forceps
TroGARD Finesse dilating trocar system
troglitazone
Troisier sign
Trömner (Troemner) percussion hammer
Tronolane (pramoxine HCl)
Tronzo elevator
TrophAmine total parenteral nutrition
trophic effect
trophic lesion
tropical sprue
tropical steatorrhea
tropisetron
trospectomycin
Trousseau esophageal bougie
Trousseau sign
Trousseau test
Trousseau trachea dilator
Troutman needle
Troutman rectus forceps
trovafloxacin
Trovan (trovafloxacin)
Trovax
troxacitabine
Tru-Area Determination wound-measuring device
Tru-Close wound drainage system
Tru-Cut cutting biopsy needle
Tru-Cut liver biopsy needle
Tru-Cut needle (TCNB) biopsy
true diverticulum (pl. diverticula)
true lateral view
True/Fit femoral intramedullary rod system
TruJect auto-injector drug delivery system
Trulife silicone breast prosthesis
Trumbull suture
trumpet, Core reposable
Trumpet needle guide
trumpet valve
truncal obesity
truncal vagotomy and gastroenterostomy
truncal vagotomy and pyloroplasty
trunk, celiac

TruPulse CO_2 laser
Truquant BR radioimmunoassay
Truquant BR RIA test
Tru-Scint AD imaging agent
truss for groin hernia
Tru-Support EW (elastic wrap) bandage
Tru-Support SA (self-adhering) bandage
Trypanosoma cruzi
trypanosomiasis
trypsin, crystallized
tryptophan malabsorption
TSH (thyroid-stimulating hormone)
TSH immunoassay test
TSH-01 transdermal tape
TSH receptor stimulation
TSH secretion
TSH suppression
TSRH (Texas Scottish Rite Hospital) hook
TSRH (Texas Scottish Rite Hospital) rod
TSS (toxic shock syndrome)
T-tack gastropexy
TTC (T-tube cholangiogram)
TTS (through-the-scope) catheter
TUBA (transumbilical breast augmentation)
tube (see also *stent; tubing*)
  Abbott-Miller
  Abbott-Rawson double-lumen
  Activent antimicrobial ventilation myringotomy
  Adson brain suction
  Adson suction
  Andrews Pynchon suction
  angled 24F pleural
  angled pleural
  Argyle chest
  Argyle-Salem sump
  Argyle Sentinel Seal chest
  ascites drainage
  Atkinson silicone rubber
  Axiom double sump
  baby Poole suction

tube *(cont.)*
  baby Yankauer suction
  Baker decompression
  Baker intestinal decompression
  Baker jejunostomy
  Baron suction
  Baylor sump
  bent inner
  bilateral pleural
  Biosystems feeding
  Bivona TTS (tight-to-shaft) tracheostomy
  Blakemore
  Blakemore-Sengstaken
  blocked shunt
  blue line Murphy tracheal
  Boyce modification of Sengstaken-Blakemore
  brain suction
  Brochman suction
  Broncho-Cath endobronchial
  Broncho-Cath endotracheal
  Buie rectal suction
  Buie suction
  calibration
  Caluso PEG (percutaneous endoscopic gastrostomy) tube
  Cantor
  Cattell gallbladder
  Celestin esophageal
  Celestin intraluminal
  Celestin latex rubber
  cement
  chest
  Ciaglia Blue Rhino
  Cole
  colonic
  Combitube
  cone suction
  Cooley graft suction
  Cooley intracardiac suction
  Corflo-Ultra jejunostomy
  Corpak feeding
  Cottle suction

tube *(cont.)*
crystal tracheostomy
cuffed endotracheal
cuffed fenestrated
Dawson-Yuhl suction
decompression
Dennis intestinal
dePezer gastrostomy
diathermy suction
directional endotracheal
Dobbhoff gastrectomy feeding
double-lumen
double-lumen endobronchial
drainage
Dreiling
Dumon-Gilliard prosthesis pushing
Edlich gastric lavage
EMT emergency medicine
endoesophageal
endotracheal
Endotrol tracheal
EntriStar PEG (percutaneous endoscopic gastrostomy)
esophageal
Ewald
Ewald evacuator
Ewald gastric lavage
Fazier modified suction
feeding
feeding gastrostomy
FELL suction
fenestrated
fenestrated tracheostomy
Ferguson brain suction
Ferguson-Frazier suction
Fergusson suction
fil d'Arion silicone
filler
Flexiflo Stomate low-profile gastrostomy
Foley catheter gastrostomy
four-lumen
Frazier Britetrac suction
Frazier-Paparella suction

tube *(cont.)*
front lifting hood rectoscope
gastric aspiration
gastric calibration
gastric lavage
gastrointestinal
gastrostomy
germination
Glasser gastrostomy
Gomco suction
Gott
grafting suction
Guibor Silastic
guide
Guilford-Wright suction
Haldane-Priestley
Hardy suction
Harris
Hemo-Drain wound
Hi-Lo Evac endotracheal
Hi-Lo Jet tracheal
Hi-Lo tracheal
Hodge intestinal decompression
Holinger open-end aspirating
Hollister gastrostomy
Holter
House suction-irrigation
Immergut suction coagulation
insulated outer
intermediate Hi-Lo tracheal
Inverta-PEG
J
Jackson laryngectomy
Jackson Open-End aspirating
Jackson trachea
Jackson Velvet eye aspirating
Jako laryngeal suction
jejunal feeding
jejunostomy
Jergesen
Jesberg aspirating
J-shaped
Kahn-Frazier suction
Kam Vac suction

tube *(cont.)*
Kaslow intestinal
Keofeed feeding
Killian suction
K-Tube
Lanz low-pressure cuff endotracheal
large-bore gastric lavage
large-caliber
laryngoflex laryngectomy
laser laryngeal suction
Laser-Flex tracheal
Lepley-Ernst
Levin
Lewis laryngeal
LGT laryngectomy
ligament sizing
Lindholm tracheal
Linton-Nachlas
Lo-Contour
Lo-Pro tracheal
long intestinal
Magill insulated suction
Malecot gastrostomy
Malis
Mallinckrodt Laser-Flex tube
Mallinckrodt Medical tracheal
Mark IV
Martin laryngectomy
Mason suction
maxillofacial
McCulloch suction
Medi-Vac bulk tubing
Medoc-Celestin pulsion
mercury-weighted
metal-weighted Silastic feeding
MIC gastroenteric
MIC jejunostomy
MIC-Key G gastrostomy
MIC-Key J gastrostomy
MIC-TJ (transgastric jejunal)
micro irrigation suction
Micron bobbin ventilation
Mik (Mikulicz) gastrostomy
Miller-Abbott

tube *(cont.)*
Miller-Abbott intestinal
Miller-Abbott long gastrointestinal
Minnesota
modified Minnesota
Molteno seton
Montgomery Safe-T-Tube
Mosher life-saving
Moss G-tube PEG kit
Moss gastrostomy
Moss nasal
Moss Suction Buster
Mousseaux-Barbin intraluminal
Mousseaux-Barbin prosthetic
mushroom gastrostomy
Nasal RAE uncuffed
nasobiliary
nasobiliary drainage
nasoduodenal feeding
nasogastric (NG) feeding
nasojejunal (NJ) feeding
nasopancreatic drainage
nasotracheal
Neo tracheal
neural
New York Glass suction
NEW Speaking Tube
Newvicon vacuum chamber pickup
NG (nasogastric) feeding
Nuport PEG
Nyhus-Nelson gastric decompression and jejunal feeding
obstructed shunt
Olympus One-Step Button gastrostomy
oral gastric (OGT)
oral gastric calibration
Oral RAE uncuffed
oroendotracheal
orogastric
Ossoff-Karlan microlaryngeal suction
ostiomeatal stent
Pacifico-type suction

tube *(cont.)*
Paul-Mixter
Pedi PEG
pediatric feeding
pediatric nasogastric
pediatric Y
PEG (percutaneous endoscopic gastrostomy)
percutaneous gastrostomy
percutaneous jejunostomy
Pitt talking tracheostomy
Plester suction
Pleur-evac suction
pleural
polyethylene
Poole
Poole abdominal suction
Precut intermediate Hi-Lo tracheal
pressure-sensitive valve in shunt
Pribham suction
Procter-Livingston
PTCS
Pynchon suction
Quinton
Radius enteral feeding
RAE endotracheal
rectal
Rehfuss
reinforced trachea
Replogle
Reuter bobbin
Rhoton-Merz suction
right-angle chest
Ring–McLean sump
Robert Shaw bronchus
Rosen suction
rubber
Rubin-Quinton small bowel biopsy
Ruschelit PVC tracheostomy
Ryle
Sachs brain suction
Sacks-Vine feeding gastrostomy
Sacks-Vine PEG (percutaneous endoscopic gastrostomy)

tube *(cont.)*
Salem duodenal sump
Sandoz suction/feeding
Sarns intracardiac suction
Saticon vacuum chamber pickup
S-B (Sengstaken-Blakemore)
Schwann cell
Scott nasal suction
Sengstaken-Blakemore (S-B)
Shah permanent
Shiley tracheal
Shiley tracheotomy
Shiner
shunt
Silastic
Simpson-Smith rectal suction
single-cannula tracheal
small bowel
Souttar
Spachmann
spring-loaded, retractable blunt inner protective
Stamm
standard with flex
stomach
straight chest
suction
Suh ventilation
sump nasogastric
Super PEG
T
tampon
Teflon
Thora-Klex chest
thumb-control suction
Tinckler rectal suction
tracheostomy
transendoscopic
transhepatic
transpyloric
triple-lumen Sengstaken-Blakemore
Tru-Arc
T-shaped silicone shunt
U

tube *(cont.)*
  uncuffed Magill endo
  Vacutainer
  Value-Line Poole abdominal suction
  Versatome laser fiber
  Vidicon vacuum chamber pickup
  Vivonex Moss
  V. Mueller-Poole suction
  Wagener-Mosher
  Walton-Poole suction
  Walton-Yankauer suction
  Wangensteen suction
  water-seal chest
  Wilson-Cook
  Wookey skin
  Wurbs-type nasobiliary
  Yankauer suction
  Yasargil suction
tube anode
tube cecostomy
tube check
tube clip
tube decompression
tube drainage
tube duodenostomy with feeding jejunostomy
tube enteroscope
tube-fed patient
tube feeding
tube flap graft
tube graft (see *graft*)
tube guide
tube-occluding clamp
tubercle of Zuckerkandl
tubercle, pubic
tuberculosis lesion
tuberculosis, peritoneal
tuberculous Addison disease
tuberculous colitis
tuberculous peritonitis
tube thoracostomy
Tubex gauze dressing
Tubigrip bandage
Tubigrip dressing
Tubigrip glove
tubing (see also *tube*)
  CO_2
  corrugated
  HI VAC
  irrigation
  Lamis
  Lamis Y
  large-bore Tygon
  Lysonics handle
  Medi-Vac bulk
  mentor
  nonconducting
  Orthotec handpiece and
  Pennsylvania Hospital
  PSI-TEC
  Tygon venovenous bypass
  Universal female DISS
tubing clamp
tubing connector
Tubinger gastric reconstruction
tubing forceps
tubocurarine chloride
tubogram
tubo-ovarian abscess
tubular adenocarcinoma
tubular adenoma
tubular cancer
tubular carcinoma
tubular elastic bandage
tubular esophagus
tubular lesion
tubular narrowing
tubular necrosis, acute
tubular plate
tubular polyp
tubular punch
tubular stockinette bandage
tubular vertical gastroplasty
tubulovillous adenoma
tubulovillous polyp
tubus digestorius
Tucker spindle-shaped dilator
Tucks Pads

Tudor-Edwards bone-cutting forceps
Tuffier abdominal retractor
Tuffier abdominal spatula
Tuffier laminectomy retractor
Tuffier-Raney retractor
Tuffier rib spreader
tuft, vascular
tuftsin and properdin (opsins)
tulip probe
TULIP (transurethral laser-induced prostatectomy device)
tumbler graft
tumbling obstruction
tumescent liposuction technique
tumescent technique of breast reduction
tummy tuck flap
tumor (see also *neoplasm*)
 Abrikosov
 adrenal
 AML (angiomyolipoma) solid renal
 ampullary
 anaplastic
 aneuploid
 Askin
 benign
 benign bile duct
 benign epidermal
 benign liver
 benign primary
 benign vascular (of the liver)
 beta cell (of the pancreas)
 bifurcation
 bladder
 bone
 breast
 Brenner
 brown
 bulky
 carcinoid
 CNS (central nervous system)
 colon
 cortisol secreting
 cutaneous
 D-cell

tumor *(cont.)*
 desmoid
 discrete
 ectopic cortisol-producing
 embryonal
 endocardial
 endocrine (of the pancreas)
 esophageal
 estrogen-receptor-negative (ER–)
 estrogen-receptor-positive (ER+)
 Ewing
 excision of primary
 extraluminal retrorectal
 extraparathyroid
 feminizing (of the adrenal cortex)
 fibrous
 focal
 functioning adrenocortical
 gastrin-producing
 gastrin-secreting non-beta islet cell
 gastrointestinal
 giant cell
 globular
 glucagon-producing
 glucagon-secreting
 grading
 granular cell
 granulosa cell
 gray
 GRFoma pancreatic endocrine
 gritty
 gross
 gynecologic
 highly vascular
 Hürthle (Huerthle) cell
 ileal primary
 insulin-producing
 insulin-secreting
 intracranial
 invasive
 invasive ductal
 invasive lobular
 islet cell
 kidney

tumor *(cont.)*
- Klatskin
- Krukenberg
- liposarcoma
- liver
- lobulated
- locally invasive
- lung
- lymphangiosarcoma
- lymphoid
- main
- malignant
- malignant mesenchymal
- malignant teratoma
- medullary
- MENIN
- metastatic
- mixed cell
- multifocal
- multiloculated
- myxomatous
- necrotic
- nodal
- nonadrenal
- nonislet cell
- oropharyngeal
- ovarian
- pancreatic
- pancreatic glucagonoma
- pancreatic islet cell
- pancreatic non-beta islet cell
- paraffin
- parathyroid
- periampullary
- pituitary
- polypoidal
- Pott
- presacral
- primary benign liver
- progesterone-receptor negative (PR–)
- progesterone-receptor positive (PR+)
- reddish
- retinal

tumor *(cont.)*
- sacrococcygeal
- salivary gland
- scirrhous
- small cell
- solitary
- splenic
- sporadic
- submucosal
- subserosal
- testicular
- thymic
- thyroid
- urinary
- uterine
- vascular cutaneous and hepatic
- virilizing adrenal
- Warthin (adenolymphoma)
- well-differentiated
- Wharton (cystadenoma)
- white
- Wilms

tumor ablation
tumoral calcinosis
tumor amplified protein expression therapy (TAPET)
tumor debulking
tumor embolization
tumor embolus
tumor encroachment
tumor extension
tumor-free margin of normal tissue
tumor-grasping forceps
tumoricidal solution
tumor implantation at site of specimen extraction
tumor implantation at trocar site
tumor invasion
tumor involvement
tumor localization
tumor lysis syndrome
tumor marker
- CA1-18
- CA 15-3 RIA (radioimmunoassay) serum

tumor marker *(cont.)*
  CA 19-9
  CA 72-4 cancer antigen serum
  CA 72–4 gastric cancer antigen
  CEA
  chromosome 14q
  CYFRA 21-1
  pancreatic
  sigmaS serum
tumor mass
tumor necrosis factor (TNF)
tumor necrosis factor-alpha (TNF-alpha)
tumor necrosis factor-binding protein I and II
tumor necrosis therapy (TNT)
tumorous hepatic vein invasion
tumor pseudocapsule
tumor-reductive surgery
tumor registry
tumor resection
tumor progesterone receptor
tumor suppressor gene
  APC
  DCC
  DPC4
  MTS1
  p53
  Rb
  VHL
tumor virus
Tums
tunable dye laser lithotripsy
tungsten carbide (TC) insert
tunica propria
tuning fork
tunnel
  carpal
  retrogastric-retrocolic
  retropancreatic
  subcutaneous
  subcutaneous catheter
  submucosal
  tarsal
  Witzel feeding jejunostomy
tunnel drill guide
tunneler
tunnel infection
tunnel retrogastric
tunnel view
Tuohy-Borst introducer
Tuohy-Borst valve
Tuohy Decade
Tuohy epidural needle
Tuohy lumbar puncture needle
Tuohy needle
Tuohy Perifix
Tuohy point needle
Tuohy thin-wall needle
Tupman plate
turbid bile
turbid peritoneal fluid
Turcot syndrome
turgor, poor tissue
Turnbull multiple ostomy
Turner biopsy needle
Turner pin
Turner sign
Turner syndrome
Turner Warwick diathermy scalpel handle
Turner Warwick diathermy scissors
Turner Warwick forceps
TURP (transurethral resection of prostate)
Turrell biopsy forceps
Turrell-Wittner rectal forceps
Tutofix cortical pin
Tutoplast process
Tuttle proctoscope
Tuttle thoracic forceps
tweezers, LaserTweezers 100 (LT100)
twin-blade oscillating saw
twin stomach clamps
Twin-Tip marker
Twinrix (hepatitis A inactivated and hepatitis B [recombinant] vaccine)
Twisk needle holder
Twisk forceps
Twisk scissors

twist drill
twist drill catheter
twist hook
twisted plate
twisted suture
twister, Rubio-TC wire
twisting of the colon on itself about its mesentery
TwoCal HN enteral nutritional therapy
two-channel duodenoscope
two-channel endoscope
two-hole (2-hole) plate
two-inch gauze bandage
two-layer anastomosis
two-layer closure
two-layer latex and Marlex closure technique
two-loop J-shaped ileal pouch
two-lumen catheterization
two-lumen papillotome
two-piece ostomy pouch
two-plane view
two-prong rake retractor
two-quadrant hemorrhoidectomy
two-stage triolein test
two-staged operation
two-strand suture
two-thirds rule
two-tube cuff
two-valved anoscope
two-way laparoscopic port
Tycos aneroid sphygmomanometer
Tycron suture (also Ti-Cron)
Tydings tonsil seizing/snare
Tygon venovenous bypass tubing
tying forceps
Tylenol No. 3 (or #3)
Tyler-Gigli saw
tympanites
tympanitic abdomen
tympanitic dullness
tympany, abdominal
type A, B, or C lesion
type A gastritis
type and cross blood
type and crossmatch
type B chronic gastritis
type B gastritis
type I hepatorenal syndrome
type I hiatal hernia
type 1 plasminogen activator inhibitor (PAI-1)
type II hepatorenal syndrome
type II hiatal hernia
typhlitis (appendicitis)
typhloenteritis
typhlomegaly
typhlonous debris
typhlorrhaphy
typhlostenosis
typhlostomy
typhoidal cholangiolitis
typhoidal cholecystitis
Typhoon microdebrider blade
typing and crossmatching of blood
typing system (see *classification*)
Tyrell hook
Tyrex-2 enteral nutritional therapy
tyropanoate contrast medium
tyropanoate sodium
tyrosine
tyrosinemia, hereditary
tyrosyluria
Tyson test
T–Y stent
Tzanck smear

U, u

UA (urinalysis)
UBT (urea breath test) for *Helicobacter pylori* (*H. pylori*)
UC (ulcerative colitis)
UCB (unconjugated hyperbilirubinemia)
UCLA pouch
UCP compression plate
UD-BMT (unrelated donor, bone marrow transplantation)
UDCA (ursodeoxycholic acid)
U double-barrel suture
Udranszky test
U-drape
U echovirus
UES (upper esophageal sphincter)
Uffelmann test
UFT (uracil plus tegafur)
UGI (upper gastrointestinal) tract
UGI (upper gastrointestinal) with small bowel follow-through
UGI (upper gastrointestinal) bleeding
UGI contrast study
UICC TNM staging classification
Ultrasil material

ulcer (see also *ulceration*)
  acid peptic
  active duodenal
  acute peptic
  amebic
  anastomotic
  anterior wall antral
  antral
  aphthoid
  aphthous
  atheromatous
  atrophic-hyperplastic
  Barrett
  bear claw
  benign
  benign gastric
  buccal
  bulbar peptic
  cervical
  chiclero
  chronic
  chronic peptic
  collar button-like
  corneal
  craterlike (with jagged edges)

ulcer *(cont.)*
- Cruveilhier
- Curling
- Cushing
- cutaneous
- decubitus
- Dieulafoy
- duodenal
- flask-shaped
- focal colonic mucosal
- gastric
- gastrocolic
- gastroduodenal
- gastrointestinal
- gastrojejunal
- genital
- giant peptic
- GI tract
- granulomatous
- greater curvature
- healing
- heel
- herpes
- Hunner
- hypertensive ischemic
- incised
- indolent
- indolent radiation-induced rectal
- intestinal
- intractable
- intractable leg
- ischemic skin
- jejunal
- juxtapyloric
- kissing
- Kocher dilatation
- LE arterial insufficiency
- lesser curvature
- linear
- malignant
- marginal
- Marjolin
- Martorell hypertensive
- minute bleeding mucosal

ulcer *(cont.)*
- mucosal
- oral
- painless indurated
- penetrating
- penetrating atherosclerotic aortic
- peptic
- perforated
- perforated acid peptic
- perforating
- postbulbar duodenal
- posterior perforated duodenal
- postpyloric
- postsurgical recurrent
- prepyloric
- prepyloric gastric
- punched-out
- punctate
- puncture
- pyloric channel
- rake
- recurrent
- recurring
- rodent
- Rokitansky-Cushing
- rose thorn
- round
- sea anemone
- secondary jejunal
- serpiginous
- shallow mucosal
- stasis
- stercoral
- stomal
- stress
- subcutaneous
- surgical
- toe
- urinary
- varicose
- venereal
- venous stasis
- V-shaped

ulcerated lesion

ulcerating adenocarcinoma
ulceration (see also *ulcer*)
  anastomotic
  collar-button
  duodenal
  esophageal
  frank
  gastric
  gastrointestinal
  necrotic
  patchy colonic
  radiation-induced
  serpiginous
  stress
ulcerative colitis (UC)
ulcerative dermatosis
ulcerative enteritis
ulcerative enterocolitis
ulcerative esophagitis
ulcerative gastritis
ulcerative ileocolitis
ulcerative inflammation
ulcerative lymphoma
ulcerative proctitis
ulcerative stomatitis
ulcer base
ulcer bed
ulcer crater
ulcerlike dyspepsia
ulcer of the nipple
ulcer perforation
ulcer-prone personality
ulcer refractory to medical management
ulcer with heaped-up edges
Uldall (not Udall) subclavian hemodialysis catheter
Ulrich bone-holding clamp
Ulrich bone-holding forceps
Ulrich-St. Gallen forceps
Ultec hydrocolloid dressing
Ultima spatula
Ultimax distal femoral intramedullary rod system
ultimobranchial pouch
ultimobronchial body
UltrAblator
Ultracal enteral nutritional therapy
Ultracision Harmonic Scalpel
Ultracision ultrasonic knife
UltraClean electrosurgical blade
Ultracot sponge
Ultra 8 balloon catheter
ultrafast CT
ultrafast electron beam tomography
Ultrafera wound dressing
ultrafiltration, continuous arteriovenous (CAVU)
UltraFine erbium laser
UltraFix MicroMite suture anchor
Ultraflex stent
Ultraject prefilled syringe
UltraKlenz wound cleanser dressing
ultra-rapid pharyngeal phase of swallowing
Ultralase MT 20 digestive enzymes
UltraLite flow-directed microcatheter
Ultramark 4 ultrasound
UltraPulse CO_2 laser
Ultra Robertazzi nasopharyngeal airways
Ultrashear electrocautery
ultrasonic dissector
ultrasonic lithotripsy
ultrasonic probe
ultrasonic surgical aspirator
ultrasonographer
ultrasonography, ultrasound (see also *imaging*)
  abdominal
  Acuson Aspen ultrasound system
  Aloka 650 ultrasound system
  Aspen ultrasound system
  ATL UM 9 HDI Colorflow ultrasound system
  Atlas 2.0 diagnostic ultrasound system
  AU5 Harmonic ultrasound system
  AutoSonix system

ultrasonography *(cont.)*
Bak-Pac portable
Bisound AP 3000 Colorflow ultrasound system
B-mode
Bruel & Kjaer 3535 ultrasound system
endoanal
endoscopic
endoscopic (EUS) Doppler
GE RT 3200 ADV II ultrasound system
graded compression
gray-scale
HDI 3000
Hewlett-Packard ultrasound system
HIFU (high-intensity focused)
high-intensity focused (HIFU)
high-resolution
intraoperative
intrarectal
laparoscopic contact (LCU)
laparoscopic intracorporeal (LICU)
laparoscopic ultrasound system (LUS)
Mammotome ultrasound system
Perception 5000 PC-based ultrasound scanner
PowerVision
pulsed
real-time
sagittal
Sequoia ultrasound system
Site ~ Rite 3
SonoCT Real-Time Compound Imaging
Sonopsy 3-D
SonoSite 180 handheld
Synergy system
Technos
thyroid
Toshiba 270 ultrasound system
Toshiba EccoCee ultrasound system

ultrasonography *(cont.)*
transabdominal
transrectal
transperineal
ultrasonography-guided fine-needle aspiration biopsy
UltraSorb reinforcement
ultrasound (see *ultrasonography*)
ultrasound biopsy needle
ultrasound diagnosis
ultrasound disruption of stone
ultrasound guidance
ultrasound-guided anterior subcostal liver biopsy
ultrasound-guided echo biopsy
ultrasound-guided needle biopsy
ultrasound-guided stereotactic biopsy
ultrasound probe, Versadopp 10 Doppler
ultrasound scan
ultrathin section
ultraviolet phototherapy
ultraviolet radiation
ultravirus
Ultrex hydrogel wound dressing
Ultzmann test
U Luque vertebral rod
umbilectomy
umbilical artery (UAC) catheter
umbilical cord scissors
umbilical fissure
umbilical fossa
umbilical hernia
umbilical hernia rupture
umbilical ligament
umbilical region
umbilical ring
umbilical ring closure, delayed
umbilical scissors
umbilical tape
umbilical tape suture
umbilical trocar
umbilical vein
umbilication

umbilicus
  everted
  inverted
  Richet fascia
UMI needle
unattended death
unbanded gastroplasty
uncinate process of pancreas
uncompensated acidosis
uncomplicated acute cholecystitis
unconjugated bilirubin
unconjugated hyperbilirubinemia
uncuffed Magill endotracheal tube
uncuffed tube
underlying hematologic disorder
underlying motor neuron disease
underlying structure
undermine
undermining of muscle
undermining of skin edges
undermining of tissue
undernourished
undernutrition
underperfusion
Undies (trademark)
undifferentiated adenocarcinoma
undifferentiated adenoma
undifferentiated carcinoma
undifferentiated carcinoma of thyroid gland
undifferentiated cell
undifferentiated pattern
undifferentiated squamous cell carcinoma
undigested food in stool
undigested lactose
undyed braided polyglycolic acid suture
undyed suture
undyed Vicryl suture
unenhanced scan
unexplained abdominal pain
unexplained diarrhea
unformed stool
unguided bougie
unguided sound
Unica CO_2 laser
unicellular organism
Uniflex intramedullary nail
Uniflex polyurethane adhesive surgical dressing
uniform uptake throughout
Uni-Gold test for *H. pylori*
Unigraft bone graft material
Unilab Surgibone graft
unilateral adrenalectomy
unilateral anesthesia
unilateral breath sounds
unilateral groin dissection
unilateral hernia
unilateral hyperplasia
unilateral injury
unilateral pleural effusion
unilateral renal parenchymal disease
Unilax (phenolphthalein; docusate sodium)
unilobar location
unilobular cirrhosis
Unimar J-Needle
Uni-Matic infiltration syringe
uninodular goiter
uniplane
Uniqcot sponge
UNI-SHUNT hydrocephalus shunt
Uni-Site breathable transparent dressing
UniSpec disposable anoscope
unit (see *device*)
United Bongort Lifestyle pouch
United Max-E drainable pouch
United Network for Organ Sharing (UNOS)
United Ostomy Association (UOA)
United Ostomy irrigation set
United Skin Barrier XL Soft-Guard
United States Public Health Service (USPHS)
United States Surgical Corporation (USSC) devices (see *USSC*)
United Surgical Bongort Lifestyle pouch

United Surgical Convex Insert
United Surgical Featherlite ileostomy pouch
United Surgical Hypalon faceplate
United Surgical Seal Tite Gasket
United Surgical Shear Plus drainable pouch
United Surgical Soft and Secure pouch
United XL 14 Skin Barrier
Unithroid (levothyroxine sodium)
Uni-trac biliary stent
universal colitis
universal critical measurement unit
universal donor cells
Universal female DISS tubing
Universal Plus multi-function laparoscopic handpiece
universal retractor
universal ulcerative colitis
University of Minnesota retractor
University of Wisconsin (UW) solution for donor organ preservation
unmitigated
Unna boot
Unna-Flex (compressive Unna boot) dressing
Unna-Pak compression dressing and wrap
unopposed PTH secretion
UNOS (United Network for Organ Sharing)
UNOS Liver and Intestinal Organ Transplantation Committee
unrelenting diarrhea
unrelenting pain
unrelenting right upper quadrant pain or tenderness
unrelieved pain
unremitting pain
unresectable malignancy
unresolving pancreatitis
unroofing of cyst
unsaturated blood
unstable lesion
unstable patient
unsuspected cause of death
Untied Skin Prep for ostomy skin
UOA (United Ostomy Association)
UOS tonic pressure
up-biting biopsy cup forceps
up-biting cup forceps
up-biting rongeur
upper endoscopy
upper esophageal sphincter (UES)
upper gastrointestinal (UGI)
upper gastrointestinal bleeding (UGIB)
upper gastrointestinal endoscopy
upper gastrointestinal tract
upper GI atresia
upper GI bleed
upper GI endoscopy
upper GI with small bowel follow-through
upper-hand retractor
Upper Hands self-retaining retractor used in liver transplantation
upper inner quadrant
upper motor neuron lesion
upper outer quadrant
upper panendoscopy
upper respiratory infection (URI) infection
upper respiratory tract infection (URTI)
UPPP (uvulopalatopharyngoplasty)
upright abdominal film
upright chest x-ray
upright film
upright view
upset stomach
upside-down stomach
uracil plus tegafur (UFT)
Urban operation
urea breath test (UBT)
urea, hepatic
Ureaplasma urealyticum
urease breath test
urease-producing organism
Ureflex catheter

uremia
Uresil laparoscopic cholangiography catheter
ureteral or ureteric orifice
ureteral reimplantation
ureteric stone
ureteroileocutaneous anastomosis
ureteroileostomy, Bricker
ureteroscope, flexible
urethral injury
urethral meatus
urethral orifice
urethral papilla
urethropexy, Schwartz-Pregenzer
urethrovaginal fistula
URF-P2 choledochoscope
urgent splenectomy
urge to defecate
uric acid level
uridine diphosphate glucuronosyltransferase deficiency
urinalysis (UA)
urinary aldosterone
urinary amylase
urinary calcium excretion
urinary electrolytes
urinary free cortisol
urinary metanephrine
urinary mucosa
urinary potassium
urinary 17-hydroxycorticosteroid
urinary stone
urinary 3-methylhistidine
urinary tract infection (UTI)
urinary tumor
urinary ulcer
urinary VMA
urine 5-HIAA
urine bilirubin
urine cortisol
URINELISA for *Helicobacter pylori*
urine output variations
urine potassium
urine smear
urine urobilinogen
urine vanillylmandelic acid and catecholamine excretion
urine-free cortisol
UriSite microalbumin/creatinine urine test
Uri-Test
urobilinogen
  fecal
  urine
UroCoil self-expanding stent
UROD (uroporphyrinogen decarboxylase)
urogenital region
Urografin 290 contrast medium
Urolase fiber laser
UroLume stent
UroMax II catheter
urosepsis
urp (to retch; vomit)
urpiness
urpy
Urschel first rib rongeur
Urso (ursodiol)
ursodeoxycholic acid
ursodiol
urticaria pigmentosa with systemic mastocytosis
USA pattern chisel
USA pattern gouge
USA retractor
U.S. Army bone chisel
U.S. Army gouge
U.S. Army pattern bone chisel
U.S. Army retractor
USCI cannula
U.S. Food and Drug Administration (FDA)
U-shaped incision
U-shaped retractor
U-sheet
U.S. retractor
U.S. Surgical GIA-30 stapler
Uslenghi plate

USSC (United States Surgical Corporation) devices, including:
ABBI system
CEEA stapler (21, 25, 28, 31)
Endo Babcock clamp
Endo Catch
Endo Close Stapler
Endo Cinch stapler
Endo Dissect
Endo GIA 60 stapler
Endo GIA II stapler
Endo Grasp
Endo Lung
Endo Stitch
Endo Suture
Ento Retract
Endo Universal
MiniSite laparoscope system
Multifire Endo Hernia
Premium CEEA stapler
Premium Plus CEEA stapler
Protack
Purstring (no *e*) device
Surgiview multiple-use disposable laparoscope
USSC *(cont.)*
USSC suture
VCS clip applier
Versaport trocar
USS-Trex Universal advanced radiology technology
uterine cannulas and forceps
uterine cervix carcinoma
uterine corpus carcinoma
uterine forceps
uterine polyp
uterine tumor
uterovesical pouch
uterus, enlarged
utility and sterilizer forceps
utility shears
U tube
U-tube hepaticoenterostomy
U-tube stent
uveal melanoma
uvulectomy
uvulopalatopharyngoplasty (UPPP)
uvulopharyngoplasty
U wave
UW (University of Wisconsin) solution

V, v

V-A alignment rod
VABES (vasoablative endothelial
  sarcoma)
vaccine (see also *medications*)
  Arilvax yellow fever
  Avicine therapeutic cancer
  Bio-Hep-B
  Campyvax
  Certiva
  COLO-Vax
  Comvax (*Haemophilus* b purified
    capsular polysaccharide;
    Neisseria meningitidis OMPC;
    hepatitis B virus vaccine)
  CTP37
  DISC (disabled infectious
    single cycle)
  edible
  Engerix-B (hepatitis B vaccine
    [recombinant])
  FluMist
  Gastrimmune
  Havrix (hepatitis A vaccine,
    inactivated)
  Helivax
  Hepagene
  Hepagene hepatitis B
  hepatitis A, inactivated

vaccine *(cont.)*
  hepatitis B surface antigen
  hepatitis B virus
    inactivated
    recombinant
  hepatitis C
  HIB polysaccharide vaccine
  ImuLyme
  Infanrix
  LYMErix
  Nabi-Altastaph
  Nabi-HB (hepatitis B immune
    globulin [human])
  Nabi NicVAX
  Nabi-StaphVAX
  Oncophage
  OncoVax-P
  Ostavir
  Quilimmune-M
  Recombivax HB (hepatitis B virus
    vaccine, recombinant)
  rhesus rotavirus-tetravalent vaccine
    (RRV-TV)
  Rotamune
  RotaShield
  RRV-TV (rhesus rotavirus-
    tetravalent)
  theraccine

vaccine *(cont.)*
  Theratope
  Theratope-STn
  Trovax
  Twinrix (hepatitis A inactivated and hepatitis B [recombinant] vaccine)
  Vaqta (hepatitis A, inactivated)
vaccinia virus
V.A.C. Plus pump
Vac-Rite suction canister
VAC smoke evacuation unit
VACTERL (vertebral anomalies; anal atresia; congenital cardiac disease; tracheoesophageal fistula; renal anomalies; radial dysplasia; and other limb defects) syndrome
Vaculance
Vacutainer tube
vacuum manifold
vagal afferent
vagal efferent tonic response
vagal fibers
vagal innervation
vagal input
vagal stimulation
vagal stimulation of stomach
vagal trunk
vagina
vaginal enterocele
vaginal lengthening
vaginal mucosa
vaginal orifice
vaginal pessary
vagotomy
  bilateral
  highly selective
  medical
  parietal cell (PCV)
  proximal gastric (PGV)
  selective proximal (SPV)
  superselective
  surgical
  total bilateral
  truncal
vagotomy and antrectomy
vagotomy and antrectomy with gastro-duodenostomy
vagotomy and pyloroplasty
vague gastrointestinal dysfunction
vagus nerve
vagus nerve stimulation (VNS)
Valeo lifting glove
Valin hemilaminectomy retractor
valinemia
vallecula (pl. valleculae)
vallecular dysphagia
vallecular pooling
Valleix probe
Valleylab electrocautery
Valleylab electrocautery interchange-able hook
Valleylab SSE-2 cautery unit
Valleylab trigger instrument
Valpin 50
valproic acid
Valsalva maneuver
valsavagenic COPD
Value-Line Poole abdominal suction tube
value, serum glucose
valve
  anal
  antireflux
  aortic
  Bard-Davol trumpet
  Bauhin
  bicuspid
  blunting of
  bulb and air-flow control
  Cabot trumpet
  competent
  competent ileocecal
  CPAP
  failed nipple
  Heister valve
  Holter
  Houston
  ileocecal
  incompetent

valve *(cont.)*
- Kerckring
- LeVeen
- lipomatous ileocecal
- mitral
- nipple
- popoff
- pig
- porcine heart
- pressure-sensitive
- rectal
- shunt
- spiral
- Spivack
- Stryker trumpet
- tricuspid
- Tuohy-Borst

valve hook
valve of Bauhin
valve of Houston
valve of Kerckring
valve scissors
valvular heart disease
valvular regurgitant lesion
Vamin amino acid solution
VanAlyea antrum trocar and wash tube
Van Andel catheter
Van Bogaert disease
Van Buren catheter guide
Van Buren sequestrum forceps
Van Buren urethral bougie
Van Buren urethral sound
vancomycin-resistant enterococci (VRE)
vancomycin-resistant *Enterococcus faecium* (VREF) infection
van den Bergh test
Van Doren biopsy forceps
Vanguard splinter probe
van Heuven anatomic classification of diabetic retinopathy
van Sonnenberg sump drain
vanillylmandelic acid (VMA)
vanishing lung
Vannas micro scissors
Vansil (oxamniquinel)
vanSonnenberg sump
vanSonnenberg-Wittich catheter
Vantage first aid shears
Vantage Graves vaginal speculum
Vantage iris scissors
Vantage Knowles bandage scissors
Vantage Lister bandage scissors
Vantage Metzenbaum scissors
Vantage needle holder
Vantage operating scissors
Vantage Spencer stitch scissors
Vantage strabismus scissors
Vantex central venous catheter
VaporTrode
vapreotide
Vaqta (hepatitis A vaccine, inactivated)
Varco gallbladder forceps
variable-dose patient-controlled anesthesia
variable in location
variable stiffness endoscope
variable stiffness colonoscope
Vari-angle clip applier
variceal bleeding, gastroesophageal
variceal column
variceal decompression
variceal hemorrhage
variceal sclerosis
variceal sclerotherapy in esophagus
variceal wall
varicella-zoster virus (VZV)
varices (pl. of varix) (also varicosity, varicosities)
- actively bleeding
- alcoholic
- bleeding esophageal
- bleeding esophagogastric
- bleeding from esophageal
- bleeding gastric
- colonic
- downhill esophageal
- esophageal
- esophagogastric

varices *(cont.)*
  fundal
  gastric
  ileal
  isolated gastric
  paraesophageal
  radius of
  rectal
  transesophageal ligation of
varices on varices
varicocele
varicose ulcer
varicose vein
varicosity (pl. varicosities) (see *varices*)
variegated uptake of radioiodine
Vari/Moist wound dressing
varioliform gastritis
varix (see *varices*)
Varney pin
Vas-Cath catheter
Vascoray (iothalamate meglumine; iothalamate sodium)
Vascu-Guard bovine pericardial surgical patch graft
Vascufil suture
vascular anastomosis
vascular anomaly
vascular apron
vascular autoregulation
vascular bruit
vascular bundle
vascular cirrhosis
vascular clamp
vascular collapse
vascular compromise
vascular congestion
vascular cutaneous and hepatic tumor
vascular ectasia
vascular encasement
vascular endothelial cell
vascular endothelium
vascular forceps
vascular goiter
vascular hemangioma
vascular injury
vascularized bed
vascularized fibula graft
vascularized gastric tissue
vascular lesion
vascular load
vascular mediator
vascular pedicle
vascular polyp
vascular proliferation
vascular tape
vascular tuft
vasculature of the thyroid gland
vasculitic lesion
vasculitis
  hepatic capsular
  necrotizing bowel
Vascutek graft
vas deferens
Vaseline gauze
Vaseline gauze dressing
Vaseline petrolatum gauze dressing
vasoablative endothelial sarcoma (VABES)
vasoactive intestinal peptide (VIP)
vasoactive intestinal polypeptide (VIP)
vasoactive peptide
vasoconstriction of the mesenteric vessel
vasoconstriction, splanchnic
vasodilation of skeletal and mesenteric vascular beds
vasomotor instability
vasopermeation enhancement (VE)
vasopressin
vasopressin analog
vasopressin deficiency
vasopressin with nitroglycerin
Vasotrax blood pressure/heart rate sensor
vasovagal episode
vasovagal reflex
vasovagal response
VasoView balloon dissection system

Vater
ampulla of
papilla of
vaterian segment
VATER (vertebral and/or vascular defects; anorectal malformation; transesophageal fistula; radial, ray, or renal anomaly) syndrome
vault
rectal
vaginal
Vayre suturing technique
Vbeam laser
VBG (vertical-banded gastroplasty)
V blade plate
VCARE vaginal-cervical Ahluwalia retractor-elevator
VCS clip adapter
VCS clip applier
VDS (ventral derotating spinal) compression rod
VE (vasopermeation enhancement)
Vector and VectorX large-lumen guiding catheter
vector-borne infection
Vectra VAG (vascular access graft)
vecuronium bromide
vegetarian diet
vegetative lesion
VEGF (vascular endothelial growth factor)
vein (see Table of Veins in Appendix)
Veingard transparent dressing
vein graft
vein of Retzius
vein of Sappey
vein retractor
vein stone
vein stripper
Velban (vinblastine sulfate)
Velogene rapid VRE assay
velopharyngeal closure
Velosulin Human BR (insulin)
Velpeau bandage
Velpeau dressing
vena cava compression
vena cava sampling
Venable plate
Venable-Stuck nail
Venable-Stuck pin
venacavography
Venaflow vascular graft
venereal proctocolitis
venereal ulcer
venereal wart
Veni-Gard I.V. stabilization dressing
venocavography, inferior
venodilation
venogram, hepatic
venography (see *imaging*)
veno-occlusive disease (VOD)
veno-occlusive liver disease
venous blood
venous blood gas
venous catheterization
venous drainage
venous hum
venous oozing
venous patency
venous pattern
venous phase of selective splenic arteriography
venous plexus
venous return
venous sampling for PTH
venous stasis ulcer
venous supply
venous web disease
venovenous bypass
Ventex wound dressing
ventilated patient
ventilation
decreased alveolar
excessive mechanical
mechanical
minute
positive pressure
ventilation-perfusion mismatch

ventilator mode
ventilator settings (mode, tidal volume, ventilator rate, FiO_2, PEEP)
venting aortic Bengash-type needle
vent settings
vent the bowel
Ventra catheter
ventral hernia
ventral herniorrhaphy
ventral pancreas
ventral surface
ventricle of larynx appendix
ventricular cannula
ventricular catheter
ventricular needle
ventricular septal defect
ventriculoatrial (VA) shunt
ventriculojugular (VJ) shunt
ventriculoperitoneal (VP)
ventriculoperitoneal drain
ventriculoperitoneal shunt (VPS)
ventriculostomy drain
ventriculostomy needle
ventriculosubarachnoid (VS) shunt
ventriculovenous shunt
ventrolateral hernia
ventroptosis
Ventureyra ventricular catheter
Verbatim balloon catheter
Verbatim balloon probe
Verbrugge bone clamp
Verbrugge bone-holding forceps
Verbrugge clamp
Verbrugge-Hohmann bone retractor
Verbrugge needle
Veress (*not* Verres) needle
Veress cannula
Veress needle
verge, anal
Veridien clamp
Veripath peripheral guiding catheter
Verluma (nofetumobab)
vermicide
vermicular colic
vermiform appendix
vermiform body
vermifuge
vermilionectomy
Vermox (mebendazole)
Verner-Morrison syndrome
vernier calipers
Vernon-David rectal speculum
VerreScope microlaparoscopic entry
verrucous carcinoma
Versabran
Versadopp 10 Doppler ultrasound probe
VersaLight laser
Versalon dressing
Versaport obturator
Versaport Plus reducer
VersaPort trocar
VersaPulse holmium laser
VersaPulse Select holmium laser
Versatack surgical stapler
VersaTack stapler
Versatome laser
Versatrac lumbar retractor
Versed (midazolam HCl)
vertebral body biopsy
vertebral body plate
vertebral body retractor
vertebral pleural reflection
vertical-banded gastroplasty (VBG)
vertical bipedicle flap technique reduction
vertical incision
vertical mattress suture
vertical midline incision
vertical pedicle technique in breast reduction mammoplasty
vertical reduction mammoplasty
vertical retractor
vertical ring gastroplasty (VRG)
vertical Silastic ring gastroplasty
vertical stapled small gastric pouch
vertical suture
very low-calorie diet (VLCD)
very low-density lipoprotein (VLDL)

Vesely-Street split nail
vesical fistula
vesicle, herpetic
vesicoenteric fistula
vesicoureteral reflux
vesicoureterine pouch
vesicouterine fistula
vesicovaginal fistula
vesicular appendix
vesicular pattern
vesiculocolic perforation
VESS (videoendoscopic swallowing study)
vessel
  aberrant
  abnormal feeding blood
  afferent
  atypical
  blood
  chyliferous
  cremasteric
  deep epigastric
  epigastric
  gastroepiploic
  great
  hemorrhoidal
  hypogastric
  ileocolic
  iliac
  inferior epigastric
  intercostal
  lacteal
  lymph
  mesocolonic
  perforating
  portal
  short gastric (SGV)
  splenic
  spermatic
  telangiectatic
  testicular
  thoracic
  thoracic great
vessel constriction
vessel hook
vessel knife
vessel loop
vessel retractor
vessel-sizing catheter
vessel transection
vessels were clamped, divided, and ligated
vessels were skeletonized
vest-over-pants hernia repair
vestibule of mouth
vestibuloplasty, anterior or posterior
vestigial fold
V-excision
Vezien abdominal scissors
viable omentum
vial decanter
Vianain (ananain; comosain; bromelains)
Viasorb wound dressing
Vibra-Surge ultrasonic instrument
Vibrio cholerae
Vibrio jejuni
Vibrio parahaemolyticus
Vickers needle holder
Vickers ring tip forceps
Vicryl knitted mesh
Vicryl Rapide suture
Vicryl Rapide synthetic absorbable suture
Vicryl suture
Vicryl woven mesh
vide supra (L. "see above")
video-assisted thoracic surgery (VATS)
video barium swallow
video camera
videoendoscope
videoendoscope-assisted microsurgery
videoendoscopic augmentation mammoplasty
videoendoscopic surgical equipment
videoendoscopic swallowing study (VESS)

videofluoroscopic swallowing
  evaluation
VideoHydro laparoscope
video image
videolaparoscopic cardiomyotomy
videolaparoscopy
videolaseroscopy
video optical intubation stylet
videorectoscope
videoresectoscope
videoscope (see *endoscope*)
videoscopic fundoplication
video signal enhancer
videothoracoscopy
Vidicon vacuum chamber pickup tube
Vi-Drape
Vienna nasal speculum
view (see also *position, projection*)
  abdominal
  anterior
  AP (anteroposterior)
  AP supine
  apical
  apical lordotic
  axial sesamoid
  axillary
  baseline
  Beath
  Boehler (Böhler) calcaneal
  Boehler lumbosacral
  Breuerton
  Broden x-ray
  brow-down skull
  brow-up skull
  Bucky
  carpal tunnel
  Carter-Rowe
  cine
  clenched fist
  close-up
  coalition
  cone
  coned-down
  cranial angled

view *(cont.)*
  craniocaudad
  craniocaudal
  cross-table
  CTLV (cross-table lateral view)
  decubitus
  dens (cervical spine)
  dorsiflexion
  dorsoplantar
  Dunlop-Shands
  dynamic stress x-ray
  erect
  FCS (full cervical spine)
  Ferguson
  flexion
  fluoroscopic stress x-ray
  frog-leg
  frog-leg lateral
  frontal
  full length
  Harris
  Harris-Beath axial hindfoot
  hemiaxial
  hepatoclavicular
  hip-to-ankle
  Hobb
  Hughston
  infrapatellar view of knee
  intraoperative
  inversion ankle stress
  Jones
  Judet radius
  Knuttsen bending
  LAO (left anterior oblique)
  lateral
  lateral anterior drawer stress
  lateral bending
  lateral decubitus
  lateral oblique
  lateral tilt stress ankle
  limited
  long axial oblique
  long axis
  long-axis parasternal

view *(cont.)*
lordotic
mediolateral
mediolateral oblique
Merchant
mortise
mucosal
multiplanar fluoroscopic stress
navicular
Neer lateral
Neer transscapular
no-angulation
nonstanding lateral oblique
nonweightbearing
notch
oblique
occipital
odontoid
open-mouth odontoid
orthogonal
outlet
overhead
overhead oblique
PA (posteroanterior)
parasternal long-axis
parasternal short-axis
patellar skyline
plain
planar
plantar axial
plantar flexion
plantar flexion stress
portable
postevacuation
postoperative
preliminary
preoperative
prereduction
prone
prone lateral
Puddu
push-pull ankle stress
push-pull hip
RAO (right anterior oblique)

view *(cont.)*
recumbent
right lateral decubitus
routine magnification
Schüller (Schueller)
serendipity
short-axis
short-axis parasternal
ski-jump
skyline
spot
standing dorsoplantar
standing lateral
standing weightbearing
steep LAO (left anterior oblique)
Stenver
stress
stress Broden
stress eversion
stress inversion
Stryker notch
submental vertex
submentovertex
subxiphoid
sunrise
sunset
supine
supine full
suprasternal notch
swimmer's
tangential
tangential scapular
tomographic
true lateral
tunnel
two-plane
upright
von Rosen
Waters
weightbearing
weightbearing dorsoplantar
West Point
White leg-length
x-ray

Viewing Wand (surgical digitizer), The
Vigilon dressing
Vigilon primary wound dressing sheets
vigorous achalasia
villi (see *villus*)
villin protein
villoglandular adenoma
villoglandular polyp
villous adenoma
villous atrophy
villous carcinoma
villous epithelium
villous papilloma
villous polyp
villus (pl. villi)
  colonic
  duodenal
  finger-like
  gallbladder
  intestinal
  leaflike
  ridged-convoluted
  tongue-shaped
Vim-Silverman liver biopsy technique
Vim-Silverman needle
Vim-Silverman needle biopsy
Vim-Silverman technique for liver biopsy
VIMRxyn (synthetic hypericin)
vinblastine sulfate
Vincent angina
Vincent infection
vincristine sulfate
vindesine sulfate
Vinson syndrome
vinyl chloride
Viokase
violin-string adhesion
Vioxx (rofecoxib)
VIP (vasoactive intestinal peptide)
VIP (vasoactive intestinal polypeptide)
VIPoma (vasoactive intestinal polypeptide tumor)
VIP secretion
viral cholangitis
viral diarrhea
viral enteritis
viral gastritis
viral gastroenteritis
viral hepatitis (VH)
viral infection
viral load
virally encoded RNA polymerase
viral persistence
viral population
viral respiratory infection (VRI)
viral thyroiditis
Virchow gland
Virchow knife
Virchow node
Virchow sentinel node
Virchow skull breaker
Virchow-Troisier node
viremia
Virgo antimitochondrial antibody kit
viridans streptococci
virilization
virilizing adrenal tumor
virilizing tumor of the adrenal cortex
Virilon (methyltestosterone)
virologic response
virtual colonoscopy
virulent diarrhea
virulent organism
Virulizin
virus
  AIDS
  Andes
  anti-HA, anti-HAV (antibody to hepatitis A virus)
  arbovirus (arthropod-borne)
  ARV (AIDS-related)
  avian influenza A (H5N1)
  Bayou (BAY)
  Black Creek Canal
  Colorado tick fever
  cytomegalovirus (CMV)
  delta

virus *(cont.)*
epidemic gastroenteritis
Epstein-Barr (EBV)
fecal-oral route of transmission
gastroenteritis virus type A, type B
HAV (hepatitis A)
HBV (hepatitis B)
HBV (hepatitis B)
HDV (hepatitis D)
hematogenous dissemination of
hepadna (hepatitis B-like DNA)
hepatitis A
hepatitis B (HBV)
hepatitis C (HCV) (formerly non-A, non-B)
hepatitis D
hepatitis E (HEV)
herpes simplex virus (HSV)
herpes zoster virus (HZV)
H5N1
HGV (hepatitis G)
HHV-8 (human herpesvirus-8)
HIV (human immunodeficiency)
HMTV (human mammary tumor)
human herpesvirus 6 (HHV-6)
human mammary tumor (HMTV)
Juquitiba
KSHV (Kaposi sarcoma-associated virus)
Laguna Negra
lymphocytic choriomeningitis (LCMV)
Marburg
MCV (molluscum contagiosum)
mutant
Nipah
nonsyncytium-inducing (NSI) variant of AIDS virus
Norwalk
respiratory syncytial (RSV)
RNA
rotavirus
Rous sarcoma
Sin Nombre (SNV)

virus *(cont.)*
Theradigm-HBV (hepatitis B)
varicella zoster (VZV)
West Nile
wild-type hepatitis
virus-host interaction
virus-like infectious agent (VLIA)
virus-like particle (VLP) of non-A, non-B hepatitis
Visa II PTCA catheter
viscera (see *viscus*)
visceral anesthesia
visceral edema
visceral neuropathy
visceral pain
visceral peritoneum
visceral surface of liver
visceromegaly
visceroptosis
viscid bile
viscous (adj.)
viscous bile
viscous fluid
viscous lidocaine
viscous Xylocaine gargle
viscus (pl. viscera)
abdominal
abdominopelvic
hollow
intra-abdominal
intraperitoneal
perforated
strangulated
Visi-Black surgical needle
visible peristalsis
visibly and palpably normal
Visicath endoscopic instrument
Visick grading system for dysphagia
Visick grading system for postgastrectomy carcinoma recurrence
Visicol (sodium phosphate) bowel prep
Visidex II blood glucose testing strips
Visilex polypropylene mesh
Vision PTCA catheter

Visipaque (iodixanol)
Visistat stapler
Visitec circular knife
Visitec crescent knife
Visitec EdgeAhead knife
Visitec stiletto knife
Vistaflex biliary stent
Vistaril
Vistec x-ray detectable sponge
visualization
  direct
  excellent
  good
  inadequate
  poor
Visulas Nd:YAG laser
VISX excimer laser
VISX Star S2 excimer laser
VitaClip clip applier
Vitacuff dressing
Vital Cooley microvascular needle holder
Vital-Duval forceps
Vital forceps
Vital High Nitrogen enteral nutritional therapy
Vital Ryder microvascular needle holder
Vital stapler
Vitallium Küntscher (Kuentscher) nail
Vitallium plate
Vitallium staple
vitamin, ADEKs
vitamin B_{12} absorption test
vitamin, fat-soluble
vitamin K
vitamin, water-soluble
Vita-PMS Plus
vitelline duct
vitelline fistula
vitellointestinal cyst
vitellointestinal duct
Vitesse Cos laser catheter
Vitesse E-II catheter
Vitex tissue adhesive
VITEX fibrin sealant
vivax malaria
Vivonex elemental powdered feeding
Vivonex HN (high-nitrogen) powdered feeding
Vivonex jejunostomy catheter
Vivonex Moss tube
Vivonex T.E.N.
V-Lax (psyllium hydrophilic mucilloid)
VLCD (very low calorie diet)
VLDL (very low density lipoprotein)
VLDL cholesterol
V+Loop electrode
VLP (virus-like particle)
V-medullary nail
V. Mueller bulldog clamp
V. Mueller laparoscope
V. Mueller-Poole suction tube
V. Mueller rigid laparoscope
V nail plate
VNS (vagus nerve stimulation)
VNUS Restore catheter
VOD (veno-occlusive disease)
Voges-Proskauer test
volar incision
volar plate
Volkmann bone hook
Volkmann curette
Volkmann hook
Volkmann pancreatic calculus spoon
Volkmann rake retractor
Volkmann retractor
Volkmann spoon for pancreatic calculus
volume
  blood
  circulating blood
  colonic balloon
  end-diastolic
  excess fluid
  fluid
  increased tidal
  intravascular
  mean corpuscular (MCV)

volume *(cont.)*
  shrinking liver
  stroke (SV)
  tidal
volume acquisition (MRI)
volume analysis (MRI)
volume displacement transducer
volume rendering of helical CT data
volume replacement
voluming artifact (MRI)
voluntarily stopping eating and drinking (VSED)
voluntary guarding
volvulated Meckel diverticulum
volvulus
  bascule
  cecal
  colonic
  compound
  decompression of
  gastric
  gastric dilatation
  large-bowel
  midgut
  Onchocerca
  recurrent
  sigmoid
  splenic flexure
  transverse colon
  "traveling"
volvulus of splenic flexure
volvulus of transverse colon
Vom Saal pin
vomiting (also emesis)
  bile-stained
  bilious
  bloody
  bright red
  chemotherapy-induced
  coffee-grounds
  concealed
  cyclic
  dry
  epidemic
vomiting *(cont.)*
  episodic
  erotic
  fecal
  feculent
  hysterical
  intractable
  ipecac-induced
  nausea and (N&V)
  nervous
  nonbilious
  periodic
  perioperative
  pernicious
  postoperative
  postprandial
  post-tussive
  profuse
  projectile
  prolonged
  psychogenic
  recurrent bouts of
  self-induced
  stercoraceous
  surreptitious
  vomitus (also emesis)
  winter
vomiting center
vomitus (see *vomiting*)
Von Andel catheter
Von Gierke disease
Von Haberer-Finney anastomosis
Von Haberer gastroenterostomy
von Hippel-Lindau disease
von Jaksch test
von Kupffer test
von Langenbeck periosteal elevator
von Meyenburg complex
Von Petz suturing apparatus
von Recklinghausen disease
von Rokitansky disease
von Rosen view
voodoo death

Vorse-Webster clamp
Vozzle Vacu-Irrigator
VPI ileostomy system
VPI nonadhesive open-end pouch
VPI nonadhesive pouch
VRE (vancomycin-resistant enterococcus)
VRG (vertical ring gastroplasty)
V-scan test kit
VSED (voluntarily stopping eating and drinking)
VSF (Vermont spinal fixator) clamp
VSF (Vermont spinal fixator) rod
V-shaped incision
V-shaped laceration
V-shaped ulcer
VSP (variable screw placement) plate
V-to-Y closure
vulnerary (agent that promotes wound healing)
vulvar lesion
vulvar vestibulitis syndrome
VX-497
Vygon Nutricath S catheter
V-Y plasty

W, w

Wagener-Mosher tube
Wagner acetabular reamer
Wagner closed pin
Wagner retractor
Wagner skin incision
Wagner test
Wainwright plate
Waldenstrom macroglobulinemia
Waldeyer fascia
Waldeyer fossa
Waldmann disease
Waldmann scissors
Walker gallbladder retractor
wall
    abdominal
    anorectal
    anterior abdominal
    axial
    body
    bowel
    carotid
    cavity
    cell
    chest
    entire bowel
    gallbladder
    intra-abdominal
    midabdominal

wall *(cont.)*
    posterior abdominal
    thickened gallbladder
    thoracic
    variceal
wall akinesis
Wallstent
Wallstent biliary endoprosthesis
Wallstent enteral endoprosthesis
Walter-Carmalt splinter forceps
Walter-Liston forceps
Walton biopsy forceps
Walton cartilage clamp
Walton-Liston bone rongeur
Walton meniscus clamp
Walton-Poole suction tube
Walton ribbon retractor
Walton-Ruskin bone rongeur
Walton-Ruskin forceps
Walton scissors
Walton wire-pulling forceps
Walton-Yankauer suction tube
wand
    AccESS
    CLO (Cool Laser Optics)
    CollagENT
    collection
    flexible

wand *(cont.)*
  Hummingbird
  image-guided
  irrigation
  Kaye Lap-Wand
  Lap-Wand with Kittner tip
  laser
  Microblater ArthroWand
  ReFlex
  stereotactic
  surgical
  The Wand
  Viewing Wand
wandering gallbladder
wandering goiter
wandering kidney
wandering liver
wandering spleen
Wangensteen anastomosis clamp
Wangensteen drain
Wangensteen forceps
Wangensteen needle
Wangensteen needle holder
Wangensteen patent ductus clamp
Wangensteen suction
Wangensteen suction tube
Wangensteen tissue forceps
Wangensteen trocar
Wangensteen tube
Ward approximating forceps
Ward needle holder
Ward periosteal elevator
warfarin potassium
warfarin sodium
warm saline solution
Warren splenorenal shunt
wart
  intra-anal
  perianal
  venereal
Warthin (adenolymphoma) tumor
warty papilloma
Was-Cath catheter
washed clot
washing catheter
washing
  bronchial
  gastric
  peritoneal
washings and brushings
Wassmund retractor
wasting, muscle
wasting syndrome
watchful waiting (monitoring tumor growth while deferring treatment)
water-borne gastroenteritis
water-borne infection
water brash
waterfall stomach
Waterfield needle
water-filled pouch
water-gurgle test
Waterhouse-Friderichsen syndrome
water-infusion esophageal manometry catheter
watermelon stomach
Water Pik, endoscopic
water probe
water recovery test
water retention
water-seal chest tube
watershed area
water-sipping test
water-soluble bilirubin
water-soluble contrast enema
water-soluble contrast esophageal swallow
water-soluble vitamins
Waterston's stratification for tracheo-esophageal fistula
Waters view
water swallows
water-trap stomach
watery diarrhea
watery diarrhea syndrome
watery secretion
watery stools
Watson-Alagille syndrome

Watson-Cheyne dissector
Watson-Cheyne probe
Watson-Jones bone gouge
Watson-Jones incision
Watson-Jones nail
Watson knife
Watson-Williams intervertebral disk rongeur
wattage
Waugh-Clagett pancreaticoduodenostomy
Waugh diathermy forceps
Waugh dissecting forceps
wave
  abdominal fluid
  flattened T
  fluid
  gastric slow
  inverted T
  peaked T
  peristaltic
  primary peristaltic
  secondary peristaltic
  tetrahertz
  U
WaveWire guidewire
wax pattern
waxy kidney
waxy liver
WBC (white blood cell) count
  bands
  basos (basophils)
  blasts
  differential
  eos (eosinophils)
  immature forms
  leukocytes
  lymphs (lymphocytes)
  monos (monocytes)
  neutrophils
  polys or PMN (polymorphonuclear leukocytes)
  segs (segmented neutrophils)
  stabs
WBC, elevated
WBCs (white blood cells)
WDE (wound dressing emulsion)
WDHA (watery diarrhea, hypokalemia, achlorhydria) syndrome
weaning, immunosuppressive steroid
Weary cordotomy knife
Weary nerve hook
Weary nerve root retractor
Weaveknit vascular graft
web
  duodenal
  esophageal
  hepatic
  intestinal
  postcricoid
  venous
Webb-Balfour abdominal retractor
Webb-Balfour self-retaining retractor
Weber aortic clamp
Weber-Christian disease
Weber-Christian panniculitis
Weber gland
Weber rectal catheter
Webb nail
Webril bandage
Webril dressing
web space incision
Webster abdominal retractor
Webster meniscectomy scissors
Webster needle
Webster needle holder
Webster-TC needle holder
Weck-Baggish rigid laparoscope
Weck-cel sponge dressing
Weck clamp
Weck clip and applicator
Weck knife
Weck laparotomy pad
Weck microsuture cutting scissors
Weck operating laparoscope
Weck 110405 0° 5 mm rigid laparoscope
Weck 110800 rigid laparoscope

wedge biopsy of liver
wedged hepatic venous pressure
(WHVP)
wedge hepatic biopsy
wedge liver biopsy
wedge resection
weekend drinker
weeping willow appearance
on venogram
Weibel-Palade granule
weightbearing dorsoplantar view
weightbearing view
weighing, underwater
weight gain
weight, ideal body (IBW)
weight loss, significant long-term
weight loss with hyperphagia
weight-reduction operation
weight-relieving calipers
weights, daily
Weil-Blakesley intervertebral disk
rongeur
Weil disease
Weil syndrome
Weinberg modification of pyloroplasty
Weinberg pyloroplasty
Weinberg vagotomy retractor
Weiss amputation saw
Weitlaner-Beckman retractor
Weitlaner retractor
Welch Allyn anoscope
Welch Allyn flexible sigmoidoscope
Welch Allyn KleenSpec sigmoidoscope
Welch Allyn upper GI videoendoscope
Welchol (formerly Cholestagel)
welder's lung
welding of suture
well-circumscribed neoplasm
well-differentiated adenoma
well-differentiated carcinoma
Weller cartilage forceps
Weller cartilage scissors
Wellferon (interferon alfa-n1)
Wells posterior rectopexy
Welt syndrome
Wenger plate
Wermer syndrome
Wernicke encephalopathy
Wernicke-Korsakoff syndrome
Wernicke syndrome
Wertheim clamp
Wertheim-Cullen clamp
Wertheim retractor
Wertheim scissors
Wesolowski vascular graft
Wesselsbron virus
Wesson perineal retractor
West bone chisel
West bone gouge
Westcott cutting biopsy needle
Westcott dissecting scissors
Westerman-Jensen needle
WEST (Weinstein Enhanced Sensory
Test) for diabetic neuropathy
West gouge
West Nile virus
Weston rectal snare
Westphal forceps
Westphal gall duct forceps
Westphal-Strümpell (Struempell) disease
West Point view
West retractor
Westscott scissors
wet colostomy
wet-field cautery
wet lung
wet smear
wet swallow (on esophageal
manometry)
wet-technique reduction mammoplasty
wetting agent
wet-to-dry dressing
Wharton (cystadenoma) tumor
wheat gliadin
Wheeless surgical construction of J
rectal pouch
whiplash technique for repositioning
a catheter

Whipple disease
Whipple pancreatectomy
Whipple pancreaticoduodenectomy
Whipple pancreaticoduodenostomy
Whipple test
Whipple triad
Whipple triad test
whipstitch suture
whipworm
whistle-tip ureteral catheter
Whitacre spinal needle
Whitcomb-Kerrison laminectomy rongeur
white bile
white blood cells (WBCs)
White classification for diabetes mellitus
white cotton umbilical tape
white fatty stool
White leg-length view
white line of Toldt
white lung
white patch
white phenolphthalein
white pulp of spleen
white silk suture
white suture
Whitehead deformity
Whitehead hemorrhoidectomy
Whitman plate
Whitmore bag
WHO (World Health Organization) classification of gastric carcinoma
whole blood
whole transplantation
whorled appearance
WHVP (wedged hepatic venous pressure)
Wiberg periosteal elevator
wide excision
wide glucose excursions
wide-mesh petroleum gauze dressing
wide-mouth sac
wide periosteal elevator
widespread bleeding
width of tumor invasion
Wiedemann-Beckwith syndrome
Wiet cup forceps
Wiet otologic scissors
Wigmore plaster saw
Wikstroem artery forceps
Wiktor GX Hepamed coated
Wiktor Prime
Wiktor stent
Wilberg bone staple
wild daisy
Wilde dressing forceps
Wilde ethmoid forceps
wild-type hepatitis virus
Wilde forceps
Wilde incision
Wilde intervertebral disk rongeur
Wilde rongeur forceps
Wilfred Adams diathermy artery forceps
Wilkinson abdominal retractor
Wilkinson-Deaver retractor
Willauer abdominal scissors
Willauer-Gibbon periosteal elevator
Willauer thoracic scissors
Williams intestinal forceps
Williams overtube sleeve
Williger bone mallet
Williger curette
Williger periosteal elevator
Willis pancreas
Willis pouch
Willy Meyer incision for mastectomy
Wilmer dissecting scissors
Wilmer scissors
Wilms tumor
Wilson bone graft
Wilson-Cook endoprosthesis
Wilson-Cook esophageal balloon dilator
Wilson-Cook forceps
Wilson-Cook French stent
Wilson-Cook mechanical lithotriptor
Wilson-Cook prosthesis introducer

Wilson-Cook snare
Wilson-Cook tube
Wilson-Cook wire-guided sphincterotome
Wilson disease
Wilson gonad retractor
Wilson plate
Wiltse rod
Wiltse-Bankart retractor
Wiltse-Gelpi retractor
Winckler test
wind, passing (flatus)
window
 acoustic
 dilating
 gastric
 gastroesophageal
 jejunal
 mesocolic
 subxiphoid
wing plate
wing suture
WinGel
Wink retractor
Winslow, foramen of
Winslow pancreas
Winston-Acland clamp
Winston clamp
winter gastroenteritis
winter vomiting
winter vomiting disease
wire (also see *guidewire*)
 chisel-tip
 diathermy
 Director biliary guide
 fixation
 Glide Wire
 guidewire
 Hawkins localization
 high torque
 infusion
 J
 loop
 monofilament

wire *(cont.)*
 preoperative placement of needle
 localization
 ProStream infusion
 Sadowsky hook
 Sippy pusher
 snare
 stainless steel
 suture
 Teflon-coated guided
 Thiersch
wire-circling needle
wire-crimping forceps
wire-cutting forceps
wire-cutting pliers
wire-cutting scissors
wire cutter, double-action
wire drill
wire-extracting forceps
wire fixation clamp
wire forceps
wire guide
 HIC
 soft-tipped
wire-guided probe
wire-holding forceps
wire-loop lesion
wire-pass drill
wire-pulling forceps
wire pullout suture
wire saw
wire scissors
wire suture
wire-tightening forceps
wire-twisting forceps
Wirsung, duct of
Wirthlin splenorenal clamp
Wisap laparoscope
Wiscott-Aldrich syndrome
Wise areola mastopexy breast
 augmentation (WAMBA)
Wise pattern for reduction mammoplasty
wishbone retractor

Wissinger rod
Wister vascular clamp
within normal limits (WNL)
without harm (commensally)
Wittner biopsy forceps
Witz test
Witzel duodenostomy
Witzel enterostomy catheter
Witzel feeding jejunostomy tunnel
Witzel gastrostomy
Witzel jejunostomy
Witzel tunnel for feeding jejunostomy
Wizard balloon replacement device
WNL (within normal limits)
Woelfler gland
Woldman test
Wolf 10/5 (L-angle) operative laparoscope
Wolf 170 12 mm rigid laparoscope
Wolf 7732 rigid laparoscope
Wolf 8934.40 rigid laparoscope
Wolf 8937.31 0° 10 mm rigid laparoscope
Wolfe-Boehler mallet
Wolfe full-thickness free graft
Wolfe hand surgery graft
Wolfe-Kawamoto bone graft
Wolff-Junghans test
Wolff telescope
Wolf Lumina rigid laparoscope
Wolfram syndrome
Wolf rigid laparoscope
Wolfson gallbladder retractor
Wolfson intestinal clamp
Wolf trocar
Wolf videoresectoscope
Wolman disease
Wolman xanthomatosis
Wolson gallbladder retractor
Womack procedure
womb stone
Wood lamp
Woodson elevator
Woodward esophagogastrostomy
Woodward hemostat
Wookey skin tube
Workhorse percutaneous transluminal angioplasty balloon catheter
working diagnosis
working in a clockwise direction
World Health Organization (WHO) classification of gastric carcinoma
worm
  roundworm (nematode)
  tapeworm (cestode)
wound
  abraded
  abscess
  aseptic
  avulsed
  ballistic
  blowing
  burn
  clean
  closed
  contaminated
  contused
  craniocerebral penetrating
  crease
  cross-irrigation of
  cutaneous
  depth of
  exit
  gaping
  glancing
  gunshot (GSW)
  gutter
  high-energy gunshot
  high-velocity gunshot
  incised
  lacerated
  nonpenetrating
  open
  parasternal gunshot
  parasternal stab
  penetrating
  perforating
  plantar puncture

wound *(cont.)*
  puncture
  septic
  seton
  stab
  subcutaneous
  sucking
  sucking chest
  tangential
  tetanus-prone
  traumatopneic
wound adhesive
wound approximation
wound care
wound cleanser (see *cleanser*)
wound closure
wound debridement enzymes
wound debriding agent
wound dehiscence
wound drain
wound dressing emulsion (WDE)
Wound-Evac drain
wound healing agent
wound healing, impaired
wound hematoma
wound infection
wound laceration
wound management
wound protector
wound repair
Woun'Dres hydrogel dressing
Wound Stick probe
wound towels
wound was steri-stripped
W pouch, ileal
wrap
  Ace
  bias stockinette
  gastric fundus
  Nissen fundoplication
  surgical
  total gastric
  270-degree (270°)
  360-degree (360°)
wrap-around flap bone graft
wrap-around ghosting artifact
wrench pin
Wright needle holder
Wright plate
Wright stain of stool
Wrigley forceps
W-shaped forceps
W-shaped ileal pouch
W-sitting position
W-stapled urinary reservoir
Wullstein retractor
Wurbs-type nasobiliary tube
Wurd catheter
Wurzburg plate
WuScope endoscope
Wyanoids
Wyanoids Relief Factor (cocoa butter; shark liver oil)
Wylie carotid artery clamp
Wylie hypogastric clamp
Wylie splanchnic retractor

X, x

Xanar 20 Ambulase CO_2 laser
xanthelasma
xanthogranulomatous cholecystitis
xanthography
xanthoma cell
xanthoma
  gastric
  skin
xanthomatosis
  biliary hypercholesterolemia
  cerebrotendinous
  Wolman
xanthomatous biliary cirrhosis
Xcytrin (motexafin gadolinium)
XeCl (xenon-chloride) laser
Xeloda (capecitabine)
Xenical (orlistat) capsules
XenoDerm graft
xenograft
XenoMouse Technology
xenon endoscopic light source
xenon flash endoscopic light source
xenon light source
xenon 127 (^{127}Xe)
xenon 133 (^{133}Xe)
xenotransplant with genetically engineered pig organ
xenotransplantation
Xeroflo dressing
Xeroform dressing
Xeroform gauze
Xeroform gauze dressing
Xillix LIFE-GI fluorescence endoscopy system
Xillix LIFE-Lung GI fluorescence endoscopy system
xiphoid appendix
xiphoid-to-umbilicus incision
XL-11 catheter
X-linked infantile agammaglobulinemia (Bruton-type)
X-linked lymphoproliferative (XLP) syndrome
XLP (X-linked lymphoproliferative) syndrome
XMB tibial reaming guide
XMG (x-ray mammogram)
Xomed drill
Xomed Kartush insulated retractor
Xpeedior catheter
Xplorer 1000 digital x-ray imaging system
Xplorer imaging system
X-Prep (senna extract; alcohol)
X-Prep bowel prep
X-PRESS vascular closure system

XPS Sculpture System
XPS Straightshot
XQ230 Olympus gastroscope
x-ray view
X-shaped micro plate
X-shaped plate
XT coronary stent (radiopaque)
X-trode electrode catheter
X-trode stent
Xylocaine (lidocaine)
Xylo-Pfan (xylose)
xylose absorption test
xylose tolerance test

Y, y

YAG (yttrium-aluminum-garnet) laser
YagLAZR or YagLazr laser
Yale SK poliovirus
Yamada myelotomy knife
Yankauer periosteal elevator
Yankauer punch
Yankauer suction tube
Yasargil arachnoid knife
Yasargil artery forceps
Yasargil bayonet scissors
Yasargil carotid clamp
Yasargil clip-applying forceps
Yasargil elevator
Yasargil hypophyseal forceps
Yasargil knotting forceps
Yasargil ligature guide
Yasargil micro forceps
Yasargil micro rasp
Yasargil micro scissors
Yasargil microvascular knife
Yasargil pituitary rongeur
Yasargil spring hook
Yasargil suction tube
Yasargil tumor forceps
Y bone plate
year, quality-adjusted life (QALY)
yellow atrophy
yellow fever
yellow fever hepatitis
yellow fever virus
yellow jaundice
yellow phenolphthalein
Yeoman biopsy forceps
Yeoman rectal biopsy forceps
Yeoman-Turrell rectal biopsy forceps
Yeoman-Wittner rectal forceps
Yersinia enterocolitica colitis
Yersinia pseudotuberculosis
yersiniasis
YETSS (yuppie executive tight
sphincter syndrome)
Y incision
yolk sac carcinoma
Yorke-Mason incision
Young forceps
Young intestinal forceps
Young-Millin boomerang needle holder
Yours Truly breast prosthesis
yo-yo dieting
yo-yo weight fluctuation phenomenon
Y-shaped graft
Y-shaped incision
Y-shaped microplate
Y-shaped plate

yttrium-aluminum-garnet (YAG) laser
yuppie executive tight sphincter
syndrome (YETSS)
Yu pyloroplasty
Y-V anoplasty
Y-V plasty

Z, z

Zachary Cope-DeMartel clamp
zacopride
Zacutex (lexipafant)
Zadaxin (thymosin alpha-1)
zamifenacin
Zanosar (streptozocin)
Zantac 75 (ranitidine)
Zappacosta test
Zaufel-Jansen bone rongeur
Z clamp
Z-clamp forceps
Zebra exchange guidewire
Zeffix (lamivudine)
Zeiss Endolive endoscope
Zeiss operating microscope
Zeiss OPMI surgical microscope
Zeiss Visulas 690s laser
Zellweger cerebrohepatorenal syndrome
Zelmac (tegaserod)
Zemplar (paricalcitol)
Zenapax (daclizumab)
Zenith AAA (abdominal aortic aneurysm) endovascular graft
Zenker artery forceps
Zenker diverticulum
Zenker fluid
Zenker necrosis
Zenker pouch
Zenker retractor
Zenotech graft
Zephiran Chloride (benzalkonium chloride)
Zeppelin clamp
zero-degree (0°) forward optic laparoscope
ZES (Zollinger-Ellison syndrome)
ZEUS robotic system
Z fixation nail
Zickel intramedullary nail
Zickel rod
Zickel subtrochanteric nail
Zickel supracondylar medullary nail
Ziegler head mirror
Ziehl-Neelsen stain
Zielke gouge
Zielke hook
Zielke rod
Zieve syndrome
zigzag finger incision
zigzag incision
Zika virus
Zimaloy staple
Zimmer caudal hook
Zimmer femoral condyle blade plate
Zimmer gouge
Zimmer hand drill

Zimmer low-viscosity adhesive
Zimmer micro saw
Zimmer oscillating saw
Zimmer pin
Zimmer rigid laparoscope
Zimmer side plate
Zimmer Statak suture/suturing device
Zimmer Y plate
Zimmon papillotome
zinc acetate
Zinca-Pak (zinc sulfate) intravenous nutritional therapy
Zinnanti Z-clamp
Zinn retractor
zipper scar
zipper sphincterotomy
zipper stitch
Zipzoc stocking compression dressing
Zipzoc stocking compression wrap
Zixoryn (flumecinol)
Z line
Z-Med catheter
Zoellner rasp
Zofran ODT (ondansetron)
Zoladex (goserelin acetate)
zoledronic acid
Zollinger classification of groin hernias
Zollinger-Ellison syndrome (ZES)
Zometa (zoledronic acid)
zona (pl. zonae)
zonal gastritis
zonal necrosis
zone
  abdominal
  anal transitional (ATZ)
  arcuate
  barrier
  basement membrane
  bloodless, of necrosis

zone *(cont.)*
  calcification
  cloacogenic
  echo
  entry
  hemorrhoidal
  high-pressure (HPZ)
  marginal, of spleen
  medullary
  mucosal
  "no-trocar"
  pectinate
  portal
  proliferation
  transformation
  vascular
Zone Specific II meniscal repair system
zopolrestat
Zosyn (piperacillin sodium; tazobactam sodium)
Z-plasty incision
Z-plasty local flap graft
Z-Scissors
Z-shaped plate
ZstatFlu test
Z stent for bile duct and esophageal stenosis
Z-stitch suture
Z suture
Zuelzer awl
Zuelzer hook
Zuelzer hook plate
Zuma guiding catheter
Zydone (hydrocodone bitartrate/acetaminophen)
zygomycetous fungus
zymogenic cell
Zyoptix laser
Zyvox (linezolid)

Appendix

Table of Arteries

artery	arteria (pl. arteriae)
Abbott's artery	
abdominal aorta artery	arteria aorta abdominalis
aberrant artery	
aberrant obturator artery	
accessory meningeal artery	arteria meningea accessoria
accessory obturator artery	arteria obturatoria accessoria
accessory pudendal artery	arteria pudenda accessoria
accompanying artery of ischiadic nerve	arteria comitans nervi ischiadici
accompanying artery of median nerve	arteria comitans nervi mediani
acetabular artery	ramus acetabularis arteriae circumflexae femoris medialis
acromial artery	
acromiothoracic artery	
Adamkiewicz, artery of	arteria radicularis magna
adipose arteries of kidney	rami capsulares arteriae renis
adrenal artery, middle	arteria suprarenalis media
afferent artery of glomerulus	vas afferens glomeruli
alar artery of nose	
alveolar artery, inferior	arteria alveolaris inferior
alveolar arteries, superior, anterior	arteriae alveolares superiores anteriores
alveolar artery, superior, posterior	arteria alveolaris superior posterior
anastomotic atrial artery	ramus atrialis anastomoticus arteriae coronariae sinistrae
angular artery	arteria angularis
angular gyrus artery	arteria gyri angularis
anonymous artery	
anterior auricular artery	arteria auricularis anterior
anterior cecal artery	arteria cecalis anterior
anterior cerebellar artery	arteria cerebelli anterior
anterior cerebral artery	arteria cerebri anterior
anterior choroidal artery	arteria choroidea anterior
anterior ciliary artery	arteria ciliaris anterior

artery	arteria (pl. arteriae)
anterior circumflex humeral artery	arteria circumflexa humeri anterior
anterior communicating artery	arteria communicans anterior
anterior conjunctival artery	arteria conjunctivalis anterior
anterior descending artery	
anterior ethmoidal artery	arteria ethmoidalis anterior
anterior humeral circumflex artery	
anterior inferior cerebellar artery	arteria cerebelli inferior anterior
anterior inferior segmental artery of kidney	arteria segmenti anterioris inferioris renis
anterior intercostal arteries	rami intercostales anteriores
anterior interosseous artery	arteria interossea anterior
anterior interventricular artery	ramus interventricularis anterior arteriae coronariae sinistrae
anterior labial arteries	arteriae labiales anteriores
anterior lateral malleolar artery	arteria malleolaris anterior lateralis
anterior medial malleolar artery	arteria malleolaris anterior medialis
anterior mediastinal arteries	rami mediastinales arteriae thoracicae internae
anterior meningeal artery	arteria meningea anterior
anterior parietal artery	arteria parietales anterior
anterior peroneal artery	ramus arteriae fibularis anterior
anterior radial carpal artery	arteria radialis carpalis
anterior spinal artery	arteria spinalis anterior
anterior superior alveolar arteries	arteriae alveolares superiores anteriores
anterior superior dental artery	arteria alveolaris anterior superior
anterior superior segmental artery of kidney	arteria segmenti anterioris superioris renis
anterior temporal artery	arteria temporalis anterior
anterior tibial artery	arteria tibialis anterior
anterior tibial recurrent artery	arteria recurrens tibialis anterior
anterior tympanic artery	arteria tympanica anterior
anterolateral central arteries	arteriae centrales anterolaterales
anterolateral striate arteries	arteriae centrales anterolaterales
anterolateral thalamostriate arteries	arteriae centrales anterolaterales
apicoposterior artery	
appendicular artery	arteria appendicularis
arch of aorta	arteria arcus aortae

artery	**arteria** (pl. **arteriae**)
arciform arteries	arteriae arcuatae renis
arcuate artery of foot	arteria arcuata pedis
arcuate arteries of kidney	arteriae arcuatae renis
articular artery, proper, of little head of fibula	ramus circumflexus fibulae arteriae tibialis posterioris
ascending artery	arteria ascendens
ascending aorta	arteria aorta ascendens
ascending cervical artery	arteria cervicalis ascendens
ascending palatine artery	arteria palatina ascendens
ascending pharyngeal artery	arteria pharyngea ascendens
atrial anastomotic artery	ramus atrialis anastomoticus arteriae coronariae sinistrae
atrial arteries	arteriae atriales
atrioventricular node, artery to	ramus nodi atrioventricularis
atrioventricular nodal artery	ramus nodi atrioventricularis arteriae coronariae dextrae
auditory artery, internal	arteria labyrinthina
auricular arteries, anterior	rami auriculares anteriores arteriae temporalis superficialis
auricular artery	arteria auricularis
axillary artery	arteria axillaris
axis thoracic artery	arteria thoracica axillaris
azygos arteries of vagina	vaginales arteriae uterinae
basilar artery	arteria basilaris
brachial artery	arteria brachialis
brachiocephalic artery	truncus brachiocephalicus
bronchial arteries	rami bronchiales
buccal artery, buccinator artery	arteria buccalis
bulbourethral artery	arteria bulbi urethrae
bulb of penis, artery of	arteria bulbi penis
bulb of vestibule of vagina, artery of	arteria bulbi vestibuli vaginae
calcaneal arteries	rami calcanei
calcarine artery	
calf, artery of	arteria sural
callosomarginal artery	arteria callosomarginalis
capsular artery	arteria suprarenalis
caroticotympanic arteries	arteriae caroticotympanicae
carotid artery	
caudal artery	arteria sacralis mediana

artery	**arteria** (pl. **arteriae**)
caudate lobe, artery of	arteria lobi caudati
cavernous artery	
cecal artery	arteria caecalis
celiac artery	
central arteries	arteriae centrales
central artery of retina, Zinn's artery	arteria centralis retinae
central sulcus artery	arteria sulci centralis
cephalic artery	arteria carotis communis
cerebellar artery	arteria cerebelli
cerebral artery, cerebral arteries	arteria cerebri, arteriae cerebrales
cervical artery	arteria cervicalis
cervicovaginal artery	arteria cervicovaginalis
Charcot's artery	
chief artery of thumb	arteria princeps pollicis
choroid artery, anterior	arteria choroidea anterior
ciliary arteries	arteriae cilliares
circle of Willis	
circumflex artery	ramus circumflexus arteriae coronariae sinistrae
circumflex artery, deep, internal	ramus profundus arteriae circumflexae femoris medialis
circumflex femoral artery, lateral	arteria circumflexa femoris lateralis
circumflex femoral artery, medial	arteria circumflexa femoris medialis
circumflex humeral artery, anterior	arteria circumflexa anterior humeri
circumflex humeral artery, posterior	arteria circumflexa posterior humeri
circumflex iliac artery, deep	arteria circumflexa iliaca profunda
circumflex iliac artery, superficial	arteria circumflexa iliaca superficialis
circumflex scapular artery	arteria circumflexa scapulae
clavicular artery	
clitoris, artery of, deep	arteria profunda clitoridis
clitoris, artery of, dorsal	arteria dorsalis clitoridis
coccygeal artery	arteria sacralis mediana
cochlear artery	ramus cochlearis arteriae labyrinthi
Cohnheim's artery	arteria terminalis
coiled artery	
colic artery	arteria colica
collateral artery	arteria collateralis
common carotid artery	arteria carotis communis
common hepatic artery	arteria hepatica communis

artery	arteria (pl. arteriae)
common iliac artery	arteria iliaca communis
common interosseous artery	arteria interossea communis
common palmar digital artery	arteria digitalis palmaris communis
common plantar digital artery	arteria digitalis plantaris communis
communicating artery of cerebrum	arteria communicans cerebri
companion artery	
conducting artery	
conjunctival artery	arteria conjunctivalis
conus artery	ramus coni arteriosi arteriae coronariae
copper-wire artery	
corkscrew artery	
coronary artery of heart	arteria coronaria
coronary artery of stomach	arteria gastrica
corpus cavernosum	
cortical artery	
costocervical trunk artery	
cremasteric artery	arteria cremasterica
cricothyroid artery	ramus cricothyroideus
crural artery	
cystic artery	arteria cystica
deep artery of clitoris	arteria profunda clitoridis
deep artery of penis	arteria profunda penis
deep artery of thigh	arteria profunda femoris
deep auricular artery	arteria auricularis profunda
deep brachial artery	arteria profunda brachii
deep cervical artery	arteria cervicalis profunda
deep circumflex iliac artery	arteria circumflexa iliaca profunda
deep epigastric artery	arteria epigastrica profunda
deep external pudendal artery	arteria pudenda profunda externa
deep femoral artery	arteria femoralis profunda
deep iliac circumflex artery	arteria circumflexa iliaca superficialis
deep lingual artery	arteria profunda linguae
deep palmar arch	arcus palmaris profundus
deep penis artery	arteria profunda penis
deep plantar artery	ramus plantaris profundus
deep temporal artery	arteria temporalis profunda
deep volar branch of ulnar artery	arteria ulnaris
deferential artery	arteria ductus deferentis
deltoid artery	ramus deltoideus arteriae profundae brachii

artery	arteria (pl. arteriae)
dental artery	arteria alveolaris
descending branch of occipital artery	arteria occipitalis descendens
descending genicular artery	arteria anastomotica magna
descending palatine artery	arteria palatina descendens
descending scapular artery	arteria scapularis descendens
diaphragmatic arteries	arteriae phrenicae inferiores
digital arteries	arteriae digitales
digital collateral artery	arteria digitalis palmaris propria
distributing artery	
dorsal artery of clitoris	arteria dorsalis clitoridis
dorsal artery of foot	arteria dorsalis pedis
dorsal artery of great toe	arteria dorsalis hallucis
dorsal artery of nose	arteria dorsalis nasi
dorsal artery of penis	arteria dorsalis penis
dorsal carpal artery	arteria dorsalis carpal
dorsal digital artery	arteria digitalis dorsalis
dorsal interosseous artery	arteria interossea dorsalis
dorsal metacarpal artery	arteria metacarpalis dorsalis
dorsal nasal artery	arteria dorsalis nasi
dorsalis pedis artery	arteria dorsalis pedis
dorsalis penis artery	arteria dorsalis penis
dorsal metacarpal artery	arteria metacarpea dorsalis
dorsal metatarsal artery	arteria metatarsea dorsalis
dorsal nasal artery	arteria nasi externa
dorsal pancreatic artery	arteria pancreatica dorsalis
dorsal scapular artery	arteria dorsalis scapulae
Drummond, artery of (marginal artery of colon)	
ductus deferens, artery of	arteria ductus deferentis
duodenal arteries	arteriae pancreaticoduodenales inferiores
efferent artery of glomerulus	vas efferens glomeruli
elastic artery	
emulgent artery	arteria renalis
end artery (terminal artery)	
epigastric artery	arteria circumflexa iliaca
epiphyseal artery	
episcleral arteries	arteriae episclerales
esophageal arteries	rami esophagei arteriae gastricae

artery	arteria (pl. arteriae)
ethmoidal artery	arteria ethmoidalis
external carotid artery	arteria carotis externa
external iliac artery	arteria iliaca externa
external mammary artery (lateral thoracic artery)	arteria thoracica lateralis
external maxillary artery (facial artery)	arteria maxillaris externa
external pudendal arteries	arteriae pudendae externae
external spermatic artery (cremasteric artery)	
facial artery	arteria facialis
fallopian artery	areria uterina
femoral artery	arteria femoralis
fibular artery (peroneal artery)	arteria fibularis
foot, artery of, dorsal	arteria dorsalis pedis
frontal artery (supratrochlear artery)	arteria supratrochlearis
frontobasal artery, lateral	arteria frontobasalis lateralis
funicular artery	arteria testicularis
gastric artery	arteria gastrica
gastroduodenal artery	arteria gastroduodenalis
gastroepiploic artery	arteria gastro-omentalis
gastro-omental artery	arteria gastro-omentalis
genicular artery	arteria genicularis
glaserian artery (anterior tympanic)	arteria tympanica anterior
glomerular artery	
gluteal artery	arteria glutealis
great anastomotic artery	arteria radicularis magna
greater palatine artery	arteria palatina major
great pancreatic artery	arteria pancreatica magna
great radicular artery	arteria radicularis magna
great superior pancreatic artery (dorsal)	arteria pancreatica magna superior
helicine arteries of penis	arteriae helicinae penis
hemorrhoidal artery	arteria rectalis
hepatic artery	arteria hepatica
Heubner, artery of (medial striate artery)	
highest intercostal artery (superior)	rami intercostales superiores
highest thoracic artery (superor)	arteria thoracica superior
humeral artery (brachial artery)	arteria humeri
hyaloid artery	arteria hyaloidea
hyoid artery	ramus suprahyoideus arteriae lingualis

artery	arteria (pl. arteriae)
hypogastric artery (internal iliac artery)	arteria iliaca interna
hypophysial artery	arteria hypophysialis
ileal arteries	arteriae ileales
ileocolic artery	arteria ileocolica
iliac artery	arteria iliaca
iliolumbar artery	arteria iliolumbalis
inferior alveolar artery	arteria alveolaris inferior
inferior cerebellar artery	arteria cerebelli inferior
inferior dental artery	arteria alveolaris inferior
inferior epigastric artery	arteria epigastrica inferior
inferior gastroduodenal artery	arteria gastroduodenalis inferior
inferior genicular artery	arteria genicularis inferior
inferior gluteal artery	arteria glutea inferior
inferior hemorrhoidal artery	arteria rectalis inferior
inferior hypophysial artery	arteria hypophysialis inferior
inferior labial artery	arteria labialis inferior
inferior laryngeal artery	arteria laryngea inferior
inferior lateral genicular artery	arteria genus inferior lateralis
inferior medial genicular artery	arteria genus inferior medialis
inferior mesenteric artery	arteria mesenterica inferior
inferior pancreatic artery	arteria pancreatica inferior
inferior pancreaticoduodenal artery	arteria pancreaticoduodenalis inferior
inferior phrenic artery	arteria phrenica inferior
inferior profunda artery	arteria profunda inferior
inferior rectal artery	arteria rectalis inferior
inferior segmental artery of kidney	arteria segmenti inferioris renis
inferior suprarenal artery	arteria suprarenalis inferior
inferior thyroid artery	arteria thyroidea inferior
inferior tympanic artery	arteria tympanica inferior
inferior ulnar collateral artery	arteria collateralis ulnaris inferior
inferior vesical artery	arteria vesicalis inferior
infracostal artery	ramus costalis lateralis arteriae thoracicae internae
infrahyoid artery	arteria infrahyoideus
infraorbital artery	arteria infraorbitalis
infrascapular artery	arteria infrascapularis
innominate artery	truncus brachiocephalicus
inguinal arteries	rami inguinales arteriae femoralis
innominate artery	truncus brachiocephalicus

artery	arteria (pl. arteriae)
insular arteries	arteriae insulares
intercostal arteries	rami intercostales arteriae thoracicae
interlobar arteries of kidney	arteriae interlobares renis
interlobular arteries of kidney	arteriae interlobulares renis
interlobular arteries of liver	arteriae interlobulares hepatis
intermediate atrial artery	ramus atrialis intermedius
intermediate temporal artery	arteria temporalis intermedia
intermetacarpal arteries	arteriae metacarpales palmares
internal auditory artery (labyrinthine)	arteria labyrinthi
internal carotid artery	arteria carotis interna
internal iliac artery	arteria iliaca interna
internal malleolar artery	arteria malleolaris interna
internal mammary artery (thoracic)	arteria thoracica interna
internal maxillary artery	arteria maxillaris interna
internal palpebral artery	arteria palpebralis interna
internal plantar artery	arteria plantaris interna
internal pubic artery	arteria pubicus interna
internal pudendal artery	arteria pudenda interna
internal spermatic artery (testicular)	arteria testicularis interna
internal thoracic artery	arteria thoracica interna
interosseous artery	arteria interossea
interosseous palmar artery	arteria palmaris interossea
intersegmental artery	
interventricular artery	ramus interventricularis
intestinal arteries (ileal or jejunal)	arteriae intestinales
jejunal arteries	arteriae jejunales
kidney, arteries of (segmental arteries of kidney)	arteriae renis
Kugel's anastomotic artery	arteria anastomotica auricularis magna
labial arteries of vulva	rami labiales arteriae femoralis
labyrinthine artery	arteria labyrinthi
lacrimal artery	arteria lacrimalis
laryngeal artery	arteria laryngea
lateral calcaneal artery	arteria calcanei lateralis
lateral circumflex femoral artery	arteria circumflexa femoris lateralis
lateral circumflex artery of thigh	arteria circumflexa femoris lateralis
lateral costal artery	
lateral frontobasal artery	arteria frontobasalis lateralis
lateral inferior genicular artery	arteria genicularis lateralis inferior

artery	arteria (pl. arteriae)
lateral malleolar arteries	rami malleolares laterales
lateral nasal artery	arteria nasi lateralis
lateral occipital artery	arteria occipitalis lateralis
lateral palpebral artery	arteria palpebralis lateralis
lateral plantar artery	arteria plantaris lateralis
lateral sacral artery	arteria sacralis lateralis
lateral striate arteries	arteriae centrales anterolaterales
lateral tarsal artery	arteria tarsea lateralis
lateral thoracic artery	arteria thoracica lateralis
left anterior descending coronary artery	ramus interventricularis anterior arteriae coronariae sinistrae
left colic artery	arteria colica sinistra
left coronary artery	arteria coronaria sinistra
left gastric artery	arteria gastrica sinistra
left gastroepiploic artery	arteria gastro-omentalis sinistra
left gastro-omental artery (left gastroepiploic artery)	
left hepatic artery	ramus sinister arteriae hepaticae propriae
left pulmonary artery	arteria pulmonalis sinistra
lenticulostriate arteries (Charcot's artery) (lateral striate arteries)	
lesser palatine artery	arteria palatina minor
lienal artery (splenic artery)	
lingual artery	arteria lingualis
lingual artery, dorsal	arteria lingualis dorsalis
lobar artery	
long central artery (medial striate artery)	
long ciliary artery	arteria ciliaris longa
long posterior ciliary artery	arteria ciliaris posterior longa
long thoracic artery (lateral)	arteria thoracica lateralis
lowest lumbar arteries	arteriae lumbales imae
lowest thyroid artery	arteria thyroidea ima
lumbar artery	arteria lumbalis
macular arteries	
malleolar artery	arteria malleolaris
mammary artery	arteria thoracica
mandibular artery	arteria alveolaris inferior
marginal artery	ramus marginalis

artery	arteria (pl. arteriae)
marginal artery of colon (artery of Drummond, Riolan's arc)	arteria marginalis coli
masseteric artery	arteria masseterica
mastoid artery	rami mastoidei arteriae auricularis posterioris
maxillary artery	arteria maxillaris
medial artery of foot, superficial	ramus superior arteriae plantaris medialis
medial circumflex femoral artery	arteria circumflexa femoris medialis
medial frontobasal artery	arteria frontobasalis medialis
medial malleolar arteries	arteriae malleolares posteriores mediales
medial palpebral artery	
medial striate artery	
medial tarsal artery	
median artery	arteria comitans nervi mediani
median sacral artery	arteria sacralis mediana
mediastinal arteries, anterior	rami mediastinales arteriae thoracicae internae
mediastinal arteries, posterior	rami mediastinales aortae thoracicae
medullary artery	arteria nutriens
meningeal artery, accessory	ramus meningeus accessorius arteriae meningeae mediae
meningeal artery, anterior	ramus meningeus anterior arteriae ethmoidalis anterioris
meningeal artery, middle	arteria meningea media
meningeal artery, posterior	arteria meningea posterior
mental artery	arteria mentalis
mesencephalic arteries	arteriae mesencephalicae
mesenteric artery	arteria mesenterica
metacarpal arteries	arteriae metacarpales
metaphyseal artery	
metatarsal artery	arteria metatarsae
middle capsular artery	arteria suprarenalis media
middle cerebral artery	arteria cerebri media
middle colic artery	arteria colica media
middle collateral artery	arteria collateralis media
middle genicular artry	arteria articularis azygos
middle hemorrhoidal artery	

artery	arteria (pl. arteriae)
middle meningeal artery	arteria meningea media
middle rectal artery	arteria rectalis media
middle sacral artery	arteria sacralis media
middle suprarenal artery	arteria suprarenalis media
middle temporal artery	arteria temporalis media
middle vesical artery	arteria vesicalis media
Mueller, arteries of	arteriae helicinae penis
musculophrenic artery	arteria musculophrenica
mylohyoid artery	ramus mylohyoideus arteriae alveolaris inferioris
myomastoid artery	ramus occipitalis arteriae auricularis posterioris
nasal artery, dorsal	arteria dorsalis nasi
nasopalatine artery	arteria sphenopalatina
Neubauer's artery	arteria thyroidea ima
nodal artery	
nose, dorsal artery of	arteria dorsalis nasi
nutrient artery	arteria nutricia
obliterated hypogastric artery	
obliterated umbilical artery	
obturator artery	arteria obturatoria
occipital artery	arteria occipitalis
omental artery	
omphalomesenteric artery	
ophthalmic artery	arteria ophthalmica
orbital artery	
orbitofrontal artery (lateral frontobasal)	
ovarian artery	arteria ovarica
palatine artery	arteria palatina
palmar metacarpal artery	arteria metacarpea palmaris
palpebral arteries	arteriae palpebrales
pancreatic artery	arteria pancreatica
pancreaticoduodenal artery	arteria pancreaticoduodenalis
paracentral artery	arteria paracentralis
parietal arteries, anterior and posterior	arteriae parietales anterior et posterior
parieto-occipital artery	arteria parieto-occipitalis
parieto-temporal artery	
pectoral artery	
pelvic artery, posterior	arteria iliaca interna

artery	arteria (pl. arteriae)
penis, deep artery of	arteria profunda penis
penis, dorsal artery of	arteria dorsalis penis
perforating arteries	arteriae perforantes
pericallosal artery	arteria pericallosa
pericardiac arteries, posterior	rami pericardiaci aortae thoracicae
pericardiacophrenic artery	arteria pericardiacophrenica
perineal artery	arteria perinealis
periosteal artery	
peroneal artery, fibular artery	arteria peronea, arteria fibularis
pharyngeal artery, ascending	arteria pharyngea ascendens
phrenic arteries	arteriae phrenicae
plantar artery	arteria plantaris
plantar metatarsal artery	arteria metatarsea plantaris
pontine arteries	arteriae pontis
popliteal artery	arteria poplitea
postcentral sulcal artery	arteria sulci postcentralis
posterior alveolar artery	arteria alveolaris posterior
posterior auricular artery	arteria auricularis posterior
posterior cecal artery	arteria cecalis posterior
posterior cerebral artery	arteria cerebri posterior
posterior choroidal artery	arteria choroidea posterior
posterior circumflex humeral artery	arteria circumflexa humeri posterior
posterior communicating artery	
posterior descending coronary artery	ramus interventricularis posterior arteriae coronariae dextrae
posterior humeral circumflex	artria circumflexa humeri posterior
posterior inferior cerebellar artery	arteria cerebelli posterior inferior
posterior intercostal artery	
posterior interosseous artery	arteria interossea posterior
posterior pancreaticoduodenal artery	arteria pancreaticoduodenalis posterior
posterior scapular artery	arteria scapulae posterior
posterior scrotal artery	arteria scrotalis posterior
posterior septal artery of nose	arteria nasalis posterior septi
posterior spinal artery	arteria spinalis posterior
posterior superior alveolar artery	arteria alveolaris superior posterior
posterior temporal artery	arteria temporalis posterior
posterior tibial artery	arteria tibialis posterior
posterior tibial recurrent artery	arteria recurrens tibialis posterior
posterior tympanic artery	arteria tympanica posterior

artery	arteria (pl. arteriae)
posterolateral central artery	arteriae centrales posterolaterales
posteromedial central arteries	arteriae centrales posteromediales
precentral sulcal artery	arteria sulci precentralis
princeps pollicis artery	arteria princeps pollicis
precuneal artery	arteria precunealis
prepancreatic artery	arteria prepancreatica
presegmental artery	arteria presegmenti
prevertebral artery	arteria prevertebralis
principal artery of thumb	arteria princeps pollicis
profunda brachii artery	arteria profunda brachii
profunda femoris artery	arteria profunda femoris
proper hepatic artery	arteria hepatica propria
proper palmar digital artery	arteria digitalis palmaris propria
proper plantar digital artery	arteria digitalis plantaris propria
pterygoid arteries	rami pterygoidei
pterygoid canal, artery of	arteria canalis pterygoidei
pubic artery	ramus pubicus arteriae epigastricae inferioris
pudendal arteries	arteriae pudendae externae
pulmonary artery	truncus pulmonalis
pyloric artery	arteria gastrica dextra
quadriceps artery of femur	ramus descendens arteriae circumflexae femoris lateralis
radial artery	arteria radialis
radial artery of index finger	arteria volaris radialis indicis
radial carpal artery	
radial collateral artery	arteria collateralis radialis
radial recurrent artery	arteria recurrens radialis
radiate arteries of kidney	arteriae interlobulares renis
radicular arteries	rami spinales arteriae vertebralis
ranine artery	arteria profunda linguae
rectal artery	arteria rectalis
recurrent artery	arteria centralis longa
recurrent artery, radial	arteria recurrens radialis
recurrent artery, tibial, anterior	arteria recurrens tibialis anterior
recurrent artery, tibial, posterior	arteria recurrens tibialis posterior
recurrent artery, ulnar	arteria recurrens ulnaris
recurrent interosseous artery	arteria interossea recurrens
recurrent radial artery	arteria recurrens radialis

artery	arteria (pl. arteriae)
recurrent ulnar artery	arteria recurrens ulnaris
renal artery, renal arteries	arteria renalis, arteriae renales
retinal artery	
retrocostal artery	ramus costalis lateralis arteriae thoracicae internae
retroduodenal artery	arteria retroduodenalis
retroesophageal subclavian artery	artery subclavia retroesophagei
revehent artery	vas efferens glomeruli
right colic artery	arteria colica dextra
right coronary artery	arteria coronaria dextra
right gastric artery	arteria gastrica dextra
right gastroepiploic artery	arteria gastro-omentalis dextra
right hepatic artery	ramus dexter arteriae hepaticae propriae
right pulmonary artery	arteria pulmonalis dextra
round ligament of uterus, artery of	arteria ligamenti teretis uteri
sacral arteries	arteriae sacrales
sacrococcygeal artery	arteria sacralis mediana
saphenous artery	
scapular artery	arteria scapulare
sciatic artery	arteria comitans nervi ischiadici
scrotal arteries, anterior	rami scrotales anteriores arteriae femoralis
scrotal arteries, posterior	rami scrotales posteriores arteriae pudendae internae
segmental artery	arteria segmenti
semilunar ganglion artery	
septal arteries, anterior	rami interventriculares septales
septal arteries, posterior	rami interventricularis posterioris
short central artery	arteria centralis brevis
short ciliary artery	arteria ciliaris brevis
short gastric artery	arteriae gastricae breves
short posterior ciliary artery	arteria ciliaris posterior brevis
sigmoid arteries	arteriae sigmoideae
sinoatrial nodal artery, sinuatrial (S-A) node artery	ramus nodi sinuatrialis arteriae coronaria dextra
somatic artery	
spermatic artery, external	arteria cremasterica
spermatic artery, internal	arteria testicularis
sphenopalatine artery	arteria sphenopalatina

artery	**arteria** (pl. **arteriae**)
spinal arteries	rami spinales arteriae vertebralis
spiral artery	
splanchnic artery	
splenic artery	arteria splenica
stapedial artery	
sternal arteries, posterior	rami sternales arteriae thoracicae internae
sternocleidomastoid artery, superior	ramus sternocleidomastoideus arteriae thyroideae superioris
straight arteries of kidney	arteriolae rectae renis
striate arteries	arteriae centrales anterolaterales
stylomastoid artery	arteria stylomastoidea
subclavian artery	arteria subclavia
subcostal artery	arteria subcostalis
sublingual artery	arteria sublingualis
submaxillary glandular artery	
submental artery	arteria submentalis
subscapular artery	arteria subscapularis
sulcal artery	
superficial brachial artery	arteria brachialis superficialis
superficial cervical artery	arteria cervicalis superficialis
superficial circumflex iliac artery	arteria circumflexa iliaca superficialis
superficial epigastric artery	arteria epigastrica superficialis
superficial external pudendal artery	arteria pudenda superficialis externa
superficial iliac circumflex artery	arteria circumflexa iliaca superficialis
superficial palmar arch artery	arteria arcus palmaris superficialis
superficial perineal artery	arteria perinealis superficialis
superficial petrosal artery	
superficial temporal artery	arteria temporalis superficialis
superficial volar artery	
superficial volar arch artery	
superior cerebellar artery	arteria cerebelli superior
superior epigastric artery	arteria epigastrica superior
superior gluteal artery	arteria glutea superior
superior hemorrhoidal artery	arteria rectalis superior
superior hypophysial artery	arteria hypophysialis superior
superior intercostal artery	arteria intercostalis suprema
superior labial artery	arteria labialis superior
superior laryngeal artery	arteria laryngea superior
superior lateral genicular artery	arteria genus superior lateralis

artery	arteria (pl. arteriae)
superior medial genicular artery	arteria genus superior medialis
superior mesenteric artery	arteria mesenterica superior
superior pancreaticoduodenal artery	arteria pancreaticoduodenalis superior
superior phrenic artery	arteria phrenica superior
superior profunda artery	arteria profunda superior
superior rectal artery	arteria rectalis superior
superior segmental artery of kidney	arteria segmenti superioris renis
superior suprarenal arteries	arteriae suprarenales superiores
superior thoracic artery	arteria thoracica superior
superior thyroid artery	arteria thyroidea superior
superior tympanic artery	arteria tympanica superior
superior ulnar collateral artery	arteria collateralis ulnaris superior
superior vesical artery	arteria vesicalis superior
supraduodenal artery	arteria supraduodenalis
suprahyoid artery	arteria superhyoideus
supraorbital artery	arteria supraorbitalis
suprarenal artery, aortic	arteria suprarenalis media
suprascapular artery	arteria suprascapularis
supratrochlear artery	arteria supratrochlearis
sural artery	arteria suralis
sylvian artery	arteria cerebri media
tarsal artery	arteria tarsalis
temporal artery	arteria temporalis
terminal artery (Cohnheim's artery)	
testicular artery	arteria testicularis
thalamostriate arteries, anterolateral	arteriae centrales anterolaterales
thoracic artery	arteria thoracica
thoracicoacromial artery	arteria thoracoacromialis
thoracodorsal artery	arteria thoracodorsalis
thymic arteries	rami thymici arteriae thoracicae internae
thyroid artery	arteria thyroidea
thyroid artery, inferior, of Cruveilhier	ramus cricothyroideus arteriae thyroideae superioris
thyroid ima artery	arteria thyroidea ima
tibial artery	arteria tibialis
tonsillar artery	ramus tonsillaris arteriae facialis
tracheal artery	
transverse artery of neck	arteria transversa cervicis
transverse cervical artery	arteria transversa cervicis

artery	arteria (pl. arteriae)
transverse facial artery	arteria transversa faciei
transverse perineal artery	arteria transversa perinealis
transverse scapular artery	arteria transversa scapulae
trunk artery	
tubo-ovarian artery	arteria ovarica
tympanic artery	arteria tympanica
ulnar artery	arteria ulnaris
ulnar carpal artery	
ulnar collateral artery, inferior	arteria collateralis ulnaris inferior
ulnar collateral artery, superior	arteria collateralis ulnaris superior
umbilical artery	arteria umbilicalis
upper limb, arteries of	arteriae membri superioris
ureteric artery	
urethral artery	arteria urethralis
urethral bulb artery	
uterine artery	arteria uterina
uterine artery, aortic	arteria ovarica
vaginal artery	arteria vaginalis
venous arteries	venae pulmonales
ventricular arteries	arteriae ventriculares
vermiform artery	arteria appendicularis
vertebral artery	arteria vertebralis
vesical artery, inferior	arteria vesicalis inferior
vesical arteries, superior	arteriae vesicales superiores
vestibular arteries	rami vestibulares arteriae labyrinthi
vidian artery	arteria canalis pterygoidei
visceral artery	
vitelline artery	arteria vitellina
volar carpal artery	
volar interosseous artery	arteria interossea volaris
Zinn, artery of	arteria centralis retinae
zygomatic artery	
zygomatico-orbital artery	arteria zygomatico-orbitalis

Table of Muscles

muscle	musculus (pl. musculi)
abdominal muscles	musculi abdominis
abdominal external oblique muscle	musculus obliquus externus abdominis
abdominal internal oblique muscle	musculus obliquus internus abdominis
abductor digiti minimi muscle of foot (abductor muscle of little toe)	musculus abductor digiti minimi pedis
abductor digiti minimi muscle of hand (abductor muscle of little finger)	musculus abductor digiti minimi manus
abductor hallucis muscle (great toe)	musculus abductor hallucis
abductor pollicis brevis muscle (abductor muscle of thumb, short)	musculus abductor pollicis brevis
abductor pollicis longus muscle (abductor muscle of thumb, long)	musculus abductor pollicis longus
accessory flexor muscle of foot (quadratus plantae muscle)	musculus flexor accessorius
adductor muscle, short	musculus adductor brevis
adductor muscle of great toe	musculus adductor hallucis
adductor muscle, long	musculus adductor longus
adductor muscle, great	musculus adductor magnus
adductor minimus muscle (adductor muscle, smallest)	musculus adductor minimus
adductor pollicis muscle (thumb)	musculus adductor pollicis
Aeby's cutaneomucous muscle	
agonistic muscles	
Albinus' muscle	
anconeus muscle	musculus anconeus
antagonistic muscles	
anterior auricular muscle	musculus auricularis anterior
anterior cervical intertransverse muscles	musculi intertransversarii anteriores cervicis
anterior rectus muscle of head	musculus rectus capitis anterior
anterior scalene muscle	musculus scalenus anterior

muscle	musculus (pl. musculi)
anterior serratus muscle	musculus serratus anterior
anterior tibial muscle	musculus tibialis anterior
antigravity muscles	
antitragus muscle	musculus antitragicus
arrector pili muscles (erector muscles of hairs)	musculi arrectores pilorum
articular muscle	musculus articularis
articular muscle of elbow	musculus articularis cubiti
articular muscle of knee	musculus articularis genus
articular muscle of knee	articularis genu musculus
aryepiglottic muscle	musculus aryepiglotticus
auditory ossicles, muscles of	musculi ossiculorum auditus
axillary arch muscle	pectorodorsalis musculus
back muscles	musculi dorsi
Bell's muscle (ureteric bridge)	
biceps brachii muscle (biceps muscle of arm)	musculus biceps brachii
biceps femoris muscle (biceps muscle of thigh)	musculus biceps femoris
bipennate muscle	musculus bipennatus
Bochdalek's muscle	musculus triticeoglossus
Bovero's muscle ("sucking muscle")	musculus cutaneomucosus
Bowman's muscle (ciliary muscle)	musculus ciliaris
brachial muscle (brachialis)	musculus brachialis
brachiocephalic muscle	musculus brachiocephalicus
brachioradial muscle (brachioradialis)	musculus brachioradialis
Braune's muscle	musculus puborectalis
broadest muscle of back	musculus latissimus dorsi
bronchoesophageal muscle	musculus bronchoesophageus
Brücke's muscle (Crampton's muscle)	
buccinator muscle	musculus buccinator
buccopharyngeal muscles (also, constrictor muscles of pharynx, superior)	musculi pars buccopharyngea
bulbocavernous muscle	musculus bulbospongiosus
canine muscle	musculus levator anguli oris
cardiac muscle	
Casser's perforated muscle (casserian muscle)	musculus coracobrachialis (ligamentum mallei anterius)

muscle	musculus (pl. musculi)
ceratocricoid muscle	musculus ceratocricoideus
cervical iliocostal muscle	musculus iliocostalis cervicis
cervical interspinal muscles	musculi interspinalis cervicis
cervical longissimus muscle (neck)	musculus longissimus cervicis
cervical muscles	musculi colli
cervical rotator muscles	musculi rotatores cervicis
Chassaignac's axillary muscle	
chin muscle	musculus mentalis
chondroglossus muscle	musculus chondroglossus
chondropharyngeal muscles (constrictor muscle of pharynx, middle)	musculi pars chondropharyngea (constrictor pharyngis medius)
ciliary muscle	muscularis ciliaris
coccygeal (coccygeus) muscle(s)	musculus coccygeus, musculi coccygei
Coiter's muscle	musculus corrugator supercilii
compressor muscle of naris	
congenerous muscles	
constrictor muscle of pharynx, inferior	musculus constrictor pharyngis inferior
constrictor muscle of pharynx, middle	musculus constrictor pharyngis medius
constrictor muscle of pharynx, superior	musculus constrictor pharyngis superior
coracobrachial muscle (coracobrachialis)	musculus coracobrachialis
corrugator muscle	corrugator supercilii musculus
corrugator cutis muscle of anus	musculus corrugator cutis ani
corrugator supercilii muscle	musculus corrugator supercilii
Crampton's muscle (Bruecke's muscle)	
cremaster muscle (Riolan's muscle)	musculus cremaster
cricoarytenoid muscle, lateral	musculus crico-arytenoideus lateralis
cricoarytenoid muscle, posterior	musculus crico-arytenoideus posterior
cricopharyngeal muscle	musculus cricopharyngeus
cricothyroid muscle	musculus cricothyroideus
cruciate muscle	musculus cruciatus
cutaneomucous muscle (the "sucking muscle," also called Aeby's muscle, Bovero's muscle, Klein's muscle, Krause's muscle, mucocutaneous muscle)	musculus cutaneomucosus
cutaneous muscle	musculus cutaneus
dartos muscle of scrotum	musculus tunica dartos
deep muscles of back (true back muscles)	musculi dorsi
deep flexor muscle of fingers	musculus flexor digitorum profundus

muscle	musculus (pl. musculi)
deep transverse perineal msucle	musculus transversus perinei profundus
deltoid muscle	musculus deltoideus
depressor muscle of angle of mouth	musculus depressor anguli oris
depressor muscle of epiglottis	musculus thyroepiglottic
depressor muscle of eyebrow	musculus depressor supercilii
depressor muscle of lower lip	musculus depressor labii inferioris
depressor muscle of septum of nose	musculus depressor septi
depressor superciliary muscle	musculus depressor supercilii
detrusor muscle of urinary bladder	musculus detrusor urinae (musculus detrusor vesicae)
diaphragm, diaphragmatic muscle	diaphragma
digastric muscle	musculus digastricus
dilator muscle	musculus dilatator
dilator muscle of ileocecal sphincter	musculus dilator pylori ilealis
dilator muscle of pupil	musculus dilator pupillae
dilator muscle of pylorus	musculus dilator pylori gastro-duodenalis
dorsal interosseous muscles of foot	musculi interossei dorsalis pedis
dorsal interosseous muscles of hand	musculi interossei dorsalis manus
dorsal muscles (muscles of back)	musculi dorsi
dorsal sacrococcygeal muscle	musculus sacrococcygeus dorsalis
Dupré's muscle	musculus articularis genu
Duverney's muscle	musculus orbicularis oculi
elevator muscle of anus	musculus levator ani
elevator muscle of prostate	musculus levator prostatae
elevator muscles of rib	musculi levatores costarum
elevator muscle of scapula	musculus levator scapulae
elevator muscle of soft palate	musculus levator veli palatini
elevator muscle of upper eyelid	musculus levator palpebrae superioris
elevator muscle of upper lip	musculus levator labii superioris
elevator muscle of upper lip and wing of nose	musculus levator labii superioris alaeque nasi
emergency muscles	
epicranial muscle	musculus epicranius
epimeric muscle	
epitrochleoanconeus muscle	musculus epitrochleoanconaeus
erector muscles of hairs (arrector pili)	musculi arrectores pilorum
erector muscle of penis	musculus ischiocavernosus
erector muscle of spine	musculus erector spinae

muscle	musculus (pl. musculi)
eustachian muscle	musculus tensor tympani
expression, muscles of	musculi faciales
extensor muscle of fingers	musculus extensor digitorum
extensor muscle of great toe, long	musculus extensor hallucis longus
extensor muscle of great toe, short	musculus extensor hallucis brevis
extensor muscle of hand, short (Pozzi's muscle)	musculus extensor digitorum brevis manus
extensor muscle of index finger	musculus extensor indicis
extensor muscle of little finger	musculus extensor digiti minimi
extensor muscle of thumb, long	musculus extensor pollicis longus
extensor muscle of thumb, short	musculus extensor pollicis brevis
extensor muscle of toes, long	musculus extensor digitorum longus
extensor muscle of toes, short	musculus extensor digitorum brevis
extensor muscle of wrist, radial, long	musculus extensor carpi radialis longus
extensor muscle of wrist, radial, short	musculus extensor carpi radialis brevis
extensor muscle of wrist, ulnar	musculus extensor carpi ulnaris
external intercostal muscles	musculi intercostales externi
external oblique muscle	musculus obliquus externus abdominis
external obturator muscle	musculus obturator externus
external pterygoid muscle	lateral pterygoid musculus
external sphincter muscle of anus	
extraocular muscles	musculi bulbi
extrinsic muscles	
eyeball muscles (extraocular muscles)	
facial and masticatory muscles	musculi faciales et masticatores
facial expression, muscles of	musculi faciales
facial muscles	musculi faciales
fast muscle (white muscle)	
fauces (the throat), muscles of	musculi palati et faucium
femoral muscle	musculus vastus intermedius
fibular muscle, long	musculus peroneus longus
fibular muscle, short	musculus peroneus brevis
fibular muscle, third	musculus peroneus tertius
fixation muscles, fixator muscles	
fixator muscle of base of stapes	musculus fixator baseos stapedis
flexor muscle of fingers, deep	musculus flexor digitorum profundus
flexor muscle of fingers, superficial	musculus flexor digitorum superficialis
flexor muscle of great toe, long	musculus flexor hallucis longus
flexor muscle of great toe, short	musculus flexor hallucis brevis

muscle	musculus (pl. musculi)
flexor muscle of little finger, short	musculus flexor digiti minimi brevis manus
flexor muscle of little toe, short	musculus flexor digiti minimi brevis pedis
flexor muscle of thumb, short	musculus flexor pollicis brevis
flexor muscle of thumb, long	musculus flexor pollicis longus
flexor muscle of toes, short	musculus flexor digitorum brevis
flexor muscle of toes, long	musculus flexor digitorum longus
flexor muscle of wrist, radial	musculus flexor carpi radialis
flexor muscle of wrist, ulnar	musculus flexor carpi ulnaris
Folius' muscle	ligamentum mallei laterale
fusiform muscle (spindle-shaped muscle)	musculus fusiformis
Gantzer's muscle	
gastrocnemius muscle	musculus gastrocnemius
Gavard's muscle	
gemellus muscle, inferior	musculus gemellus inferior
gemellus muscle, superior	musculus gemellus superior
genioglossal muscle	musculus genioglossus
geniohyoid muscle	musculus geniohyoideus
glossopalatine muscle (palatoglossus)	musculus palatoglossus
glossopharyngeal muscle	pars glossopharyngea musculi constrictoris pharyngis superioris
gluteal muscle, greatest	musculus gluteus maximus
gluteal muscle, least	musculus gluteus minimus
gluteal muscle, middle	musculus gluteus medius
gracilis muscle	musculus gracilis
great adductor muscle	musculus adductor magnus
greater pectoral muscle	musculus pectoralis major
greater posterior rectus muscle of head	musculus rectus capitis posterior major
greater psoas muscle	musculus psoas major
greater rhomboid muscle	musculus rhomboideus major
greater zygomatic muscle	musculus zygomaticus major
Guthrie's muscle	sphincter urethrae
hamstring muscles	
head, muscles of	musculi capitis
Hilton's muscle	musculus aryepiglotticus
Horner's muscle	musculus orbicularis oculi
Houston's muscle	compressor venae dorsalis penis
hyoglossal (hyoglossus) muscle	musculus hyoglossus

muscle	**musculus** (pl. **musculi**)
iliac muscle	musculus iliacus
iliacus minor muscle	musculus iliacus minor
iliococcygeal muscle	musculus iliococcygeus
iliocostal muscle	musculus iliocostalis
iliocostal muscle of neck	musculus iliocostalis cervicis
iliocostal muscle of loins	musculus iliocostalis lumborum
iliocostal muscle of thorax	musculus iliocostalis thoracis
iliopsoas muscle	musculus iliopsoas
incisive muscles of inferior lip	musculi incisivi labii inferioris
incisive muscles of lower lip	musculi incisivi labii inferioris
incisive muscles of superior lip	musculi incisivi labii superioris
incisive muscles of upper lip	musculi incisivi labii superioris
index extensor muscle	musculus extensor indicis
inferior constrictor muscle of pharynx	musculus constrictor pharyngis inferior
inferior gemellus muscle	musculus gemellus inferior
inferior longitudinal muscle of tongue	musculus longitudinalis inferior
inferior oblique muscle	musculus obliquus inferior
inferior oblique muscle of head	musculus obliquus capitis inferior
inferior posterior serratus muscle	serratus posterior inferior musculus
inferior rectus muscle	musculus rectus inferior
inferior tarsal muscle	musculus tarsalis inferior
infrahyoid muscles	musculi infrahyoidei
infraspinous muscle	musculus infraspinatus
innermost intercostal muscle	musculus intercostalis intimus
inspiratory muscles	
intercostal muscles	musculi intercostales
interfoveolar muscle	ligamentum interfoveolare
intermediate great muscle	musculus vastus intermedius
internal intercostal muscle	musculus intercostalis internus
internal oblique muscle	musculus obliquus internus abdominis
internal obturator muscle	musculus obturator internus
internal pterygoid muscle	musculus pterygoideus medialis
interosseous muscles	musculi interossei
interspinal muscles	musculi interspinales
intertransverse muscles	musculi intertransversarii
intra-auricular muscles	
intraocular muscles	
intrinsic muscles	
intrinsic muscles of foot	

muscle	musculus (pl. musculi)
involuntary muscles	
iridic muscles	
ischiocavernous muscle	musculus ischiocavernosus
Jarjavay's muscle	
Jung's pyramidal auricular muscle	
Klein's cutaneomucous muscle	
Kohlrausch's muscle	
Koyter's muscle	musculus corrugator supercilii
Krause's cutaneomucous muscle	musculus cutaneomucosus
Landstrom's muscle (umlaut o)	
Langer's axillary arch muscle	
larynx, muscles of	musculi laryngis
lateral cricoarytenoid muscle	musculus cricoarytenoideus lateralis
lateral great muscle	musculus vastus lateralis
lateral lumbar intertransversarii muscles	musculi intertransversarii laterales lumborum
lateral pterygoid muscle	musculus pterygoideus lateralis
lateral rectus muscle	musculus rectus lateralis
lateral rectus muscle of the head	musculus rectus capitis lateralis
lateral vastus muscle	musculus vastus lateralis
latissimus dorsi muscle	musculus latissimus dorsi
lesser rhomboid muscle	musculus rhomboid minor
lesser zygomatic muscle	musculus zygomaticus minor
levator ani muscle	musculus levator ani
levator muscles (see *elevator muscles*)	
lingual muscles	musculi linguae
long abductor muscle of thumb	musculus abductor pollicis longus
long adductor muscle	musculus adductor longus
long extensor muscle of great toe	musculus extensor hallucis longus
long extensor muscle of thumb	musculus extensor pollicis longus
long extensor muscle of toes	musculus extensor digitorum longus
long fibular muscle	musculus peroneus longus
long flexor muscle of great toe	musculus flexor hallucis longus
long flexor muscle of thumb	musculus flexor pollicis longus
long flexor muscle of toes	musculus flexor digitorum longus
long muscle of head	musculus longus capitis
longissimus muscle	musculus longissimus
longissimus muscle of back (thorax)	musculus longissimus thoracis
longissimus muscle of head	musculus longissimus capitis

muscle	musculus (pl. musculi)
longissimus muscle of neck	musculus longissimus cervicis
longitudinal muscle of tongue, inferior	musculus longitudinalis inferior linguae
longitudinal muscle of tongue, superior	musculus longitudinalis superior linguae
long muscle of head	musculus longus capitis
long muscle of neck	musculus longus colli
long palmar muscle	musculus palmaris longus
long peroneal muscle	musculus peroneus longus
long radial extensor muscle of wrist	musculus extensor carpi radialis longus
lumbar iliocostal muscle	musculus interspinalis lumborum
lumbar interspinal muscles	musculus interspinalis lumborum
lumbar quadrate muscle	musculus quadratus lumborum
lumbar rotator muscles	musculi rotatores lumborum
lumbrical muscles of foot	musculi lumbricales pedis
lumbrical muscles of hand	musculi lumbricales manus
Marcacci's muscle	
masseter muscle	musculus masseter
medial great muscle	musculus vastus medialis
medial lumbar intertransverse muscles	musculi intertransversarii mediales lumborum
medial pterygoid muscle	musculus pterygoideus medialis
medial rectus muscle	musculus rectus medialis
medial vastus muscle	musculus vastus medialis
mentalis muscle	musculus mentalis
Merkel's muscle	musculus ceratocricoideus
mesothenar muscle	musculus adductor pollicis
middle constrictor muscle of pharynx	musculus constrictor pharyngis medius
middle scalene muscle	musculus scalenus medius
mucocutaneous muscle	
Mueller's muscle	musculus orbitalis
multifidus muscles (intermediate layer of transversospinalis muscles)	musculi multifidi
multipennate muscle	musculus multipennatus
mylohyoid muscle	musculus mylohyoideus
nasal muscle	musculus nasalis
neck, muscles of	musculi colli
nonstriated muscle (smooth muscle)	
notch of helix, muscles of	musculus incisurae helicis
oblique arytenoid muscle	musculus arytenoideus obliquus
oblique auricular muscle	musculus obliquus auriculae

muscle	musculus (pl. musculi)
oblique muscle of abdomen, external	musculus obliquus externus abdominis
oblique muscle of abdomen, internal	musculus obliquus internus abdominis
oblique muscle of head, inferior	musculus obliquus capitis inferior
oblique muscle of head, superior	musculus obliquus capitis superior
obturator muscle, external	musculus obturator externus
obturator muscle, internal	musculus obturator internus
occipitofrontal muscle	musculus occipitofrontalis
Ochsner's muscles	
ocular muscles	musculi bulbi
Oddi's muscle (sphincter)	
Oehl's muscles	
omohyoid muscle	musculus omohyoideus
opposing muscle of little finger	musculus opponens digiti minimi
opposing muscle of thumb	musculus opponens pollicis
orbicular muscle	musculus orbicularis
orbicular muscle of eye	musculus orbicularis oculi
orbicular muscle of mouth	musculus orbicularis oris
orbital muscle	musculus orbitalis
organic muscle (visceral musscle)	
palate and fauces, muscles	musculi palati et faucium
palatine muscles	musculi palati
palatoglossus muscle	musculus palatoglossus
palatopharyngeal muscle	musculus palatopharyngeus
palmar interosseous muscle	musculus interosseus palmaris
palmar muscle, short	musculus palmaris brevis
palmar muscle, long	musculus palmaris longus
papillary muscle	musculus papillaris
pectinate muscles	musculi pectinati
pectineal muscle	musculus pectineus
pectoral muscle, greater	musculus pectoralis major
pectoral muscle, smaller	musculus pectoralis minor
pectorodorsalis muscle (axillary arch)	
penniform muscle	musculus unipennatus
perineal muscles	musculi perinei
peroneal muscle, long	musculus fibularis longus
peroneal muscle, short	musculus fibularis brevis
peroneal muscle, third	musculus fibularis tertius
pharyngopalatine muscle	musculus palatopharyngeus
Phillips' muscle	

muscle	musculus (pl. musculi)
piriform muscle	musculus piriformis
plantar interosseous muscle	musculus interosseus plantaris
plantar muscle	musculus plantaris
plantar quadrate muscle	musculus quadratus plantae
platysma muscle	musculus platysma
pleuroesophageal muscle	musculus pleuroesophageus
popliteal muscle	musculus popliteus
posterior auricular muscle	musculus retrahens aurem
posterior cervical intertransverse muscles	musculi intertransversarii posteriores cervicis
posterior cricoarytenoid muscle	musculus cricoarytenoideus posterior
posterior scalene muscle	musculus scalenus posterior
posterior tibial muscle	musculus tibialis posterior
Pozzi's muscle (extensor digitorum brevis muscle of hand)	musculus extensor digitorum brevis manus
procerus muscle	musculus procerus
pronator muscle, quadrate	musculus pronator quadratus
pronator muscle, round	musculus pronator teres
psoas muscle, greater	musculus psoas major
psoas muscle, smaller	musculus psoas minor
pterygoid muscle	musculus pterygoideus
pubococcygeal muscle	musculus pubococcygeus
puboprostatic muscle	musculus puboprostaticus
puborectal muscle (Braune's muscle)	musculus puborectalis
pubovaginal muscle	musculus pubovaginalis
pubovesical muscle	musculus pubovesicalis
pyloric sphincter muscle	musculus sphincter pyloricus
pyramidal auricular muscle (Jung's m.)	musculus pyramidalis auriculae
quadrate (four-sided) muscle	musculus quadratus
quadrate muscle of loins	musculus quadratus lumborum
quadrate muscle of lower lip	musculus depressor labii inferioris
quadrate muscle of sole	musculus quadratus plantae
quadrate muscle of thigh	musculus quadratus femoris
quadrate muscle of upper lip	musculus quadratus labii superioris
radial flexor muscle of wrist	musculus flexor carpi radialis
rectococcygeus muscle	musculus rectococcygeus
rectourethral muscle	musculus recto-urethralis
rectouterine muscle	musculus recto-uterinus
rectovesical muscle	musculus rectovesicalis

muscle	musculus (pl. musculi)
rectus abdominis muscle (rectus muscle of abdomen)	musculus rectus abdominis
rectus muscle of head, anterior	musculus rectus capitis anterior
rectus muscle of head, lateral	musculus rectus capitis lateralis
rectus muscle of head, greater posterior	musculus rectus capitis posterior major
rectus muscle of head, smaller posterior	musculus rectus capitis posterior minor
rectus femoris muscle (rectus muscle of thigh)	musculus rectus femoris
red muscle (slow muscle)	
Reisseisen's muscles	
rhomboid muscle, greater	musculus rhomboideus major
rhomboid muscle, lesser	musculus rhomboideus minor
ribbon muscles	musculi infrahyoidei
rider's muscles (adductor muscles of thigh)	
Riolan's muscle (cremaster muscle)	musculus cremaster
risorius muscle (Albinus' muscle, Santorini's muscle)	musculus risorius
rotator muscles	musculi rotatores
rotator muscles of neck	musculi rotatores cervicis
rotator muscles of back	musculi rotatores lumborum
rotator muscles of thorax	musculi rotatores thoracis
Rouget's muscle	
round pronator muscle	musculus pronator teres
Ruysch's muscle	
sacrococcygeal muscle	musculus sacrococcygeus
salpingopharyngeal muscle	musculus salpingopharyngeus
Santorini's muscle	musculus risorius
sartorius muscle (tailor's muscle)	musculus sartorius
scalene muscle, anterior	musculus scalenus anterior
scalene muscle, middle	musculus scalenus medius
scalene muscle, posterior	musculus scalenus posterior
scalene muscle, smallest (Albinus' m., Sibson's m.)	musculus scalenus minimus
scalp muscle (epicranius muscle)	
Sebileau's muscle	
second tibial muscle	musculus tibialis secundus
semimembranous muscle	musculus semimembranosus
semispinal muscle	musculus semispinalis
semispinal muscle of head	musculus semispinalis capitis

muscle	musculus (pl. musculi)
semispinal muscle of neck	musculus semispinalis cervicis
semispinal muscle of thorax	musculus semispinalis thoracis
semitendinous muscle	musculus semitendinosus
serratus anterior muscle	musculus serratus anterior
serratus posterior inferior muscle	musculus serratus posterior inferior
serratus posterior superior muscle	musculus serratus posterior superior
shawl muscle (trapezius muscle)	
short adductor muscle	musculus adductor brevis
short extensor musscle of great toe	musculus extensor hallucis brevis
short extensor muscle of thumb	musculus extensor pollicis brevis
short extensor muscle of toes	musculus extensor digitorum brevis
short fibular muscle	musculus peroneus brevis
short flexor muscle of great toe	musculus flexor hallucis brevis
short flexor muscle of little finger	musculus flexor digiti minimi brevis
short flexor muscle of little toe	musculus flexor digiti minimi brevis
short flexor muscle of thumb	musculus flexor pollicis brevis
short flexor muscle of toes	musculus flexor digitorum brevis
short palmar muscle	musculus palmaris brevis
short peroneal muscle	musculus peroneus brevis
short radial extensor muscle of wrist	musculus extensor carpi radialis brevis
Sibson's muscle	musculus scalenus minimus
skeletal muscles	musculi skeleti
slow muscle (red muscle)	
smaller muscle of helix	musculus helicis minor
smaller pectoral muscle	musculus pectoralis minor
smaller posterior rectus muscle of head	musculus rectus capitis posterior minor
smaller psoas muscle	musculus psoas minor
smallest scalene muscle	musculus scalenus minimus
smooth muscle (unstriated, unstriped, visceral)	
Soemmerring's muscle (levator muscle of thyroid gland)	
soleus muscle	musculus soleus
somatic muscles	musculi skeleti
sphincter muscle of anus	musculus sphincter ani
sphincter muscle of bile duct	musculus sphincter ductus choledochi
sphincter muscle of hepatopancreatic ampulla	musculus sphincter ampullae hepatopancreaticae
sphincter muscle of pupil	musculus sphincter pupillae

muscle	musculus (pl. musculi)
sphincter muscle of pylorus	musculus sphincter pyloricus
sphincter muscle of urethra	musculus sphincter urethrae
sphincter muscle of urinary bladder	musculus sphincter vesicae urinariae
spinal muscle	musculus spinalis
spinal muscle of head	musculus spinalis capitis
spinal muscle of neck	musculus spinalis cervicis
spinal muscle of thorax	musculus spinalis thoracis
spindle-shaped muscle	musculus fisiform
splenius muscle of head	musculus splenius capitis
splenius muscle of neck	musculus splenius cervicis
stapedius muscle	musculus stapedius
sternal muscle	musculus sternalis
sternochondroscapular muscle	musculus sternochondroscapularis
sternoclavicular muscle	musculus sternoclavicularis
sternocleidomastoid muscle	musculus sternocleidomastoideus
sternocostal muscle	musculus transversus thoracis
sternohyoid muscle	musculus sternohyoideus
sternomastoid muscle (sternocleidomastoid)	
sternothyroid muscle	musculus sternothyroideus
strap muscles	
striated muscle	
styloauricular muscle	musculus styloauricularis
styloglossus muscle	musculus styloglossus
stylohyoid muscle	musculus stylohyoideus
stylopharyngeal muscle	musculus stylopharyngeus
subanconeus muscle	musculus articularis cubiti
subclavian muscle	musculus subclavius
subcostal muscle	musculus subcostalis
subcrural muscle	musculus articularis genu
suboccipital muscles	musculi suboccipitales
subquadricipital muscle	musculus articularis genu
subscapular muscle	musculus subscapularis
subvertebral muscles	musculi hypaxial
superficial back muscles	
superficial flexor muscle of fingers	musculus flexor digitorum superficialis
superficial lingual muscle (of tongue)	
superficial transverse perineal muscle (Theile's muscle)	musculus transversus perinei superficialis
superior auricular muscle	musculus auricularis superior

muscle	**musculus** (pl. **musculi**)
superior constrictor muscle of pharynx	musculus constrictor pharyngis superior
superior gemellus muscle	musculus gemellus superior
superior longitudinal muscle of tongue	musculus longitudinalis superior
superior oblique muscle	musculus obliquus superior
superior oblique muscle of head	musculus obliquus capitis superior
superior posterior serratus muscle	musculus serratus posterior superior
superior rectus muscle	musculus rectus superior
superior tarsal muscle (Mueller's muscle)	musculus tarsalis superior
supinator muscle	musculus supinator
supraclavicular muscle	musculus supraclavicularis
suprahyoid muscles	musculi suprahyoidei
supraspinalis muscle	musculus supraspinalis
supraspinous muscle	musculus supraspinatus
suspensory muscle of duodenum (Treitz' ligament)	musculus suspensorius duodeni
synergic or synergistic muscles	
tailor's muscle (sartorius muscle)	
temporal muscle	musculus temporalis
temporoparietal muscle	musculus temporoparietalis
tensor muscle of fascia lata	musculus tensor fasciae latae
tensor muscle of soft palate	musculus tensor veli palati
tensor tarsi muscle	musculus orbicularis oculi
tensor muscle of tympanic membrane (Toynbee's muscle)	musculus tensor tympani
teres major muscle	musculus teres major
teres minor muscle	musculus teres minor
Theile's muscle (superficial transverse perineal muscle)	
third peroneal muscle	musculus peroneus tertius
thoracic interspinal muscle	musculi thoracic interspinalis
thoracic intertransverse muscles	musculi intertransversarii thoracis
thoracic longissimus muscle	musculus longissimus thoracis
thoracic rotator muscles	musculi rotatores thoracis
thorax, muscles of	musculi thoracis
thyroarytenoid muscle	musculus thyroarytenoideus
thyroepiglottic muscle (depressor muscle of epiglottis)	musculus thyroepiglotticus
thyrohyoid muscle	musculus thyrohyoideus

muscle	musculus (pl. musculi)
tibial muscle, anterior	musculus tibialis anterior
tibial muscle, posterior	musculus tibialis posterior
Tod's muscle (oblique auricular muscle)	
tongue, muscles of	musculi linguae
Toynbee's muscle	musculus tensor tympani
tracheal muscle	musculus trachealis
tracheloclavicular muscle	musculus tracheloclavicularis
trachelomastoid muscle	musculus longissimus capitis
tragicus muscle (Valsalva's muscle)	musculus tragicus
transverse arytenoid muscle	musculus arytenoideus transversus
transverse muscle of abdomen	musculus transversus abdominis
transverse muscle of auricle	musculus transversus auriculae
transverse muscle of chin	musculus transversus menti
transverse muscle of nape	musculus transversus nuchae
transverse muscle of neck	musculus transversus nuchae
transverse muscle of thorax	musculus transversus thoracis
transverse muscle of tongue	musculus transversus linguae
transversospinal muscle	musculus transversospinalis
trapezius muscle	musculus trapezius
Treitz' muscle (suspensory muscle of duodenum)	
triangular muscle	musculus triangularis
triceps muscle of arm	musculus triceps brachii
triceps muscle of hip	musculus triceps coxae
triceps muscle of calf	musculus triceps surae
trigonal muscle	
true (deep) muscles of back	musculi dorsi
two-bellied muscle (digastric muscle)	musculus digastricus
ulnar extensor muscle of wrist	musculus extensor carpi ulnaris
ulnar flexor muscle of wrist	musculus flexor carpi ulnaris
unipennate muscle	musculus unipennatus
unstriated muscle, unstriped muscle (smooth muscle)	
urogenital diaphragm, muscles of	musculi diaphragmatis urogenitalis
uvula, muscle of	musculus uvulae
Valsalva's muscle	
vastus intermedius muscle (intermediate great muscle)	musculus vastus intermedius

muscle	musculus (pl. musculi)
vastus lateralis muscle (lateral great muscle)	musculus vastus lateralis
vastus medialis muscle (medial great muscle)	musculus vastus medialis
ventral sacrococcygeal muscle	musculus sacrococcygeus ventralis
vertical muscle of tongue	musculus verticalis linguae
visceral muscle (smooth)	
vocal muscle	musculus vocalis
voluntary muscle	
white muscle (fast muscle)	
Wilson's muscle (urethral sphincter)	musculus sphincter urethrae
wrinkler muscle of eyebrow	musculus corrugator supercilii
yoked muscles	
zygomatic muscle, greater	musculus zygomaticus major
zygomatic muscle, lesser	musculus zygomaticus minor

Table of Veins

vein	vena (pl. venae)
accessory cephalic vein	vena cephalica accessoria
accessory hemiazygos vein	vena hemiazygos accessoria
accessory saphenous vein	vena saphena accessoria
accessory vertebral vein	vena vertebralis accessoria
accompanying vein	vena comitans
accompanying vein of hypoglossal nerve	vena comitans nervi hypoglossi
adrenal veins	venae suprarenales
afferent veins	
anastomotic vein, inferior	vena anastomotica inferior
anastomotic vein, superior	vena anastomotica superior
angular vein	vena angularis
anonymous veins	venae brachiocephalicae
antebrachial vein, median	vena intermedia antebrachii
anterior auricular vein	vena auricularis anterior
anterior cardiac veins	venae cordis anteriores
anterior cardinal veins	
anterior cerebral vein	vena cerebri anterior
anterior facial vein	
anterior intercostal veins	venae intercostales anteriores
anterior jugular vein	vena jugularis anterior
anterior labial veins	venae labiales anteriores
anterior pontomesencephalic vein	vena pontomesencephalica anterior
anterior scrotal veins	venae scrotales anteriores
anterior vein of septum pellucidum	vena septi pellucidi anterior
anterior veins of heart	venae ventriculi dextri anteriores
anterior veins of right ventricle	venae ventriculi dextri anteriores
anterior tibial veins	venae tibiales anteriores
anterior vertebral vein	vena vertebralis anterior
appendicular vein	vena appendicularis
aqueduct of cochlea, vein of	vena aqueductus cochleae
aqueduct of vestibule, vein of	vena aqueductus vestibuli

vein	vena (pl. venae)
aqueous veins	
arciform veins of kidney	
arcuate veins of kidney	venae arcuatae renis
arterial vein	vena arteriosa, truncus pulmonalis
arterial vein of Soemmering	vena portae hepatis
articular veins	venae articulares
ascending veins of Rosenthal	venae inferiores cerebri
ascending lumbar vein	vena lumbalis ascendens
atrial veins of heart, left	venae atriales sinistrae
atrial veins of heart, right	venae atriales dextrae
atrial vein, lateral	vena lateralis atrii
atrial vein, medial	vena medialis atrii
atrioventricular veins of heart	venae atrioventriculares cordis
auditory veins, internal	venae labyrinthinae
auricular veins, anterior	venae auriculares anteriores
auricular veins, posterior	vena auricularis posterior
axillary vein	vena axillaris
azygos vein	vena azygos
basal vein, Rosenthal's	vena basalis
basilic vein	vena basilica
basivertebral vein	vena basivertebralis
Baumgarten's veins	
Boyd communicating perforation veins	
brachial veins	venae brachiales
brachiocephalic veins	venae brachiocephalicae
Breschet's vein	venae diploicae
bronchial veins	venae bronchiales
Browning's vein	
bulb of penis, vein of	vena bulbi penis
Burow's vein	
canaliculus of cochlea, vein of	vena aqueductus cochleae
capillary vein	
cardiac veins	venae cordis
cardiac veins, anterior	venae ventriculi dextri anteriores
cardiac vein, great	vena cardiaca magna
cardiac vein, middle	vena cardiaca media
cardiac vein, small	vena cardiaca parva
cardiac veins, smallest	venae cardiacae minimae
cardinal veins	

vein	vena (pl. venae)
carotid vein, external	vena retromandibularis
caudate nucleus, veins of	venae nuclei caudati
cavernous veins of penis	venae cavernosae penis
central veins of liver	venae centrales hepatis
central vein of retina	vena centralis retinae
central vein of suprarenal gland	vena centralis glandulae suprarenalis
cephalic vein	vena cephalica
cerebellar veins	venae cerebelli
cerebral veins	venae cerebri
cervical vein, deep	vena cervicalis profunda
choroid vein	vena choroidea
choroid veins of eye	
ciliary veins	venae ciliares
circumflex veins	venae circumflexae
cochlear aqueduct, vein of	vena aqueductus cochleae
cochlear canaliculus, vein of	vena aqueductus cochleae
Cockett communicating perforating veins	
colic vein, left	vena colica sinistra
colic vein, middle	vena colica media
colic vein, right	vena colica dextra
common basal vein	vena basalis communis
common cardinal veins (ducts of Cuvier)	
common facial vein	vena facialis communis
common iliac vein	vena iliaca communis
communicating veins (perforating veins)	
companion vein, companion veins	vena comitans, venae comitantes
condylar emissary vein	vena emissaria condylaris
conjunctival veins	venae conjunctivales
coronary vein, left	vena coronaria sinistra
coronary vein, right	vena coronaria dextra
corpus callosum, vein of, dorsal	vena dorsalis corporis callosi
corpus callosum, vein of, posterior	vena posterior corporis callosi
corpus striatum, vein of	
costoaxillary veins	venae costoaxillares
cubital vein, median	vena intermedia cubiti
cutaneous vein	vena cutanea
cutaneous vein, ulnar	vena basilica
Cuvier's veins	
cystic vein	vena cystica

vein	vena (pl. venae)
deep cerebral veins	venae cerebri profundae
deep cervical vein	vena cervicalis profunda
deep circumflex iliac vein	vena circumflexa iliaca profunda
deep veins of clitoris	venae profundae clitoridis
deep dorsal vein of clitoris	vena dorsalis clitoridis profunda
deep dorsal vein of penis	vena dorsalis penis profunda
deep epigastric vein	
deep facial vein	vena faciei profunda
deep femoral vein	vena profunda femoris
deep lingual vein	vena profunda linguae
deep middle cerebral vein	vena cerebri media profunda
deep vein of penis	vena profunda penis
deep temporal veins	venae temporales profundae
digital veins	venae digitales
diploic vein	vena diploica
dorsal callosal vein	vena corporis callosi dorsalis
dorsal veins of clitoris	venae dorsales clitoridis
dorsal vein of corpus callosum	vena corporis callosi dorsalis
dorsal digital veins of foot	venae digitales dorsales pedis
dorsal digital veins of toes	
dorsal lingual vein	venae dorsales linguae
dorsal metacarpal veins	venae metacarpeae dorsales
dorsal metatarsal veins	venae metatarseae dorsales
dorsal veins of penis, deep	vena dorsalis profunda penis
dorsal scapular vein	vena scapularis dorsalis
dorsispinal veins	
emissary vein	vena emissaria
emulgent vein	
epigastric veins, superior	venae epigastricae superiores
episcleral veins	venae episclerales
esophageal veins	venae esophageae
ethmoidal veins	venae ethmoidales
external iliac vein	vena iliaca externa
external jugular vein	vena jugularis externa
external nasal veins	venae nasales externae
external pudendal veins	venae pudendae externae
eyelids, veins of	
facial vein	vena facialis
femoral vein	vena femoralis

vein	vena (pl. venae)
fibular veins	venae fibulares
frontal veins	venae frontales
Galen, veins of	venae internae cerebri
gastric veins	venae gastricae
gastroepiploic vein, left	vena gastro-omentalis sinistra
gastroepiploic vein, right	vena gastro-omentalis dextra
gastro-omental vein, left	vena gastro-omentalis sinistra
gastro-omental vein, right	vena gastro-omentalis dextra
genicular veins	venae geniculares
gluteal veins, inferior	venae gluteae inferiores
gluteal veins, superior	venae gluteae superiores
great cardiac vein	vena cordis magna
great cerebral vein	
great cerebral vein of Galen	vena cerebri magna
great vein of Galen	
great saphenous vein	vena saphena magna
hemiazygos vein	vena hemiazygos
hemorrhoidal veins	venae rectales
hepatic veins	venae hepaticae
hepatic portal vein	
highest intercostal vein	vena intercostalis suprema
hypogastric vein	vena iliaca interna
ileal veins	venae ileales
ileocolic vein	vena ileocolica
iliac vein, common	vena iliaca communis
iliac vein, external	vena iliaca externa
iliac vein, internal	vena iliaca interna
iliolumbar vein	vena iliolumbalis
inferior anastomotic vein	vena anastomotica inferior
inferior basal vein	vena basalis inferior
inferior cardiac vein	
inferior veins of cerebellar hemisphere	venae hemispherii cerebelli inferiores
inferior cerebral veins	venae cerebri inferiores
inferior choroid vein	vena choroidea inferior
inferior epigastric vein	vena epigastrica inferior
inferior eyelid veins	
inferior gluteal veins	venae gluteae inferiores
inferior hemorrhoidal veins	
inferior labial vein	vena labialis inferior

vein	vena (pl. venae)
inferior laryngeal vein	vena laryngea inferior
inferior mesenteric vein	vena mesenterica inferior
inferior ophthalmic vein	vena ophthalmica inferior
inferior palpebral veins	venae palpebrales inferiores
inferior phrenic vein	vena phrenica inferior
inferior rectal veins	venae rectales inferiores
inferior thalamostriate veins	venae thalamostriatae inferiores
inferior thyroid vein	vena thyroidea inferior
inferior ventricular vein	vena ventricularis inferior
inferior vein of vermis	vena vermis inferior
innominate veins	venae brachiocephalicae
innominate cardiac veins (Vieussens' veins)	
insular veins	venae insulares
intercapitular veins	venae intercapitales
intercostal veins	venae intercostales
interlobar veins of kidney	venae interlobares renis
interlobular veins of kidney	venae interlobulares renis
interlobular veins of liver	venae interlobulares hepatis
intermediate antebrachial vein	
intermediate basilic vein	vena intermedia basilica
intermediate cephalic vein	vena intermedia cephalica
intermediate colic vein	vena colica media
intermediate cubital vein	
intermediate vein of forearm	
internal auditory veins	
internal cerebral veins	venae cerebri internae
internal iliac vein	vena iliaca interna
internal jugular vein	vena jugularis interna
internal pudendal vein	vena pudenda interna
internal thoracic vein	vena thoracica interna
interosseous veins	venae interosseae
intersegmental veins	pars intersegmentalis
intervertebral vein	vena intervertebralis
intrasegmental veins	pars intrasegmentalis
jejunal and ileal veins	venae jejunales et ilei
jugular veins	venae jejunales
key vein	
kidney, veins of	venae renis
knee, veins of	venae genus

vein	vena (pl. venae)
Krukenberg's veins	venae centrales hepatis
Labbe's vein (acute e)	vena anastomotica inferior
labial veins	venae labiales
labyrinthine veins	venae labyrinthi
lacrimal vein	vena lacrimalis
large vein	vena magna
large saphenous vein	vena saphena magna
laryngeal vein, superior	vena laryngea superior
Latarget's vein	
lateral atrial vein	vena atrii lateralis
lateral circumflex femoral veins	venae circumflexae femoris laterales
lateral direct veins	venae directae laterales
lateral vein of lateral ventricle	vena atrii lateralis
lateral recess of fourth ventricle, vein of	vena recessus lateralis ventriculi quarti
lateral sacral veins	venae sacrales laterales
lateral thoracic vein	vena thoracica lateralis
left colic vein	vena colica sinistra
left coronary vein	vena coronaria sinistra
left gastric vein	vena gastrica sinistra
left gastroepiploic vein	vena gastro-omentalis sinistra
left gastro-omental vein	vena gastro-omentalis sinistra
left hepatic veins	venae hepaticae sinistrae
left inferior pulmonary vein	vena pulmonalis inferior sinistra
left ovarian vein	vena ovarica sinistra
left superior intercostal vein	vena intercostalis superior sinistra
left superior pulmonary vein	vena pulmonalis superior sinistra
left suprarenal vein	vena suprarenalis sinistra
left testicular vein	vena testicularis sinistra
left umbilical vein	vena umbilicalis sinistra
levoatrio-cardinal vein	
lingual vein	vena lingualis
long saphenous vein	vena saphena longus
long thoracic vein	vena thoracica longus
lumbar veins	venae lumbales
Marshall's oblique vein	
masseteric veins	venae massetericae
mastoid emissary vein	vena emissaria mastoidea
maxillary vein	vena maxillaris
Mayo's vein	

vein	vena (pl. venae)
medial atrial vein	vena atrii medialis
medial circumflex femoral veins	venae circumflexae femoris mediales
medial vein of lateral ventricle	vena atrii medialis
median antebrachial vein	vena intermedia antebrachii
median basilic vein	vena intermedia basilic
median cephalic vein	vena intermedia cephalica
median cubital vein	vena intermedia cubiti
median vein of forearm	vena intermedia antebrachii
median vein of neck	vena mediana colli
median sacral vein	vena sacralis mediana
mediastinal veins	venae mediastinales
median vein	vena intermedia
medulla oblongata, veins of	venae medullae oblongatae
meningeal veins	venae meningeae
mesencephalic veins	venae mesencephalicae
mesenteric vein, inferior	vena mesenterica inferior
mesenteric vein, superior	vena mesenterica superior
metacarpal veins	venae metacarpales
middle cardiac vein	vena cordis media
middle colic vein	vena colica media
middle hemorrhoidal veins	venae rectales mediae
middle hepatic veins	venae hepaticae mediae
middle meningeal veins	venae meningeae mediae
middle rectal veins	venae rectales mediae
middle temporal vein	vena temporalis media
middle thyroid vein	vena thyroidea media
musculophrenic veins	venae musculophrenicae
nasofrontal vein	vena nasofrontalis
oblique vein of left atrium	vena obliqua atrii sinistri
obturator vein	vena obturatoria
occipital vein	vena occipitalis
occipital cerebral veins	venae occipitales
occipital emissary vein	vena emissaria occipitalis
olfactory gyrus, vein of	vena gyri olfactorii
ophthalmic vein, inferior	vena ophthalmica inferior
ophthalmic vein, superior	vena ophthalmica superior
ovarian vein, left	vena ovarica sinistra
ovarian vein, right	vena ovarica dextra
palatine vein	vena palatina

vein	vena (pl. venae)
palmar digital veins	venae digitales palmares
palmar metacarpal veins	venae metacarpeae palmares
palpebral veins	venae palpebrales
pancreatic veins	venae pancreaticae
pancreaticoduodenal veins	venae pancreaticoduodenales
paraumbilical veins	venae paraumbilicales
parietal veins	venae parietales
parietal emissary vein	vena emissaria parietalis
parotid veins	venae parotidea
pectoral veins	venae pectorales
peduncular veins	venae pedunculares
perforating veins	venae perforantes
pericardiac veins	venae pericardiales
pericardiacophrenic veins	venae pericardiacophrenicae
pericardial veins	venae pericardiacae
peroneal veins	venae peroneae
petrosal vein	vena petrosa
pharyngeal veins	venae pharyngeae
phrenic veins	venae phrenicae
plantar digital veins	venae digitales plantares
plantar metatarsal veins	venae metatarseae plantares
pontine veins	venae pontis
popliteal vein	vena poplitea
portal vein	vena portae hepatis
posterior anterior jugular vein	vena jugularis posterior anterior
posterior auricular vein	vena auricularis posterior
posterior cardinal veins	
posterior facial vein	vena retromandibularis
posterior horn, vein of	vena cornus posterioris
posterior intercostal veins	venae intercostales posteriores
posterior labial veins	venae labiales posteriores
posterior vein of left ventricle	vena posterior ventriculi sinistri
posterior marginal vein	vena corporis callosi dorsalis
posterior parotid veins	venae parotideae posterioreae
posterior pericallosal vein	vena corporis callosi dorsalis
posterior scrotal veins	venae scrotales posteriores
posterior vein of left ventricle	vena ventriculi sinistri posterior
posterior vein of septum pellucidum	vena septi pellucidi posterior
posterior tibial veins	venae tibiales posteriores

vein	vena (pl. venae)
precardinal veins	
precentral cerebellar vein	vena precentralis cerebelli
prefrontal veins	venae prefrontales
prepyloric vein	vena prepylorica
pterygoid canal, vein of	vena canalis pterygoidei
pudendal veins	venae pudendae
pulmonary veins	venae pulmonales
pyloric vein	vena gastrica dextra
radial veins	venae radiales
ranine vein	vena sublingualis
rectal veins	venae rectales
renal veins	venae renales
retromandibular vein	vena retromandibularis
Retzius' veins	
right colic vein	vena colica dextra
right gastric vein	vena gastrica dextra
right gastroepiploic vein	vena gastro-omentalis dextra
right gastro-omental vein	vena gastro-omentalis dextra
right hepatic veins	venae hepaticae dextrae
right inferior pulmonary vein	vena pulmonalis inferior dextra
right ovarium vein	vena ovarica dextra
right superior intercostal vein	vena intercostalis superior dextra
right superior pulmonary vein	vena pulmonalis superior dextra
right suprarenal vein	vena suprarenalis dextra
right testicular vein	vena testicularis dextra
Rosenthal's vein	
Ruysch's veins	
sacral veins	venae sacrales
Santorini's vein	
saphenous veins	venae saphenae
Sappey's veins	venae paraumbilicales
scleral veins	venae sclerales
scrotal veins	venae scrotales
septum pellucidum, vein of, anterior	vena anterior septi pellucidi
septum pellucidum, vein of, posterior	vena posterior septi pellucidi
short gastric veins	venae gastricae breves
short saphenous vein	vena saphena breve
sigmoid veins	venae sigmoideae
small vein of heart	vena cardiaca parva

vein	vena (pl. venae)
small cardiac vein	vena cordis parva
smallest cardiac veins	venae cordis minimae
small saphenous vein	vena saphena parva
spermatic vein	vena spermatica
spinal veins	venae spinales
spiral vein of modiolus	vena spiralis modioli
splenic vein	vena splenica
stellate veins of kidney	venulae stellatae renis
Stensen's veins	venae vorticosae
sternocleidomastoid vein	vena sternocleidomastoidea
striate veins	venae thalamostriatae inferiores
stylomastoid vein	vena stylomastoidea
subclavian vein	vena subclavia
subcostal vein	vena subcostalis
subcutaneous veins of abdomen	venae subcutaneae abdominis
sublingual vein	vena sublingualis
sublobular veins	
submental vein	vena submentalis
superficial vein	vena superficialis
superficial cerebral veins	venae cerebri superficiales
superficial circumflex iliac ven	vena circumflexa iliaca superficialis
superficial dorsal veins of clitoris	venae dorsales clitoridis superficiales
superficial dorsal veins of penis	venae dorsales penis superficiales
superficial epigastric vein	vena epigastrica superficialis
superficial middle cerebral vein	vena cerebri media superficialis
superficial temporal veins	venae temporales superficiales
superior anastomotic vein	vena anastomotica superior
superior basal vein	vena basalis superior
superior veins of cerebellar hemisphere	venae hemispherii cerebelli superiores
superior cerebral veins	venae cerebri superiores
superior choroid vein	vena choroidea superior
superior epigastric veins	venae epigastricae superiores
superior eyelid, veins of	
superior gluteal veins	venae gluteae superiores
superior hemorrhoidal vein	vena rectales superior
superior intercostal vein	vena intercostalis superior
superior labial vein	vena labialis superior
superior laryngeal vein	vena laryngea superior
superior mesenteric vein	vena mesenterica superior

vein	vena (pl. venae)
superior ophthalmic vein	vena ophthalmica superior
superior palpebral veins	venae palpebrales superiores
superior phrenic veins	venae phrenicae superiores
superior rectal vein	vena rectalis superior
superior thalamostriate vein	vena thalamostriata superior
superior thyroid vein	vena thyroidea superior
superior vein of vermis	vena vermis superior
supraorbital vein	vena supraorbitalis
suprarenal veins	venae suprarenales
suprascapular vein	vena suprascapularis
supratrochlear veins	venae supratrochleares
supreme intercostal vein	vena intercostalis suprema
sural veins	venae surales
surface thalamic veins	venae directae laterales
sylvian vein, vein of sylvian fossa	vena mediae superficiales cerebri
temporal veins	venae temporales
temporomandibular joint, veins of	venae articulares temporomandibulares
temporomaxillary vein	vena temporomaxillaris
terminal vein	vena thalamostriata superior
testicular veins	venae testiculares
thalamostriate veins	venae thalamostriatae
thebesian veins	venae cordis minimae
thoracic veins	venae thoracicae
thoracoacromial vein	vena thoracoacromialis
thoracoepigastric vein	vena thoracoepigastrica
thymic veins	venae thymicae
thyroid veins	venae thyroideae
tibial veins	venae tibiales
trabecular veins	
tracheal veins	venae tracheales
transverse cervical veins	venae transversae colli
transverse facial vein	vena transversa faciei
transverse veins of neck	venae transversae cervicis
transverse vein of scapula	venae transversae scapulae
Trolard's vein	vena anastomotica superior
tympanic veins	venae tympanicae
ulnar veins	venae ulnares
umbilical vein	vena umbilicalis
uncus, vein of	vena unci

vein	vena (pl. venae)
upper limb, veins of	venae membri superioris
uterine veins	venae uterinae
varicose veins	
vena cava, inferior	vena cava inferior
vena cava, superior	vena cava superior
ventricular veins of heart	venae ventriculares cordis
vermis, inferior vein of	vena inferior vermis
vertebral vein	vena vertebralis
vertebral column, veins of	venae columnae vertebralis
vesalian vein	
Vesalius' vein	
vesical veins	venae vesicales
vestibular veins	venae vestibulares
vestibular aqueduct, vein of	vena aqueductus vestibuli
vestibular bulb, vein of	vena bulbi vestibuli
vidian veins	venae canalis pterygoidei
Vieussens' veins	venae cardiacae anteriores
vitelline vein	vena vitellina
vortex veins (vorticose veins)	venae vorticosae